To ...spital.

Novem...

Alternatives to Blood Transfusion in Transfusion Medicine

Alternatives to Blood Transfusion in Transfusion Medicine

EDITED BY

Alice Maniatis, MD
Professor Emeritus
Director, Hematology Division
Henry Dunant Hospital
Athens, Greece

Philippe Van der Linden, MD, PhD
Chief, Department of Anesthesiology
Centre Hospitalier Universitaire (CHU) Brugmann
Brussels, Belgium

Jean-François Hardy, MD, FRCPC
Professor of Anesthesiology
University of Montreal
CHUM-Notre-Dame Hospital
Montréal, Québec, Canada

SECOND EDITION

WILEY-BLACKWELL
A John Wiley & Sons, Ltd., Publication

NATA
Network for Advancement of Transfusion Alternatives

Blackwell Publishing was acquired by John Wiley & Sons in February 2007. Blackwell's publishing program has been merged with Wiley's global Scientific, Technical and Medical business to form Wiley-Blackwell.

Registered office: John Wiley & Sons Ltd, The Atrium, Southern Gate, Chichester, West Sussex, PO19 8SQ, UK

Editorial offices: 9600 Garsington Road, Oxford, OX4 2DQ, UK
The Atrium, Southern Gate, Chichester, West Sussex, PO19 8SQ, UK
111 River Street, Hoboken, NJ 07030-5774, USA

For details of our global editorial offices, for customer services and for information about how to apply for permission to reuse the copyright material in this book please see our website at www.wiley.com/wiley-blackwell

Library of Congress Cataloging-in-Publication Data

Alternatives to blood transfusion in transfusion medicine / edited by Alice Maniatis, Philippe Van der Linden, Jean-François Hardy. – 2nd ed.
p. ; cm.
Rev. ed. of: Transfusion medicine and alternatives to blood transfusion / NATA (Network for Advancement of Transfusion Alternatives). c2000.
Includes bibliographical references.
ISBN 978-1-4051-6321-7
1. Blood–Transfusion. 2. Blood–Transfusion–Complications. 3. Blood substitutes–Therapeutic use. I. Maniatis, Alice. II. Linden, Philippe Van der. III. Hardy, Jean-François. IV. Transfusion medicine and alternatives to blood transfusion.
[DNLM: 1. Blood Transfusion, Autologous–trends. 2. Blood Substitutes–therapeutic use. 3. Hemostasis, Surgical–trends. WB 356 A466 2010]
RM171.A623 2010
615′.39–dc22

2009038757

ISBN: 978-1-4051-6321-7

A catalogue record for this book is available from the British Library.

Set in 9/12pt Meridien by Aptara® Inc., New Delhi, India
Printed in Singapore by Markono Print Media Pte Ltd

1 2011

Contents

Contributors List

Philippe L. Baele
Department of Anesthesiology
Cliniques Universitaires Saint-Luc
Brussels, Belgium

John A.J. Barbara
Emeritus Consultant to National Health Service Blood and Transplant; Visiting Professor University of the West of England, Bristol, UK

Charles H. Baron
Boston College Law School
Newton Centre, MA, USA

Sylvain Bélisle
Department of Anesthesiology
University of Montreal
Québec, Canada

Javad Bidgoli
Department of Anesthesiology
CHU Brugmann-HUDERF
Université Libre de Bruxelles,
Brussels, Belgium

Elvira Bisbe
Department of Anesthesiology
University Hospital Mar-Esperanza
Barcelona, Spain

Joachim Boldt
Department of Anesthesiology and Intensive Care Medicine
Klinikum der Stadt Ludwigshafen
Ludwigshafen, Germany

Anneke Brand
Department of Immunohematology and Blood Transfusion
Leiden University Medical Centre;
Sanquin Blood Bank South West Region
Leiden, The Netherlands

Mark E. Brecher
Department of Pathology Laboratory Medicine
McLendon Clinical Laboratories;
University of North Carolina
Chapel Hill, USA

Christian Breymann
Obsterics, Gynecology and Feto Maternal Medicine
Feto Maternal Haematology Research Group,
Obstetric Research
University Hospital Zurich
Zurich, Switzerland

Edward Burdett
National Hospital for Neurology and Neurosurgery
London, UK

Pedro Cabrales
La Jolla Bioengineering Institute
La Jolla, California, USA

Rebecca Cardigan
NHS Blood and Transplant
Cambridge, UK

Marcela Contreras
Royal Free & University College Hospitals Medical School;
Chair of Blood Transfusion International (BTI)
London, UK

Jorge Cuenca
Department of Orthopedic Surgery
University Hospital Miguel Servet
Zaragoza, Spain

Brian Custer
Blood Systems Research Institute
San Francisco, USA

G. Deby-Dupont
Centre of Oxygen Research and Development
University of Liege
Liege, Belgium

Ann Dierick
Department of Anesthesiology
CHU Brugmann-HUDERF
Université Libre de Bruxelles
Brussels, Belgium

Wulf Dietrich
Institute for Research in Cardiac Anesthesia and Working Group of Perioperative Hemostasis
Departments of Anesthesiology and Transfusion Medicine
University of Munich, Munich, Germany

Ronald E. Domen
Department of Pathology
Division of Clinical Pathology;
Penn State College of Medicine
Milton S. Hershey Medical Center
Hershey, PA, USA

Michael A. Dubick
US Army Institute of Surgical Research
San Antonio, TX, USA

Richard P. Dutton
University of Maryland School of Medicine;
R Adams Cowley Shock Trauma Center
University of Maryland Medical System
Baltimore, Maryland, USA

Dean Fergusson
Ottawa Health Research Institute
University of Ottawa Faculty of Medicine
Ottawa, Ontario, Canada

José Antonio García-Erce
Department of Hematology
University Hospital Miguel Servet
Zaragoza, Spain

Hans Gombotz
Department of Anesthesiology and Intensive Care
General Hospital Linz
Linz, Austria

Lawrence T. Goodnough
Departments of Medicine and Pathology
Stanford University School of Medicine
Stanford, CA, USA

A. Gerson Greenburg
Brown University School of Medicine
Providence, USA;
Medical Affairs
Biopure Corporation
Cambridge, USA

Bertrand Guidet
UMR-S 707, Pierre-et-Marie-Curie University (Paris 6), Paris, France;
Department of Intensive Care
Saint-Antoine Hospital, Assistance Publique–Hôpitaux de Paris, Paris, France

Kristine J. Guleserian
Cardiothoracic Surgery
Children's Medical Center
UT Southwestern Medical Center
Dallas, USA

Oliver Habler
Clinic of Anesthesiology, Intensive Care Medicine, and Pain Control
Nord-West Hospital
Frankfurt, Germany

Hengo Haljamäe
Department of Anaesthesiology and Intensive Care
Sahlgrenska University Hospital
Göteborg, Sweden

Ernil Hansen
Department of Anesthesiology
Regensburg University Medical Center
Regensburg, Germany

Jean-François Hardy
Department of Anesthesiology
University of Montreal
Québec, Canada

Nicholas Heming
Department of Anesthesiology and Intensive Care, Saint-Louis Hospital
Assistance Publique–Hôpitaux de Paris, Paris, France

Brian Hutton
Ottawa Health Research Institute
University of Ottawa Faculty of Medicine
Ottawa, Ontario, Canada

Yalcin Inel
Department of Anesthesiology and Intensive Care
Friedrich Schiller University Hospital
Jena, Germany

Laurent Jacob
Department of Anesthesiology and Intensive Care, Saint-Louis Hospital
Assistance Publique–Hôpitaux de Paris, Paris, France

Michael F.M. James
Department of Anaesthesia
University of Cape Town

Faculty of Health Sciences
Western Cape, Cape Town, South Africa

Hae W. Kim
Brown University, School of Medicine
Providence, RI, USA

Alan D. Kitchen
National Transfusion Microbiology Reference Laboratory,
National Health Service Blood and Transplant,
London, UK

Spyridon Koulouris
First Department of Cardiology
Evangelismos General Hospital of Athens
Athens, Greece

Sibylle A. Kozek-Langenecker
Department of Anesthesiology and Pain Management
Medical University of Vienna
Vienna, Austria

Maurice Lamy
Department of Anaesthesia and Intensive Care Medicine
University Hospital
Domaine universitaire du Sart Tilman,
Liège, Beligum

Philippe Van der Linden
Department of Anesthesiology, CHU Brugmann-HUDERF
Université Libre de Bruxelles, Brussels, Belgium

Francesco Locatelli
Department of Nephrology, Dialysis, and Renal Transplantation
Alessandro Manzoni Hospital
Lecco, Italy

Sheila Maclennan
NHS Blood and Transplant (NHSBT)
Leeds, UK

Alice Maniatis
Hematology Department
Henry Dunant Hospital, Athens, Greece

Antonis S. Manolis
First Department of Cardiology
Evangelismos General Hospital of Athens
Athens, Greece

Jens Meier
Department of Anesthesiology
Intensive Care Medicine and Pain Control
Johann Wolfgang Goethe-University
Frankfurt, Germany

Helen Melita
Central Laboratories
Onassis Cardiac Surgery Center
Athens, Greece

Konrad Messmer
Institute for Surgical Research
Ludwig-Maximilians-University
Munich, Germany

Manuel Muñoz
GIEMSA, Transfusion Medicine
University of Málaga
Málaga, Spain

Cristina Navarrete
National Head of Histocompatibility & Immunogenetic Services, National Health Service Blood & Transplant (NHSBT), London

Sokratis Pastromas
First Department of Cardiology
Evangelismos General Hospital of Athens
Athens, Greece

Bruce Pearce
Biopure Corporation
Cambridge, MA, USA

Michael Piagnerelli
Department of Intensive Care
Erasme Hospital
Université Libre de Bruxelles
Brussels, Belgium

Arkadiy Pitman
Biopure Corporation
Cambridge, MA, USA

Chris Prowse
Scottish National Blood Transfusion Service
Edinburgh, UK

Bernadette Rémy
Department of Anaesthesia and Intensive Care Medicine
University Hospital
Domaine universitaire du Sart Tilman
Liège, Beligum

L. Ressler
University of Ottawa Heart Institute
Ottawa, Ontario, Canada

Fraser Rubens
Division of Cardiac Surgery
University of Ottawa Heart Institute
Ottawa, Ontario, Canada

Dimitris Sakellariou
First Department of Cardiology
Evangelismos General Hospital of Athens
Athens, Greece

Yasser Sakr
Department of Anesthesiology and Intensive Care
Friedrich-Schiller-University Hospital
Jena, Germany

Marc Samama
Hôtel-Dieu de Paris
Paris, France

Eva Schaden
Department of Anesthesiology and Pain Management
Medical University of Vienna
Vienna, Austria

Gisela Scharbert
Department of Anesthesiology and Pain Management
Medical University of Vienna
Vienna, Austria

Davide Simion
Department of Intensive Care, Erasme Hospital
Université Libre de Bruxelles, Brussels, Belgium

Neil Soni
Consultant ITU and Anaesthetics
Chelsea and Westminster Hospital
London, UK

Ronald G. Strauss
University of Iowa College of Medicine
DeGowin Blood Center
University of Iowa Hospitals
Iowa City, IA, USA

Stefan Suttner
Department of Anesthesiology and Intensive
Care Medicine
Klinikum der Stadt Ludwigshafen
Ludwigshafen, Germany

He Tao
Division of Cardiac Surgery
University of Ottawa Heart Institute
Ottawa, Ontario, Canada

Clare Taylor
SHOT Medical Director, NHSBT, London, UK

Pongdhep Theerawit
Department of Intensive Care, Erasme Hospital
Université Libre de Bruxelles, Brussels, Belgium

Benjamin Thomas
SpR Anaesthesia
St Mary's Hospital
Paddington, London, UK

Dafydd Thomas
Intensive Therapy Unit, Morriston Hospital
Abertawe Bro Morgannwg University NHS Trust and
Welsh Blood Service
Swansea, Wales, UK

Kostas Triantafyllou
First Department of Cardiology
Evangelismos General Hospital of Athens
Athens, Greece;
Hôpital Bichat Paris, France

Leo van de Watering
Sanguin Blood Bank South West Region
Leiden, The Netherlands

Lucia Del Vecchio
Department of Nephrology, Dialysis, and Renal
Transplantation
Alessandro Manzoni Hospital
Lecco, Italy

Andre Vercueil
King's College Hospital
London, UK

Jean-Louis Vincent
Department of Intensive Care, Erasme Hospital
Université Libre de Bruxelles, Brussels, Belgium

Marloes Waanders
Department of Immunohematology and Blood Transfusion,
Leiden
University Medical Center;
Sanquin Blood Bank South West
Region, Leiden, The Netherlands

Charles E. Wade
US Army Institute of Surgical Research
San Antonio, TX, USA

Tim Walsh
Anaesthetics, Critical Care and Pain Medicine
New Edinburgh Royal Infirmary
Edinburgh, Scotland, UK

PART 1

History and Development of Transfusion Medicine

CHAPTER 1

From Blood Transfusion to Transfusion Medicine

Alice Maniatis
Hematology Department, Henry Dunant Hospital, Athens, Greece;
Network for Advancement of Transfusion Alternatives (NATA)

Attempts at using blood transfusion for the treatment of bleeding and anemia were made centuries ago mostly with disastrous effects, and although James Blandell (1818) is granted with the first successful transfusion, it was only during the twentieth century that blood transfusion came of age. The first half of the century was the era of pioneers and ingenious, hardworking individuals who made major breakthroughs.

The second half saw the organization of large institutions charged with developing methods of procurement of safe and effective blood products.

During this time, developments occurred in quick succession in a variety of fields like immunology, biochemistry, microbiology, genetics, molecular biology, and biotechnology, all impacting on transfusion and leading to today's complex therapeutic intervention and the new specialization of transfusion medicine.

"The history of blood transfusion is marked by numerous bright pages but also some dark moments" as pointed out by Douglas Starr.

The surgical phase

Blood transfusion was introduced by surgeons, as theirs was the main need of finding a method of transferring blood from donor to patient. Alexis Carrel became famous for accomplishing a transfusion through suturing of vessels of the donor to those of the patient, in this case, the father to his baby daughter.

The technique underwent numerous modifications with the use of cannulae and tubes but remained difficult and cumbersome, so as to be used only infrequently. By the end of the first decade of the twentieth century, surgeons were performing some 20 transfusions a year at Mount Sinai hospital, New York.

New York had become home to a number of prominent physicians and scientists like Carrel, Landsteiner, Lindemann (the first full time specialist in transfusion, who introduced the multiple syringe method of transfusion), and others.

Direct donor–patient transfusions performed by surgeons continued to be practiced for decades and even as late as the early 1940s, though as described by Douglas Starr, "nobody liked transfusion as it existed, not the patient or the donor not even the doctors, who spent more time performing the transfusion, than the operation they were using it for." In addition to being cumbersome, transfusions were resulting in severe reactions in more than 30% of instances.

The laboratory phase

By the end of the first decade, Landsteiner's discovery of ABO blood groups dating to 1900 began to enter the transfusion field through the efforts,

Alternatives to Blood Transfusion in Transfusion Medicine, 2nd edition. Edited by A. Maniatis, P. Van der Linden, J.-F. Hardy.

to a large extent, of Ottenberg, who was also the first to use compatibility testing before transfusion; he was thus able to reduce the posttransfusion accidents concluding that "accidents can be absolutely excluded by careful preliminary tests."

The next problem to be addressed was clotting of the blood which necessitated either suturing of donor to patient vessels or very rapid removal and reinjection of the blood, which presented technical difficulties.

The syringe technique introduced by Lindemann eliminated the need for suturing blood vessels, as he inserted needles into the veins of donor and patient, and withdrew and reinjected blood with syringes; nevertheless, the method required quick action and clotting was not always prevented. So the next hero proved to be Lewisohn who introduced sodium citrate as the anticoagulant, publishing his method in 1915.

Surgeons, however, were apparently reluctant to accept the simplified procedure offered by anticoagulation (namely the collection of blood in a vessel containing sodium citrate); they wanted to maintain transfusion as "a complicated and lucrative operation."

Donor recruitment

Despite the use of anticoagulants, blood could not be stored for any length of time, hence the need for proximity of donor and patient. Compatible donors had to be recruited by the doctor, either from the patient's family or the environment, so the donor supply was difficult and unreliable. In London, donor recruitment techniques were developed similar to those used to this day; donors were tested for ABO group and called by telephone when needed. Through the efforts of Percy Oliver, 2500 nonremunerated donors were made available to London hospitals by 1930. Oliver's example was followed in other countries as well.

Meantime in Russia, Dr Alexander Bogdanov in 1926 established the "Central Institute of Hematology" where research in transfusion was carried out; experimenting with transfusion on himself, he eventually died of a massive intravascular hemolysis. In 1930, cadaver blood for transfusion was used for the first time in Russia by Dr Serge Yudin.

Blood banking

It was in Russia that the idea of storing blood was originated by Dr Yudin, leading to the institution of blood banks. Blood storage facilities spread throughout the country and blood was being stored for weeks resulting in a high percentage of reactions. Blood bank establishments were followed in Europe and the United States. In 1937, Bernard Fantus in Chicago established what was initially called Blood Preservation Laboratory changing the name later to Blood Bank as it operated with deposits and withdrawals of blood! This, in my opinion, unfortunate name, lingers until today throughout the world, giving false messages to potential donors.

Eventually with the improvement of storage vessels, anticoagulants, and preservatives, longer storage periods became possible, and in the 1940s, blood collection and transfusion stopped being a surgical enterprise and came into the hands of blood bankers. The year 1940 also marks the separation of plasma from whole blood. With regard to the volume of blood to be collected, based on experiments carried out in the 1930s and 1940s, it was decided that it should not exceed 13% of the donor's estimated blood volume; the 70 mL/kg rule may not be very accurate as pointed out by Frank Boulton, but has prevailed ever since as has the addition of 120 mL of anticoagulant to each blood unit.

World wars

The need for blood transfusion skyrocketed during World War II leading to a series of developments; glass bottles for blood collection, acid citrate dextrose developed by Patrick Mollison for blood anticoagulation, and separation and fractionation of plasma by Cohn with the production of albumin. Dried plasma and albumin were used as volume expanders on the battlefields during World War II. "By the end of 1943, the military had received more than two and a half million packages of dried plasma and nearly 125,000 ampoules of albumin" as mentioned by Starr.

In parallel with these developments, blood group serology was progressing thus increasing the safety of transfusion. The Coombs test introduced in 1945 for pretransfusion testing reduced significantly the risk of immune hemolysis of transfused RBCs. New methods of antibody detection led to the recognition of blood group systems, an endeavor that continues until today.

Blood collection—blood centers versus hospital blood banks

Blood collection from volunteers was relatively easy during the war but became increasingly difficult after the end of the war. Some countries like France and England managed to proceed to the development of National Blood Transfusion Centers and adopt the idea that blood should be voluntarily given without payment to donors. They developed networks of smaller and larger blood banks for collection and distribution of blood to hospitals.

In other countries such as Switzerland and Canada, it was the Red Cross that assumed the responsibility to recruit volunteer donors and supply blood products. In the United States, the American Association of Blood Banks formed in 1947 emphasized individual responsibility for blood procurement, asking patients to replace transfused units or else reimburse the blood bank; in contrast, the Red Cross supported community responsibility.

In many countries, a multitude of small blood banks collecting blood from paid blood donors prevailed in the 1950s and 1960s. By the late 1960s, it became apparent that most deaths by transfusion worldwide were because of viruses, bacteria, or parasites in the blood, and that the incidence was higher from paid donor blood leading to pressures to eliminate paid blood donation. In some instances, this led to substitution of paid donors by friends and relatives of patients, the so-called "replacement donors." Replacement donors are safer than paid but not as safe as truly volunteer donors.

Even until today, very few countries have achieved 100% collections from truly volunteer donors.

Blood components: hemapheresis

Progress in the technology of blood collection allowed the separation of whole blood into cellular components and plasma, making it possible to cover the transfusion needs of more than one patient with one unit of blood. The terms "component therapy" or "blood economy" were coined by Edwin Cohn. In developed countries, whole blood transfusion is a rarity nowadays as each unit is separated into red cells, plasma, and platelets.

Plasmapheresis, a term coined in 1914 by John Jacob Abel, described the removal of plasma while returning the cells to the donor. It was initially conceived as treatment to remove toxic substances from blood but evolved into a component production technique to provide plasma for transfusion and also for fractionation. Initially, it was carried out manually but it expanded, as automation became available in the 1960s. Blood cell separators made the procedure faster, safer, and yielding a better product. The need for albumin, gamma globulins, and coagulation factors encouraged the expansion of the fractionation industry with numerous companies becoming active throughout the world.

Therapeutic plasmapheresis or rather plasma exchange has contributed significantly in the treatment of hematologic, autoimmune, and metabolic diseases by the removal of antibodies of immune complexes, monoclonal proteins, or cholesterol.

Selective removal of cells, platelets, granulocytes, erythrocytes, and hemopoietic progenitor cells with discontinuous or continuous cell separators are carried out today in blood banks around the world. Platelet apheresis available since the 1970s is gaining ground, replacing gradually the recovery of random platelets for transfusion. Peripheral blood stem cell collection is also replacing bone marrow harvesting for bone marrow transplantation. Red cell apheresis is the most recent development with advantages to both donors and patients, but is limited to larger donors.

Blood safety

The 1970s were marked by progress in the safety of blood through the introduction of screening for hepatitis B virus, which reduced the incidence of posttransfusion hepatitis (PTH), followed by documentation of residual PTH, and the identification of hepatitis C, for which testing was developed in the early 1990s. Unfortunately, the 1980s were marked by the AIDS epidemic, which caused a tremendous amount of grief to both patients and blood providers.

Pathogens continued to emerge calling for constant vigilance; West Nile virus and Chikungunya are the most recent invaders of the blood supply, but such epidemics are quickly brought under control nowadays.

Transfusion risks are not limited to infectious agents; alloimmunization and transfusion reactions, platelet refractoriness due to HLA and antiplatelet-specific antibodies, immunosuppression, transfusion-associated graft versus host disease, and TRALI (transfusion-related acute lung injury) have all received attention in the last 20 years, and measures to prevent them are continuously being studied.

Since a number of risks are attributed to the leukocytes in blood units, leukodepletion, or reduction of leukocytes in blood units by filtration, was introduced some 20 years ago and has proven to be effective in reducing febrile reactions, platelet refractoriness, cytomegalovirus transmission, red cell alloimmunization, and transfusion-induced immunosuppression.

The latest weapon in enhancing the safety of blood products is the inactivation of pathogens.

Solvent detergent treatment of plasma disrupts lipid-enveloped viruses and has been used in pooled plasma since the 1990s, whereas methylene blue, a photoactive virucidal agent, can be added to single units as it has proven to be safe especially since it is being removed before transfusion. Inactivation of pathogens in cellular components is proving more difficult although for platelets, psoralen and UVA light activation are proving feasible and effective. Although screening for viruses will continue, treatment of blood components could be added to reduce the risk of pathogens that we cannot test for.

Information technology (IT) is also adding to the safety of blood transfusion; electronic medical records, electronic blood donor records, computer crossmatch, and virtual blood inventories are beginning to change the way transfusion medicine is practiced.

Alternatives to allogeneic transfusion

The realization that blood can never become 100% safe gave impetus to the development of transfusion alternatives.

Autologous transfusion

- Autologous transfusion, initially by predeposit autologous blood collection before surgery took off mainly in the 1980s after the AIDS epidemic; its advantages (safety, economy of allogeneic blood) were soon counteracted by disadvantages, mainly cost, and its practice is now limited to selective indications.
- Intraoperative hemodilution, the removal of two units immediately preoperatively replacing the volume with crystalloid, proved feasible and had the advantage of decreasing the loss of red cells during surgery but concerns over cardiac ischemia have limited its application to experienced centers.
- Intraoperative red cell salvage particularly with automated centrifugation and washing machines introduced in the late 1980s, is gaining ground. The method is safe but is suitable mainly for major procedures with significant predicted blood loss such as cardiovascular, vascular, and orthopedic operations.
- Postoperative red cell salvage, namely blood collected from drains in the first 6 hours following surgery and reinfused without manipulation, is simple and is adopted mainly by orthopedic

teams, but concerns regarding reinfusion of activated plasma proteins and wound debris remain.

Pharmacologic alternatives

Hemopoietic growth factors became available in the 1990s as a result of progress in recombinant technology.

Erythropoietin was the first one to be used in renal disease resulting in drastic decrease in transfusions for these patients. The indications for rhEPO have expanded reducing the need for transfusion in hematologic disease and cancer patients as well as in the anemia of chronic disease and of prematurity.

Colony stimulating factors (CSFs), granulocyte G-CSF, and granulocyte-macrophage GM-CSF for chemotherapy-induced neutropenia, chronic, and neonatal neutropenia are widely used and have resulted in decreased mortality from infection.

The use of thrombopoietin for the treatment of thrombocytopenia has been under investigation for the past 10 years but has not yet had an impact in reducing platelet transfusions.

Hemostatic agents

Almost 50% of blood units are transfused during surgical procedures, so, if perioperative blood loss could be reduced, transfusions would also be reduced.

Antifibrinolytic agents like tranexamic acid, epsilon-aminocaproic acid, and aprotinin have all been used in the last 20 years and have resulted in significant decreases in the need for transfusions, mainly in cardiovascular surgery; unfortunately, aprotinin was recently implicated in thrombosis and myocardial infarction and has been removed from circulation.

Fibrin sealants

Topical agents made of fibrinogen and thrombin or platelet gel applied on surgical surfaces to accelerate hemostasis have been developed in the last 10 years and are used mainly in cardiovascular and orthopedic surgery.

Red cell substitutes

The greatest hope for reducing the need for transfusions was the development of red cell substitutes; perfluorocarbons and hemoglobin-based oxygen carriers have been the subject of intense investigation for more than 20 years but safety problems are still limiting them to clinical studies.

Hemovigilance quality systems

Systematic surveillance of adverse transfusion effects begun in the 1990s; France was the first country to implement such a system in 1993, followed by the United Kingdom in 1996. Today, most European countries have a hemovigilance system, although it is not obligatory in all of them. In addition to disease transmission and reactions, these systems document errors occurring in the entire transfusion chain; by far, the most frequent adverse events were those resulting from errors in the transfusion process leading to the transfusion of ABO incompatible blood. Implementation of hemovigilance has led to establishment of new guidelines for a number of procedures.

In the last 15–20 years, emphasis was given to the application of quality systems principles; good manufacturing practices (GMPs) and quality management systems have been implemented in blood centers, leading to better standardization of blood products and reduction of errors and accidents.

Transfusion medicine

Blood transfusion started out as a relatively simple replacement therapy for bleeding or anemic subjects. The last 20 years, however, have seen a tremendous progress in the development of a number of blood products and in their safety; at the same time, emphasis was placed on the proper indications for transfusion and on the choice of available specialized blood products to cover the needs of patients. Hemotherapy acquired a complexity that necessitated specialized knowledge, and studies began to show the deficiencies in such knowledge of clinicians in making transfusion decisions. The effectiveness of transfusion came under scrutiny, while the risks remained significant. Blood bank personnel used to dealing with normal subjects such as the blood donors, with the emergence of therapeutic apheresis and stem cell collection for transplantation, have to deal now with patients; clinical laboratory training is not sufficient any more. These developments created the need for a new medical discipline, namely transfusion medicine. Transfusion specialists trained in laboratory medicine, pharmaceutical production, clinical medicine, epidemiological aspects, stem cell transplantation, legal, ethical, and administrative aspects could bridge the gap between the blood bank and the clinicians, be it internists, anesthesiologists, or surgeons. Clinician education and audits of transfusion practice are the tools by which transfusion specialists are aiming at improving the use of blood products.

In 1989, Dr Sacket coined the term evidence-based medicine (EBM), defined as the integration of the best research evidence with the best clinical expertise for good clinical decision making.

Transfusion medicine had to follow the principles and research methodologies that support EBM in order to develop transfusion guidelines based on such evidence, by performing Randomized Controlled Trials (RCTs). As per the McCarthy et al.'s study, 1000 RCTs on transfusion and apheresis and 70 meta-analyses were published by 2006.

Borzini et al. in an article published 10 years ago pointed out that "transfusion medicine had become a self-sufficient autonomous discipline." He went on to say that in order for TM to be "a stand alone discipline," self-recognition of such autonomy was necessary but not recognition by other disciplines!

I would argue that the latter recognition is important but unfortunately 10 years later the specialty of TM is still not widely recognized. Mueller and Seifried questioned recently why European directives, recognizing professional qualifications of European doctors, do not include TM, blood transfusion, or immunohematology at all, although TM is recognized as a specialty by a number of EU member states.

Efforts to this end should continue in order to attract young doctors to the specialty of TM and secure not only the safety and economy of blood but most importantly the continued research in the particular field.

Further reading

Aubuchon JP. The role of transfusion medicine physicians. Arch Pathol Lab Med 1999;123:663–7.

Borzini P, Nembri P, Biffoni F. The evolution of transfusion medicine as a stand alone discipline. Transfus Med Rev 1997;11:200–208.

Daniels G. Red cell immunohematology. Vox Sang (ISBT Science Series) 2007;9–13.

Douglas S. *Blood: An Epic History of Medicine and Commerce*. Alfred Knopf, New York, 1998.

McCarthy LG, Emmett TW, Smith DS, et al. Evidence-based medicine in transfusion medicine: an update. Vox Sang (ISBT Science Series) 2007;35–40.

Mueller MM, Seifried E. Blood transfusion in Europe: basic principles for initial and continuous training in transfusion medicine: an approach to an European harmonization. Transf Clin Biol 2006;13:282–5.

Oberman HA. The history of transfusion medicine. In: Lawrence P. (ed.) *Clinical Practice of Transfusion Medicine*. Churchill Livingstone, New York, 1996.

Shoos LK, Wolf E. Legal issues in transfusion medicine. In: Macpherson CR, Domen RE, Perlin T (eds) *Ethical Issues in Transfusion Medicine*. AABB Press, Bethesda, MD, 2001.

Slichter SJ. Evidence based platelet transfusion guidelines. Am Soc Hematol Educ Program 2007;172–8.

PART 2

Allogeneic Blood Usage—Risks and Benefits

CHAPTER 2

Allogeneic Blood Components

Rebecca Cardigan[1] *& Sheila Maclennan*[2]
[1]NHS Blood and Transplant, Cambridge, UK
[2]NHS Blood and Transplant, Leeds, UK

Donor selection and testing

Blood in Europe and America is collected from nonremunerated volunteer donors who undergo donor selection procedures designed to protect the health of both donor and recipient. A health questionnaire aims to identify any underlying illness in the donors which may put their health at risk when making a donation and identifies any factors (such as foreign travel or promiscuous sexual behavior) which may indicate an increased risk of carrying a potentially transfusion-transmissible infection. All donations are tested for mandatory microbiological markers (hepatitis B and C, HIV, syphilis, and HTLV; see the chapter by Kitchen and Barbara [1] in this volume) and ABO and Rh blood groups. A proportion of donations also undergo testing for other viruses (e.g., CMV) and additional typing, such as extended blood grouping and human leukocyte antigen (HLA) typing, for patients with specific requirements.

Whole-blood collection, storage, and processing

European and American guidelines recommend that the volume of whole blood collected is between 450 and 500 mL ± 10 % [2–4]. Blood is collected into an anticoagulant composed of citrate, phosphate, and dextrose designed to prevent blood from clotting and maintain cellular function during storage. Adenine may also be added to the anticoagulant to improve the quality of red cells during storage if other solutions are not added during later processing steps. It is generally accepted that there are very few clinical indications for transfusion of whole blood, and the vast majority of blood is therefore processed into its basic components: red cells, platelets, and plasma. This is achieved by centrifugation of whole blood in the primary collection pack, followed by manual or automated extraction of the components into satellite packs.

The initial storage temperature of whole blood determines which components can be produced from it (Figure 2.1). Because platelet function rapidly deteriorates at 4°C, whole blood must be processed on the day of blood collection or stored overnight at 22°C for platelet production. However, for the production of red cells, whole blood can be stored at 4°C for 48–72 hours prior to separation. Plasma is generally separated from whole blood on the day of collection or from blood that has been stored at 22°C for up to 24 hours, as these methods have been shown to preserve plasma quality. In the United States, "liquid plasma" (which has not been frozen) and thawed plasma are also available for use when transfusion of labile clotting factors (e.g., factors V and VIII) is not required. The storage temperature, media, and shelf life of blood components is tailored to each type of component, so that there is preservation of component quality while affording the maximal usable shelf life.

Alternatives to Blood Transfusion in Transfusion Medicine, 2nd edition. Edited by A. Maniatis, P. Van der Linden, J.-F. Hardy.

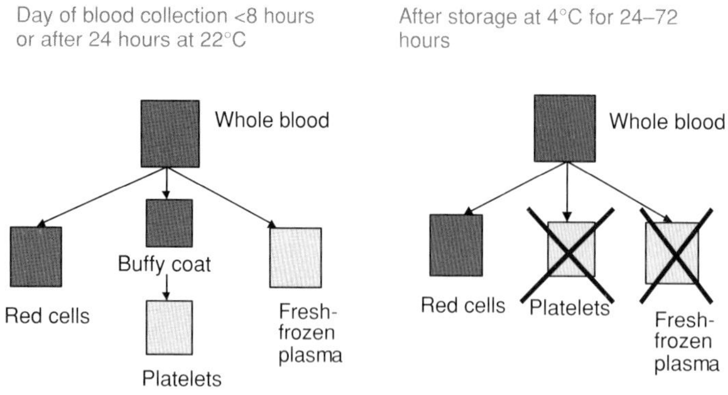

Figure 2.1 Production of components from whole blood.

Collection of blood components by apheresis

Apheresis, from a Greek word meaning "to take away," is an alternative to producing blood components from whole-blood donations by selectively collecting one or more components directly from donors and returning the rest to the circulation. Automated apheresis can be used to collect platelets, plasma, red cells, or granulocytes, and more specialized products, such as stem cells. The main emphasis in the past has been the collection of platelets and plasma components, with red cells being returned to the donor. The size and complexity of the equipment, as well as welfare of the donor, has previously necessitated this activity to take place in static clinics. However, smaller portable machines are now available that can be used on mobile sessions to collect red cells, platelets, and plasma. The main advantage of apheresis collections are that more than one dose of platelets or red cells can be collected from one donor per donation, thus reducing patient exposure to multiple donors. In addition, the hematocrit and hemoglobin content of red cells is much more consistent than those produced from whole-blood donations, which vary considerably because of the variation in hematocrit of whole blood in different donors.

Leukocyte depletion

Many countries have implemented universal leukocyte depletion (LD) of blood components, whereas in others leukocyte-depleted components may be issued for selected patient groups only. In the UK, a perceived benefit in terms of reduction in the risk of variant Creutzfeldt-Jakob disease (vCJD) transmission was a major contributory factor in the decision to introduce universal LD in 1998. Other benefits of LD, such as the potential for reduced immune complications and transfusion transmission of some cell-associated viruses (e.g., CMV), were considered more important by other countries.

Although in the past LD was performed at the bedside, the preference is now, because of quality reasons, for LD to be performed prior to component storage, usually within 48 hours of donation. For whole-blood donations, this is achieved by filtration, whereas an LD step by centrifugation/elutriation is integral to some apheresis technologies. Most whole-blood LD filters remove >2 logs of platelets in addition to >4 logs leukocytes. Therefore, only fresh-frozen plasma (FFP) and red cells can be produced from whole blood that has been leukocyte depleted. To produce platelet concentrates, each component (red cells, plasma, or platelets) must be filtered after their separation from whole blood. However, a second generation of whole-blood filters is becoming available that permit platelets to pass through the filter, although these are not yet in widespread use. LD results in a 10–15% loss of volume of whole blood or processed component but has minimal adverse effects on the quality of blood components.

The specification for leukocyte-depleted blood components varies between countries (Table 2.1), but all reflect the current capability of LD systems,

Table 2.1 Specifications for leukocyte-depleted blood components.

	UK	Council of Europe/ European directive	AABB
Level of residual leukocytes	$<5 \times 10^6$/U	$<1 \times 10^6$/U	5×10^6/U for red cells and apheresis platelets $<8.3 \times 10^5$/U for platelet-rich plasma platelets
Percentage of components in which this must be attained	99	90	95
Statistical confidence that this is attained	95%	Not stated	Not stated

Adapted from Cardigan and Williamson [5].

the fact that only a fraction of components are tested for residual leukocytes and that the limit of sensitivity of current counting methods is around 0.3×10^6/U. Recent studies have demonstrated >3.8 log reduction in all leukocyte subtypes by whole-blood filtration and >3.1 log reduction by platelet filtration and one platelet-apheresis technology [6].

Despite advances in technology, LD systems occasionally fail. The risk that an LD system will result in blood components being issued that fail to meet the required specification for residual leukocytes is dependent upon a number of factors: the capability of the ID system, potential manufacturing defects in the LD filter or pack system, the proportion of components that are tested for residual leukocytes, and donor-related causes. An estimation of the likelihood of components is issued that exceed certain levels of residual leukocytes are illustrated (Table 2.2). Although most donor-related causes of filter failure are poorly understood, it is known that donors with sickle cell trait are more likely to either block LD filters or fail to leukocyte deplete; 100% of donations from such donors are therefore usually assessed for residual leukocytes [7].

Preparation and storage of red-cell components

Red cells are transfused to treat clinically significant anemia or blood loss. They are produced by removing the majority of plasma from whole blood by centrifugation (Figure 2.2). Red cells produced from blood where the buffy coat has been removed to make platelets will contain slightly lower volume and hemoglobin content because of loss of some red cells into the buffy coat (Table 2.3).

Table 2.2 Estimation of the residual risk of a leukocyte-depleted component being issued containing residual leukocytes above defined levels.

	$>1 \times 10^6$/U	$>5 \times 10^6$/U	$>100 \times 10^6$/U
Apheresis platelets	1:175	1:1352	1:6381
Pooled platelets	1:202	1:2028	<1:22304
Red cells in additive	1:160	1:1522	1:7250
Fresh-frozen plasma	1:1072	1:18251	<1:14783

Figures are taken from UK quality monitoring data for an 18-month period.
Residual risk = number of units issued/(number of units not tested/number of units tested) × number of units that have residual leukocytes above defined level.
Adapted from Cardigan and Williamson [5].

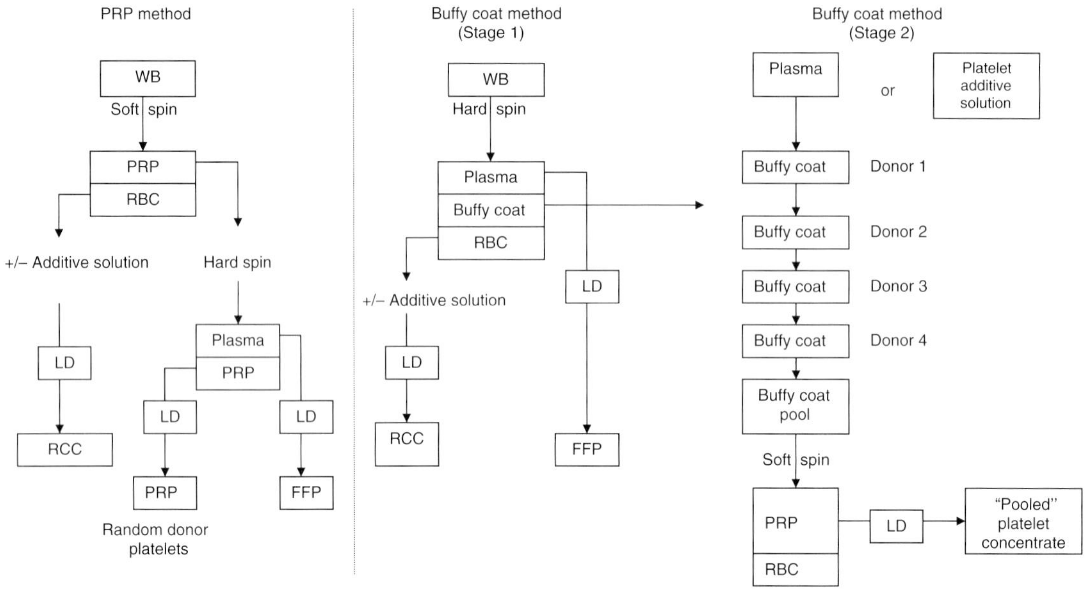

Figure 2.2 Production of platelet components from whole blood. WB, whole blood; LD, leukocyte depletion; PRP, platelet-rich plasma. Reproduced from Williamson and Cardigan [8], with permission.

Table 2.3 Specification and typical values for volume and hemoglobin content for leukocyte-depleted red-cell components.

	Specification						Typical values		
	Volume (mL)			Hb content (g/unit)					
	UK	EU	AABB	UK	EU	AABB	Volume (mL)	Hb (g/unit)	Plasma volume (mL)
Red cell in additive solution, LD all methods	>75%, 220–340 mL	NS	NS	>75%, >40 g	>40 g	NS	284 ± 25	56 ± 7	17
Red cell in additive solution, LD, apheresis	>75%, 220–340 mL	NS	>95%, >128 mL red cells	>75%, >40 g	>40 g	>95%, >42.5	273 ± 17	53 ± 4	22
Red cells in plasma, LD for exchange	NS	>75%, >40 g	NS				321 ± 27	60 ± 6	116
Red cells in additive solution, LD buffy coat removed	As above						250 ± 19	49 ± 6	6
Red cells in additive solution, LD	As above						304 ± 17	58 ± 5	28

LD, leukocyte depletion; NS, not stated.
Adapted from Cardigan and Williamson [5].

Red-cell components are stored at 4 ± 2°C for a maximum of 35–49 days in additive solution or 28–35 days in plasma. The shelf life depends upon the combination of anticoagulant, storage medium, blood pack, and whether any further processing steps are performed on the red-cell component (e.g., irradiation of the component).

For the vast majority of red-cell units processed, an additive solution containing adenine is added following separation to achieve a hematocrit of 50–70% and maintain red-cell quality during storage. The amount of residual plasma in a red-cell unit in additive solution is dependent on the hematocrit of the donor and how hard red cells have been centrifuged; it is between 5 and 30 mL. Red cells used for intrauterine transfusions (IUTs) and exchange or large-volume transfusion to neonates are normally stored or reconstituted in 100% plasma because of concerns over potential toxic effects of some of the constituents of additive solutions.

For patients with immunoglobulin A deficiency or severe allergic or anaphylactoid reactions to red cells, it may be necessary to remove >90% of plasma by washing and resuspending red cells in saline. Red cells from donors with rare phenotypes may be stored frozen for up to 30 years and are washed prior to transfusion to remove the cryoprotectant used to store them.

Preparation and storage of platelet components

Platelets are transfused to patients who have an inherited or acquired deficiency of platelet number or platelet function [9]. There are two basic methods for producing platelets from whole-blood donations: the "buffy-coat" method favored in Europe or the platelet-rich plasma (PRP) method favored in North America (Figure 2.2). Specifications for platelet components are given in Table 2.4. In the PRP method, whole blood is separated into PRP and red cells following a "soft spin." The PRP is then subjected to a "hard spin" to remove plasma and concentrate the platelets. In the buffy-coat method, whole blood is subjected to a "hard spin"

Table 2.4 Specification and typical values for volume and platelet content for leukocyte-depleted platelet components.

Platelet processing method	Number of donors per dose	Specification						Typical values†	
		Volume (mL)*			Platelet content ($\times 10^9$/unit)				
		UK	EU	AABB	UK	EU	AABB	Volume (mL)	Platelet content
Platelet-rich Plasma	5–10	—	>40 mL per 60×10^9 platelets	Not specified	—	>60	>55‡		
Apheresis	1–2	Locally defined	>40 mL per 60×10^9 platelets	Not specified	>240§	>200	>300‡	198 ± 15	288 ± 38
Buffy-coat-derived pooled	4–8	Locally defined	>40 mL per 60×10^9 platelets	Not specified	>240§	>60 per single unit equivalent	—	297 ± 38	330 ± 52

*The volume is also partly dictated by a requirement to keep the pH of platelet components within specified limits during storage.

†Typical values are taken from national quality monitoring data from the English National Blood Service and are likely to vary between countries.

‡More that 90% of components must meet this criterion.

§More than 75% of components must meet this criterion.

Adapted from Cardigan and Williamson [5].

and separated into plasma, red cells, and a buffy coat that contains most of the platelets but also some leukocytes and red cells. Buffy coats from four to six donations are then pooled with a unit of plasma from one of the donations (or PAS, platelet additive solution), subjected to a "soft spin" and the PRP removed. The main difference between platelet concentrates collected by apheresis and PRP or buffy-coat platelets is that one or more adult therapeutic doses can be collected by apheresis from a single donor, which is not possible from one whole-blood donation.

For either buffy-coat-derived or apheresis platelets, the majority of plasma (70%) in the platelet concentrate can be replaced with an artificial PAS designed to maintain platelet function during storage. PAS differ in their composition; key elements are the use of acetate or glucose as a substrate for platelet metabolism, phosphate that buffers lactate production, citrate to prevent coagulation and lactate production and the inclusion of potassium and magnesium to improve platelet function during storage. Three different PAS are CE marked in Europe for platelet storage, and some European blood centers routinely produce and store platelets in PAS. Platelets are stored with agitation at 22 ± 2°C for up to 5 days, although in some countries this is extended to 7 days, provided platelets are screened for bacterial contamination. For some patients with severe anaphylactic reactions to platelets because of contaminating plasma proteins, platelets can be re-suspended in 100% additive solution. However, these "washed" platelets have a reduced shelf life of 24 hours because of the rapid deterioration of platelet quality in the complete absence of plasma, and a proportion of the platelets may be lost during the process.

Preparation and storage of frozen-plasma components

Plasma from whole-blood donations or apheresis is used to either prepare plasma components for clinical transfusion or fractionate to produce pure plasma proteins.

FFP is produced by rapidly freezing the plasma removed from a whole-blood donation or collected by apheresis. This is usually performed within 8 hours of donation to preserve the activity of coagulation factors V and VIII, which are relatively labile. However, FFP can be produced from whole blood that has been stored at 4°C or 22°C for 24 hours. FFP is now only used to replace congenital single coagulation factor deficiencies where purified factor concentrates are not available (factors V and XI). Most FFP is used to treat acquired multiple coagulation factor deficiencies, usually in a clinical setting of massive transfusion, liver disease or disseminated intravascular coagulation [10]. Specifications of frozen-plasma component are given in Table 2.5.

Cryoprecipitate is produced by slowly thawing FFP at 4°C. This causes the so-called cryoproteins to precipitate out: factor VIII, fibrinogen, von Willebrand factor (VWF), fibronectin, and factor XIII. By centrifuging and removing the supernatant plasma, the cryoprecipitate left is a rich source of these proteins in a small volume of plasma. Because of the widespread availability of purified or recombinant concentrates of factor VIII and VWF, cryoprecipitate is rarely used in the developed world to replace these factors and is mainly used in the treatment of hypo- or dysfibrinogenemia. Because of its high fibrinogen content, cryoprecipitate is also used as a starting material for the production of fibrin glue.

The supernatant plasma removed from cryoprecipitate (CDP, cryoprecipitate-depleted plasma) has been used as a replacement fluid for plasma-exchange treatment of patients with thrombotic thrombocytopenic purpura (TTP), as an alternative to FFP. There are theoretical advantages of using CDP as it contains lower levels of high-molecular-weight multimers of VWF, but this benefit has not been proven clinically. In the UK, however, solvent-detergent-treated FFP is now recommended for the treatment of TTP because it is subject to pathogen inactivation during its manufacture and carries a lower risk of transfusion-related acute lung injury (TRALI) because of plasma pooling, which dilutes down the donor antibodies.

Frozen-plasma components can be stored for up to 36 months depending on the storage temperature, which is usually below −30°C. Once thawed, FFP should be used immediately but can be stored for up to 24 hours at 4°C.

Table 2.5 Specifications and typical values for residual cellular and coagulation factor content of frozen-plasma components.

	Residual cellular content (× 10^9/L)*			Coagulation factor content		
Specification	UK	EU	AABB	UK†	EU	AABB
Fresh-frozen plasma	Platelets <30	Platelets <50 Red cells <6	None	Factor VIII >0.70 IU/mL	Factor VIII >0.70 IU/mL	None
Cryoprecipitate	None	Platelets <50 Red cells <6	None	Fibrinogen >140 mg/unit Factor VIII >70 IU/unit	Fibrinogen >140 mg/unit Factor VIII >70 IU/unit	Fibrinogen >150 mg/unit Factor VIII >80 IU/unit
Cryoprecipitate-depleted plasma	None	Platelets <50 Red cells <6	None	None	None	None

Typical values‡	Residual cellular content	Coagulation factor content	Total volume (mL)
Fresh-frozen plasma	Platelets <3 × 10^9/L Red cells 0.63 ± 0.50 × 10^9/L	Factor VIII 1.19 ± 0.40 IU/mL	272 ± 17
Cryoprecipitate	—	Factor VIII 182 ± 71 IU/unit Fibrinogen 471 ± 199 mg/unit	40 ± 5
Cryoprecipitate-depleted plasma	—	—	305 ± 31

*Specifications for residual leukocytes are as per Table 2.1.
†More than 75% of components must meet these criteria.
‡Typical values are taken from national quality monitoring data from the English National Blood Service and are likely to vary between countries.
Adapted from Cardigan and Williamson [5].

Preparation and storage of granulocytes

Granulocytes may be transfused to patients with a severe deficiency or dysfunction of neutrophils which have developed or are at risk of developing life-threatening infections. There is anecdotal evidence of benefit, but few randomized controlled trials (RCTs) have been performed, and a recent systematic review found that there is inconclusive evidence from RCTs to support or refute the generalized use of granulocyte transfusion therapy in neutropenic patients [11]. Granulocytes are normally collected by apheresis and contain mainly neutrophils but also significant numbers of lymphocytes, red cells, and platelets; hence, they need to be crossmatched prior to transfusion. Preadministration of steroids and granulocyte-colony stimulating factor (G-CSF) to donors can considerably increase the yields collected ($1-10 \times 10^{10}$), but this is not permitted in volunteer donors in some countries. Yields in unstimulated donations rarely exceed 0.5×10^{10}, which is below the dose generally considered adequate for adults ($>1 \times 10^{10}$). Because of the logistical and ethical constraints in providing apheresis granulocytes, some countries issue buffy coats as a source of granulocytes. Ten to twelve buffy coats are transfused to provide a dose of 1×10^{10} neutrophils.

Granulocytes should be transfused as soon as possible after collection or preparation but can be stored at 22°C for up to 24 hours without agitation and are irradiated prior to transfusion to prevent transfusion-associated graft-versus-host disease (TA-GVHD) (see below).

Irradiation

Patients with congenital or acquired cellular immunodeficiency are at risk of development of TA-GVHD, an almost universally fatal condition caused by seeding of donor lymphocytes in the immunodeficient recipient. This condition can be prevented by irradiation of blood components prior to transfusion. A dose of 25–50 Gy is administered, usually using purpose-built gamma irradiation chambers; however, newer X-irradiation devices are now coming on the market, which do not carry the security risks of a gamma irradiation source.

Irradiation of red cells results in increase in extracellular potassium levels and hemolysis. For this reason, it is recommended that components only up to 14 days following collection are irradiated, and the shelf life is limited to 14 days post irradiation. Potassium levels are more critical in neonatal transfusions, and therefore the shelf life of large-volume transfusions for neonates (e.g., for exchange transfusion) is reduced to 24 hours post irradiation. There is no change to the shelf life of platelets postirradiation. Frozen components (FFP, cryoprecipitate) do not require irradiation as they do not contain live lymphocytes, and TA-GVHD has not been reported following transfusion of these components.

Patients at risk of TA-GVHD, who should receive irradiated cellular components, include hemopoietic stem-cell-transplant recipients, children with congenital cellular immunodeficiency, patients with Hodgkin's disease, and those treated with purine analog drugs and fetuses receiving IUT. Subsequent transfusions to IUT recipients should also receive irradiated components during the neonatal period. Some immunocompetent patients are also at risk, namely those receiving HLA-matched platelets, transfusions from first- or second-degree relatives, or therapeutic granulocytes.

Quality monitoring of blood components

Blood establishments manufacture blood components to meet agreed specifications [2–4]. However, because of biological variation of the starting material (i.e., the donor), not all components produced can be expected to meet specification. Quality monitoring is therefore performed on a proportion of components (usually 1% of components of which a large number are made; 10 per day when small numbers are made) to assess conformance. For some parameters, e.g., LD performance, statistical process monitoring is used to detect any drift in process capability before overt failures to specification are found.

Prion removal

At the time of writing, there have been four cases of possible transmission of vCJD by transfusion [12], all from nonleukocyte-depleted red cells. Recently, studies using hamster scrapie models have shown that LD reduces infectivity by 42% [13]. As LD alone is unlikely to render units non-infectious, there is considerable interest in alternative methods to reduce infectivity. Several companies are developing technology to remove prion protein from blood. PRDT/Macopharma has developed a filter that removes prion protein from LD red-cell concentrates. As this is an additional filtration step to LD, it is associated with a further loss of hemoglobin. On the basis of current Spongiform Encephalopathy Advisory Committee (SEAC) working assumptions on levels of infectivity, it is predicted that at least 3 log removal of infectivity (in addition to LD) would be needed to provide clinical benefit in terms of preventing transmission of vCJD. The PRDT device removes 3–4 logs of infectivity from red cells spiked with scrapie infected hamster brain [14] and >1.2 log (to below the limit of detection) of infectivity from the blood of hamsters infected with scrapie [15].

The PRDT/Macopharma P-Capt™ Prion Capture filter (Pathogen Removal and Diagnostic Technologies, Inc., New York, NY, USA, and Macopharma Tourcoring, France) has been shown in vitro to have negligible effect on the quality of red cells or on the expression of common red cell antigens. Studies in healthy volunteers examining the recovery of red cells filtered using P-Capt have been completed with satisfactory results, and a clinical study in patients designed to detect increased rates of adverse events or red-cell alloimmunization has commenced. Furthermore, the UK transfusion services have commissioned an independent assessment of the efficacy of prion reduction which is being performed by the Health Protection Agency.

A combined LD and prion removal filter is being developed by Pall (Ann Arbor, MI, USA). As yet, there are no prion removal filters for whole blood, platelets, or single unit plasma.

Prion removal technologies would therefore appear to offer great promise in reducing the risk of vCJD by transfusion; however, their implementation will require careful consideration of the costs and benefits involved and what role they will play if and when it becomes possible to test donors for vCJD. In October 2009, the Advisory Committee on the Safety of Blood Tissues and Organs recommended this to UK adopt prior filtration of red cells for patients born after 1st January 1996 (who will not have been exposed to BSE through diet). The UK Blood services are awaiting a decision in the Departments of Health as to whether this recommendation will be enacted.

Components for IUT and for neonatal transfusion

IUT and exchange or large-volume transfusions to neonates

Red cells are transfused in utero to treat severe fetal anemia. In order to keep the volume transfused to a minimum, they are prepared by removing some of the plasma from whole blood to achieve a high hematocrit of 0.70–0.90. Platelets may also need to be transfused in utero in cases of severe thrombocytopenia because of fetomaternal alloimmunization to platelet antigens (e.g., HPA-la). A hyperconcentrated platelet for this purpose can be produced using apheresis technology from geno-typed donors.

Exchange transfusions are performed on neonates to treat hyperbilrubinemia. As for red cells for IUT, those for exchange transfusion are prepared by removing some of the plasma from whole blood, but to achieve a lower hematocrit of 0.50–0.55. Red cells for IUT/exchange transfusion are limited to a 5-day shelf life and should be used within 24 hours of irradiation.

Because of concerns over the potential toxicity of adenine and mannitol in red cell additive solutions, red cells for IUT and exchange transfusion are prepared and stored in plasma. The same concerns apply to other clinical situations where large volumes of red cells are transfused to neonates, such as cardiac surgery or extracorporeal membrane oxygenation. However, some countries use red cells in additive for exchange and large volume transfusion without apparent problem. In the UK, there is a move toward the use of red cells in additive for large-volume transfusion where possible to reduce the unnecessary exposure of neonates to plasma and therefore risk of TRALI and vCJD.

Top-up red-cell transfusions to neonates

These are usually given to replace blood taken repeatedly for laboratory analysis in premature babies. They are prepared by splitting red cells in additive solution into multiple smaller packs, which can be stored up to the normal shelf life of red cells in additive (35 days in the UK) and reserved for individual recipients. This reduces the exposure of the recipient to different donors considerably. These need not be irradiated unless there has been a previous IUT, or the blood donation is from a family member.

Platelets and FFP

These are generally given to extremely sick babies with multiple defects in hemostasis. They can be prepared by splitting a full size unit into multiple aliquots or in the case of platelets by preparing them from a single donor by the PRP or buffy-coat method. They have the same shelf life as standard platelet and plasma components. In the UK, plasma for FFP and cryoprecipitate production for those under the age of 16 is imported from the USA as a precautionary measure to reduce the risk of vCJD transmission.

References

1. Kitchen AD, Barbara AJ. Current information on the infectious risks of allogeneic blood transfusion. In: Maniatis A, Van der Linden P, Hardy J-F (eds). *Alternatives to Blood Transfusion in Transfusion Medicine*. Wiley-Blackwell, Oxford, 2010, pp. 21–30.
2. American Association Blood Banks. *Guidelines and Standards for Blood Banks and Transfusion Services*, 24th edn. AABB Press, Bethesda, MD, 2006.
3. Council of Europe. *Guide to the Preparation, Use and Quality Assurance of Blood Components*, 13th edn. Council of Europe Publishing, Strasbourg, 2007.
4. James V. (ed.) *Guidelines for the Blood Transfusion Services in the United Kingdom*, 7th edn. The Stationery Office, London, 2005.
5. Cardigan R, Williamson L. Component procurement and processing strategies to reduce vCJD transmission risk. In: Turner ML (ed.) *Creutzfeldt-Jakob Disease: Managing the Risk of Transmission by Blood, Plasma and Tissues*. AABB Press, Bethesda, MD, 2006.
6. Pennington J, Garner SF, Sutherland J, Williamson LM. Residual subset population analysis in leucocyte depleted blood components using real-time quantitative RT-PCR. Transfusion 2001;41:1591–600.
7. Beard MJ, Cardigan R, Seghatchian J, et al. Variables determining blockage of leucocyte depleting filters by haemoglobin sickle cell donations. Transfusion 2004; 44:422–30.
8. Williamson LM, Cardigan R. Production and storage of blood components. In: Murphy ME, Pamphilon DH (eds) *Practical Transfusion Medicine*, 3rd edn. Blackwells Publishing, Oxford, 2009; pp. 259–73.
9. British Committee for Standards in Haematology. Blood transfusion task force. Guidelines for the use of platelet transfusions. Brit J Haematol 2003;122:10–23.
10. O'Shaughnessy DF, Atterbury C, Bolton Maggs P, et al. Guidelines for the use of fresh-frozen plasma, cryoprecipitate and cryosupernatant. Brit J Haematol 2004; 126:11–28.
11. Stanworth S, Massey E, Brunskill S, et al. *Granulocyte Transfusions for Treating Infections in Patients with Neutropenia or Neutrophil Dysfunction Cochrane Review. The Cochrane Library, Issue 1.* John Wiley & Sons, Ltd., Chichester, 2004.
12. Health Protection Agency. 2006. vCJD and Blood Products. Accessed at http://www.hpa.org.uk/infections/topics_az/cjd/blood_products.htm (accessed August 12, 2008).
13. Gregori L, McCombie N, Palmer D, et al. Effectiveness of leucoreduction for removal of infectivity of transmissible spongiform encephalopathies from blood. Lancet 2004;364:529–31.
14. Gregori L, Lambert BC, Gurgel PV, et al. Reduction of transmissible spongiform encephalopathy infectivity from human red blood cells with prion protein affinity ligands. Transfusion 2006;46:1152–61.
15. Gregori L, Gurgel PV, Lathrop JT, et al. Reduction in infectivity of endogenous transmissible spongiform encephalopathies present in blood by adsorption to selective affinity resins. Lancet 2006;368:2226–30.

CHAPTER 3

Current Information on the Infectious Risks of Allogeneic Blood Transfusion

Alan D. Kitchen[1] *& John A. J. Barbara*[2]
[1]National Transfusion Microbiology Reference Laboratory, National Blood Service, London, UK
[2]National Blood Service, London; University of the West of England, Bristol, UK

Introduction

Although transfusion services globally strive to ensure the microbial safety of the products they provide, even in developed countries there remains a residual, albeit small, risk of transfusion-related infection. However, it is also important to recognize that any invasive clinical procedure carries a finite risk. The key issues are to understand the principles of risk and risk assessment in the transfusion context, to determine the specific infection risks associated with allogeneic transfusion, to determine the consequences of any transmission and then to quantify those risks. This is complicated to some degree by the fact that transmission of infection may not always lead to clinical disease, and in such a situation there are no signs and symptoms of infection and therefore any infectious events are unlikely to be identified. This raises the question whether the transmission of an infectious agent that does not result in clinical disease, and when the recipient is not harmed in any way, should be considered to be an "infectious risk" of transfusion or not. Although the issue of transfusion-transmitted infection may seem to be fairly clear-cut—the transfusion transmission of any infectious agent is always a serious situation—the resultant pathological outcomes must be considered. In the absence of any resultant identifiable pathology, it could be hard to justify introducing screening.

This review will consider the overall infectious risks of allogeneic transfusion, the agents most commonly involved and their prevalence and incidence, how donations are screened to minimize the risk of infection, the concept and quantification of residual risk, new infectious "threats," and the importance of ensuring the appropriate clinical use of blood to minimize unnecessary exposure to human-sourced products.

The infectious risks of allogeneic transfusion

There are perhaps two main areas that can contribute to "risk" in terms of transfusion-transmitted infection: first, the risk of not identifying those transmissible infectious agents present in the donor population and for which donations need to be screened; second, the risk of then failing to detect an infectious donation with the screening program in use.

The first "risk" reflects the fundamental need to ensure that the right infectious agents have been identified and are being screened for in the first place. Although simple in concept, resolution of this can be complex. While most transfusion services globally would consider that all donations should, as a minimum, be screened for hepatitis B virus (HBV), hepatitis C virus (HCV), human immunodeficiency virus (HIV), and syphilis, there then remains the issue of additional agents that

Alternatives to Blood Transfusion in Transfusion Medicine, 2nd edition. Edited by A. Maniatis, P. Van der Linden, J.-F. Hardy.

may need to be screened for. This is largely dependent upon the incidence and prevalence of other transmissible infectious agents present in the donor population. These "other" transmissible agents include, for example, malaria, Chagas disease, human T-cell lymphotropic virus, agents that are restricted geographically, by continent, region, or even country, and thus present with wide ranging incidence and prevalence, and for which universal screening is not appropriate. Infrastructure of blood services and financial resources are also important issues in developing a screening policy.

The second risk is one of the most critical in transfusion practice today—the failure of the screening program to detect an infectious donation. There are a number of reasons for this, ranging from human error to biological variability, and a significant proportion of the resource of national transfusion services is allocated to reduction of this risk. While the reliability of the infectious disease screening of donated blood is critical to ensuring a blood supply that is as safe as possible, there are areas where this may fail. Although most national transfusion services tend to automate as much as possible the screening of donations, and also have fairly robust and comprehensive quality systems, there is always a reliance on staff to ensure that the systems are used correctly and effectively. Because neither the staff nor the systems in place are totally infallible, errors may still occur. However, it is probably true to say that in any well-developed and managed blood transfusion service the risks associated with failing to detect an infectious donation are more scientific/biological; this will be discussed in more detail in a later section.

In most countries with developed healthcare systems and developed blood transfusion services, the transfused blood is rarely the source of infection. More often either the patient was already infected or there was a different source. Nonetheless it is still crucial that the transfusion be ruled out as the source of infection as soon as possible.

Table 3.1 Infectious agents transmissible by blood transfusion.

Viruses
Hepatitis viruses
Hepatitis A virus (HAV)
Hepatitis B virus (HBV)
Hepatitis C virus (HCV)
Hepatitis D virus (HDV) (requires co-infection with HBV)
Hepatitis E virus (HEV)
Retroviruses
Human immunodeficiency virus (HIV) 1 and +2 (+ + other subtypes)
Human T-cell leukemia virus (HTLV) I and II
Herpes viruses
Human cytomegalovirus (HCMV)
Epstein–Barr virus (EBV)
Human herpesvirus 8 (HHV-8)
Parvoviruses
Parvovirus B19
Miscellaneous viruses
GBV-C [previously referred to as hepatitis G virus (HGV)]
TTV
West Nile virus
Bacteria
Endogenous
Treponema pallidum (syphilis)
Borrelia burgdorferi (Lyme disease)
Brucella melitensis (brucellosis)
Yersinia enterocolitica
Salmonella spp.
Exogenous (environmental species and skin commensals)
Staphyloccocal spp.
Pseudomonads
Serratia spp.
Rickettsiae
Rickettsia rickettsii (Rocky Mountain spotted fever)
Coxiella burnettii (Q fever)
Protozoa
Plasmodium spp. (malaria)
Trypanosoma cruzi (Chagas disease)
Toxoplasma gondii (toxoplasmosis)
Babesia microti/divergens (babesiosis)
Leishmania spp. (leishmaniasis)
Prions
Variant Creutzfeldt–Jakob disease (vCJD)

Transfusion-transmissible agents

There are a number of infectious agents that are known, because of documented cases, to be transmitted by transfusion. Table 3.1 provides a current listing.

Although the list may appear long, the bulk of the risk is centered on a small number of infectious agents, mainly those giving rise to persistent infections, for which it is generally considered that all donations should be screened: hepatitis B and C, HIV, and syphilis. Although for many years, "clinically," risk has been associated more with the persistent viral agents causing a carrier state, acute (short viremia) agents can be a risk, especially if at a high incidence.

Additionally, there are other agents such as plasmo-dium spp. (malaria), *Trypanosoma cruzi* (Chagas disease), and T-cell lymphotropic virus for which donors and/or donations may be screened in nonendemic areas such as Europe, but which may not be considered as such a universal threat as the specific infection risks associated with donors are more clearly defined, and thus the donor selection process can play a major role in screening for such infections.

Finally, there are those infectious agents such as *Borrelia burgdorferi* (Lyme disease), *Brucella melitensis* (brucellosis), *Babesia microti,* and *divergens,* and *Rickettsia rickettsii* (Rocky Mountain spotted fever), which are very restricted in their distribution/risk, and which may only present a risk in specific countries or even specific regions/localities within individual countries.

New/emerging infectious "threats"

In addition to the "existing" infectious risks, the threat of either new or emerging infection is always present. These "threats" may be newly identified infectious agents, known agents not previously identified as a threat to transfusion and known transmissible agents when the incidence of infection has increased both significantly and rapidly. Whatever the threat, it is obviously important to identify it as soon as possible.

A major problem for transfusion services is that very often the first knowledge of a "new" infectious threat comes from the report of an infection identified in the transfusion recipient. In some countries there is monitoring of transfusion recipients, and this is a way in which possible transfusion-related infections can be identified, hopefully as early as possible following the development of infection. However, this is very expensive, time-consuming, and fraught with problems, and therefore only performed in a small number of countries (and even then often only on a percentage of recipients). Additionally there are specific studies of cohorts of transfused patients, often looking for evidence of infection with "known" infectious agents, but sometimes looking for specific agents to determine if transfusion transmission occurs or has occurred. However, although such studies are valuable, they do not provide a systematic approach to the identification of transfusion-transmitted infectious agents.

Although many countries do have surveillance programs that monitor infectious disease outbreaks and their spread in the population for both new and existing infectious diseases, this may not always be related to any resultant risk of transfusion-related infection. The West Nile virus epidemic in the United States is such an example. Although the spread of infection in the population was being monitored and West Nile virus fitted the category of potentially transfusion-transmissible infectious agents, it still took transfusion transmissions to trigger interventions to reduce the transfusion risk. Additionally the risk of transmission of even a low-risk infectious agent may increase as the level of infection rises. Thus it is not just the monitoring of the prevalence of infection that is needed, but also the monitoring of the incidence of infection. Increasing incidence of a transmissible infectious agent in the general population almost always translates into an increased risk of infection in donors and thus potentially increased risk of the agent entering the blood supply [1].

Probably the most significant emerging threats to transfusion safety are the mosquito-borne infections, notably viruses such as Chikungunya, Dengue, Zika virus. Dengue is a well known and characterized virus and although always a potential threat it has rarely been reported to have compromised blood safety probably because it gives rise to an acute and highly symptomatic infection. Similarly Chikungunya is another well characterized threat, and although generally uncommon in actually compromising blood safety, it has caused specific problems following a major outbreak on the island of Reunion in 2005/6. Zika virus is a more recently identified flavivirus that effectively appears as a milder form of Dengue. As it is has relatively mild clinical sequelae, its actual significance in terms of transfusion transmission is unclear. Transfusion-transmitted infections may be more clinically significant, or alternatively mild infections following transfusion may not be identified in the absence of clinical symptoms and transmissions may be missed. However, in all such cases the emerging threat is primarily because of spread of the disease either through increased travel to endemic places or through the spread of infected mosquitoes to previously uninfected areas. Globally there would appear to be a slow but continuing spread of infectious agents from endemic areas into nonendemic areas or areas from where the infectious agents had been eradicated. There are a number of factors at play here, including increased global travel, the changing global climatic patterns, and failure or cessation of national/regional eradication programs. Although increasing the potential for transfusion transmission, in nonendemic countries at least, "at-risk" donors can be identified through travel/residency history (most risks in nonendemic countries come from travelers or migrants) and deferred or screened accordingly. There is an emerging issue, but in most cases there is also a viable solution.

Screening to reduce risk

The key to minimizing infectious risk is screening of both donors and donations. Screening is thus a two-stage approach: the donor selection process is the first stage of the screening process, and laboratory screening/testing the second stage.

Donor selection and screening

At the outset, the donor selection/deferral process determines whether the donor himself/herself represents a risk. If so a donation should not be collected from that donor. The definition of "risk" as far as donor selection is concerned revolves around the likelihood of the donor having been exposed to any infectious agent that is likely to be transmitted by transfusion. This risk is normally assessed by identifying particular activities/behavior, which could have resulted in the transmission of infection, i.e., unprotected sex, intravenous drug use, tattooing, travel, and so on, although this approach is not effective if exposure is common, e.g., eating beef in the United Kingdom.

Information is usually provided to donors in advance of donation so that self-exclusion can take place. This approach can be very effective as it reduces the issues surrounding obtaining the right information from donors in the "open" environment of a collection session. If potential donors have sufficient information ahead of time, they can elect not to attend a session if they are an "infection risk" in any way.

At the collection session, donors are normally then interviewed further and in more detail to ensure that they meet the selection criteria. These include medical conditions that may actually result in risk to the donors themselves if they donate.

Donation screening

Once the donor has been cleared for donation, laboratory screening/testing of the donation collected is the next step in the process. For most products this is also the final step. A screen negative result releases the product for clinical use. Thus there is a heavy reliance on the screening program to ensure that any donation from an infected donor is detected and removed from inventory as soon as possible. The effectiveness of any screening program is dependent upon a number of individual factors: the incidence and prevalence of the infectious diseases being screened for, the performance of the screening assays used, the screening algorithm, and the overall breadth and effectiveness of the quality system.

Understanding the infectious agents present in the donor population is critical—not just which agents are present, but their incidence and prevalence. In the context of transfusion safety, it is the incidence of infection in the donor population that is generally more relevant than prevalence as this represents the greatest risk in terms of encountering recent infections. Populations with a high incidence of infection are a greater risk, as at any point in time, there is a greater likelihood that a recently infected donor may present to donate; in most countries with developed transfusion services, it is these donations that represent the greatest infectious threat to blood safety today. Although high prevalence populations do also present a risk, if the incidence is low, the risk may be different. Depending upon the specific circumstances, it would be expected that most infected individuals would have (long) past infections, and any infected donations would therefore be detected easily on screening. In addition, if on resolution of infection immunity is conferred, then history of previous resolved infection would not exclude donation (c.f. HBV screening).

The screening assays in use must be selected carefully, ensuring the highest possible sensitivity and specificity. To achieve this, formal scientific evaluation of the assays is required, and their performance must be well characterized [2]. This includes evaluating the performance of assays in the detection of the different types and subtypes of the specific infectious agents, and importantly the ability to detect any mutants that either already exist or may appear. Thus the assay evaluation process plays a major part in ensuring safety. However, such evaluations are expensive and time-consuming, and even today there are limited numbers of high-quality in-depth evaluations performed globally. However, most of the evaluation data are subsequently made available in the public domain and so are accessible to most countries. The only proviso is that the data generally have a slight bias toward the specific needs of the country that performed the evaluation, its donor population, disease levels, and transfusion risks, and therefore may need supplementing in countries with significantly different disease prevalence and incidence. In addition to sensitivity, specificity assessment is also important to ensure that donations are not wasted unnecessarily. Even today, this still involves a degree of mutual exclusivity: increasing sensitivity results in decreasing specificity, and vice versa. Thus, assay sensitivity is not the sole performance marker.

The screening algorithm adopted plays an important role in the overall effectiveness of any screening program. The algorithm defines how the assay is used and the actions to be taken as a consequence of the results obtained. The simplest algorithm involves screening with the selected assay and then acting directly on the results obtained, i.e., releasing the screen negative donations and discard the reactives. This provides safety, but at the expense of sufficiency. Although safety is important, sufficiency is also important. A more balanced algorithm, for example, would be to screen with the selected assay, release the screen negative donations, and repeat the screening test (in duplicate) on all initially reactive donations. Donations with both repeat tests negative are released and repeat reactives discarded. There are other algorithms that can be used depending upon the circumstances. The rationale behind all of the algorithms is to ensure that the screening being performed is as effective as it can be given the particular situation. This is a function of the expectation of the screening, i.e., in the blood transfusion service context it is expected that the population being screened is a low-risk population and therefore the majority of screen reactives reflect nonspecific reactivity rather than true infection.

Finally, the overall quality of the laboratory screening performed obviously plays an important role in assuring safety. The effectiveness of the quality system is critical here. No matter how good the assays used, if they are not used correctly and effectively, there is a risk that an infected donation could be missed. The quality system ensures that the screening is performed effectively and consistently so that the results generated can be relied upon. There are numerous specific elements of any laboratory quality system, too many to cover adequately in this text. However, key elements of the quality system include the effective training of staff, documents and document control systems, evaluation and validation, and the ongoing monitoring of results; all of these drive toward process control and the aim of "error-free" testing. With these in place, the overall quality of the screening outcomes—the reliability of the results—increases.

Residual risk

Overall, well-designed laboratory screening programs are very effective in ensuring that donations with evidence of infection are identified. Nonetheless, there are limitations, and even the best screening programs may not prevent all instances of failure to detect an infectious donation. Probably the main reason today for any failure of the screening program within a well-organized and well-managed blood transfusion service is the situation where a donor has been recently (unknowingly) infected and then donates—although "incorrect" donor selection (for whatever reason) may also result in potentially infectious donations being collected. At that time the donation may be infectious, but the particular circulating marker of infection screened for, for that particular agent is not yet present at a detectable level. The donation will be "screen negative" although potentially infectious. This situation is described as the "window period" of infection, that period when a donor may be infectious, yet undetectable on screening. All blood screening strategies therefore aim to reduce the window period as much as possible. Whether the window period can be closed totally is a matter of debate, but good screening strategies can certainly reduce it significantly. However, to understand how this can be achieved, and the limitations, the factors that give rise to the window period must be considered and understood, and then the probability of collecting a donation from a donor in the window period must be quantified in some way.

Importantly, the window period is not simply a result of poor assay sensitivity; further factors are involved. The window period exists due to the combination of the biology of the infectious agent, the immunocompetence of the donor, the incidence of infection, the screening marker chosen, and the sensitivity of the screening assay used. Following exposure to an infectious agent, it takes some time, variable according to the agent, before replication has generated sufficient target, or the immune response has produced enough antibodies, to appear in the circulation and be detectable in a given test. Even then, there is a finite level at which it is detectable, although this may be greater than the level required to transmit infection. This is then dependent upon the particular marker of infection screened for—the agent itself (nucleic acid or antigen) or the host's immune response to the agent (antibody). Detection of the marker is then a function of its presence in the circulation, its level, and the sensitivity of the screening performed. Thus, the complexity of the window period and its importance in blood screening can be seen clearly.

The topic of residual risk, definition, calculation, and minimization, is one that has been of particular interest to transfusion services for over 10 years now. Residual risk (of transfusion-transmitted infection) is, very simply, the risk of an infectious donation being present in the blood supply after all of the donor and donation screening activities have taken place and the unsuitable donations have been removed and discarded. Although to "complete the circle" it would be useful to extend this definition to include the risk of the recipient then becoming infected, this clearly involves several factors and cannot be calculated exactly and reproducibly. However, the risk of failing to detect an infectious donation can be calculated with some degree of accuracy by using basic data generated through the screening program. In general, the data help to establish, by measurement, the overall effectiveness of the screening program. More specifically, however, the data can be used in a number of ways to both provide a baseline for the "current screening strategy" and predict the impact of changes to screening programs, for example, of introducing an additional assay or changing an assay. In addition, the data can be extrapolated to help calculate the potential risk of a "new" or "emerging" infectious agent by comparing data for a similar existing agent.

The estimates of residual risk are calculated by using the original formula of Schreiber et al. [3] and are based upon knowing the incidence of each transmissible infection in the donor population in question, the window period for each infectious agent, and the inter-donation interval. Although these data are general estimates in themselves, they are largely based upon clear measurables that can be obtained by transfusion services from within their own screening systems. The residual risk decreases as the incidence and the window period decrease and the inter-donation interval increases.

Residual risk estimates are now available from a number of countries. However, the nature of some of the data required (incidence of infection, interdonation intervals) is such that not all

Table 3.2 UK data on residual risk of transfusion-transmitted viral infections 2003–2004* [4].

Risk due to	HBV	HCV	HIV	HTLV I
Window period donation				
Per million	1.03	0.01	0.17	0.03
1 per × million	0.97	79.05	5.8	30.39
All causes				
All donations				
Per million	1.09	0.01	0.19	0.04
1 per × million	0.91	71.92	5.38	23.89
Donations from new donors				
Per million	4.38	0.05	0.27	0.15
1 per × million	0.23	18.39	3.65	6.65
Donations from repeat donors				
Per million	0.73	0.01	0.18	0.03
1 per × million	1.36	105.57	5.67	33.36

*Data include additional risk because of test sensitivity and testing errors.

transfusion services have the organization and structure to have accurate figures for these data. In these cases, it is very hard to generate accurate and meaningful data. Nonetheless, countries are starting to report residual risk data. Tables 3.2 and 3.3 provide residual risk data: detailed data from the United Kingdom (Table 3.2) and data from a number of countries (Table 3.3).

Bacterial contamination

A further, and important "risk" aspect of transfusion, although most commonly of platelet products, is bacterial contamination. The contamination of blood and components by bacteria has been a persistent problem for many years, although the advent of single use disposable collection systems has helped reduce significantly the incidence of contamination. However, platelet products, because of their storage temperature at 20–22°C and the nutrients in the plasma, provide the ideal conditions for bacterial growth. Over the years the numbers of reported cases of bacterial contamination have increased [12, 13] partly because of the development of coordinated reporting systems and partly because of an increased awareness and improved monitoring of patients. The risk of contamination effectively arises from either endogenous bacteremia in the donor, or from exogenous bacteria

Table 3.3 Data on residual risk of transfusion-transmitted viral infections from seven countries 2000–2005.

Country	Tests in addition to HBs Ag, HCV Ab, HIV Ab or Ag/Ab	Years	Risks per 10^6 donations		
			HIV	HCV	HBV
Germany [5]	HIV/HCV RNA, HBV DNA (pools)	2000–2002	0.22	0.37	1.51
France [6]	HIV/HCV RNA (pools)	2001–2003	0.32	0.1	1.57
Switzerland [7]	HIV/HCV RNA (pools) (2002)	2001–2003	1.35	1.5	5.36
Italy [8]	HIV/HCV RNA (pools)	2001–2003	1.1	0.5	
Spain [9]	HCV RNA (pools)	2000–2002	2.48	3.94	9.78
UK [10]	HCV RNA + HIV RNA (pools)	2002–2003	0.22	0.05	2.2
Canada [11]	HIV/HCV RNA	2001–2005			

entering the blood from the environment at some point in the donation process. Bacterial contamination from bacteremic donors is uncommon. Either levels are very low, such as after recent dental work and there may be automatic temporary deferral after such interventions, or the donor would be too unwell to donate. The major cause of bacterial contamination is because of exogenous contamination at some stage during the collection, processing, storage, or even use of the product. At the point of donation there is the greatest risk, as bacteria are present on the skin of the donor. Donor arm cleansing techniques have been refined over the years to minimize this risk, but some bacteria sit deep in the skin and may enter the donation in the plug of skin that is excised by the collection needle. Blood bag manufacturers have assisted in reducing the risk of contamination at the point of collection by adding a small pouch to the collection set into which the first 20–30 mL of blood is diverted. This should then capture any bacteria associated with the plug of skin. This, together with the improved arm cleansing methods, should reduce significantly contamination because of bacteria introduced at the time of donation [14]. In addition, although poor cleanliness and care during the subsequent processing of donations may result in the introduction of bacteria into one or more of the products, closed systems and improvements in hygiene and cleanliness in processing areas have reduced this risk also. Today, although bacterial contamination still occurs, improved practices have reduced the incidence of events. Monitoring of bacterial contamination of platelets has also been introduced in some countries to try to reduce the risk further still [15].

Identifying transfusion-transmitted infections

As discussed above, information about transfusion-transmitted infection incidents may come from a variety of sources. However, although prospective screening of recipients can be highly effective, it is not a highly practical approach. Thus, in terms of ensuring that any infections resulting from transfusion are identified, national hemovigilance programs are essential for capturing this information. Many countries now have such programs, which aim to identify nationally adverse outcomes of transfusions, and to collate and analyze the information. In the United Kingdom, this is achieved through the national Serious Hazards of Transfusion system [13], which requires all users of blood and blood components to report any adverse incidents in transfusion practice. Individual hospitals report to a central point any adverse incidents arising directly from transfusion. The information reported includes a full description of the incident and surrounding circumstances, the clinical outcome, possible causes, and the outcome of any local investigation. This information is then analyzed in a standardized way that enables incidents to be grouped according to underlying cause, outcome, and so on. The data obtained not only provide a good overview of the outcomes of blood transfusion, but also provide the essential information to enable a transfusion service to change/develop its strategies in response to identified issues and clinical outcomes.

However, it is also just as important to determine as accurately as possible whether a reported case of transfusion transmission of infection is genuine or not. This applies equally to known agents as well as new/emerging agents. For any reported transmission, it is crucial to investigate and determine (i) whether the recipient is truly infected; (ii) whether the recipient was infected before the transfusion event; and (iii) whether the infectious agent was actually present in one or more of the donations transfused. The acid test is to determine whether the reported infection event fulfills Koch's postulate, i.e., the proven detection of the infectious agent in both the transfused product and the recipient. Clearly, without demonstrating the presence of the agent in any of the products transfused, it is unlikely that the transfusion would be confirmed as the source of the infection.

Appropriate clinical use of blood

One of the most obvious ways to reduce the risk of posttransfusion infection is to transfuse only when it is necessary, and then only what is actually needed to obtain and maintain the desired clinical outcome. Thus, blood should only be used and transfused when clinically indicated. The use of alternatives, e.g., crystalloids and colloids when simple volume expansion is required, must be encouraged. It is only when either red cells, platelets, or plasma are specifically indicated that they should be transfused. This is a key element of medical education and is now being incorporated into medical training at undergraduate and graduate levels. It is also becoming increasingly emphasized by national departments of health as an important aspect of clinical governance.

Other interventions to reduce risk

Although screening today is still the mainstay of ensuring the microbiological safety of the blood supply, there are other interventions that can be applied to the products themselves to help reduce risk even further. Pathogen inactivation, the post-processing treatment of blood products by using combinations of chemical and physical treatments, has been in use for some years now, for specific, largely fractionated plasma products [16, 17], and more recently for ID products [18]. The effectiveness of such approaches on cellular products is limited, primarily as many of the approaches adopted so far are incompatible with cellular products, rendering them ineffective. There are a number of companies now working on more broadly applicable systems, and it should be expected that the use of pathogen inactivation technology would increase. However, this approach will not replace laboratory screening as the cornerstone of blood safety until it can be applied to all blood components.

Leukodepletion, although not intended to be an intervention solely to reduce microbial risk, may now also be considered to play a role in helping to reduce infection risk [19, 20]. There are some transmissible infectious agents that are essentially cell (leukocyte) associated, and removal of a significant percentage of the leukocytes may reduce any risk of their transmission. However, it must also be remembered that leukodepletion does not remove all leukocytes, and even with the expected 3–4 $\log_{10}$ removal there are still large numbers remaining. Leukodepletion has been considered to be a way to reduce the risk of variant Creutzfeldt–Jakob disease because of its association with leukocytes. In addition to leukodepletion, nanofiltration of red cell products to remove prions is also under evaluation, but the costs are high and the net benefit yet to be determined.

Although there are approaches and interventions that are aiming to reduce risk by replacing human-derived materials with artificial ones or by applying postprocessing procedures to inactivate/remove pathogens, these approaches leave gaps such that laboratory screening is still the keystone of the removal of infectious risk from transfusion.

Conclusion

Although blood transfusion is not without infection risk, in most countries with developed healthcare systems and transfusion services this risk is extremely small, almost negligible, and certainly well below the level of the general risk associated with invasive clinical procedures and other aspects of health care in general. The vast majority of patients are not at risk of infection from the blood and products that they receive. However, it is also important that transfusion services are vigilant and ensure that risks are kept low and that any threats to safety are identified and dealt with as soon as possible. Notwithstanding this, there is a real threat to blood safety—that of maintaining the right balance between cost and benefit. There is no question that there is a cost to ensuring safe blood and also a clear need. However, a problem arises when the costs spiral out of all proportion to the benefit obtained. This is an emerging consequence of the (over) use of the precautionary principle, applied increasingly to blood safety. Of course, measurement of the benefit is important, and then the issue arises of an expectation of absolute safety of all blood and products. Clearly, for those of us working in the field, no matter how much we may strive for it, we know this is unrealistic.

Nevertheless, patients, politicians, and some clinicians seem to have this expectation.

References

1. Brant LJ, Bukasa A, Davison KL, Newham J, Barbara JAJ. Increase in recently acquired syphilis infection in English, Welsh and Northern Irish blood donors. Vox Sang 2007;93:19–26.
2. Barbara JAJ, Ramskill S, Perry K, Parry J, Nightingale M. The National Blood Service (England) approach to evaluation of kits for detecting infectious agents. Transfus Med Rev 2007;21:147–58.
3. Schreiber GB, Busch MP, Kleinman SH, Korelitz JJ. The risk of transfusion-transmitted viral infections. The retrovirus epidemiology donor study. N Engl J Med 1996;334:1685–90.
4. NBS/HPA Surveillance Unit. Bloodborne infections in blood donors (BIBD). Available at: http://www.hpa.org.uk/ infections/topics_az/BIBD/est_freq_uk.htm (last accessed August 7, 2008).
5. Offergeld R, Faensen D, Ritter S, Hamouda O. Human immunodeficiency virus, hepatitis C and hepatitis B infections among blood donors in Germany 2000–2002: risk of virus transmission and the impact of nucleic acid amplification testing. Euro Surveill 2005;10:8–11.
6. Pillonel J, Laperche S. Etablissement Français du sang. Trends in risk of transfusion-transmitted viral infections (HIV, HCV, HBV) in France between 1992 and 2003 and impact of nucleic acid testing (NAT). Euro Surveill 2005;10:5–8.
7. Niederhauser C, Schneider P, Fopp M, Ruefer A, Lévy G. Incidence of viral markers and evaluation of the estimated risk in the Swiss blood donor population from 1996 to 2003. Euro Surveill 2005;10:14–16.
8. Velati C, Fomiatti L, Baruffi L, Romanò L, Zanetti A. Gruppo Italiano per lo Studio delle Malattie Trasmissibili con la Trasfusione. Impact of nucleic acid amplification technology (NAT) in Italy in the three years following implementation (2001–2003). Euro Surveill 2005;10:12–14.
9. Alvarez do Barrio M, González Díez R, Hernández Sánchez JM, Oyonarte Gòmez S. Residual risk of transfusion-transmitted viral infections in Spain, 1997–2002, and impact of nucleic acid testing. Euro Surveill 2005;10:20–22.
10. Soldan K, Davison K, Dow B. Estimates of the frequency of HBV, HCV, and HIV infectious donations entering the blood supply in the United Kingdom, 1996 to 2003. Euro Surveill 2005;10:17–19.
11. O'Brien SF, Yi QL, Fan W, et al. Current incidence and estimated residual risk of transfusion-transmitted infections in donations made to Canadian Blood Services. Transfusion 2007;47:316–25.
12. Wagner SJ. Transfusion-transmitted bacterial infection: risks, sources and interventions. Vox Sang 2004;86:157–63.
13. Stainsby D, Jones H, Asher D, et al. Serious Hazards of Transfusion: a decade of hemovigilance in the UK. Transfus Med Rev 2006;20:273–82.
14. McDonald CP, Roy A, Mahajan P, et al. Relative values of the interventions of diversion and improved donor-arm disinfection to reduce the bacterial risk from blood transfusion. Vox Sang 2004;86: 178–82.
15. Eder AF, Kennedy JM, Dy BA, et al. Bacterial screening of apheresis platelets and the residual risk of septic transfusion reactions: the American Red Cross experience (2004–2006). Transfusion 2007;47: 1134–42.
16. Bryant BJ, Klein HG. Pathogen inactivation: the definitive safeguard for the blood supply. Arch Pathol Lab Med 2007;131:719–33.
17. Klein HG, Anderson D, Bernardi MJ, et al. Pathogen inactivation: making decisions about new technologies – preliminary report of a consensus conference. Vox Sang 2007;93:179–82.
18. Irsch J, Pinkoski L, Corash L, Lin L. INTERCEPT plasma: comparability with conventional fresh-frozen plasma based on coagulation function an – in vitro analysis. Vox Sanguinis 2010; 98:47–55.
19. van de Watering L. What has universal leucodepletion given us: evidence from clinical trials? Vox Sang 2004;87(Suppl. 2):139–42.
20. Williamson LM, Cardigan R. Production and storage of blood components. In: Murphy MF, Pamphilon DH (eds) *Practical Transfusion Medicine*, 2nd edn. Blackwell: Oxford, 2005, pp. 259–73.

CHAPTER 4
Immunological Complications of Blood Transfusion

Clare Taylor[1], *Cristina Navarrete*[2] *&* *Marcela Contreras*[3]

[1]SHOT Medical Director, NHSBT, London, UK

[2]National Head of Histocompatibility & Immunogenetic Services, National Health Service Blood & Transplant (NHSBT), London, UK

[3]Royal Free & University College Hospitals Medical School; Chair of Blood Transfusion International (BTI), London, UK

Introduction

It is impossible to attain zero risk from blood transfusion, as indeed it is from any therapeutic intervention in medicine. There is increasing public awareness of the possible complications of blood transfusion with intense media attention focusing particularly on the risk of transfusion transmitted infections. The result is that the public perceive that blood transfusion is becoming more and more unsafe, whereas the reality is that blood transfusion has probably never been safer. This public concern is also misdirected, as the majority of potential blood recipients are aware of possible infectious complications but oblivious to the risks of incompatible transfusion. In the developed countries, transfusion transmitted infections carry an extremely low risk, while the risk of immunological complications of blood transfusion is somewhat higher. This risk tends to receive rather less media attention although some fatal cases of the wrong blood being transfused into a patient occasionally reach the newspaper headlines. However, the public and the media have a great deal of influence on blood transfusion services, resulting in demands for both improvements in the microbiological safety of blood, and for increased availability of alternatives to blood transfusion.

Alternatives to Blood Transfusion in Transfusion Medicine, 2nd edition. Edited by A. Maniatis, P. Van der Linden, J.-F. Hardy.

In this chapter, the immunological complications of blood transfusion will be discussed; the problems of viral transmission and bacterial contamination are discussed by Kitchen and Barbara [1] in this volume. In the United Kingdom, 2,250,000 of red cells are issued to hospitals in the course of 1 year, together with 300,000 units of fresh frozen plasma and 255,000 units of platelets. Between the years 1996 and 2008, the Serious Hazards of Transfusion (SHOT) report, a centralized anonymous hemovigilance data collection scheme to which all UK hospitals contribute [2, 3], included 5374 reports of transfusion related adverse incidents.

Figure 4.1 shows a pie chart illustrating the breakdown of causes of these transfusion reactions reported to the UK national hemovigilance system, SHOT. Transfusion of the incorrect blood component (IBCT) accounted for 43.8% of the cases reported (2355 cases). This underlines the fact that procedural errors resulting in the blood of the incorrect group or specification being transfused, including incorrect ABO and Rh D groups, are responsible for the majority of complications of transfusion. Incorrect prescription, administration of components, handling and storage are also included in the IBCT category. In fact, in only 24 cases in 12 years, was the transfusion of the IBCT causal or contributory to death; fortunately only 5–10% of recipients of ABO incompatible blood suffer serious morbidity of mortality. It is estimated in the United States and the United Kingdom that about 1 in 30,000 units of red cells transfused are ABO

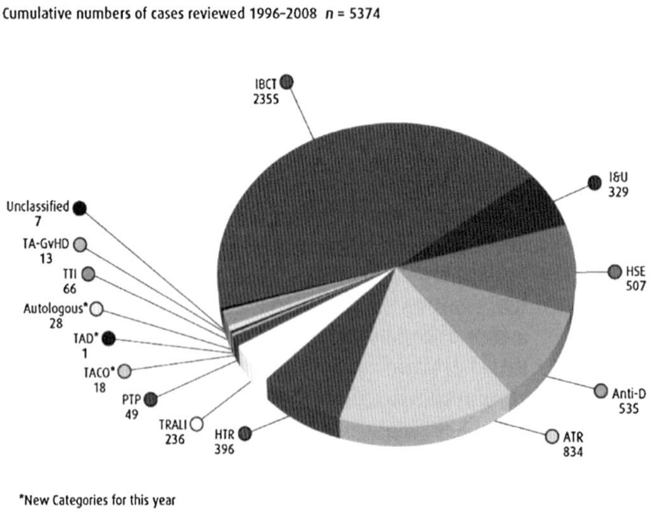

Figure 4.1 Cumulative numbers of cases reviewed by SHOT, the UK hemovigilance system 1996–2008 ($n = 5374$) (Before 2006 the HTR category was referred to as delayed transfusion reactions.) ATR, acute transfusion reaction; HSE, handling and storage errors; HTR, hemolytic transfusion reaction; IBCT, incorrect blood component transfusion; I&U, Inappropriate and unnecessary transfusion; PTP, post-transfusion purpura; TACO, transfusion associated circulatory overload; TAD, transfusion associated dyspnoea; TA-GVHD, transfusion-associated graft-versus-host disease; TRALI, transfusion-related acute lung injury; TTI, transfusion-transmitted infection.

incompatible, while deaths because of ABO incompatibility are of the order of 1 in 500,000–600,000 [3, 5]. This fatality rate, although very small, is much higher than the residual risk of acquiring HIV infection by transfusion in the United Kingdom, i.e., less than 1 in 5,000,000 units transfused (see the chapter by Kitchen and Barbara [1] in this volume).

Other immune-mediated causes of transfusion fatalities and of serious morbidity are generally less predictable or preventable. These include white cell antibody-mediated transfusion-related acute lung injury (TRALI), extravascular acute and delayed hemolytic transfusion reactions (HTR) because of non-ABO antibodies, transfusion-associated graft-versus-host disease (TA-GVHD), post-transfusion purpura (PTP), and anaphylactic reactions because of IgA in plasma transfused to IgA-deficient recipients with anti-IgA (Table 4.1).

HTR

HTR are the clinical consequence of the immune destruction of transfused red cells. This typically occurs when antigen-positive red blood cells are transfused into a patient who has a clinically significant alloantibody to that antigen. Severe acute HTR (AHTR) which occur within 24 hours of the offending transfusion are largely due to intravascular hemolysis caused by complement fixing IgM antibodies. However, less severe AHTR can be caused

Table 4.1 Immunological complications of blood transfusion.

Acute or immediate immunological complications of blood transfusion (occur within 1–2 hours)
Hemolytic transfusion reactions with symptoms (intra- or extravascular)
Febrile, nonhemolytic transfusion reactions
Uticarial reactions
Anaphylactic reactions
Transfusion-related acute lung injury
Delayed immunological complications of blood transfusion
Delayed hemolytic transfusion reactions with symptoms; always extravascular
Post-transfusion purpura
Graft-versus-host disease
Immunological refractoriness to platelet transfusions

by extravascular red cell destruction by IgG antibodies, such as, anti-D, anti-K in patients sensitized by previous transfusions, or pregnancy. The incidence of these is reported to be approximately 1 in 25,000 transfused units of blood [6]. Delayed HTR (DHTR) occur after 5–8 days following transfusion and are due to anamnestic or secondary immune responses in previously sensitized ("primed") patients in whom no antibody can be detected in the pretransfusion sample leading to extravascular hemolysis. The incidence of these is frequently reported to be 1 in 2500 transfused units [7].

The clinical presentation is a spectrum of symptoms, including fever and chills, which are the most common symptoms in both AHTR and DHTR [8]. Hypotension, tachycardia, nausea, and vomiting are more likely to occur in acute reactions, as are loin pain and chest pain, although these may also occur in delayed reactions. A leukocytosis may be noted in any HTR. The intravascular hemolysis of the AHTR produces the classic signs of hemoglobinemia and hemoglobinuria, which are pathognomonic of this condition (they may occur in extravascular HTR if very potent antibodies lead to red cell destruction by cytotoxicity). These signs are not a feature of DHTR in which the hemolysis is largely extravascular and jaundice is characteristic. Disseminated intravascular coagulation (DIC) and renal failure are much more common in AHTR but may also sometimes occur in DHTR, and death may ensue in either case, although more frequently after acute intravascular HTR. In certain circumstances, particularly in patients who are under anesthesia, the typical symptoms may be masked by the paralysis and unconsciousness of the patient. An HTR may then be first noted from the hemoglobinuria and excessive bleeding because of DIC. Biochemical tests may reveal hemoglobinemia, elevated lactic dehydrogenase, renal failure, and hyperbilirubinemia. Haptoglobin may become depressed in both kinds of reactions but is more important in intravascular cases. There is of course a danger in this situation that further blood may be transfused to keep up with blood loss, and this may be incompatible blood if the cause of the problem has not yet been fully identified.

Occasionally, an HTR may result from transfusion of non-red cell blood components such as fresh frozen plasma or platelets. In this event, the plasma, which is usually group O transfused to A, B, or AB recipients, may contain sufficient potent antibodies directed against A or B antigens on the recipient's red cells to cause hemolysis. Even more rarely, incompatibility between red cells from one donor and plasma from another donor may result in hemolysis when the two are mixed in the recipient ("interdonor" incompatibility). In some instances of DHTR, the apparent loss of circulating red cells exceeds what would be expected if only the antigen-positive transfused cells were cleared from peripheral blood. This may be because of complement deposition on autologous red cells which become positive on the direct antiglobulintest (DAT). This phenomenon has been called "bystander hemolysis" [9]. This reaction can be differentiated from autoimmune hemolytic anemia by the absence of anti-IgG reactivity in the DAT and a lack of an autoantibody in the eluate.

The characteristics of the alloantibodies and their specificity determine the course and severity of an HTR. Red cell alloantibodies are primarily IgG and less often IgM. IgM antibodies readily fix complement and it is these that classically cause the intravascular AHTR. IgG antibodies typically cause extravascular HTR which can be acute (if there is antibody present in sufficient quantity at the time of the incompatible transfusion), or delayed (if antibody is absent in the pretransfusion testing, "boosted" by the transfusion and becomes apparent 5–8 days later leading to red cell destruction). Table 4.2 shows the specificities associated with intravascular or extravascular hemolysis. Other red cell antibodies may rarely cause mild extravascular hemolysis but not intravascular hemolysis, and are very unlikely to be life-threatening.

Pathophysiology

Intravascular HTR (e.g., caused by anti-A; -B; -A,B; anti-Le^a anti-PP^k)

The most frequent cause is ABO incompatibility because of procedural errors, such as identification mistakes or laboratory errors. Most deaths because

Table 4.2 Red cell antibody specificities associated with hemolysis.

Blood group system	Intravascular hemolysis	Extravascular hemolysis
ABO, H	A, B, A_1, H	
Lewis	Le^a Le^b	
P	P + P_1+Pk(Tj^a)	P_1
I/i	I, i	
Rh		All
Duffy		Fy^a Fy^b
MNS		M, S, s, Mi, N
Lutheran		Lu^b
Kell		K, k, Kp^a Kp^b Js^a Js^b
Kidd		Jk^a Jk^b Jk^3
Vel	Vel	Vel

of incompatibility are caused by the transfusion of group A or B red cells to group O recipients, because anti-A,B is significantly more potent than anti-A or anti-B in group B or A subjects, respectively. There is activation of the full complement cascade by potent ABO IgM antibodies, leading to hemoglobinemia and hemoglobinuria. Cl to C9 activation leads to liberation of anaphylatoxins C3a and C5a, which are responsible for a significant proportion of the signs and symptoms of immune intravascular hemolysis (e.g., hypotension, shock, renal failure, DIC), and are usually far more serious than those of non-immune intravascular hemolysis or than those of immune extravascular hemolysis.

C3a and C5a act on mononuclear phagocytic cells and neutrophils to stimulate the respiratory burst and to enhance the expression of C3b receptors on these cells. As anaphylatoxins, C3a and C5a trigger the mast cell and basophilic release of mediators already preformed in their granules (e.g., histamine, platelet activating factor, tumor necrosis factor (TNF), IL-1, IL-3, 4, 5, and 6) or newly synthesized through the metabolism of arachidonic acid (e.g., leukotrienes, prostaglandins). In addition, mononuclear phagocytic cells are activated by phagocytosis per se and by C5a with the consequent secretion of mediators of the acute inflammatory response: TNF, IL-1, IL-8, PGE2, neutrophil-activating factor (NAP-1), and neutrophil chemotactic factor. Thromboplastic substances released by hemolysis and the activation of complement lead to activation of the extrinsic pathway of the coagulation cascade, contributing to DIC.

Extravascular HTR (caused by anti-Rh; -K; etc.)

Adherence of red cells coated with IgGl or IgG3 antibodies and/or C3b, to Fc receptors (FcγRl, FcγR2, and FcγR3), and to complement (CR1) receptors on mononuclear phagocytic cells or lymphocytes, leads to either phagocytosis and/or cytotoxicity of red cells. Cytotoxicity is mediated mostly by lysozymal enzymes released by the mononuclear phagocytic cells when red cells bind to them, heavily coated with IgGl and/or IgG3 antibodies. Moderate coating of red cells leads to phagocytosis. Those IgG antibodies that fix complement, such as anti-Jk^a are not as efficient as IgM antibodies and will only activate the cascade up to C3. C3b alone does not mediate cytotoxicity or phagocytosis but greatly enhances IgG-induced phagocytosis or cytotoxicity through adherence to the complement receptors (for C3b only) on mononuclear cells. Free IgG in plasma inhibits the binding of IgG red cell antibodies to Fc receptors on mononuclear phagocytic cells. Hence, red cells coated with noncomplement fixing IgGl or IgG3 antibodies (e.g., anti-D, -E, -c) are destroyed mainly in the spleen where there is hemoconcentration and large numbers of macrophages. C3b, with a very short half-life on red cells, abolishes the inhibitory effect of free IgG in plasma on Fc receptors of mononuclear cells: as there is no free C3b in plasma, cells coated with C3b will easily bind to CR1 receptors wherever they are present. For this reason, red cells coated with IgG and C3b (e.g., most anti-Jk^a, -Jk^b, many anti-K, many anti-Fy^3, etc.) are destroyed predominantly in the liver where there are abundant phagocytic cells and a good blood flow. This destruction occurs generally more rapidly and efficiently than when cells are coated only with IgG antibodies. Most clinically important IgG red cell antibodies are composed of subclasses 1 and 3, which are the subclasses with greatest destructive power as Fcγ receptors recognize only these two subclasses. Those IgM antibodies which do not activate complement do not seem to cause red cell destruction. Red cell alloantibodies composed only of IgA have not been found [8].

Clinical signs and symptoms of HTR

Fever and chills are usually the first signs of HTR, and it is impossible to distinguish them from febrile non-HTR (FNHTR). They are due to the release of anaphylatoxins and other mediators. *Back or loin pain* is very common and the cause is unknown. *Feelings of unrest* and *dyspnea* are caused by lung perivascular and peribronchial edema. *Hypotension, shock, and renal failure* occur in up to 10% of patients who have intravascular HTR but are rarely seen in extravascular reactions. Complement activation is likely to be a significant factor in these cases, and the anaphylatoxins C3a and C5a are probably the most important. In addition, the cytokines TNF and IL-1 can cause hypotension and shock. Renal failure may occur in either type of HTR although it is more common in the acute variety. Mildly affected patients may have elevated serum urea and creatinine levels but no symptoms. In more severe cases the patient may become anuric and require dialysis, with hypotension and DIC contributing to the renal impairment. Pathologically, the initial response is acute tubular necrosis, but there is also some thrombus formation in renal arterioles which may cause cortical infarction. With full supportive care, many patients regain normal renal function.

DIC is seen in intravascular AHTR but is very rare in extravascular HTR. It is probably due to complement activation and the release of thromboplastic substances caused by intravascular red cell destruction as well as by inflammatory cytokines. It may be difficult to distinguish from other causes of coagulopathy, which may occur in massive transfusion or in liver disease. Any patient who has been transfused and has microvascular bleeding must be considered to have an AHTR and be investigated accordingly. Coagulation tests and platelet counts are useful in guiding management.

Investigation of HTR based on AABB standards [10]

• Each blood bank or transfusion service must have a system for detection, reporting, and evaluation of suspected complications of transfusion. A responsible physician and the transfusion department/laboratory must be notified immediately and the reactions must be evaluated promptly.

• If there are symptoms or findings suggestive of an HTR, the transfusion must be stopped and the following must be performed:

1 Checking of all labeling on blood containers and documentation. If it is discovered at this stage that the wrong blood has been transfused, leading to an ABO incompatible transfusion, there is no need to continue investigating any further, except for inves tigating for signs of hemolysis and monitoring for severe signs and symptoms. The destination of the units of blood intended for that patient must be ascertained in order to avoid an incompatibility to another patient.

2 A properly labeled blood sample must be obtained from the patient and sent to the transfusion laboratory along with the original transfusion bag and giving set.

3 Post-reaction serum must be inspected for evidence of hemoglobinemia. A DAT must be performed and if positive must be compared with a prereaction sample.

4 Visual inspection of the urine for hemoglobinuria.

Additional testing must be carried out as necessary:

1 Repeat ABO and Rh testing on pre- and post-transfusion samples and on donor units.

2 Repeat the crossmatches on pre- and posttransfusion samples using the antiglobulin technique.

3 Repeat antibody screen on pre- and post-transfusion samples with antibody identification. Supplementary immunohematological tests may be necessary.

• Hematology tests for confirming hemolysis:

1 Red cell osmotic fragility.

2 Peripheral blood film.

Table 4.3 Differential diagnosis of hemolytic transfusion reactions.

Autoimmune hemolytic anemia
Cold hemagglutinin disease
Non-immune hemolysis
Incompatible fluids
Improper storage
Malfunctioning blood-warmer
Hereditary hemolytic anemias
G6PD deficiency
Hereditary spherocytosis
Hemoglobinopathies, e.g. sickle cell disease
Drug-induced hemolysis
Microangiopathic hemolytic anemia
Thrombotic thrombocytopenic purpura
Hemolytic uremic syndrome
HELLP syndrome
Mechanical heart valve dysfunction
Paroxysmal nocturnal hemoglobinuria
Bacterial contamination
Clostridium welchii
Malaria
Babesiosis

G6PD, glucose-6-phosphate dehydrogenase; HELLP, hemolysis, elevated liver enzymes and low platelets syndrome.

3 Reticulocyte count.

• Biochemical tests to confirm hemolysis:

1 Haptoglobins.

2 Methemalbumin.

3 Lactate dehydrogenase.

4 Bilirubin.

5 Tests for hemoglobinuria and hemosiderinuria.

If none of these tests are positive and involvement of the local reference laboratory yields no further information, then one must consider non-immunological causes of hemolysis. These include bacterial contamination, physical damage to transfused cells or recipient's cells, destruction of recipient's abnormal cells, e.g., in G6PD deficiency or hemoglobinopathy, or infectious causes such as gram-negative sepsis or malaria (Table 4.3).

Treatment

The treatment of an HTR must be guided by the clinical manifestations in the patient. The patient with minimal symptoms may be managed by careful observation, but in a severe reaction, early vigorous intervention may save life. Generally, the severity of a hemolytic reaction is directly related to the volume of incompatible blood transfused (although some deaths have been reported after ABO-incompatible transfusions of <30 mL of blood), so early recognition and stopping the transfusion is paramount in preventing severe morbidity and mortality. If there is ABO incompatibility and severe hemolysis, exchange transfusion may be necessary to prevent death and may be considered if large quantities of incompatible red cells are known to have been transfused. However, it is not always appropriate to expose the patient to further donated units with the associated risks of transfusion-transmitted disease if the hemolytic process is being well tolerated. Renal failure may be prevented by maintaining urine output with intravenous fluids and diuretics such as frusemide, and pressor support may be necessary for hypotension. Care must be taken to avoid fluid overload, especially in oliguric renal failure or patients with cardiac impairment.

DIC should be treated according to local protocols as there is still some controversy in the management of this condition. Plasma, cryoprecipitate, and platelets may be necessary; they should be prescribed against the clinical condition of the patient and the results of frequent monitoring of the coagulation screen, fibrinogen, FDP (fibrinogen degradation products) levels, and platelet count. Some authors advocate the use of heparin in the management of DIC. Intravenous immunoglobulin (IVIg) has occasionally been used as a pretreatment for a patient when incompatible blood has had to be given to an alloimmunized patient, because the IgG antibody is acting against a very common antigen and no compatible blood can be found promptly. This has successfully prevented extravascular haemolytic transfusion reactions [11]. Selection of red cells for a patient bleeding severely following an extravascular HTR may be very difficult. It is of course paramount that no patient is allowed to bleed to death for lack of red cells in the face of serological incompatibility. If possible, red cells should be obtained which lack the known antigens to which the patient has developed clinically significant antibodies.

Prevention

Proper patient identification is of ultimate importance in the prevention of AHTR because of ABO incompatibility, as the vast majority of these are the result of errors [2, 3].

These generally occur at the bedside before administration of the blood component or when taking samples for pretransfusion testing [2, 3,12]. Laboratory errors are less common. The majority of serious transfusion errors arise from breaches of current and established codes of practice in each institution. Human error is inevitable, but systems must be in place to minimize the possibility of harm to the recipient. Current standard operating procedures for accurate identification of patients must be in place both for taking of blood for pretransfusion testing and for bedside documentation immediately before transfusion [13]. Staff must be fully trained in the recognition of transfusion reactions and in taking prompt and appropriate action. Simple protocols should be established, implemented, and adhered to at all hospitals administering blood transfusions [14].

FNHTR

FNHTR are the most common adverse effect of blood transfusion and have a plethora of causes. When non-leukoreduced or -leukodepleted red cells or platelets are transfused, they occur with an incidence of 1% and 5–10%, respectively [10]. This reaction is usually immune mediated, because of the reaction of white cell antibodies in the recipient's plasma with the leukocytes in the transfused component. However, some evidence suggests that plasma proteins may also have an etiological role in FNHTR [15].

Definition and differential diagnosis

The definition of FNHTR includes a rise in temperature of at least 1°C (sometimes 1.5–2°C), which is not accounted for by the patient's clinical condition. The fever occurs in association with the transfusion and may be accompanied by chills, rigors, and a feeling of discomfort. It usually responds to antipyretic medication and hemolysis does not occur. FNHTR are not life-threatening, but repeated episodes may make the patient very apprehensive and reluctant to have subsequent blood components. To avoid these problems, premedication (with paracetamol) is often used to prevent febrile reactions [8]. However, in many multitransfused patients, premedication will not be sufficient and the white cell load of cellular components will need to be reduced. The differential diagnosis may be difficult, especially when comorbid disorders such as infection or malignancy, and certain treatments, may cause a similar spectrum of symptoms. Fever may also accompany other acute transfusion reactions, including AHTR, infusion of a bacterially contaminated blood component, or TRALI. The diagnosis of FNHTR must therefore be a diagnosis of exclusion. If in doubt, a direct antiglobulin (Coombs) test and a test for the presence of free hemoglobin in plasma may be performed. Bacterially contaminated blood components usually cause a rapid and profound febrile hypotensive reaction occurring much earlier than FNHTR. On the other hand, TRALI, which can be severe and life-threatening, is associated with dyspnea and cyanosis as well as hypotension and therefore a clinical diagnosis may be possible.

Antibody-mediated reactions

Evidence has been available since the 1950s to support the hypothesis that FNHTR are associated with the presence of white cell antibodies in the recipient reacting with leucocytes in the transfused component [16]. Also, it was noted that many patients who developed FNHTR had received previous blood transfusions or had been pregnant. Such white cell antigen–antibody interactions result in the stimulation and release of endogenous pyrogens, e.g., IL-1β, IL-6, and TNF cytokines, from the donor leukocytes. FNHTR may also result from cytokines released by the activation of the recipient's macrophages rather than the donor leukocytes. In these cases, the antibody–white cell interaction leads to the activation of complement and it is the antigen–antibody–complement interaction that may cause activation of macrophages in the recipient resulting in the production of endogenous pyrogens [17].

Antibodies against white cells are found in 70% or more of patients who suffer from FNHTR [18]. These include HLA and granulocyte antibodies. Leukodepletion or leukoreduction of blood components to below a threshold of 5×10^6 leukocytes per component significantly reduces the incidence of FNHTR. However, not all FNHTR are due to leukocyte antibodies. In 30% of patients experiencing these reactions, no white cell antibodies are in fact demonstrable. Although white cell antibodies are the main type of antibody implicated, anecdotal cases of strong FNHTR because of the presence of HPA antibodies reacting with incompatible platelets have been reported.

Reactions mediated by accumulation of biological response modifiers during storage

Among recipients of platelet transfusions, over 20% of patients suffer FNHTR on the very first exposure, while 55% experience their first reaction within their first three transfusion episodes. The occurrence of reactions to the first ever platelet transfusion in a patient means that such individuals could not have been previously alloimmunized to leukocytes, and therefore some FNHTR are not antibody-mediated. It has become clear from studies following up these data that component storage is an important factor in the occurrence of FNHTR. Also, it has been noted that the frequency of FNHTR is much greater with platelets than with red cells, even though the absolute number of leucocytes being transfused with each component is similar.

Increased concentrations of cytokines, either endogenous or exogenous, are harmful to the host, acting as endogenous pyrogens [19]. Cytokines such as IL-1β, IL-6, IL-8, and TNFα are actively synthesized and released during platelet and red cell storage. Linear correlations exist between cytokine level, white cell content, and duration of storage. Cytokines accumulate more at 22°C than at 4°C [20]. Prestorage leukocyte reduction prevents accumulation of cytokines and is associated with significantly fewer FNHTR. The removal of the buffy coat from red cells or the preparation of platelet concentrates by the "top-and-bottom" system or buffy-coat method will be sufficient to significantly reduce the production of cytokines in stored blood components; thus, it is not necessary to aim at leukodepletion when leukoreduction will be sufficient for this purpose. The effects of IL-1 include its potent pyrogenic activity, possibly mediated by IL-6 or PGE-2, stimulation of hemopoiesis, and activation of neutrophils and platelets. TNF is also a potent pyrogen, enhances B cell proliferation, and activates the extrinsic pathway of coagulation via tissue factor. IL-6 is a pyrogen and also enhances antibody responses and stimulates B cell proliferation and differentiation. IL-8 is a chemokine and a chemotactic factor for neutrophils and T cells. It stimulates neutrophil oxidative bursts and basophil histamine release. These findings support the concept that proinflammatory cytokines play a role in FNHTR, although the strong association is not necessarily proof of causation.

When plasma is exposed to plastic surfaces, complement is activated through the alternative pathway. C3 activation has been detected in both random donor and single donor apheresis platelets after storage for 5 days at room temperature with agitation. The mechanism of C3 activation is not cell-dependent as leukocyte-depleted platelets still have high C3 activation levels. C3a has multiple pathophysiological effects: it promotes mast cell histamine release, it is a vasodilator increasing microvascular permeability and it enhances in vitro platelet aggregation and serotinin release. It has been suggested that complement activation may stimulate monocytes in platelet concentrates to produce cytokines thereby contributing to the characteristic symptoms of FNHTR. Some of the newer leukodepletion filters appear to absorb C3a from platelet concentrates and may therefore be able to help reduce the incidence of FNHTR.

Prevention of FNHTR

The most effective way of preventing the majority of FNHTR is by prestorage leukodepletion of cellular blood components, i.e., red cells and platelet concentrates. Leukodepletion can be achieved by filtration of blood components or by modern apheresis techniques during the collection of platelets. In addition, as a proportion of reactions are mediated by biological response modifiers released by white cells and accumulating in the blood component over the period of storage, interventions to prevent this accumulation will decrease the frequency of FNHTR [15]. Poststorage (bedside) leukocyte reduction is not as effective as prestorage leukodepletion, as it is not well quality-controlled and cannot remove mediators and biological response modifiers such as IL-1β, IL-6, and TNF. Several groups have demonstrated that removal of leukocytes to a threshold of 5×10^6 per component before storage prevents the accumulation of IL-8 and proinflammatory cytokines such as IL-1β, IL-6, and TNF in both red cell and platelet components [21]. The administration of an antipyretic such as paracetamol may be useful in damping down the symptoms of FNHTR.

Allergic and anaphylactic reactions

These reactions occur in response to plasma proteins in the blood components administered, and represent a type 1 hypersensitivity response, i.e., an immediate allergic reaction following a second or further contact with an antigen which may vary on a scale from urticaria to anaphylaxis [8]. Hypersensitivity responses occur very rapidly following contact with the relevant antigens and recur on subsequent occasions. The primary antigen exposure stimulates plasma cells to produce specific IgE. This IgE binds to mast cells via its Fc receptor and sensitizes them. Representation of the antigen causes crosslinking of surface IgE stimulating degranulation of mast cells. The organ systems affected include skin, and the mucosa of the gastrointestinal and respiratory tracts, which are where mast cells are normally distributed. Stimulation of the sensory nerves causes itch and flare reactions while smooth muscle contraction causes vascular leakage and tissue edema. Arterial dilatation may cause headache and hypotension, while bronchoconstriction can cause respiratory distress. The mediators of this response from endogenous sources include histamine, serotonin and bradykinin, the analphylatoxins C3a and C5a, lymphokines, and leukotrienes [22]. Cutaneous allergic transfusion reactions occur in 1–3% of plasma-containing blood components, including red cells and platelets. The cardinal signs and symptoms are local erythema, urticaria, and pruritus. Soluble proteins in donor plasma are generally responsible but specific etiologies are rarely identified. Occasionally it has been discovered that the donor has ingested a food allergen or drug to which the recipient is sensitized [22]. Treatment includes antihistamines and occasionally hydrocortisone; antihistamines may be used prophylactically 1 hour before transfusion, to prevent future episodes.

Anaphylactic transfusion reactions are much less common, occurring once per 20,000–400,000 units of blood or components transfused. The cause is generally an IgG anti-IgA in an IgA-deficient recipient who is transfused with IgA-containing blood products. The formation of IgG/IgA immune complexes leads to the activation of complement and the subsequent release of C3a and C5a anaphylotoxins [23]. The signs and symptoms include a feeling of apprehension and impending doom, generalized flushing, nausea, vomiting, diarrhea and abdominal cramps, laryngeal edema, bronchospasm and dyspnea, profound hypotension, shock, and potential cardiopulmonary arrest. The transfusion should be stopped immediately and adrenaline 1 in 1000 (0.3–0.5 mL) given immediately. Supportive therapy for the circulation and respiratory system may be necessary. The differential diagnosis for such an acute and severe transfusion reaction must include ABO-incompatibility with an AHTR, TRALI, and perhaps bacterial contamination. IgA deficiency occurs in approximately 1 in 700 of the population in the United Kingdom and is defined as less than 0.05 mg/dL of IgA. The frequency of IgA deficiency with IgA antibodies is 1 in 1200; often anti-IgA is found in subjects who have never been pregnant or received a blood transfusion. Less than 20% of suspected cases of anti-IgA in a recipient reveal this to be the cause of the reaction.

Diagnosis must be made by reliably demonstrating deficiency of IgA and the detection of an anti-IgA. Once the diagnosis has been made, the patient must be clearly identified both on the hospital notes and on a wrist band or bracelet, and he/she must be fully informed of the implications. In future such patients should receive only IgA-deficient components which are collected from a special panel of IgA-deficient donors. In the absence of IgA-deficient donors, washed red cells may be administered with appropriate prophylactic measures taken beforehand in case of a mild reaction. Autologous transfusion may be considered in appropriate circumstances.

TRALI

TRALI is a life-threatening complication of transfusion which may have a very dramatic clinical presentation indistinguishable from adult respiratory distress syndrome [24]. In most cases it begins within 2 hours of transfusion but may be up to 4 or 6 hours following administration of a plasma-containing blood component. Symptoms generally include fever, hypotension, chills, cyanosis, non-productive cough, and dyspnea. Chest X-ray shows severe bilateral pulmonary edema or perihilar and lower lung field infiltration, without cardiac enlargement or involvement of the vessels. The X-ray findings may be much more severe than the auscultatory changes on examination. Severe hypoxia is usual, with very low arterial oxygen tensions, and the patient frequently requires mechanical ventilation. In contrast to patients with circulatory overload, those with TRALI have normal central venous pressure and normal or low pulmonary wedge pressure. It is possible that milder cases of TRALI may occur and not be recognized. Approximately 80% of patients with TRALI improve both clinically and physiologically within 2 or 3 days with adequate supportive care. Overall mortality appears to be in the region of 5–8%, in contrast to ARDS (adult respiratory distress syndrome), which has a mortality rate of 40–50%. Differential diagnosis includes circulatory overload, anaphylactic transfusion reaction, and bacterial contamination [8,10].

The true incidence of TRALI is unknown although there is a much quoted figure of 1 in 5000 plasma-containing transfusions [25]. This figure is likely to be an underestimate as milder cases may pass relatively unnoticed and severe cases may still be misdiagnosed, being attributed to circulatory overload. The precise mechanism involved in the development of TRALI is not clear, but two possible mechanisms have been postulated: an antibody-mediated and a soluble mediator-mediated. These mechanisms both involve the activation of granulocytes and the triggering of an inflammatory process, leading to the sequestration of neutrophils in the lung. In the vast majority of cases, investigators have demonstrated the presence of HLA class I and class II or granulocyte-specific antibodies in the donor [26]. In about half the cases studied, the HLA antibodies in the implicated donor correspond with one or more of the HLA antigens in the recipient. In other cases, neutrophil-specific antibodies (HNA1, HNA-3a) have been identified in the plasma of implicated units [26, 27]. These antibodies are most commonly found in the donations of multiparous women. It seems that the granulocytes interact with activated complement causing aggregation and blockage of the pulmonary microvasculature. Pulmonary leuko-sequestration leads to transient changes in vascular permeability and pulmonary edema. In a small number of reported cases, similar antibodies are found in the pretransfusion serum of the recipient and in such cases TRALI is more frequent after granulocyte transfusions [28]. In some cases clinically diagnosed as TRALI, no antibody has been identified. It has been suggested that in these cases the granulocyte activation is mediated by a soluble lipid substance, which accumulates during the storage of the products [29]. In any case, it is likely that a number of factors determine the final clinical response of a patient and these may include the characteristics of the antibody, nature and distribution of the related antigen, the extent of complement activation (in particular liberation of C5a) and the immune status of the recipient.

Diagnosis and treatment

There is no diagnostic test or pathognomonic finding for TRALI, so the diagnosis is one of exclusion. Other causes of respiratory distress and pulmonary edema in the transfusion setting must be fully investigated, including myocardial infarction, circulatory overload, and bacterial infection. The measuring of central venous and pulmonary wedge pressures is very helpful. A proper work-up of TRALI should include testing of the donor and recipient sera for granulocyte (HNA) and lymphocyte (HLA) antibodies.

Antibody specificity can be determined and HLA or HNA typing of the recipient's or donors' cells can also be carried out. The presence of a positive reverse lymphocyte crossmatch between donor serum and patient lymphocytes provides further supportive evidence. The treatment of TRALI includes intensive respiratory and circulatory support [24]. In almost all cases, oxygen supplementation is necessary, although mechanical ventilation may not always be required. Some reports suggest that the administration of corticosteroids may be beneficial.

Prevention

It is recommended that donors who have been implicated in TRALI and who are found to have granulocyte or lymphocyte antibodies should be withdrawn from the donor panel unless their components are to be issued as deglycerolized or washed red cells [24]. Exclusion of all multiparous women from the donor panel would result in a huge (5–30%) loss of blood donors, but it is advisable not to use their plasma for the manufacture of FFP or for suspension of platelet concentrates. Routine donor testing for HLA and granulocyte antibodies is time-consuming and much too costly to be implemented. In the United Kingdom, efforts are made to use only male donations for the preparation of FFP and for suspension of pooled platelets.

TA-GVHD

Acute GVHD is a recognized complication of allogeneic hemopoietic progenitor cell transplantation. It results from the presence of viable lymphocytes in the allograft recognizing the host HLA antigen type as foreign, resulting in a characteristic immune response [30]. The clinical syndrome includes fever, diarrhea, abnormal liver function tests, and a characteristic rash particularly affecting the palms. A similar picture may result from the transfusion of viable lymphocytes into immunosuppressed recipients in the absence of an allogeneic stem immunosuppressed cell transplant. In this situation, bone marrow aplasia and pancytopenia also result.

TA-GVHD is typically evident from 8–10 days post-transfusion. It is almost uniformly fatal, with death occurring within 1 month in over 90% of cases. The features discussed above are not substantially different from those of a variety of viral illnesses or drug reactions [31]. Comorbid conditions may obscure the clinical features of TA-GVHD, particularly if the clinician has a low index of suspicion. Cases are most certainly under-reported because of lack of recognition or the absence of definitive diagnostic studies in many cases. Cases were originally recognized in patients with severe combined immunodeficiency or Wiskott–Aldrich syndrome, neonates with hydrops fetalis, and in patients with Hodgkin's disease. The incidence is unknown, but TA-GVHD is estimated to occur in up to 1% of patients with hematological malignancies or lymphoproliferative diseases.

In addition to defined populations at risk as in Table 4.4, TA-GVHD has also been reported in non-immunocompromized hosts, particularly pregnant women, people undergoing cardiovascular and abdominal surgery, patients with active rheumatoid arthritis, and trauma cases [32]. Clearly not all immunocompromized individuals develop TA-GVHD and there must be additional risk factors predisposing patients to this condition. The main requirements for the development of GVHD are the following: shared HLA types between the recipient and donor but with other differences that will make the donor recognize the recipient as foreign, the presence of immunocompetent cells in the transfused blood components, and inability of the host to reject the immunocompetent donor lymphocytes. In a normal recipient, immune cells will far outnumber donor-derived T cells, which are therefore eliminated by a host-versus-graft reaction. However, if a small number of functional T lymphocytes are transfused which derive from a donor who is homozygous for one of the recipient's HLA

Table 4.4 Patient groups at risk of transfusion-associated graft-versus-host disease (TA-GVHD).

Patient groups at risk of TA-GVHD
Congenital immune-deficiency disorders
Hodgkin's disease
Neonates with erythroblastosis fetalis
Recipients of intrauterine transfusions
Recipients of stem cell transplants
Recipients of blood components donated by relatives
Recipient-donor pairs from genetically homogeneous populations
Recipients of HLA-matched cellular products
Premature neonates
Patients possibly at risk
Non-Hodgkin's B cell lymphomas
Solid tumors
Potential at-risk group
Full term neonates
Patients with AIDS
Patients receiving immunosuppressive medication

HLA, human leukocyte antigen.

haplotypes, the recipient will not recognize these cells as foreign. The donor T cells will, however, recognize the host as foreign, undergo clonal expansion and establish TA-GVHD. This situation is referred to as a one-way HLA match and TA-GVHD may be expected to occur regardless of the host immune status [33]. Recent experiments in selective depletion of recipients' CD4+, CD8+, and NK cells have suggested that CD4+ cells may be involved in the pathogenesis of TA-GVHD, while CD8+ and NK cells appear to be protective. This may explain why TA-GVHD is not reported in patients suffering from AIDS.

Diagnosis

Only the documentation of donor-derived lymphocytes in a recipient's circulation or tissues can confirm the presence of TA-GVHD. Characteristic histological changes may be seen in a skin biopsy which may reveal degeneration of the basal cell layer with vacuolization, dermal epithelial layer separation, and bulla formation. Liver biopsy may reveal degeneration and eosinophilia, and bone marrow aspiration may reveal aplasia with lympocytic infiltration. Several methods are used to make a positive diagnosis of TA-GVHD, and these are based on demonstrating donor cells or DNA in the patient, as shown in Table 4.5 [34–36].

Table 4.5 Diagnostic techniques for graft-versus-host disease.

HLA typing of donor and recipient, ideally using DNA-based techniques
Molecular genetic evaluation using short tandem repeats probes
Identification of donor T cells using the above techniques in skin biopsy samples

HLA, human leukocyte antigen.

Treatment

There is no effective treatment of TA-GVHD and the mortality rate is extremely high. Immunosuppressive therapies have been used with little success, including steroid therapy, antithymocyte globulin, cyclosporin, cyclophosphamide, and anti-T cell monoclonal antibodies. These treatments are sometimes useful in GVHD after stem cell transplantation but are ineffective in TA-GVHD. In the light of the absence of any effective treatment, the prevention of this condition is essential. This is particularly demonstrated by the UK hemovigilance reports (SHOT), which show that TA-GVHD has been a significant cause of mortality from transfusion. The incidence has been reduced by the introduction of universal leukodepletion, but not eliminated while other causes are gradually being eliminated [2].

Prevention

The irradiation of cellular blood components renders the donor lymphocytes non-viable and protects the recipient from potentially developing TA-GVHD. Guidelines have been produced by the American Association of Blood Banks in the United States and the British Committee for Standards in Haematology in the United Kingdom recommending for which patients gamma-irradiated products should be available [37–39]. At the moment, because of the low incidence of TA-GVHD in immunocompetent patients receiving donated blood from unrelated donors, gamma irradiation is not applied to all transfused cellular blood components. This decision is based upon the extremely low risk in such recipients, and the costs and logistics of universal irradiation, plus the effect on other measurable parameters in components such as potassium content and shelf life. Leukocyte reduction to a level of less than 5×10^6 residual leukocytes per unit is not an effective way of preventing the occurrence of TA-GVHD, as sufficient viable lymphocytes are still present to cause this syndrome. The introduction of universal leukodepletion in the United Kingdom has resulted in a significant reduction in the number of reported cases in the past years [25].

PTP

PTP is characterized by the development of severe, sudden and self-limiting thrombocytopenia occurring 5–10 days after a blood transfusion. The recipients always have a history of sensitization, mostly by pregnancy, and occasionally by blood transfusion. The diagnosis rests on the demonstration of potent antiplatelet reactivity in the patient's serum for a specific platelet antigen, usually HPA-la. PTP therefore is a disease of adults, with no patients younger than 16 years of age being reported in the literature [40]. The female-to-male ratio is 5:1. The epidemiological findings are due to the requirement that a patient has previously been exposed to platelet-specific antigens before PTP can develop following a subsequent transfusion.

Clinical presentation

In the majority of cases (over 80%), the platelet count drops around 1 week following the transfusion to less than 10×10^9 per liter. If random platelets or specific antigen-negative platelets are transfused, the increment is generally very poor or nonexistent [41]. One or two reports suggest that HPA-la-negative platelets may be beneficial, and in cases of severe bleeding platelet transfusion should be considered [42]. Hemorrhage may occur from the gastrointestinal tract and epistaxis is common. Intracranial hemorrhage is responsible for the mortality rate which is around 9%. The differential diagnosis of PTP includes immune thrombocytopenic purpura (ITP), sepsis and DIC, bone marrow failure, drug-induced thrombocytopenia, and thrombotic thrombocytopenic purpura (TTP). Drugs, infection, and DIC are common causes of thrombocytopenia and these must be excluded. In straightforward alloimmunization to platelet, red cell, or lymphocyte antigens, only the incompatible cells bearing the relevant alloantigen are destroyed by the reaction. The unique feature of PTP is destruction of autologous antigen-negative platelets in the presence of a platelet-reactive alloantibody. A source of indirect evidence of PTP as opposed to straightforward alloantibody-mediated platelet destruction is the response to therapy. IVIg infusion or plasma exchange has little effect on simple alloantibody-mediated platelet destruction, but these therapies are effective in PTP. The difficulty in proving a diagnosis of PTP means that the incidence of PTP is unclear, especially in the group of long-term platelet-dependent patients. The clinical spectrum of PTP may be very broad and mild cases may also not be noticed. Calculations of the theoretical frequency of occurrence of PTP based on the incidence of HPA-la and other platelet antigens in the population, and on the frequency of alloimmunization through pregnancy, suggest a high incidence of PTP. In fact, it is quite rare, and it may be that other immune response factors may be necessary for individuals exposed to incompatible platelet antigens to develop the syndrome whereby autologous platelets are destroyed.

Mechanism

Several theories have been put forward to explain the destruction of autologous antigen-negative platelets in PTP. The first suggests that immune complexes are formed by the interaction of soluble platelet-specific antigen in donor plasma and platelet antibody in the patient [43]. These complexes then bind to autologous platelets through a high affinity Fc receptor mediating platelet destruction. A second theory maintains that an autoantibody is developed in response to exposure to an incompatible platelet antigen and this antibody reacts not only with HPA-1a-positive cells but also with antigen-negative cells in the recipient. A third suggestion is that the soluble platelet antigen in donor plasma adsorbs onto the recipients' platelets, converting them to antigen-positive targets which are then destroyed by the alloantibody [44]. Soluble HPA-1a substances have certainly been identified in the plasma of HPA-1a-positive donors; however, platelet antigen–antibody complexes have not been demonstrated in the serum of PTP patients. In support of the auto-antibody theory, platelet-associated IgG is increased in PTP. In addition, acute-phase PTP serum contained reactivity against a protein present in both HPA-1a-positive and HPA-1a-negative platelets. This reactivity occurred concurrently with anti-HPA-1a activity and disappeared after the acute phase of the illness, although the anti-HPA-1a persisted. Certainly, the response to therapy of PTP is similar to that of ITP, in which steroids, IVIg, and splenectomy may be associated with elevations of the platelet count and decreases in platelet-associated IgG.

The diagnosis of PTP depends upon the finding of severe thrombocytopenia of less than 10×10^9 per liter approximately a week to 10 days post-transfusion. Normal red cell morphology rules out the possibility of TTP. Platelet antibody assays reveal serum antibody with HPA-1a specificity in most cases, although antibodies to other platelet-specific antigens are sometimes implicated [45]. Such patients frequently have antibodies to red cell and white cell antigens as well, and it may be that some individuals mount a generalized immune response encompassing a number of targets.

Therapy

Treatments for PTP are hard to evaluate as the condition is generally self-limiting and untreated patients recover in approximately 2 weeks. Most patients with PTP are treated with corticosteroids during the acute phase at a dose of 2 mg/kg of prednisolone, or an equivalent dose of an alternative preparation [46]. There is little evidence of the efficacy of this treatment, although steroids may inhibit reticuloendothelial cell function or alternatively may result in a decreased antibody production. The most effective therapy for PTP is plasma exchange using some fresh frozen plasma as a replacement [47]. Recently, infusions of IVIg have become the first line in therapy for PTP, and a large proportion of patients respond well [48]. Only those unresponsive to IVIg now go on to plasma exchange. Recovery from PTP occurs 3–4 days after initiation of treatment with IVIg 0.5 g/kg for 2 days.

Prognosis

Prognosis is good with spontaneous recovery occurring in all cases. Mortality rates relate to the incidence of intracranial hemorrhage in a few patients. The incidence of recurrence of PTP with subsequent transfusions in an individual patient is extremely low, although, because of the potential severity of the reaction, patients with a documented history of PTP should receive antigen-negative blood products when at all possible.

Immunological refractoriness to platelet transfusions

Platelet transfusions play a major role in the management of thrombocytopenia in hematological and onco-logic patients. However, a proportion of these patients become refractory to the transfusion of platelets from random donors, because of immunological and/or nonimmunological causes. Immunological refractoriness is primarily caused by HLA antibody-mediated destruction of transfused platelets, although HPA and high-titer ABO alloantibodies have occasionally been implicated. The nonimmunological causes of platelet refractoriness, because of the destruction/consumption of transfused platelets, include sepsis, disseminated intravascular coagulation in the patient and certain drugs, such as amphotericin B, vancomycin, and ciprofloxacin. Patients with confirmed immunological refractoriness because of the presence of HLA antibodies require transfusions of HLA-matched or HLA compatible platelets.

The laboratory investigations to identify these cases involve an HLA antibody screening of the patient's serum, and if positive, the identification of antibody specificity. This is followed by the HLA typing of patients and the selection and issue of HLA compatible platelets. An alternative approach, in the absence of a panel of HLA-typed donors, is to provide crossmatch-compatible platelets. It is important to document the posttransfusion increments in order to evaluate the efficacy of the transfusion and the donor. Although platelets express HLA-A, -B, and -C antigens, only matching at the HLA-A and -B locus antigens is considered to be relevant.

References

1. Kitchen AD, Barbara AJ. Current information on the infectious risks of allogeneic blood transfusion. In: Maniatis A, Van der Linden P, Hardy J-F (eds). *Alternatives to Blood Transfusion in Transfusion Medicine*. Wiley-Blackwell, Oxford, 2010, pp. 21–30.
2. Taylor C (Ed.), Cohen H, Mold D, Jones H, et al. on behalf of the Serious Hazards of Transfusion (SHOT) Steering Group. The 2008 Annual SHOT Report (2009). Available at: http://www.shotuk.org
3. Stainsby D, Jones H, Asher D, et al. Serious hazards of transfusion: a decade of hemovigilance in the UK. Transfus Med Rev 2006;20:273–82.
4. Sazama K. Reports of 355 transfusion-associated deaths: 1976–1985. Transfusion 1990;30:583–90.
5. Schmidt PJ. The mortality from in compatible transfusion. In: Sandier SG, Nussbacher J, Schanfield MS (eds). *Immunobiology of the Erythrocyte*. Alan R. Liss, Inc., New York, 1980, pp. 251–61.
6. Walker RH. Noninfectious risks and new trends in transfusion practice. J Fla Med Assoc 1993;80:37–8.
7. Ness PM, Shirey RS, Thoman SK, Buck SA. The differentiation of delayed serologic and delayed hemolytic transfusion reactions: incidence, long-term serologic findings, and clinical significance. Transfusion 1990;30:688–93.
8. Mollison PL, Engelfriet CP, Contreras M. *Blood Transfusion in Clinical Medicine*, 10th edn. Blackwell Science, Oxford, 1997.
9. Salama A, Mueller-Eckhardt C. Delayed hemolytic transfusion reactions. Evidence for complement activation involving allogeneic and autologous red cells. Transfusion 1984;24:188–93.
10. Vengelen-Tyler V. *Technical Manual*, 12th edn. American Association of Blood Banks, Bethesda, MD, 1996.
11. Kohan Al, Niborski RC, Rey JA, et al. High-dose intravenous immunoglobulin in non-ABO transfusion incompatibility. Vox Sang 1994;67:195–8.
12. Linden JV, Paul B, Dressier KP. A report of 104 transfusion errors in New York State. Transfusion 1992;32:601–6.
13. National Patient Safety Agency. *Right Patient – Right Blood*. 2006. Available at: http://npsa.nhs.uk
14. Murphy M, Pamphilon DH. *Practical Transfusion Medicine*. Blackwell Publishing, Oxford, 2005.
15. Heddle MM, Klama LN, Griffith L, et al. A prospective study to identify the risk factors associated with acute reactions to platelet and red cell transfusions. Transfusion 1993;33:794–7.
16. Payne R. The association of febrile transfusion reactions with leuko-agglutinins. Vox Sang 1957;2:233–41.
17. Dzik WH. Is the febrile response to transfusion due to donor or recipient cytokine? Transfusion 1992;32:594.
18. Brubaker DB. Clinical significance of white cell antibodies in febrile non-hemolytic transfusion reactions. Transfusion 1990;30:733–7.
19. Heddle NM, Klama L, Singer J, et al. Febrile nonhemolytic transfusion reactions to platelets. Curr Opin Hematol 1995;2:478–83.
20. Heddle N, Tan M, Klama L, Shroeder J. Factors affecting cytokine production in platelet concentrates. Transfusion 1994;34(Suppl.):675 (abstract).
21. Shimizu T, Uchigiri C, Mizuno S, Kamiya T, Kokubo Y. Adsorption of anaphylatoxins and platelet-specific proteins by filtration of platelet concentrates with a polyester leukocyte reduction filter. Vox Sang 1994;66:161–5.
22. Greenberger PA. Plasma anaphylaxis and immediate type reactions. In: Rossi EC, Simon TL, Moss GS, Gould SA (eds). *Principles of Transfusion Medicine*, 2nd edn. Williams & Wilkins, Baltimore, 1996, pp. 765–71.
23. Sandier SG, Mallory D, Malamut D, Eckrich R. IgA anaphylactic transfusion reactions. Transfus Med Rev 1995;9:1–8.
24. Popovsky MA, Chaplin HC Jr, Moore SB. Transfusion-related acute lung injury: a neglected, serious complication of hemotherapy. Transfusion 1992;32:589–92.
25. Chapman CE, Stainsby D, Jones H, et al. Ten years of hemovigilance reports of transfusion-related acute lung injury in the UK, and the impact of preferential use of male donor plasma. Transfusion 2009;49:440–452.
26. Win N, Massey E, Lucas G, et al. Ninety-six suspected transfusion related acute lung injury cases: investigation findings and clinical outcome. Hematology 2007;12:461–9.
27. Yomtovian R, Kline W, Press C, et al. Severe pulmonary hypersensitivity associated with passive

transfusion of a neutrophil-specific antibody. Lancet 1984;1:244–6.

28. Levy GJ, Shabot MM, Hart ME, Mya WW, Goldfinger D. Transfusion-associated noncardiogenic pulmonary edema. Report of a case and a warning regarding treatment. Transfusion 1986;26:278–81.
29. Silliman CC, Ambruso DR, Boshkov LK. Transfusion-related acute lung injury. Blood 2005;105:2266–73.
30. Ferrara JL, Deeg HJ. Graft-versus-host disease. N Engl J Med 1991;324:667–74.
31. Shivdasani RA, Anderson KC. Transfusion-associated graft-versus-host disease: scratching the surface. Transfusion 1993;33:696–7.
32. Ohto H, Anderson KC. Survey of transfusion-associated graft-versus-host disease in immunocompetent recipients. Transfus Med Rev 1996;10:31–43.
33. Shivdasani RA, Haluska FG, Dock NL, et al. Brief report: graft-versus-host disease associated with transfusion of blood from unrelated HLA-homozygous donors. N Engl J Med 1993;328:766–70.
34. Kunstmann E, Bocker T, Roewer L, et al. Diagnosis of transfusion-associated graft-versus-host disease by genetic fingerprinting and polymerase chain reaction. Transfusion 1992;32:766–70.
35. Wang L, Juji T, Tokunaga K, et al. Brief report: polymorphic microsatellite markers for the diagnosis of graft-versus-host disease. N Engl J Med 1994;330:398–401.
36. Sage D, Stanworth S, Turner D, Navarrete C. Diagnosis of transfusion-associated graft-vs.-host disease: the importance of short tandem repeat analysis. Transfus Med 2005;15:481–5.
37. Klein H. *Standards for Blood Banks and Transfusion Services*, 17th edn. American Association of Blood Banks, Bethesda, MD, 1996.
38. BCSH Blood Transfusion Task Force. Guidelines on gamma irradiation of blood components for the prevention of transfusion-associated graft-versus-host disease. Transfus Med 1996;6:261–71.
39. Williamson LM, Stainsby D, Jones H, et al. The impact of universal leukodepletion of the blood supply on hemovigilance reports of posttransfusion purpura and transfusion-associated graft-versus-host disease. Transfusion 2007;47:1455–67.
40. von dem Borne AE, van der Plas-van Dalen CM. Further observation on post-transfusion purpura (PTP). Br J Haematol 1985;61:374–5.
41. Gerstner JB, Smith MJ, Davis KD, Cimo PL, Aster RH. Posttransfusion purpura: therapeutic failure of PlAl-negative platelet transfusion. Am J Hematol 1979; 6:71–5.
42. Win N, Peterkin MA, Watson WH. The therapeutic value of HPA-1 a-negative platelet transfusion in post-transfusion purpura complicated by life-threatening haemorrhage. Vox Sang 1995;69: 138–9.
43. Shulman NR, Aster RH, Leitner A, Killer MC. Immunoreactions involving platelets. V. Posttransfusion purpura due to a complement-fixing antibody against a genetically controlled platelet antigen. A proposed mechanism for thrombocytopenia and its relevance in 'autoimmunity'. J Clin Invest 1961; 40:1597–620.
44. Kickler TS, Ness PM, Herman JH, Bell WR. Studies on the pathophysiology of posttransfusion purpura. Blood 1986;68:347–50.
45. Christie DJ, Pulkrabek S, Putnam JL, Slatkoff ML, Pischel KD. Posttransfusion purpura due to an alloantibody reactive with glycoprotein Ia/IIa (anti-HPA-5b). Blood 1991;77:2785–9.
46. Weisberg LJ, Linker CA. Prednisone therapy of posttransfusion purpura. Ann Intern Med 1984;100:76–7.
47. Cimo PL, Aster RH. Post-transfusion purpura: successful treatment by exchange transfusion. N Engl J Med 1972;287:290–2.
48. Becker T, Panzer S, Maas D, et al. High-dose intravenous immunoglobulin for post-transfusion purpura. Br J Haematol 1985;61:149–55.

CHAPTER 5
Immunomodulation and Allogeneic Blood Transfusion

Marloes Waanders[1,2], *Leo Van De Watering*[2] *& Anneke Brand*[1,2]
[1]Department of Immunohematology and Blood Transfusion, Leiden University Medical Center, Leiden, The Netherlands
[2]Sanquin Blood Bank South West Region, Leiden, The Netherlands

Introduction

Most symptomatic adverse effects of blood transfusion are caused by iso- and alloantibodies. The discovery of the antiglobulin test to detect irregular IgG red cell antibodies prevented most life-threatening acute and subacute hemolytic transfusion reactions. Characterization of antibody specificities after repeated erythrocyte transfusions led to preventive matching for Rh and Kell antigens for multitransfused patients at high risk. Similar milestones exist to limit the side effects of leukocyte antibodies. In the 1960s, leukocyte antibodies were identified as a cause of febrile nonhemolytic transfusion reactions [1] and, some years later, of transfusion-related acute lung injury [2] and platelet transfusion refractoriness [3]. Removal of leukocytes by filtration significantly reduced febrile nonhemolytic transfusion reactions and human leukocyte antigen (HLA) immunization by platelet transfusions, and this was widely implemented in Europe at the end of last century [4]. Most of these first observations, after (evidence-based) confirmation, changed transfusion management and improved transfusion safety.

In 1973, Opelz and Terasaki showed in a multivariate analysis of observational studies a significant enhancement of survival of kidney grafts in recipients of multiple transfusions compared with nontransfused patients [5]. The concern for wider consequences of this immunosuppressive transfusion effect on impairment of immunosurveillance against cancer was raised in 1981 by Gantt [6]. Since then, transfusion-related immunomodulation (TRIM) has been suspected of causing postoperative nosocomial infections and other complications leading to increased mortality after surgery. How transfusions affect the recipient's cellular immune response and which clinical benefit or harm can be attributed to transfusions is, however, still unraveled. The current evidence on TRIM is discussed in this review.

Alternatives to Blood Transfusion in Transfusion Medicine, 2nd edition. Edited by A. Maniatis, P. Van der Linden, J.-F. Hardy.

Immunological effects of blood transfusions

The adaptive immune response

The adaptive antigen-specific immune response, distinguishing self and nonself, is performed by lymphocytes. This immune response requires the recognition by helper T (Th) cells of foreign proteins on antigen presenting cells (APCs). In the case of a primary immune response in a naive patient, a strong stimulus by professional APCs such as dendritic cells, producing IL-12 p70 and IFN-γ, is most effective. Th cells can be activated by two pathways. Foreign APCs, bearing major histocompatibility complex (MHC)-HLA-class II antigens, induce direct stimulation of the immune response. A fairly large number of T cells can respond to this stimulus, which under physiological circumstances only occurs in fetomaternal hemorrhage in pregnancy, but also applies to blood transfusion and transplantation. The other T helper activation pathway, used for all foreign antigens, is by indirect stimulation. This process requires degradation of foreign proteins into small peptide fragments that are transported to the groove formed by HLA-class II molecules on the surface of APCs. Th cells recognizing foreign peptide in self-HLA class II are less abundant than T cells responding to direct activation by foreign MHC. The cytokines produced after APC-Th interaction determine the skewing towards particular effector Th cells (Thl, Th2, or Th3), relevant for developing cytotoxic T cells or specific antibodies. After elimination of the immunizing trigger, the response is downregulated to memory cells. The adaptive response in a naïve person (primary immune response) is rather slow, taking days to weeks before it is maximally effective.

The innate immune response

Our first line of defense, the innate nonantigen-specific immune system attacks dangerous foreign molecules. This system is represented by macrophages, granulocytes, natural killer (NK) cells, and soluble factors such as natural antibodies, the complement, and coagulation systems. The innate immune system uses receptors (Toll-like receptors), which are triggered by a wide range of structures present on various pathogens. Activation of the innate immune system leads to release of cytokines and chemokines which attract neutrophils and macrophages leading to inflammation, usually locally at the site of microbial invasion or tissue damage. This inflammatory process also provides accessory factors essential for activation of the adaptive response.

Transfusions and the immune response

Transfusions affect both the innate and the adaptive immune system. Transfusions contain many foreign antigens and always, increasing with longer storage intervals, apoptotic, and necrotic cells. Immediately after blood withdrawal, granulocytes start to deteriorate, followed by macrophages, although viable lymphocytes can be detected after more than 25 days of storage.

Apoptotic cells, expressing annexin V or phosphatidylserine, immediately engage a ligand on macrophages which start to produce anti-inflammatory cytokines such as prostaglandin E-2 and transforming growth factor-beta [7]. These factors not only suppress the innate immune response of macrophages and NK cells but impair the APC capacity as well, downregulating the adaptive antigen-specific immune response. During storage, soluble response modifiers accumulate in blood products. Factors derived from leukocytes are elastase, soluble HLA class I and II molecules, sFasL, and proinflammatory cytokines IL-1, IL-6, and IL-8. Pro inflammatory cytokines are an important cause of nonhemolytic febrile transfusion reactions [8, 9] and in particular IL-8 is associated with transient posttransfusion leukocytosis, observed in critically ill patients [10].

Beside gradual apoptosis, functional lesions occur during storage. After 3–5 days of storage, the responder capacity of T cells decreases owing to a phosphorylation defect, impairing the protein synthesis of T cells upon signaling of the T cell receptor. This reduces the proliferative response of donor lymphocytes, relevant to impaired transfusion-associated graft-versus-host disease [11]. The stimulator capacity by donor APCs of the direct pathway is irreversibly abrogated after 10–14 days of storage because of loss of costimulatory molecules, which are essential for effective APC-Th cell interaction [12].

Consequently, every blood product differs in content of soluble proinflammatory cytokines and in proportion of apoptotic cells, signaling macrophages to produce anti-inflammatory factors. With respect to adaptive immunity, during storage APCs lose costimulatory molecules impairing direct activation of Th cells. This leaves only the indirect pathway to elicit an adaptive immune response after processing of foreign donor antigens. This indirect pathway is dependent on APCs, which may be affected by pro- and/or anti-inflammatory stimuli in the blood product.

It makes a difference whether transfusions are administered to patients in stable condition or to patients after surgery or during critical illness or sepsis, as these latter conditions can cause a profound suppression of the innate immune system.

After transfusion, there is a two-way interaction between donor and recipient cells. Three to five days after transfusion, depending on the storage interval of contaminant leukocytes, proliferating lymphocyte blasts can be found in the circulation [13]. Most donor DNA disappears after a week, below the detection level of sensitive molecular methods, although haploidentical cells sharing an HLA-DR antigen can remain detectable for several weeks [14]. Persistence of donor cells for many years is observed in approximately 20% of apparently healthy transfused trauma survivors, even after transfusions of leukocyte-reduced blood stored for longer than 3 weeks. Lee et al. showed that these patients, prior to transfusion, have an impaired lymphocyte proliferative capacity against donor lymphocytes, owing to instant and profound suppression of the innate immune system induced by trauma injury [15]. This transfusion-induced chimerism is not associated with apparent clinical disease; a role for this chimerism in allogeneic (transplantation) tolerance has not yet been investigated.

Transplantation tolerance

Clinical results

The observations of Opelz et al. [5] showing better cadaver kidney graft survival in recipients of multiple blood transfusions initiated a debate as to whether this could be the result of an immunomodulating effect of transfusions or, because transfusions elicit HLA antibodies, an improved compatibility of a kidney graft selected by a negative leukocyte cross-match. The possibility that allogeneic leukocytes play a causal role in transplantation tolerance was made more likely by a study by Persijn et al. showing that a single blood transfusion, provided the blood was not leukocyte-depleted, improved graft survival [16]. The superiority of sharing at least one HLA-DR antigen between transfusion donor and recipient in order to obtain graft acceptance was proposed by several investigators [17, 18]. The beneficial effect of pretransplant blood transfusions is not restricted to cadaver kidney transplantation [5, 16, 18–30], but has been published in heart [18, 31–35], combined pancreas–kidney [36, 37] and liver transplantation [38, 39] (Tables 5.1 and 5.2.) The studies in Tables 5.1 and 5.2 span over 30 years during which new and highly effective immunosuppressive drugs to prevent or treat rejection were developed. As outcome after organ transplantation depends on several factors that cannot be controlled in a retrospective study, it is difficult to compare solely the effect of a pretransplant blood transfusion between studies with a historical control group. Multivariate analysis can control for confounding factors, but cannot change the setup of a study. Of the 26 clinical studies summarized in Tables 5.1 and 5.2, only four had a prospective, randomized controlled character [19–22]. Because these studies differ with regard to the selection of patients and to that of (third-party or organ-specific) transfusion donors, the transfusion schedule, and the immunosuppressive treatment, a combined analysis is not possible and a conclusion on the immunomodulatory effect of transfusion cannot yet be made. Although the beneficial transfusion effect seems to be present despite the use of modern immunosuppressive drugs, deliberate pretransplant transfusions are currently virtually abandoned. The main reasons are concerns about transfusion-transmitted diseases and development of alloimmunization.

On the mechanism

Pretransplant blood transfusions may contribute to immunological tolerance. Central tolerance results from intrathymic deletion of self-reactive lymphocytes. In the periphery, tolerance to self or nonself, such as allogeneic transplantation antigens, can be achieved by various mechanisms [40]. Proposed mechanisms are induction of apoptosis or deletion of effector cells [41–43] induction of anergy [12, 44–47] and active regulation of effector cells [48–51]. However, these putative mechanisms do not explain why HLA-DR sharing between blood donor and recipient would be advantageous in evoking a positive effect. Figure 5.1 shows a hypothetical model in which pretransplant blood transfusions from donors sharing an HLA class II antigen with the patient may facilitate peripheral

Table 5.1 Effect of pretransplant blood transfusions on clinical outcome after kidney transplantation.

	Blood transfusion				Clinical outcome after kidney transplantation†			
Reference	No	Yes	Blood product	Study	Acute rejection (%)		Graft survival (%)	
Opelz et al. [5]	$n = 25$	$n = 57$	BCD	Retro	n.a.		29% vs. 66%	$P = 0.003$¶
Persijn et al. [16]	$n = 74$	$n = 30$	n.a.	Retro	n.a.		32% vs. 87%	$P < 0.00001$**
Persijn et al. [16]		$n = 19$	BCD^1	Pros	n.a.		$79\%^1$ vs. $25\%^2$	$P < 0.0032$¶
		$n = 8$	FLR^2					
Sanfilippo et al. [22]		$n = 22$	RBC^1	Pros*	n.a.		$50\%^1$ vs. $50\%^2$	n.s.¶
		$n = 30$	BCD^2					
Lundgren et al. [23]	$n = 147$	$n = 334$	n.a.	Retro	0.88 vs. 0.74§	$P = 0.08$	n.a.	
Melzer et al. [24]	$n = 49$	$n = 163$	WB/RBC	Retro	n.a.		64% vs. 83%	$P < 0.03$¶
Kerman et al. [25]	$n = 220$	$n = 100$	RBC	Retro	37% vs. 36%	n.s.	79% vs. 79%	n.s.¶
Lagaaij et al. [18]	$n = 41$	$n = 32$	WB/BCD, 1 DR match^1	Retro	n.a.		45% vs. $81\%^1$	$P = 0.001$††
		$n = 30$	WB/BCD, no DR match^2				45% vs. $57\%^2$	n.s.††
							$81\%^1$ vs. $57\%^2$	$P = 0.02$††
Iwaki et al. [26]	n.a.	n.a.	n.a.	Retro	n.a.		75% vs. 71%	n.s.¶
Alexander et al. [21]	$n = 12$	$n = 10$	WB (donor-specific)	Pros*	42% vs. 50%	n.s.	n.a.	
					42% vs. 0%‡	$P = 0.04$		
Middleton et al. [27]		$n = 29$	RBC, 1 DR match^1	Pros	$48\%^1$ vs. $83\%^2$	$P = 0.04$	$97\%^1$ vs. $83\%^2$	n.s.¶
		$n = 12$	RBC, random^2					
Bayle et al. [28]		$n = 83$	WB, haplo-identical^1	Retro	$11\%^1$ vs. $32\%^2$	$P < 0.01$	n.a.	
		$n = 119$	WB, random^2					
Opelz et al. [20]	$n = 218$	$n = 205$	RBC	Pros*	55% vs. 54%	n.s.	70% vs. 79%	$P = 0.025$¶
					25% vs. 16%‡	$P = 0.028$		
Christiaans et al. [29]		$n = 44$	BCD, DR match^1	Retro	$27\%^1$ vs. $27\%^2$	n.s.	$78\%^1$ vs. $78\%^2$	n.s.††
		$n = 59$	BCD, no DR match^2					
Mariat et al. [30]		$n = 49$	RBC, haplo-identical^1	Pros	$65\%^1$ vs. $72\%^2$	n.s.	$94\%^1$ vs. $84\%^2$	$P = 0.039$‡‡
		$n = 107$	RBC, untyped^2					
Hiesse et al. [19]	$n = 36$	$n = 31$	BCD, 1 DR match^1	Pros*	33% vs. $19\%^1$	n.s.	92% vs. $90\%^1$	n.s.‡‡
		$n = 39$	BCD, no DR match^2		33% vs. $33\%^2$	n.s.	92% vs. $92\%^2$	n.s.‡‡
					$19\%^1$ vs. $33\%^2$	n.s.	$90\%^1$ vs. $92\%^2$	n.s.‡‡

*Randomized controlled trial.
†No blood transfusion vs. blood transfusion unless noted.
‡Severe, recurrent rejection episodes.
§Number of rejections/number of transplantations.
¶≤ 1-year graft survival.
**2-year graft survival.
††3-year graft survival.
‡‡5-year graft survival. BCD, buffy-coat depleted; FLR, filtration-Leukoreduced blood; n.a., no information available; n.s., not significant ($P > 0.05$); Pros, prospective study; RBC, red blood cell concentrate; Retro, retrospective study; WB, whole blood.

Table 5.2 Effect of pretransplant blood transfusions on clinical outcome after heart, pancreas–kidney, and liver transplantation.

	Blood transfusion			Clinical outcome after organ transplantation*				
Reference	No	Yes	Blood product	Study	Acute rejection (%)		1-year graft survival (%)	
Heart								
Keogh et al. [31]	$n = 21$	$n = 9$	n.a.	Retro	0.19 vs. 0.09‡	$P = 0.04$	n.a.	
Katz et al. [32]	$n = 29$	$n = 39$	RBC	Retro	n.a.		35% vs. 68%	$P = 0.01$
Kerman et al. [33]	$n = 65$	$n = 72$	n.a.	Retro	n.a.		69% vs. 81%	$P = 0.18$**
Lagaaij et al. [18]		$n = 10$	BCD, 1 DR match[1]	Pros	30%[1] vs. 90%[2]	$P = 0.0029$	n.a.	
		$n = 10$	BCD, no DR match[2]					
Van der Mast et al. [34]		$n = 45$	BCD, 1 DR match[1]	Retro	31%[1] vs. 53%[2]	$P = 0.042$	n.a.	
		$n = 55$	BCD, no DR match[2]					
SPKT								
Stratta et al. [36]	$n = 45$	$n = 61$	n.a.	Retro	64% vs. 47%	n.s.	93% vs. 93%	n.s.
Waanders et al. [37]	$n = 69$	$n = 49$	RBC	Retro	55% vs. 53%	n.s.	97% vs. 100%§	n.s.
					79% vs. 39%†	$P = 0.002$	87% vs. 94%¶	n.s.
Liver								
Koneru et al. [38]	$n = 25$	$n = 69$	n.a.	Retro	52% vs. 50%	n.s.	n.a.	
					40% vs. 22%†	$P = 0.006$		
Parker et al. [39]		$n = 30$	RBC[1]	Retro	67%[1] vs. 40%[2]	$P = 0.037$	n.a.	
		$n = 30$	FLR[2]					

*No blood transfusion vs. blood transfusion, unless noted.
†Severe, recurrent rejection episodes.
‡Number of rejections/number of transplantations.
§Kidney graft survival.
¶Pancreas graft survival.
**Fisher's exact test; original article Wilcoxon rank sum test: $P < 0.05$. BCD, buffy-coat depleted; FLR, filtration-leukoreduced blood; n.a., no information available; n.s., not significant ($P > 0.05$); Pros, prospective study; RBC, red blood cell concentrate; Retro, retrospective study; SPKT, simultaneous pancreas-kidney transplantation.

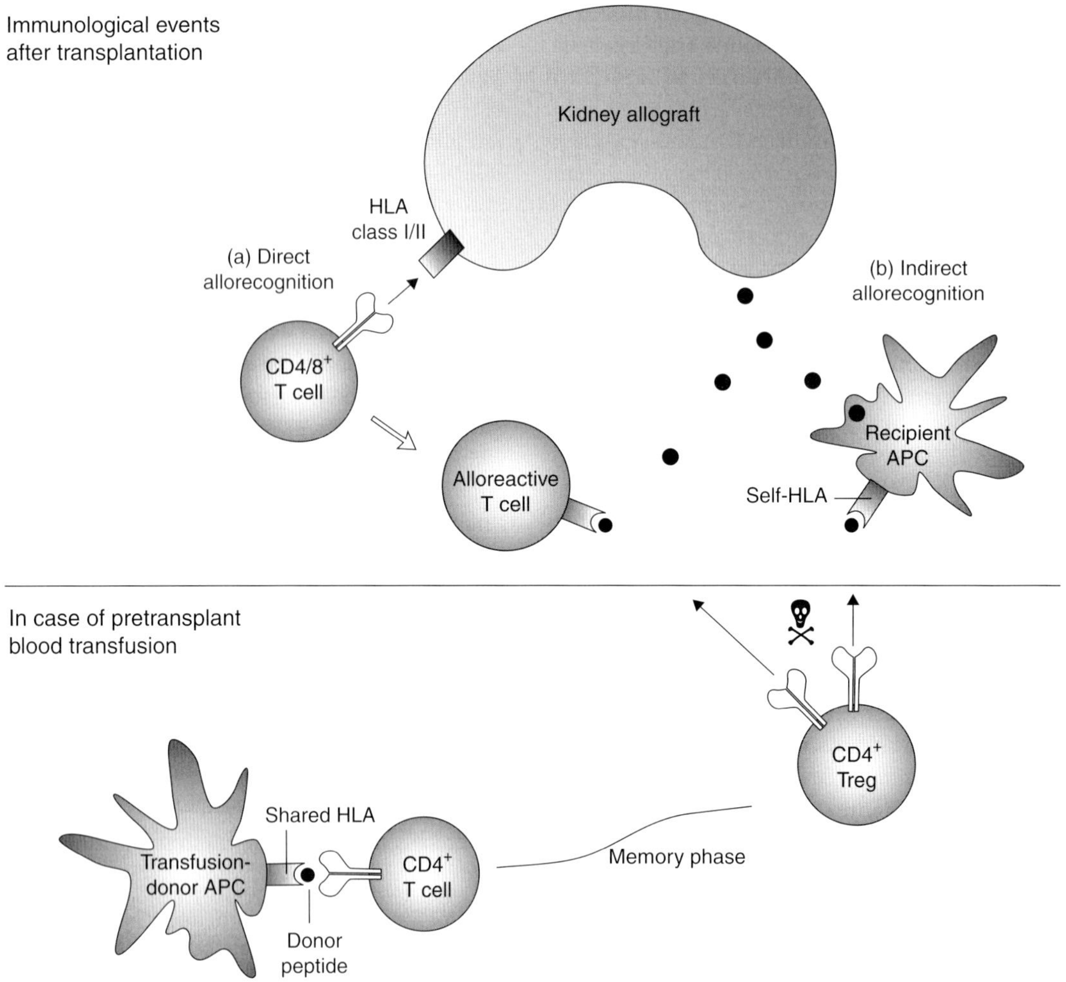

Figure 5.1 Putative mechanism of the immunomodulating effect of HLA-DR shared blood transfusions in transplantation. The upper part of the graph shows the immunological events occurring after organ transplantation in case no pre-transplant blood transfusion is given. $CD4^+$ and $CD8^+$ T cells of recipient origin may directly (a) recognize allogeneic HLA molecules on the surface of the transplanted organ. This results in upregulation of HLA class II molecules on allore-active T cells. When the transplanted organ sheds allopeptides, they may end up in the self-HLA class II molecules [109]. Triggering of recipient T cells via the indirect pathway (b) occurs as organ donor-derived peptides will be processed and presented by recipient APCs in their own HLA. T cell activation begins when T cells recognize alloantigens, either directly or indirectly. The effector phase is characterized by increased production of cytokines, activation of inflammatory cells, increased cytotoxic activity, and stimulation of B cells to produce alloantibodies, all leading to graft rejection. The lower part of the graph shows the situation after a HLA-DR shared pretransplant blood transfusion. The transfusion donor APC can trigger recipient T cells via the indirect pathway, as it expresses a HLA-DR molecule which is similar to self. After recognition of a foreign peptide in shared HLA, the primed $CD4^+$ T cells may exert effector functions, go into apoptosis or may become memory cells. It is assumed that after transplantation these memory cells can be activated again in case the same complex of allopeptide and shared/self-HLA is available as after blood transfusion. Thus the alloreactive T cell and recipient APC can trigger the $CD4^+$ Treg cell. This may result in lysis (☠) of the alloreactive T cell and recipient APC or modulation of dendritic cells by production of IL-10, leading to downregulation of the immune response towards the graft. The mechanism described above requires the sharing of HLA-DR between blood donor and recipient and sharing of a peptide between blood donor and organ donor. APC, antigen presenting cell; HLA, human leukocyte antigen.

tolerance against a third-party organ donor [52–54]. It is assumed that the recognition of an allogeneic peptide in the context of the shared HLA-DR on blood donor APC by recipient T cells, a pseudo indirect pathway of allorecognition, may lead to the induction of regulatory T cells (Tregs). Such Tregs may downregulate an immune response towards the subsequently transplanted organ sharing a peptide with the transfusion donor, which is quite likely given the multitude of shared peptides among random individuals. Subsequently, two mutually nonexclusive ways can lead to abrogation of an effector response against cells expressing this peptide. These cells are either killed by direct cytotoxicity or they may produce significant amounts of IL-10 leading to modulation of dendritic cells and less effective T helper stimulation [55, 56]. Transfusion tolerance may not only weaken graft rejection, but on the long term the presence of tolerizing cells may allow the minimization of potentially harmful immunosuppressive drugs.

Cancer immunosurveillance

A deleterious role of blood transfusions on cancer surveillance was feared because of immunological analogy between alloimmunity (such as organ graft rejection) and tumor immunity. This was further supported by in vitro studies showing transfusion-induced impaired NK functions, animal models, and hundreds of observational studies [57]. Only one randomized study investigated a role of presumed suppressive effects of leukocyte-containing transfusions compared with leukocyte-depleted filtered transfusions on recurrence of colorectal cancer after surgery with curative intent. This study found no difference in cancer recurrence after 2 and 5 years of follow-up [58, 59]. Colorectal cancer is weakly immunogenic. Most clinically manifest cancers and metastasis do not elicit an effective immune response as tumor cells can downregulate allele-specific HLA antigens, escaping T cell and NK cells [60, 61]. Blood transfusions during surgery come in a late phase of the disease, when immunosurveillance already had its chance, and failed.

Transfusions and postoperative nosocomial infections

The possible effect of blood transfusions on the incidence of postoperative infections is widely researched [58, 62–69]. So far this has lead to a large number of publications, several randomized controlled trials (RCTs) [58,62,66,67,70–75] and fierce discussions [76–80].

Observational studies

The vast majority of published studies are observational and compare transfused with nontransfused patients. This design makes them unsuitable to inform on causal relationships, as infections may be correlated to anemia and independent from the transfusions. Multivariate analyses reduced the number of significant correlations reported, but even the use of multivariate analyses can never fully correct for the inclusion bias where all patients have a clinical transfusion indication in the transfused group versus none in the nontransfused group.

Meta-analyses

Several meta-analyses [64, 76, 80–85] were performed, mainly on the RCTs, in an attempt to gain more insight in this matter. However, all were hampered by several factors:

- Different types of surgical patients were included. Bowel surgery (bowel flora), cardiac surgery (time on cardiopulmonary bypass circuit) and orthopedic surgery are all associated with different specific infection risks, and patients undergoing different types of surgery may react differently to an immunomodulatory effect by blood transfusions [80, 85].
- Different definitions were used for postoperative infections. Some studies reported on all infections fulfilling specified (e.g., CDC), criteria, some reported only on "surgical infections," others on all culture-positive infections or on all infections treated with antibiotics, and some did not specify what they reported.
- Different blood products were used. The "standard" red cell components had a leukocyte content ranging from < 0.8 to $> 3.0 \times 10^9$ per liter and was

compared with autologous or filtered blood alternatives.

• A further problem is the way study results are reported by the authors. Some only reported intention-to-treat results where others reported the results from the transfused subpopulations of the different trial arms, sometimes with the nontransfused patients combined in a control group. These differences resulted in the reporting of odds ratios ranging from <1 to >14, clearly indicating that the studies did not report on similar situations.

• Furthermore, there is some publication bias, as the smaller RCTs, reported in the literature, show more pronounced detrimental effects of leukocyte containing transfusions than the larger RCTs [76].

Authors of meta-analyses tried various ways to adjust for all these variations, resulting in different conclusions in meta-analyses based on the same studies [76, 80, 83–86]. Of the two most recently updated meta-analyses, one reports a significant odds ratio of 1.92 (95% CI, 1.22–3.01) focusing on transfused patients only, while the other one reports a nonsignificant odds ratio of 1.24 (95% CI, 0.98–1.56) following analysis according to intention-to-treat [76, 85]. With such results, an effect of transfusion on postoperative infections cannot be considered proven, but it definitely cannot be excluded either.

Transfusions and multiorgan failure and mortality

The reported higher mortality rate in transfused versus nontransfused patients can largely be explained by patient selection. However, there is an increasing amount of evidence that in specific patient groups blood transfusions may increase the incidence and/or mortality rate of multiorgan failure.

In vitro studies

We discussed earlier the proinflammatory effects of transfusing blood or blood components. Priming/activation of neutrophils [87, 88] and the transfusion and induction of proinflammatory cytokines [89–91] may all amplify an inflammatory response, thereby predisposing a patient to a systemic inflammatory response syndrome (SIRS). This SIRS may result in (multi-)organ failure and eventually death.

Clinical studies

The introduction of leukocyte reduction for all transfusions was used in several countries to perform before/after studies [92–95]. Some of these studies reported a beneficial effect of leukoreduced blood on mortality [94, 95]. Other observational studies reported transfusions as an independent risk factor for SIRS, multiorgan failure, and mortality [89, 96–99]. As for postoperative infections, the limitations of the observational design prevent any definitive conclusion on a causal relationship.

Most of the RCTs reporting on mortality investigated the effect of leukoreduction by filtration [66, 67, 71, 73–75, 100–104]. An association of nonfiltered blood transfusions with mortality was only reported in some of the cardiac surgery studies (see Figure 5.2) [66, 74, 101]. Of the RCTs investigating the use of autologous blood, none reported a beneficial effect on mortality [62, 105–107].

Meta-analyses

The meta-analysis of the before/after studies did not show a significant beneficial effect of the introduction of leukocyte reduction on mortality [81]. Meta-analyses on the RCTs also did not show significant benefits on mortality in the overall analyses [83–85, 108]. Only when the meta-analysis focused on cardiac surgery was there a significant benefit shown on mortality [85, 108].

Conclusions

On one hand, TRIM is a concept that is very attractive to exploit as specific tolerance-inducing conditioning prior to organ transplantation; on the other hand, transfusion-related immunosuppression enhancing cancer recurrence, infections and mortality is a serious concern that has led to wide implementation of universal leukocyte reduction of red blood cell transfusions. As yet, there are insufficient studies to provide solid evidence for these postulated TRIM effects. A deleterious role

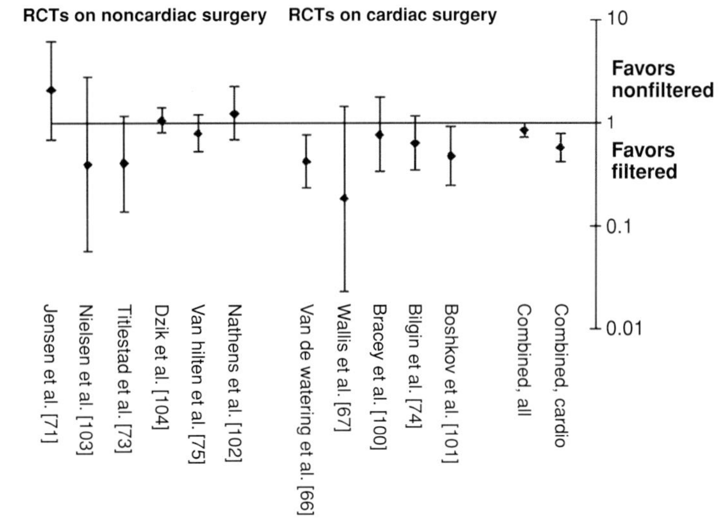

Figure 5.2 Short-term mortality (maximum 90 days) in RCTs comparing filtration-leukoreduced RBCs with nonfiltered RBCs (OR surrounded by 95% CI). RBC, red blood cell; RCT, randomized controlled trial.

of leukocyte-containing transfusions has only been demonstrated in cardiac surgery. This might be related to the effects of extracorporeal circulation and reperfusion injury leading to SIRS, with transfusions disturbing, as a second hit, the shaky balance of the recovery process.

References

1. Brittingham TE, Chaplin H, Jr. Febrile transfusion reactions caused by sensitivity to donor leukocytes and platelets. JAMA 1957;165:819–25.
2. Ward HN. Pulmonary infiltrates associated with leukoagglutinin transfusion reactions. Ann Intern Med 1970;73:689–94.
3. Yankee RA, Graff KS, Dowling R, Henderson ES. Selection of unrelated compatible platelet donors by lymphocyte HLA matching. N Engl J Med 1973;288: 760–64.
4. The TRAP Study Group. Leukocyte reduction and ultraviolet B irradiation of platelets to prevent alloimmunization and refractoriness to platelet transfusions. The Trial to Reduce Alloimmunization to Platelets Study Group. N Engl J Med 1997;337: 1861–9.
5. Opelz G, Sengar DP, Mickey MR, Terasaki PI. Effect of blood transfusions on subsequent kidney transplants. Transplant Proc 1973;5:253–9.
6. Gantt CL. Red blood cells for cancer patients. Lancet 1981;2:363.
7. Dzik S, Mincheff M, Puppo F. Apoptosis, transforming growth factor-beta, and the immunosuppressive effect of transfusion. Transfusion 2002;42:1221–3.
8. Muylle L. The role of cytokines in blood transfusion reactions. Blood Rev 1995;9:77–83.
9. Heddle NM, Klama L, Singer J, et al. The role of the plasma from platelet concentrates in transfusion reactions. N Engl J Med 1994;331:625–8.
10. Izbicki G, Rudensky B, Na'amad M, et al. Transfusion-related leukocytosis in critically ill patients. Crit Care Med 2004;32: 439–42.
11. Chang H, Voralia M, Bali M, Sher GD, Branch DR. Irreversible loss of donor blood leucocyte activation may explain a paucity of transfusion-associated graft-versus-host disease from stored blood. Br J Haematol 2000;111:146–56.
12. Mincheff MS, Meryman HT, Kapoor V, Alsop P, Wotzel M. Blood transfusion and immunomodulation: a possible mechanism. Vox Sang 1993;65: 18–24.
13. Schechter GP, Whang-Peng J, McFarland W. Circulation of donor lymphocytes after blood transfusion in man. Blood 1977;49:651–6.
14. Vervoordeldonk SF, Doumaid K, Remmerswaal EB, et al. Long-term detection of microchimaerism in peripheral blood after pretransplantation blood transfusion. Br J Haematol 1998;102:1004–9.
15. Lee TH, Paglieroni T, Utter GH, et al. High-level long-term white blood cell microchimerism after transfusion of leukoreduced blood components to patients resuscitated after severe traumatic injury. Transfusion 2005;45:1280–90.

16. Persijn GG, Cohen B, Lansbergen Q, van Rood JJ. Retrospective and prospective studies on the effect of blood transfusions in renal transplantation in The Netherlands. Transplantation 1979;28:396–401.
17. Lazda VA, Pollak R, Mozes MF, Barber PL, Jonasson O. Evidence that HLA class II disparity is required for the induction of renal allograft enhancement by donor-specific blood transfusions in man. Transplantation 1990;49:1084–7.
18. Lagaaij EL, Hennemann IP, Ruigrok M, et al. Effect of one-HLA-DR-antigen-matched and completely HLA-DR-mismatched blood transfusions on survival of heart and kidney allografts. N Engl J Med 1989;321:701–5.
19. Hiesse C, Busson M, Buisson C, et al. Multicenter trial of one HLA-DR-matched or mismatched blood transfusion prior to cadaveric renal transplantation. Kidney Int 2001;60:341–9.
20. Opelz G, Vanrenterghem Y, Kirste G, et al. Prospective evaluation of pre-transplant blood transfusions in cadaver kidney recipients. Transplantation 1997;63:964–7.
21. Alexander JW, Babcock GF, First MR, et al. The induction of immunologic hyporesponsiveness by preoperative donor-specific transfusions and cyclosporine in human cadaveric transplants. A preliminary trial. Transplantation 1992;53:423–7.
22. Sanfilippo FP, Bollinger RR, MacQueen JM, Brooks BJ, Koepke JA. A randomized study comparing leukocyte-depleted versus packed red cell transfusions in prospective cadaver renal allograft recipients. Transfusion 1985;25:116–19.
23. Lundgren G, Groth CG, Albrechtsen D, et al. HLA-matching and pretransplant blood transfusions in cadaveric renal transplantation – a changing picture with cyclosporin. Lancet 1986;2:66–9.
24. Melzer JS, Husing RM, Feduska NJ, et al. The beneficial effect of pretransplant blood transfusions in cyclosporine-treated cadaver renal allograft recipients. Transplantation 1987;43:61–4.
25. Kerman RH, Van Buren CT, Lewis RM, Kahan BD. Successful transplantation of 100 untransfused cyclosporine-treated primary recipients of cadaveric renal allografts. Transplantation 1988;45:37–40.
26. Iwaki Y, Cecka JM, Terasaki PI. The transfusion effect in cadaver kidney transplants – yes or no. Transplantation 1990;49:56–9.
27. Middleton D, Martin J, Douglas J, McClelland M. Transfusion of one HLA-DR antigen-matched blood to potential recipients of a renal allograft. Transplantation 1994;58:845–8.
28. Bayle F, Masson D, Zaoui P, et al. A haplo-identical transfusion in first renal allograft recipients: effect on alloimmunisation, acute rejection episodes, and graft survival. Transplant Proc 1995;27:2457–8.
29. Christiaans MH, van Hooff JP, Nieman F, van den Berg-Loonen EM. HLA-DR matched transfusions: development of donor-specific T- and B-cell antibodies and renal allograft outcome. Transplantation 1999;67:1029–35.
30. Mariat C, Alamartine E, De Filippis JP, et al. Effect of HLA semi-identical pretransplant blood transfusions on renal allograft outcome. Transplant Proc 2000;32:381–3.
31. Keogh A, Baron DW, Spratt P, Esmore D, Chang V. The effect of blood pretransfusion on orthotopic cardiac transplantation. Transplant Proc 1987;19: 2845–6.
32. Katz MR, Barnhart GR, Goldman MH, et al. Pretransplant transfusions in cardiac allograft recipients. Transplantation 1987;43:499–501.
33. Kerman RH, Van Buren CT, Lewis RM, et al. The impact of HLA A, B, and DR blood transfusions and immune responder status on cardiac allograft recipients treated with cyclosporine. Transplantation 1988;45:333–7.
34. van der Mast BJ, Balk AH. Effect of HLA-DR-shared blood transfusion on the clinical outcome of heart transplantation. Transplantation 1997;63: 1514–19.
35. Fernandez FG, Jaramillo A, Ewald G, et al. Blood transfusions decrease the incidence of acute rejection in cardiac allograft recipients. J Heart Lung Transplant 2005;24(Suppl. 7):S255–61.
36. Stratta RJ, Taylor RJ, Sindhi R, et al. Is there a transfusion effect in combined pancreas-kidney transplantation? Transplant Proc 1995;27:3096.
37. Waanders MM, Roelen DL, de Fijter JW, et al. Protocolled blood transfusions in recipients of a simultaneous pancreas-kidney transplant reduce severe acute graft rejection. Transplantation 2008;85: 1668–70.
38. Koneru B, Harrison D, Rizwan M, et al. Blood transfusions in liver recipients: a conundrum or a clear benefit in the cyclosporine/tacrolimus era? Transplantation 1997;63:1587–90.
39. Parker BM, Irefin SA, Sabharwal V, et al. Leukocyte reduction during orthotopic liver transplantation and postoperative outcome: a pilot study. J Clin Anesth 2004;16:18–24.
40. Golshayan D, Buhler L, Lechler RI, Pascual M. From current immunosuppressive strategies to

clinical tolerance of allografts. Transplant Int 2007;20: 12–24.

41. Puppo F, Ghio M, Contini P, Mazzei C, Indiveri F. Fas, Fas ligand, and transfusion immunomodulation. Transfusion 2001;41:416–18.
42. Rammensee HG. Veto function in vitro and in vivo. Int Rev Immunol 1989;4:175–91.
43. van Parijs L, Abbas AK. Role of Fas-mediated cell death in the regulation of immune responses. Curr Opin Immunol 1996;8:355–61.
44. Lechler R, Chai JG, Marelli-Berg F, Lombardi G. The contributions of T-cell anergy to peripheral T-cell tolerance. Immunology 2001;103:262–9.
45. Schwartz RH. T cell anergy. Sci Am 1993;269:62–71.
46. Powell JD. The induction and maintenance of T cell anergy. Clin Immunol 2006;120:239–46.
47. Alegre ML, Najafian N. Costimulatory molecules as targets for the induction of transplantation tolerance. Curr Mol Med 2006;6:843–57.
48. Sakaguchi S. Naturally arising CD4+ regulatory T cells for immunologic self-tolerance and negative control of immune responses. Annu Rev Immunol 2004;22:531–62.
49. Hutchinson IV. Suppressor T cells in allogeneic models. Transplantation 1986;41:547–55.
50. Quigley RL, Wood KJ, Morris PJ. Transfusion induces blood donor-specific suppressor cells. J Immunol 1989;142:463–70.
51. Jiang S, Lechler RI, He XS, Huang JF. Regulatory T cells and transplantation tolerance. Hum Immunol 2006;67:765–76.
52. Claas FHJ, de Koster HS, Lagaaij EL, van Rood JJ. A molecular mechanism of T cell downregulation by blood transfusion. Exp Nephrol 1993;1: 134–8.
53. Waanders MM, Roelen DL, Brand A, Claas FH. The putative mechanism of the immunomodulating effect of HLA-DR shared allogeneic blood transfusions on the alloimmune response. Transfus Med Rev 2005;19:281–7.
54. Roelen DL, van Bree S, van Hulst P, van Beelen E, Claas FHJ. Regulatory functions of human CD4(+) T cells recognizing allopeptides in the context of self-HLA class II. Hum Immunol 2002;63:902–11.
55. Claas FHJ, Roelen DL, van Rood JJ, Brand A. Modulation of the alloimmune response by blood transfusions. Transfus Clin Biol 2001;8:315–17.
56. Steinbrink K, Jonuleit H, Wölfl M, Knop J, Enk A. Induction of tolerance by interleukin-10-treated human dendritic cells. J Invest Dermatol 1997;108: 231.
57. Amato A, Pescatori M. Perioperative blood transfusions for the recurrence of colorectal cancer. Cochrane Database Syst Rev 2006;(1):CD005033.
58. Houbiers JG, Brand A, van de Watering LM, et al. Randomised controlled trial comparing transfusion of leucocyte-depleted or buffy-coat-depleted blood in surgery for colorectal cancer. Lancet 1994;344: 573–8.
59. van de Watering LM, Brand A, Houbiers JG, et al. Perioperative blood transfusions, with or without allogeneic leucocytes, relate to survival, not to cancer recurrence. Br J Surg 2001;88:267–72.
60. Natali PG, Bigotti A, Cavaliere R, Nicotra MR, Ferrone S. Phenotyping of lesions of melanocyte origin with monoclonal antibodies to melanoma-associated antigens and to HLA antigens. J Natl Cancer Inst 1984;73: 13–24.
61. Momburg F, Degener T, Bacchus E, et al. Loss of HLA-A,B,C and de novo expression of HLA-D in colorectal cancer. Int J Cancer 1986;37:179–84.
62. Heiss MM, Mempel W, Jauch KW, et al. Beneficial effect of autologous blood transfusion on infectious complications after colorectal cancer surgery. Lancet 1993;342:1328–33.
63. Braga M, Vignali A, Radaelli G, Gianotti L, Di Carlo V. Association between perioperative blood transfusion and postoperative infection in patients having elective operations for gastrointestinal cancer. Eur J Surg 1992;158:531–6.
64. Hill GE, Frawley WH, Griffith KE, Forestner JE, Minei JP. Allogeneic blood transfusion increases the risk of postoperative bacterial infection: a meta-analysis. J Trauma 2003;54:908–14.
65. Tartter PI, Driefuss RM, Malon AM, Heimann TM, Aufses AH. Relationship of postoperative septic complications and blood transfusions in patients with Crohn's disease. Am J Surg 1988;155:43–8.
66. van de Watering LM, Hermans J, Houbiers JG, et al. Beneficial effects of leukocyte depletion of transfused blood on postoperative complications in patients undergoing cardiac surgery: a randomized clinical trial. Circulation 1998;97:562–8.
67. Wallis JP, Chapman CE, Orr KE, Clark SC, Forty JR. Effect of WBC reduction of transfused RBCs on postoperative infection rates in cardiac surgery. Transfusion 2002;42:1127–34.
68. Vamvakas EC. Possible mechanisms of allogeneic blood transfusion-associated postoperative infection. Transfus Med Rev 2002;16:144–60.
69. Johnston P, Wynn-Jones H, Chakravarty D, Boyle A, Parker MJ. Is perioperative blood transfusion a risk

factor for mortality or infection after hip fracture? J Orthop Trauma 2006;20:675–9.
70. Jensen LS, Andersen AJ, Christiansen PM, et al. Postoperative infection and natural killer cell function following blood transfusion in patients undergoing elective colorectal surgery. Br J Surg 1992;79: 513–16.
71. Jensen LS, Kissmeyer-Nielsen P, Wolff B, Qvist N. Randomised comparison of leucocyte-depleted versus buffy-coat-poor blood transfusion and complications after colorectal surgery. Lancet 1996;348: 841–5.
72. Tartter PI, Mohandas K, Azar P, et al. Randomized trial comparing packed red cell blood transfusion with and without leukocyte depletion for gastrointestinal surgery. Am J Surg 1998;176:462–6.
73. Titlestad IL, Ebbesen LS, Ainsworth AP, et al. Leukocyte-depletion of blood components does not significantly reduce the risk of infectious complications. Results of a double-blinded, randomized study. Int J Colorectal Dis 2001;16:147–53.
74. Bilgin YM, van de Watering LM, Eijsman L, et al. Double-blind, randomized controlled trial on the effect of leukocyte-depleted erythrocyte transfusions in cardiac valve surgery. Circulation 2004;109: 2755–60.
75. van Hilten JA, van de Watering LM, van Bockel JH, et al. Effects of transfusion with red cells filtered to remove leucocytes: randomised controlled trial in patients undergoing major surgery. BMJ 2004;328:1281.
76. Blumberg N, Zhao H, Wang H, et al. The intention-to-treat principle in clinical trials and meta-analyses of leukoreduced blood transfusions in surgical patients. Transfusion 2007;47:573–81.
77. Vamvakas EC. Deleterious clinical effects of transfusion immunomodulation: proven beyond a reasonable doubt. Transfusion 2006;46:492–4.
78. Kunz R, Guyatt G. Which patients to include in the analysis? Transfusion 2006;46:881–4.
79. Blumberg N. Deleterious clinical effects of transfusion immunomodulation: proven beyond a reasonable doubt. Transfusion 2005;45(Suppl. 2): 33S–9S.
80. Vamvakas EC. Meta-analysis of randomized controlled trials investigating the risk of postoperative infection in association with white blood cell-containing allogeneic blood transfusion: the effects of the type of transfused red blood cell product and surgical setting. Transfus Med Rev 2002;16:304–14.
81. Vamvakas EC. White-blood-cell-containing allogeneic blood transfusion, postoperative infection and mortality: a meta-analysis of observational 'before-and-after' studies. Vox Sang 2004;86: 111–19.
82. Vamvakas EC. Transfusion-associated cancer recurrence and postoperative infection: meta-analysis of randomized, controlled clinical trials. Transfusion 1996;36:175–86.
83. McAlister FA, Clark HD, Wells PS, Laupacis A. Perioperative allogeneic blood transfusion does not cause adverse sequelae in patients with cancer: a meta-analysis of unconfounded studies. Br J Surg 1998;85:171–8.
84. Fergusson D, Khanna MP, Tinmouth A, Hébert PC. Transfusion of leukoreduced red blood cells may decrease postoperative infections: two meta-analyses of randomized controlled trials. Can J Anaesth 2004;51:417–24.
85. Vamvakas EC. White-blood-cell-containing allogeneic blood transfusion and postoperative infection or mortality: an updated meta-analysis. Vox Sang 2007;92:224–32.
86. Vamvakas EC, Blajchman MA. A proposal for an individual patient data based meta-analysis of randomized controlled trials of allogeneic transfusion and postoperative bacterial infection. Transfus Med Rev 1997;11:180–94.
87. Silliman CC, Thurman GW, Ambruso DR. Stored blood components contain agents that prime the neutrophil NADPH oxidase through the platelet-activating-factor receptor. Vox Sang 1992;63:133–6.
88. Zallen G, Offner PJ, Moore EE, et al. Age of transfused blood is an independent risk factor for postinjury multiple organ failure. Am J Surg 1999;178: 570–72.
89. Johnson JL, Moore EE, Gonzalez RJ, et al. Alteration of the postinjury hyper-inflammatory response by means of resuscitation with a red cell substitute. J Trauma 2003;54:133–9.
90. Muylle L, Joos M, Wouters E, De BR, Peetermans ME. Increased tumor necrosis factor alpha (TNF alpha), interleukin 1, and interleukin 6 (IL-6) levels in the plasma of stored platelet concentrates: relationship between TNF alpha and IL-6 levels and febrile transfusion reactions. Transfusion 1993;33:195–9.
91. Wadhwa M, Seghatchian MJ, Dilger P, Contreras M, Thorpe R. Cytokine accumulation in stored red cell concentrates: effect of buffy-coat removal and leucoreduction. Transfus Sci 2000;23:7–16.

92. Williamson LM, Murphy ME, Llewelyn C, et al. Leucocyte-depleted blood in prevention of postoperative infections following elective orthopaedic and cardiac procedures. Vox Sang 2002;83(Suppl. 1): 457–60.
93. Baron JF, Gourdin M, Bertrand M, et al. The effect of universal leukodepletion of packed red blood cells on postoperative infections in high-risk patients undergoing abdominal aortic surgery. Anesth Analg 2002;94:529–37.
94. Blumberg N, Heal JM, Cowles JW, et al. Leukocyte-reduced transfusions in cardiac surgery results of an implementation trial. Am J Clin Pathol 2002;118:376–81.
95. Hébert PC, Fergusson D, Blajchman MA, et al. Clinical outcomes following institution of the Canadian universal leuko-reduction program for red blood cell transfusions. JAMA 2003;289:1941–9.
96. Sauaia A, Moore FA, Moore EE, et al. Early predictors of postinjury multiple organ failure. Arch Surg 1994;129:39–45.
97. Tran DD, Van Onselen EB, Wensink AJ, Cuesta MA. Factors related to multiple organ system failure and mortality in a surgical intensive care unit. Nephrol Dial Transplant 1994;9(Suppl. 4):172–8.
98. Vincent JL, Baron JF, Reinhart K, et al. Anemia and blood transfusion in critically ill patients. JAMA 2002;288:1499–507.
99. Maetani S, Nishikawa T, Tobe T, Hirakawa A. Role of blood transfusion in organ system failure following major abdominal surgery. Ann Surg 1986;203:275–81.
100. Bracey AW, Radovancevic R, Nussmeier NA, et al. Leukocyte-reduced blood in open-heart surgery patients: effects on outcome. Transfusion 2002;42 (Suppl.):5S.
101. Boshkov LK, Furnary A, Morris C, et al. Prestorage leukoreduction of red cells in elective cardiac surgery: results of a double-blind randomized controlled trial. Blood 2004;104:112a.
102. Nathens AB, Nester TA, Rubenfeld GD, Nirula R, Gernsheimer TB. The effects of leukoreduced blood transfusion on infection risk following injury: a randomized controlled trial. Shock 2006;26: 342–7.
103. Nielsen HJ, Hammer JH, Krarup AL, et al. Prestorage leukocyte filtration may reduce leukocyte-derived bioactive substance accumulation in patients operated for burn trauma. Burns 1999;25:162–70.
104. Dzik WH, Anderson JK, O'Neill EM, et al. A prospective, randomized clinical trial of universal WBC reduction. Transfusion 2002;42:1114–22.
105. Busch OR, Hop WC, Hoynck van Papendrecht MA, Marquet RL, Jeekel J. Blood transfusions and prognosis in colorectal cancer. N Engl J Med 1993;328: 1372–6.
106. Farrer A, Spark JI, Scott DJ. Autologous blood transfusion: the benefits to the patient undergoing abdominal aortic aneurysm repair. J Vasc Nurs 1997; 15:111–15.
107. Wong JC, Torella F, Haynes SL, et al. Autologous versus allogeneic transfusion in aortic surgery: a multicenter randomized clinical trial. Ann Surg 2002;235:145–51.
108. Vamvakas ECWB. C-containing allogeneic blood transfusion and mortality: a meta-analysis of randomized controlled trials. Transfusion 2003;43:963–73.
109. Fast LD. Recipient elimination of allogeneic lymphoid cells: donor CD4(+) cells are effective alloantigen-presenting cells. Blood 2000;96:1144–9.

CHAPTER 6

Pathogen Inactivation of Blood Components

Chris Prowse
Scottish National Blood Transfusion Service, Edinburgh, UK

Introduction

Blood transfusion services are testing each blood donation for an ever-increasing number of pathogens. In the United Kingdom, this testing includes HIV, hepatitis B, hepatitis C, HTLV, and syphilis, with optional testing for bacteria, cytomegalovirus (CMV), and malaria (see the review by Kitchen and Barbara [1] in this volume). Elsewhere, testing for parvovirus B19, West Nile virus, Chagas' disease, and other agents is in place. Pathogen inactivation of blood components ideally offers the option of using one process to inactivate transfusion-transmitted infections and thereby potentially avoid the need to introduce further testing, and even to cease using some of the current tests. Reality is somewhat different as current technologies are not applicable to all components and are not effective against all agents.

Fractionated plasma products now have a very good safety record, based on a combination of donor questioning, donation testing, and processing (including specific pathogen inactivation steps) [2,3]. While the first two of these are also applicable to single-donation labile blood components, most pathogen-inactivation steps applied to fractionated products are incompatible with platelet and red cell viability. In recent years, *compatible* pathogen inactivation methods have become available and are now licensed, at least in Europe, for plasma and platelet products; but not yet for red cells (Table 6.1).

For those agents currently tested on all blood products, the combination of serological and nucleic acid based assays has made the residual risk of infection remarkably low—of the order of one in a million or less per donation. Benefits of pathogen inactivation technology are more likely to be realized for emerging agents for which blood is not yet tested, or where testing is only partially effective, as is the case for bacterial contamination of platelets [4].

Available and developing technologies

The first commercialized pathogen inactivation technique applied to blood components was solvent-detergent treatment of whole plasma [5]. This method relies on the disruption of virus lipid envelopes by the solvent-detergent combination and requires removal of these chemicals after processing. It is only effective against lipid-enveloped viruses (not nonlipid-enveloped viruses or bacteria), disrupts cells and is hence not applicable to platelets or red cells. It has usually been applied to pools of up to 2500 donations, but a method for single-donation plasma has also been described [6]. Other methods used in the fractionation industry have also been applied to plasma, such as nanofiltration [7] and pasteurization [8], but have not been progressed to full-scale clinical use.

Alternatives to Blood Transfusion in Transfusion Medicine, 2nd edition. Edited by A. Maniatis, P. Van der Linden, J.-F. Hardy.

Table 6.1 Status of technologies (2008).

Component	Company	Method	US status	EU status
Plasma	Octapharma	Solvent detergent	Licensed	Licensed
	Cerus	Amotosalen + UV	Phase III	Licensed
	Macopharma	Methylene blue + light	?	Licensed
	Navigant	Riboflavin + UV	?	Licensed
Platelet	Cerus	Amotosalen + UV	Phase III	Licensed
	Navigant	Riboflavin + UV	Phase II	Licensed
	Macopharma	UV (±thionine)	Preclinical	Preclinical
Red Cells	Vitex	Inactine	Abandoned	Abandoned
	Cerus	S-303 (FRALE)	Phase Ib	Phase Ib
	Navigant	Riboflavin + UV	Preclinical	Preclinical
	American Red Cross	Thiopyrilium + light	Preclinical	Preclinical

Phase 1: volunteer safety studies. Phase II: patient safety studies. Phase III: patient efficacy studies. Licensed: by FDA in USA and/or CE marked in Europe.

Recent developments have relied more on the use of combinations of visible or ultraviolet (UV) light and photosensitizers to modify nucleic acids. As therapeutic components do not require genetic material (platelets and red cells being anuclear) for function, *specific* "inactivation" of nucleic acid should have no effect on plasma, red cell, or platelet function but reduces pathogen viability (other than prion agents). As shown in Figure 6.1, pathogen inactivation can be achieved by simple use of UV or gamma irradiation, but for blood components the only practical application of this has been with UV light where specificity is dependent on the absorption characteristics of nucleic acids at this wavelength. Proteins also absorb in the UV light and damage to proteins may result at higher doses. Gamma irradiation at doses that inactivate pathogens (rather than just leukocytes) certainly causes irreversible changes to proteins and cells. More normally, specificity is achieved by use of a photosensitive compound that binds to nucleic acids. Irradiation then either results in direct cross-linking of this compound to nucleic acid (photochemical inactivation) or generation of free radicals or active oxygen species (photodynamic inactivation) that act only on molecules in the immediate vicinity owing to their short lifespan. However, the binding of such compounds (Figure 6.2) is not absolutely selective and usually some effect can be detected on other constituents. These may be minimized through the use of quenchers or reducing agents such as glutathione.

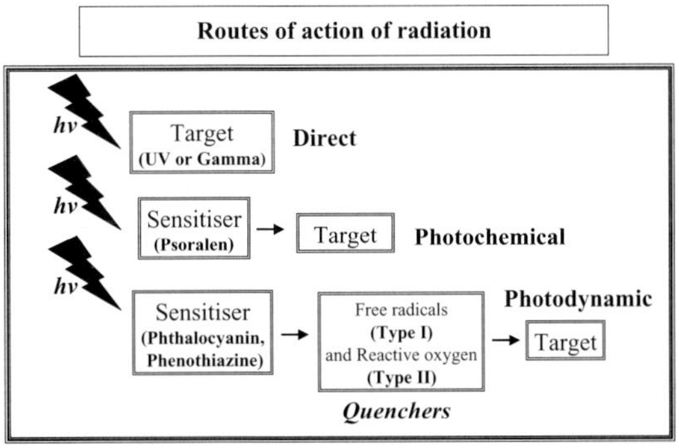

Figure 6.1 Mechanisms of pathogen inactivation by radiation.

Examples of photo-inactivation methods applied to plasma include the use of the phenothiazine dye methylene blue, in combination with visible light, [9] and the psoralen amotosalen, with UVA light [10] as well as a combination of riboflavin and UV light [11]. The latter two methods have also been developed for platelet treatment, although the amotosalen approach requires use of a platelet additive to replace two-thirds of the plasma used for platelet suspension so as to avoid excessive absorption of the UV light by plasma proteins. Macopharma are also developing the use of UV alone or in combination with thionine (a derivative of

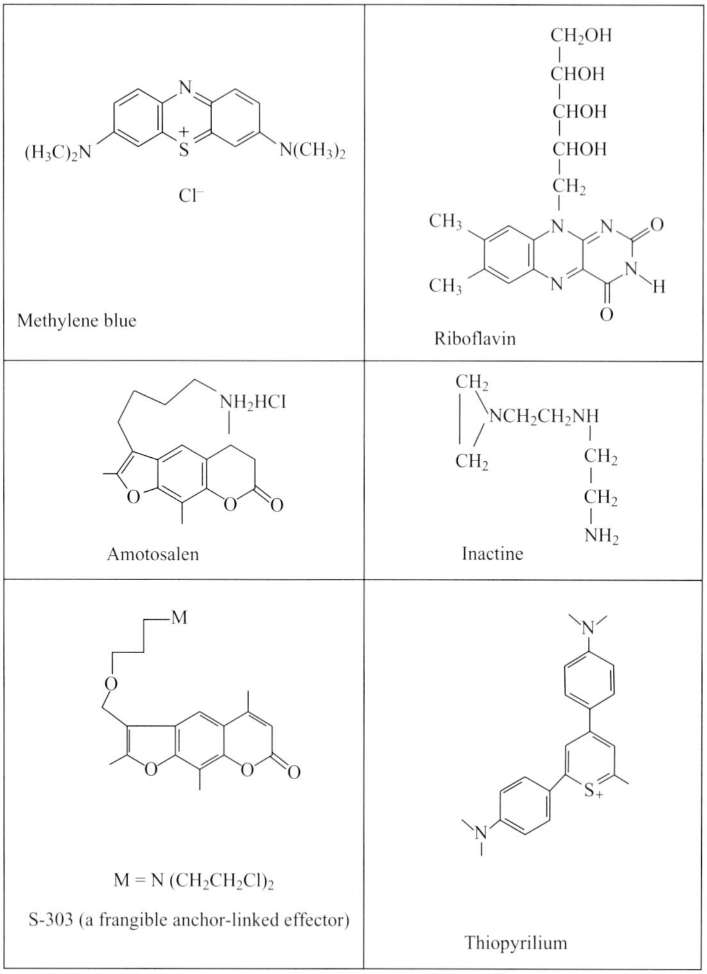

Figure 6.2 Some chemicals used in pathogen inactivation.

methylene blue) for platelet treatment [12]. The current licensing status of these technologies is shown in Table 6.1.

For red cells, photo-inactivation is less applicable owing to their high optical density, although this approach is being progressed for the riboflavin method. The alternative approach of using chemical compounds that bind specifically to nucleic acid and achieve inactivation by direct chemical action after a shift to neutral pH has been attempted by two companies using the compounds Inactine [13] and S-303 (a psoralen derivative designated as a frangible anchor-linked effector) [14]. In both cases, problems arose owing to side reactions that changed the red cell surface (see below), but Cerus are still progressing studies using a modified S-303 method. A more recent photo-inactivation approach has been to use a sensitizer that can only be activated by light when bound to nucleic acid and fixed in a certain conformation. This uses compounds such as thiopyriliums [15] and thiazole orange [16] that have yet to be assessed clinically.

Other than for riboflavin, most of the methods developed include steps to remove the residual sensitizer.

Leukodepletion may also be regarded as a pathogen removal step for those agents that primarily infect white cells, such as CMV and HTLV.

Clinical trials (plasma)

Millions of donations of methylene blue- and solvent-detergent-treated plasma have been used in patients, while many thousands of doses of amotosalen-treated platelets have been used clinically. Use on this scale is reassuring in terms of safety, but it does not address efficacy.

For trials of inactivated plasma, there is a problem in that it is uncertain what the benefits of the standard product are, other than in correcting laboratory parameters [17]. Hence, trials comparing inactivated and standard plasma may be of little value.

Nevertheless, studies on the early solvent-detergent-treated plasma demonstrated equivalence to standard plasma in a variety of disorders including coagulation deficiencies (both congenital and acquired) and in thrombotic thrombocytopenic purpura (TTP) [18, 19]. By today's standards, these trials were underpowered and are probably too small to reach definite conclusions. Soon after its widespread introduction in the United States, reports appeared of hyperfibrinolysis and even death in patients undergoing liver transplantation, [20–22] which was probably due to the reduction in protein S and antiplasmin in this product as a result of processing. A somewhat different process is used in Europe that has less impact on these proteins, and there are few if any reports of such effects with the OctaPlas product now made and licensed in Europe [21, 22].

For methylene blue-treated plasma, very few clinical trials of any size have been carried out, as licensure of this product at the time of its introduction did not require these. Such studies as exist indicate equivalent efficacy to standard plasma, [23] although there has been recent concerns over reduced efficacy in TTP despite the product containing normal levels of the von Willebrand factor cleaving enzyme ADAMTS-18, deficiency of which gives rise to this condition [24].

For amotosalen-treated plasma, a series of well-designed recent clinical trials of adequate power (except in the case of TTP) have demonstrated equivalence to standard plasma in acquired and congenital coagulation deficiency as well as in TTP [25–27].

Clinical trials (platelets)

While clinical trials on the riboflavin product have commenced with encouraging results [28, 29], the only complete trials are for the amotosalen product with one European trial using a platelet-increment endpoint [30] and a US one using a bleeding correction endpoint [31]. For the chosen endpoints, these trials showed equivalence with standard platelet products, but closer inspection suggests a somewhat reduced (around 10–15%) efficacy when using normal clinical monitoring parameters. For licensure, most platelet products are also assessed by autologous transfusion to volunteers to assess in vivo recovery and survival. The FDA has recently proposed that, at the end of their shelf life, platelet products should have 67% of fresh platelet recovery and 58% of fresh platelet survival. Against this standard, both amotosalen and riboflavin [28] platelets are close to the limit after 5 days storage, and longer storage may result in suboptimal results, particularly in the additive solution used with the amotosalen product.

Clinical trials (red cells)

Prior to full-scale clinical testing, novel red cell products are usually checked in volunteer autologous isotope-labeling studies to check that at least 75% of transfused red cells remain in the circulation 24 hours after infusion. This was done and found to be the case for both Inactine and S-303 red cell products, [32, 33] but in subsequent clinical trials both products caused the formation of antibodies to red cells, ascribed to surface modification of the red cell by the pathogen inactivation process [14]. Further work by Cerus on the S-303 method has resulted in a modified procedure with minimal effects on red cell surface structure, and this revised product is now entering early clinical testing [14].

Effects on potency and quality of product

For plasma products, conditions are usually chosen to balance the loss of potency against the level of pathogen inactivation. In practice, this usually means that there is a loss of around 30% of coagulation factor VIII potency [34]. For most products, this protein is the most susceptible to inactivation. Except in patients with moderate to severe factor VIII deficiency, who should be treated with factor VIII concentrates, this level of loss is not of concern in itself. For solvent-detergent products, it has already been mentioned that protein S and antiplasmin losses are noteworthy.

For cellular products, the process steps, including those introduced to remove sensitizer, mean that there are multiple transfers between blood packs, which can result in significant volume losses (up to 10%) and hence there is a question of yield losses as well as any resulting directly from the inactivation procedure. In routine use, the overall loss of potency can usually be limited to 15%, but can be considerably less than this for processes such riboflavin pathogen inactivation where a sensitizer removal step is not deemed necessary.

Toxicology and neoantigens

As the sensitizers or chemicals used to achieve pathogen inactivation result in modification of nucleic acids, toxic side effects are a natural concern for pathogen inactivated components. To address this, most procedures incorporate a step to remove unused chemicals or their breakdown products. Extensive testing of residual toxicity is undertaken [35]. For all licensed products, the residual toxicity is not significant, this being part of the licensing procedure [36, 37]. For those products that have been in use for some time, there is the additional reassurance of safe outcome with considerable usage over a number of years.

Separately from this, treatment may result in changes to the surface of red cells or proteins that elicit an inappropriate immune response. As already noted, formation of such "*neoantigens*" was found for the two trialed red cell methods, although whether the antibodies that formed were of clinical significance remains uncertain. For pathogen-inactivated plasmas and platelets, neoantigen formation does not seem to have been a problem to date, despite the changes in plasma proteins already described. Companies try and assess products for neoantigen formation [38], but this can only be fully assessed in human studies.

Extent of pathogen inactivation achieved and required

For bacteria, initial contamination levels in blood components are low and rare [4], although with the potential to grow during storage. For viruses, titers may rise as high as 10^{19} viruses per mL (for parvovirus B19) during the acute phase of infection, but are more normally in the range of 10^4–10^6 per mL, although for those viruses for which screening is routinely undertaken this will be reduced further (to less than 10^4) by exclusion of high-titer donations. For parasites, intermediate titers are seen.

To assess inactivation capacity, components are usually "spiked" with stocks of pathogenic or model agents before undertaking pathogen inactivation and the results expressed as a log kill, usually determined by assaying dilutions of agent in cell culture assays. The demonstrable levels of inactivation are often limited by the available titer of stock pathogens. For most lipid-enveloped viruses and for many bacteria, it is usual to find a log kill of more than 6 logs (99.9999%) [5, 9, 10, 39]. For non-lipid-enveloped viruses, more variable results are seen that range from virtually no kill to more than 6 logs. Fortunately, the viruses of most concern to date are usually lipid enveloped. Additional reassurance can be obtained by undertaking kinetic studies and showing that all the available viruses are inactivated in a period less than that usually used. Particularly, if nucleic acid testing is undertaken, these levels of inactivation are probably adequate to deal with any virus, and also with bacteria in the absence of screening.

However, where methods are known to be ineffective against nonlipid-enveloped viruses, pathogen inactivation may be inadequate, and in the case of pooled solvent-detergent-treated plasma clinical illness as a result of parvovirus B19 infection has been reported [40]. This has resulted in the introduction of nucleic acid screening both for B19 and hepatitis A, another nonlipid-enveloped virus, as part of the solvent-detergent plasma process.

As mentioned earlier, pathogen inactivation processes also inactivate white cells and may provide an alternative to gamma or X-ray irradiation in avoiding graft-versus-host disease [41, 42].

Cost-effectiveness

If only those viruses for which routine screening is in place are considered, cost-effectiveness analysis shows virus inactivation to be uneconomic, owing to the very low risks of infection already achieved. Formal analysis of this for solvent-detergent-treated plasma has given figures of at least $2,000,000 per quality-adjusted life-year (QALY) saved [43]. Assuming a cost of $50 to $100 per unit for pathogen-inactivation processing, similar results would be expected for other procedures.

For pooled solvent-detergent plasma, there are two additional variables—relating to pooling rather than infectious agents—that may influence these estimates. Both arise from the fact that pooling reduces the titer of specific antibodies that may occur in occasional donations. The result is that antibodies that may cause transfusion-related lung injury are diluted to clinically insignificant levels [44]. If the cost benefits of this are introduced, then the cost-effectiveness of solvent-detergent plasma becomes around $50,000 per QALY [45]. The second is that anti-A and anti-B antibodies may be diluted out to yield a product (UniPlas) that is universal and does not require blood-group-matched transfusion.

More interesting is to consider bacteria and emerging pathogens. For emerging infections, pathogen inactivation has the potential to avoid the delay and costs involved in introducing new tests, the value of this being dependent on the particular emerging agent. For bacteria, current testing is not fully effective [4] and, while possibly a more expensive option than testing [46], pathogen inactivation is likely to be more effective. A formal full-scale assessment of this has just commenced in France.

Conclusions and consensus

To paraphrase the conclusion of a recent consensus conference [47], pathogen inactivation of blood components cannot be justified for those transfusion [transmitted agents for which mandatory routine testing is already in place but should be given serious consideration to address the almost inevitable next emerging infection(s)].

To this I would add two points. First, no inactivation procedure is likely to be able to address prion diseases, such as variant Creutzfeldt–Jakob disease, as these are not dependent on nucleic acid. Potential screening assays for these agents are approaching field trials, as are filters that should allow removal of the infectious agent. Second, for bacterial contamination of platelets, pathogen inactivation is likely to be more effective but more expensive than bacterial screening. Ideally, one would wish to introduce the more effective technology, but whether this is affordable becomes a local political or managerial decision.

References

1. Kitchen AD, Barbara AJ. Current information on the infectious risks of allogeneic blood transfusion. In: Maniatis A, Van der Linden P, Hardy J-F (Eds). *Alternatives to Blood Transfusion in Transfusion Medicine*. Wiley-Blackwell, Oxford, 2010, pp. 21–30.
2. Bryant BJ, Klein HG. Pathogen inactivation: the definitive safeguard for the blood supply. Arch Pathol Lab Med 2007;131:719–33.
3. Prowse C. Kill and cure. The hope and reality of virus inactivation. Vox Sang 1994;67(Suppl. 3):191–6.
4. Prowse C. Zero tolerance. Transfusion 2007;47:1106–9.

5. Horowitz B, Bonomo R, Prince AM, et al. Solvent/detergent-treated plasma: a virus-inactivated substitute for fresh frozen plasma. Blood 1992;79: 826–31.
6. Burnouf T, Goubran HA, Radosevich M, et al. A process for solvent/detergent treatment of plasma for transfusion at blood centers that use a disposable-bag system. Transfusion 2006;46:2100–108.
7. Burnouf T, Radosevich M, El-Ekiaby M, et al. Nanofiltration of single plasma donations: feasibility study. Vox Sang 2003;84:111–19.
8. Burnouf-Radosevich M, Burnouf T, Huart JJ. A pasteurized therapeutic plasma. Infusionsther Transfusionsmed 1992;19:91–4.
9. Lambrecht B, Mohr H, Knüver-Hopf J, Schmitt H. Photoinactivation of viruses in human fresh plasma by phenothiazine dyes in combination with visible light. Vox Sang 1991;60:207–13.
10. Lin L, Cook DN, Wiesehahn GP, et al. Photochemical inactivation of viruses and bacteria in platelet concentrates by use of a novel psoralen and long-wavelength ultraviolet light. Transfusion 1997;37: 423–35.
11. Goodrich RP, Edrich RA, Li J, Seghatchian J. The Mirasol PRT system for pathogen reduction of platelets and plasma: an overview of current status and future trends. Transfus Apher Sci 2006;35:5–17.
12. Mohr H, Redecker-Klein A. Inactivation of pathogens in platelet concentrates by using a two-step procedure. Vox Sang 2003;84:96–104.
13. Lazo A, Tassello J, Jayarama V, et al. Broad-spectrum virus reduction in red cell concentrates using INACTINE PEN110 chemistry. Vox Sang 2002;83: 313–23.
14. Benjamin RJ, McCullough J, Mintz PD, et al. Therapeutic efficacy and safety of red blood cells treated with a chemical process (S-303) for pathogen inactivation: a Phase III clinical trial in cardiac surgery patients. Transfusion 2005;45:1739–49.
15. Wagner SJ, Skripchenko A, Cincotta L, Thompson-Montgomery D, Awatefe H. Use of a flexible thiopyrylium photosen-sitizer and competitive inhibitor for pathogen reduction of viruses and bacteria with retention of red cell storage properties. Transfusion 2005;45:752–60.
16. Skripchenko A, Wagner SJ, Thompson-Montgomery D, Awatefe H. Thiazole orange, a DNA-binding photosensitizer with flexible structure, can inactivate pathogens in red blood cell suspensions while maintaining red cell storage properties. Transfusion 2006;46:213–19.
17. Stanworth SJ, Brunskill SJ, Hyde CJ, McClelland DB, Murphy MF. Is fresh frozen plasma clinically effective? A systematic review of randomized controlled trials. Br J Haematol 2004;126:139–52.
18. Pehta JC. Clinical studies with solvent-detergent-treated products. Transfus Med Rev 1996;10:303–11.
19. Williamson LM, Llewelyn CA, Fisher NC, et al. A randomized trial of solvent/detergent-treated and standard fresh-frozen plasma in the coagulopathy of liver disease and liver transplantation. Transfusion 1999;39:1227–34.
20. Coignard BP, Colquhoun SD, Nguyen GT, et al. Intraoperative deaths in liver transplant recipients associated with the use of solvent/detergent plasma [abstract]. Hepatology 2002;36:A209.
21. Ozier Y, Rieux C. Liver transplantation, solvent-detergent-treated plasma and antifibrinolytics. Anesth Analg 2003;96:1231–2.
22. Williamson LM, Llewelyn CA. Efficacy of SD-treated plasma during liver transplantation (reply). Transfusion 2000;40:886–8.
23. Williamson L, Cardigan R, Prowse C. Methylene blue-treated fresh-frozen plasma: what is its contribution to blood safety? Transfusion 2003;43: 1322–9.
24. Alvarez-Larren A, Del Rio J, Ramirez C, et al. Methylene blue-photoinactivated plasma vs. fresh-frozen plasma as replacement fluid for plasma exchange in thrombotic thrombocytopenic purpura. Vox Sang 2004;86:246–51.
25. de Alarcon P, Benjamin R, Dugdale M, et al. Fresh frozen plasma prepared with amotosalen HC1 (S-59) photochemical pathogen inactivation: transfusion of patients with congenital coagulation factor deficiencies. Transfusion 2005;45:1362–72.
26. Mintz PD, Bass MM, Petz LD, et al. Photochemically treated fresh frozen plasma for transfusion of patients with acquired coagulopathy of liver disease. Blood 2006;107:3753–9.
27. Mintz PD, Neff A, MacKenzie M, et al. A randomized, controlled Phase III trial of therapeutic plasma exchange with fresh-frozen plasma (FFP) prepared with amotosalen and ultraviolet A light compared to untreated FFP in thrombotic thrombocytopenic purpura. Transfusion 2006;46:1693–704.
28. AuBuchon JP, Herschel L, Roger J, et al. Efficacy of apheresis platelets treated with riboflavin and ultraviolet light for pathogen reduction. Transfusion 2005;45:1335–41.

29. Goodrich RP, Li J, Pieters H, et al. Correlation of in vitro platelet quality measurements with in vivo platelet viability in human subjects. Vox Sang 2006;90:279–85.
30. van Rhenen D, Gulliksson H, Cazenave JP, et al. Transfusion of pooled buffy coat platelet components prepared with photochemical pathogen inactivation treatment: the euroSPRITE trial. Blood 2003;101:2426–33.
31. McCullough J, Vesole DH, Benjamin RJ, et al. Therapeutic efficacy and safety of platelets treated with a photochemical process for pathogen inactivation: the SPRINT Trial. Blood 2004;104:1534–41.
32. AuBuchon JP, Pickard CA, Herschel LH, et al. Production of pathogen-inactivated RBC concentrates using PEN110 chemistry: a Phase I clinical study. Transfusion 2002;42:146–52.
33. Rios JA, Hambleton J, Viele M, et al. Viability of red cells prepared with S-303 pathogen inactivation treatment. Transfusion 2006;46:1778–86.
34. Heger A, Romisch J, Svae IE. A biochemical comparison of a pharmaceutically licensed coagulation active plasma (Octaplas)(R) with a universally applicable development product (Uniplas) and single-donor FFPs subjected to methylene-blue dye and white-light treatment. Transfus Apheresis Sci 2006;35:223–33.
35. Ciaravino V, McCullough T, Cimino G. The role of toxicology assessment in transfusion medicine. Transfusion 2003;43:1481–92.
36. Chapman JR, Moore K, Butterworth BE. Pathogen inactivation of RBCs: PEN110 reproductive toxicology studies. Transfusion 2003;43:1386–93.
37. Ciaravino V, McCullough T, Cimino G, Sullivan T. Preclinical safety profile of plasma prepared using the INTERCEPT Blood System. Vox Sang 2003;85:171–82.
38. Lin L, Conlan MG, Tessman J, Cimino G, Porter S. Amotosalen interactions with platelet and plasma components: absence of neoantigen formation after photochemical treatment. Transfusion 2005;45: 1610–20.
39. Ruane PH, Edrich R, Gampp D, et al. Photochemical inactivation of selected viruses and bacteria in platelet concentrates using riboflavin and light. Transfusion 2004;44:877–85.
40. Koenigbauer UF, Eastlund T, Day JW. Clinical illness due to parvovirus B19 infection after infusion of solvent/detergent treated pooled plasma. Transfusion 2001;41:1203–6.
41. Fast LD, Semple JW, DiLeone G, et al. Inhibition of xenogeneic GVHD by PEN110 treatment of donor human PBMNCs. Transfusion 2004;44:282–5.
42. Grass JA, Wafa T, Reames A, et al. Prevention of transfusion-associated graft-versus-host disease by photochemical treatment. Blood 1999;93:3140–7.
43. Jackson BR, AuBuchon JP, Birkmeyer JD. Update of cost-effectiveness analysis for solvent-detergent treated plasma. JAMA 1999;282:329–30.
44. Sachs UJ, Kauschat D, Bein G. White blood cell-reactive antibodies are undetectable in solvent/detergent plasma. Transfusion 2005;45: 1628–31.
45. Riedler GF, Haycox AR, Duggan AK, Dakin HA. Cost-effectiveness of solvent/ detergent-treated fresh-frozen plasma. Vox Sang 2003;85:88–95.
46. Janssen MP, van der Poel CL, Buskens E, et al. Costs and benefits of bacterial culturing and pathogen reduction in the Netherlands. Transfusion 2006;46:956–65.
47. Klein HG, Anderson D, Bernardi MJ, et al. Pathogen inactivation: making decisions about new technologies – preliminary report of a consensus conference. Vox Sang 2007;93:179–82.

CHAPTER 7

The Benefits of Allogeneic Erythrocyte Transfusion: What Evidence Do We Have?

Neil Soni[1] *& Benjamin Thomas*[2]

[1]Consultant ITU and Anaesthetics, Chelsea and Westminster Hospital, London, UK

[2]SpR Anaesthesia, St Mary's Hospital, Paddington, London, UK

Introduction

Generations of doctors were taught to replace the fluid that a patient was losing—simple and sound advice that meant water was replaced with water, electrolyte solutions with similar and blood with blood, albeit from someone else. In the broadest sense, this simple advice is still pertinent and, for example, with massive blood loss there is nothing yet that will substitute for blood. The situation is made far more complex by modern medicine where there are many current and historical indications for blood where the basis for its use can, and is being, challenged. There is a rapidly growing wealth of evidence, both substantial and more commonly circumstantial, denying the usefulness and emphasizing the hazards of allogeneic blood, with few if any papers focused on demonstrating the benefits of its traditional uses. These traditional uses or indications of blood extend from its physiological value in oxygen delivery (DO_2) (see Table 7.1) through the relative benefits of replacing abnormal variants of hemoglobin and into the realms of blood as a "tonic." The intention of this paper is to address the question of what the benefits are, to necessitate a review of where and how it is used, and to assess the rationale and the available evidence.

Few textbooks list the indications for transfusion even from the era when blood was considered essential, but they all list a vast array of complications and problems. The indications of erythrocyte transfusion discussed in this review are shown in Table 7.2.

The issue of whole fresh blood

Whole fresh blood is the topic that will not go away. There have been several periods when whole blood was reputed to have almost magical properties when given hot and fresh. "Bleeding stops and the patient gets better in a way that components never get near." The potential cross-matching and infectivity problems have made this almost impossible, but leaving the question about its efficacy unanswered. There is little or no evidence to support the anecdotal reports of its efficacy, although there are theoretical arguments. These can be summed up as warm with normal 2,3-diphosphoglycerate (2,3-DPG) and with the right balance of clotting factors and fibrinogen. It also has the correct properties for volume replacement, oxygen carriage, and coagulation. It is being used in theaters of war where the risk/benefit analysis is altered by specific population screening, the nature and immediacy of the injuries and availability of supply [1–3].

Alternatives to Blood Transfusion in Transfusion Medicine, 2nd edition. Edited by A. Maniatis, P. Van der Linden, J.-F. Hardy.

Table 7.1 Oxygen availability—using the basic equation for oxygen delivery to tissues: Hb × CO × 1.34 × ER (1.34 is the hemoglobin binding constant).

Situation	Oxygen availability (mL/minute)	Oxygen delivery (mL/minute)
Hb 10, CO 6, ER 0.3	241	804
Hb 10, CO 2, ER 0.3	80	268
Hb 10, CO 2, ER 0.7	187	268
Hb 5, CO 6, ER 0.3	120	402
Hb 5, CO 6, ER 0.7	281	402
Hb 5, CO 2, ER 0.7	94	134

Sources vary as to the limits of the ER. The literature indicates that in severe exercise a ratio of 0.8 is seen if the venous saturation is used as an indicator, although it is likely that muscle oxygen consumption is exceeding its oxygen delivery at that rate, i.e. this is beyond the critical point. In most organs 0.5 is probably a more reasonable maximum ER. Here ratios of 0.3 and 0.7 are used to try to illustrate the likely oxygen availability. CO, cardiac output (L/minue); ER, extraction ratio (final saturation/initial saturation); Hb, hemoglobin concentration (g/dL).

Acute hemorrhage

In acute hemorrhage, in any scenario planned or unplanned, the sudden reduction in hemoglobin is usually linked to volume loss but also results in loss of oxygen-carrying capacity. The former is easily corrected by volume replacement. The latter is an issue that is essential to what constitutes an indication for blood transfusion. There are two key elements: first, maintaining DO_2 above the critical threshold point where tissue demand exceeds supply; and second, "dynamism," i.e., predicting the likelihood of falling below that threshold.

Oxygen delivery

The issue of oxygen supply will be dealt with below, but a brief description of the relevant features is pertinent here. Cain performed landmark studies in DO_2 in dogs rendered isovolemically anemic to see the relationship between oxygen consumption (VO_2) and DO_2 [4]. It was clearly shown that there was a point at which delivery no longer matched consumption and below which consumption fell precipitously. This was the "critical point" (CP) at which compensation failed and oxygen supply was inadequate [4]. It is from this point downward where delivery and consumption are directly related. It is important to appreciate there is a global CP but also organ-specific CPs determined by organ

Table 7.2 Indications for packed red blood cells.

Acute hemorrhage, nonsurgical	Frequently necessary
Acute hemorrhage, surgical	Necessary but use conservation methods
Acute expected hemorrhage, surgical	When conservation fails
Preoperative correction of anemia	Only if unavoidable (restrictive)
Acute hemolysis	Necessary (restrictive)
Acute hematological problems: marrow suppression and lack of red cells	Necessary (restrictive)
Critically ill: treatment of bleeding	When necessary (margin of safety threatened)
Intensive care unit: top up	Minimize need (restrictive)
Burns	Minimize need (restrictive)
Acute coronary syndrome	Confusing (see *ACUTE CORONARY SYNDROME*)
Sickle cell prophylaxis/crisis	Only when necessary
Malaria	When necessary
Chronic anemia, renal	Avoid
Chronic anemia, palliative care	Avoid
Rehabilitation	Avoid (evidence confused)
Trauma	Possibly whole fresh blood

Restrictive: apply restrictive transfusion policy.

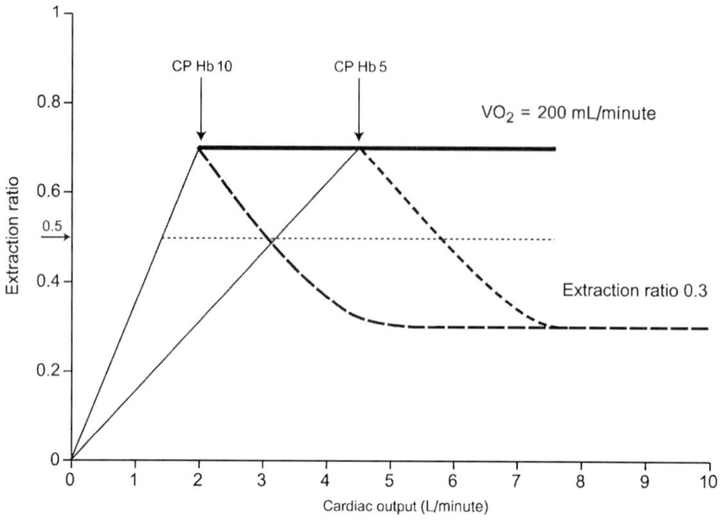

Figure 7.1 The relationship between cardia output and the extraction ratio approaching the critical point (CP) with two different hemoglobin values (5 and 10 g/dL). CP, critical point; Hb, hemoglobin concentration; VO_2, oxygen consumption. - - - Hb 5, – – Hb 10, — VO_2.

requirements and blood flow, and the two may be different.

The DO_2 is measured by the product of cardiac output and bound hemoglobin ($CO \times Hb \times 1.34 \times$ saturation). Essentially the three variables are the hemoglobin concentration, the amount of oxygen bound to hemoglobin, saturation, and the total quantity of both being delivered (Figure 7.1). Local factors such as pH, PCO_2 value, and the Bohr effect would also be relevant in terms of the absolute quantity of oxygen being unloaded from each hemoglobin molecule at tissue level. In this article the amount unloaded is described as the extraction ratio where a reasonable limit is 0.5 while up to 0.7 can occur (Figure 7.2).

This is relevant in acute hemorrhage, assuming functional lungs, as two main factors influence delivery to the blood tissue interface; cardiac output and the amount of hemoglobin saturated. DO_2 into the tissues is then determined by the amount of oxygen that can be off-loaded from the hemoglobin molecule, i.e., the fall in saturation. A decrease in any of the multiple factors that influence delivery to the tissues can then be compensated

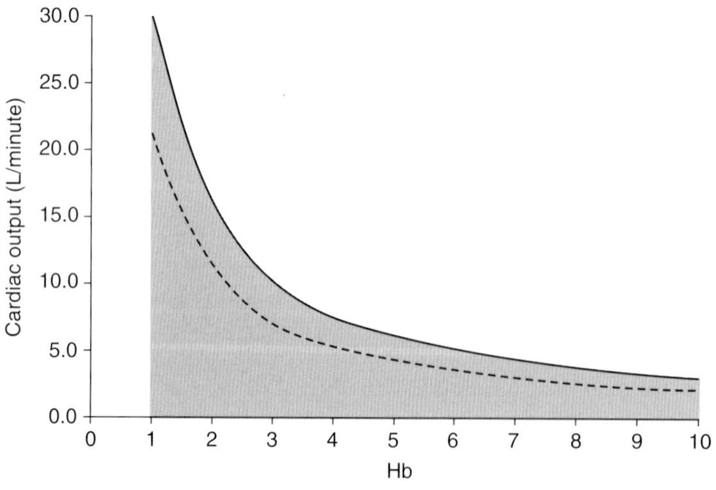

Figure 7.2 The relationship between cardiac output and hemoglobin value at the critical point at two different extraction ratios: 0.5 and 0.3. CP, critical point; ER, extraction ratio. — CP ER = 0.5, - - - CP ER = 0.7.

Table 7.3 Acute bleeding.

1. Blood loss leads to ↓ volume (cardiac output), ↓ Hb (total)
2. Compensation: Systemic: ↑ heart rate, ↑ vasoconstriction (danger; ischemic heart disease)
Local: Bohr effect, ↑ extraction ratio
3. Correction = fluid
↑ volume, ↑ cardiac output, ↓ Hb
4. Correction = blood
↑ volume, ↑ cardiac output, ↑ Hb
(but old blood = low extraction ratio)

Hb, hemoglobin concentration.

for by unloading more oxygen from the delivered hemoglobin.

Conversely, if the hemoglobin is low because of the hemorrhage, an increase in cardiac output will deliver more blood to the tissue, albeit with a lower hemoglobin concentration. The net effect is to increase DO_2. As long as the available DO_2 is above the CP, VO_2 is maintained. However, increased cardiac output from increased heart rate and vasoconstriction, which is also part of the compensatory mechanism, result in increased cardiac work, and VO_2 that may tax the potentially ischemic heart. The patient, the organ, and the cell determine what the VO_2 needs to be, and the delivery is only relevant if it is inadequate.

In acute hemorrhage, the volume depletion of bleeding reduces cardiac output and hence DO_2, while loss of hemoglobin mass will reduce potential oxygen carriage (see Table 7.3). Volume repletion will restore output that can increase to compensate for low hemoglobin. Then the hemoglobin is relatively unimportant in terms of DO_2 until the hemoglobin is extremely low. If volume status is not corrected and the cardiac output cannot compensate, then DO_2 is increasingly dependent on the oxygen unloaded from the available hemoglobin. If the latter is low, then the available oxygen is also limited.

With normovolemic anemia, improved cardiac output can provide adequate DO_2 until the hemoglobin is very low—probably considerably less than 5 g/dL. As cardiac output falls then the amount of oxygen extraction from the available hemoglobin increases dramatically. In summary, cardiac output compensates for low hemoglobin, and oxygen extraction compensates for low cardiac output. If both fall simultaneously then there is no compensatory mechanism that can increase DO_2, and the VO_2 is compromised as the CP is reached and passed.

In acute bleeding, all of the above can happen. If volume is protected then a low hemoglobin concentration can be tolerated, but if volume is compromised then a high hemoglobin concentration is protective. The real issue is how far an individual is from the CP at which DO_2 fails to match requirements.

There are other considerations. This global picture also applies to the microcosm of individual circulations, such as the coronary circulation and indeed other organs. There the flow may be determined not only by cardiac output but also by local factors, for example a stenosed vessel. Stenosis means flow limitation, irrespective of volume status. The issue is that any compensatory increases in cardiac output to improve oxygen supply will be ineffectual because of the stenosis, and the organ is increasingly dependent on oxygen extraction from the available hemoglobin.

The key is the CP, which has a global value but will also have local organ values. Identifying the CP is easy when it has been passed, in terms of signs of tissue hypoxia such as falling pH and rising lactate. In an individual organ such as the heart, overt cardiac ischemia indicates the cardiac CP has been passed. That is too late to be a useful indicator, except for rescue. There are no adequate measures of when the patient is approaching the CP, either globally or locally. Ideally the patient should not reach that point. In acute situations, both

Table 7.4 Risk factors suggesting that a patient is potentially closer to the critical point than normal.

1. Impaired ventricular function with poor cardiac output and no reserve
2. Hypovolemia
3. Hypoxemia
4. Anemia
5. Ischemic heart disease
6. Vascular disease with stenosed vessels
7. Increased metabolic activity (increased oxygen consumption)

hemoglobin and cardiac output are threatened. The cautious clinician protects both and builds in a margin of safety between the patient and their CP (see Table 7.4). "It does not matter where you are as long as you are above it."

"Dynamism"

It is important to be clear about what we know and what we do not know. This describes acute medical practice where some facts are known, several are presumed, and some are unknown. It may be known or presumed that bleeding is taking place, either from obvious overt blood loss or signs consistent with blood loss. The site may be known or presumed. What is frequently unknown is the actual bleeding rate, whether bleeding is ongoing and whether it will accelerate or decelerate. Further down the track is the uncertainty of when, by what means, and how effectively bleeding can be controlled. Frequently the estimated losses will be determined by signs and measurements, such as pulse rate, blood pressure, and hemoglobin. Some changes are immediate, but hemoglobin changes are late and indicate what has already happened, not necessarily what is currently occurring. Clinical signs that indicate a 20% loss in a normal individual may appear after a much smaller loss in a patient who is already hypovolemic and compromised from previous losses. This compote of uncertainty is what prevails in acute circumstances and represents the dynamics of the situation. In such a dynamic situation where the specific value of the CP is unknown, an approach that builds a margin of safety that protects both compensatory mechanisms (cardiac output and hemoglobin) would seem prudent. In acute bleeding, there is good evidence that both low cardiac output and low hemoglobin carry a significant morbidity and mortality. There is even better evidence that the combination is lethal.

Other considerations

Other options

In an unstable position with ongoing bleeding and a falling hemoglobin, transfusion is indicated to remain safe. In the ward environment, there may be no choices available, but in other situations such as accident and emergency, intensive care, and theaters, there are many occasions where implementation of conservation methods such as cell salvage may be feasible and may reduce transfusion requirements. This should be available to be used, if appropriate.

Efficacy of the blood

Cold stored blood with reduced 2,3-DPG content has relatively poor oxygen affinity. Increasing the hemoglobin will increase carriage, but with a low extraction rate. Paradoxically, to ensure avoiding the CP, earlier administration is necessary to allow for the relative inefficiency [5–8].

Current reports suggest that stored blood impairs nitric oxide function and thereby causes vasoconstriction. If this is correct then vasoconstriction will impair perfusion and local DO_2. The argument would then be for earlier transfusion to mitigate this side effect. In transfusing blood, reduced oxygen availability because of low 2,3-DPG will be compounded by reduced perfusion because of impaired nitric oxide. This is a microcosm of the fall in cardiac output and anemia seen on a global level [9–11].

Acute expected hemorrhage

When major bleeding is anticipated then there will be a requirement for blood, but blood transfusion with allogeneic blood should be reserved for situations where blood-conservation techniques cannot be used or where they cannot cope [12]. In many settings, means of conserving blood are available, and methods of reducing loss can be implemented prospectively. Even with good salvage and good surgery, there are situations where blood loss is large and transfusion will be necessary. A restrictive transfusion approach is feasible.

Preoperative transfusion

The patient is presenting with a low hemoglobin, losses may occur, and the margin of safety is threatened. The approach should be dictated by circumstances. In elective situations, when time is on your side, conservative means of improving a very low hemoglobin concentration should be used; and that might include iron and/or recombinant human erythropoietin. The data are confusing as in many situations there appears to be little morbidity and mortality dependent on the level of hemoglobin [13, 14]. This Halcyon approach has been challenged by a recent study in cardiac surgery [15]. In that large study, anemia was defined as less than 13 g/dL in men and 12 g/dL in women. It was quite clear that adverse outcome started increasing with preoperative hemoglobin concentrations below 10 g/dL. Given that anemia is known to be a disease marker in its own right, it is not surprising it is associated with poorer outcome. It does not mean that transfusion, fixing the number, would alter the outcome, but it would be naive to dismiss this important epidemiological finding when so many others are being accepted.

In practical terms, if there is no time to correct hemoglobin by other means, then a transfusion might be indicated to preempt heavy blood loss or just to bring the hemoglobin to a "safe" value. "Safe" means that with a corrected hemoglobin the patient has to lose both blood and volume to reach the CP. At present, in the absence of ischemic heart disease, a trigger of <8 g/dL is used by many to good effect [12–14, 16–20].

It is important to note that the transfusion studies look at populations undergoing procedures associated with very low mortality rates and low incidences of myocardial infarction, and therefore it is unsurprising that few are seen. The lack of overt morbidity has resulted in a degree of complacency about the certainty of declaring that low hemoglobin values carry little, if any, risk. Few transfusion trials are focused on the "at-risk" populations, where the preoperative cardiac surgery study of anemia indicated a problem, and so assumptions still prevail [20].

Indications in the critically ill

Acute transfusion

The same conditions apply in the critically ill as for any major hemorrhage that may result in impairment of DO_2. In the critically ill, the patient is presumably even more vulnerable as the usual compensatory mechanisms may already be compromised. For example, the hemoglobin may be partially derived from transfused blood, the cardiac output may be supported by inotropes, which incidentally increase oxygen use, or conversely the patient may be unable to produce a compensatory increase in cardiac output. The Bohr effect may already be maximally exercised. Overall the patient may reach the CP very rapidly, in terms of supporting VO_2, with blood loss. In these instances the hemoglobin has exaggerated importance. The CP is unknown but the vulnerability of organ systems in this population should indicate that a wide safety margin is desirable. It is therefore surprising to find that hemoglobin is relatively unimportant in the critically ill. Studies indicate that a restrictive approach is safe and may even be beneficial [21, 22]. A trigger of 7–8 g/dL appears to be safe.

It is very important to appreciate the context. The discussion so far has centered on acute transfusion for presumed major bleeding, and these studies did not look at this subgroup. The dynamics discussed previously are relevant in this population and the same rules apply in that keeping the patient well above the CP below which VC_2 can no longer be supported is crucial, and in these patients it is only recognizable when it has been passed. That is too late. There must be a conservative approach to restrictive triggers in unstable situations. Some authors allude to this as a tailored approach to transfusion [23].

The studies on blood conservation, the apparent safety of low hemoglobin levels, and the dangers of giving blood demonstrate some interesting details. Some studies indicate that red cell transfusion does improve DO_2 but not VO_2 [5, 24, 25]. Is this surprising? It is a physiological fact that the cells determine their oxygen requirements and take what they need. The link between delivery and consumption only occurs when there is inadequate oxygen for their needs, i.e., below the CP. Above that point, giving more than they need will not increase consumption, unless they are oxygen deprived, but will increase the margin of safety.

Various epidemiological studies indicate that mortality may be higher in patients liberally transfused, while a myriad of studies have shown that needing and receiving a blood transfusion worsens outcome. This is seen in everything from burns through cardiac surgery to intensive care in general [25–32]. Most authors claim that this is not stating the obvious—that transfusion requirement is a significant indicator of a major problem, especially in an era when blood is being used increasingly conservatively, and therefore must translate into outcome. Statistics fail dismally to separate the issue of requirement and risk. These studies are currently proliferating in the journals, but their interpretation is difficult. If blood is so bad as to cause this morbidity, it is vital to know the mechanism by which it causes damage if it is genuinely only blood related. Potential mechanisms include viscosity, microcirculation, and now the new nitric oxide findings, which suggest that a storage injury impairs nitric oxide release and hence cause vasospasm—a nice idea but currently an extrapolation too far [10, 11]. The relevance to the individual has to be set against their threshold determined by their cause of bleeding and its management but also by comorbidities. It is quite clear that high hemoglobin values cause problems. At lower hemoglobin values the issues of the efficacy of transfused stored blood may be theoretically important, but withholding blood in a patient who is close to the CP has not been subjected to trial. Observational studies in Jehovah's Witnesses indicate that at least some patients can survive despite amazingly low hemoglobin values.

Intensive care unit "top up"

Intensive care unit (ICU) patients tend to be anemic, and more than 40% of them receive blood, usually just to adjust hemoglobin. The benefits of this cannot be measured or even found [33]. Importantly, these vast numbers of minor transfusions with no apparent outcome impact must play a significant role in the studies we have to date that assess transfusion triggers [13, 22, 27]. This is a problem in that there is no differentiation between transfusions given electively and those given urgently. This is an obvious weakness in the position that needs well-designed prospective studies. In the hemoglobin "top-up" scenario, it seems at least reasonable to assume that the data fully support a restrictive approach.

There is a negative aspect to this. In Scotland, with restrictive transfusion practice about a third of patients are discharged from the ICU with a hemoglobin less than 9 g/dL [34]. To date there appears to be no problem with lower values. However, it is important to note that anemia is good indicator of poor prognosis in the critically ill [35–37]. Outside of intensive care, in practice of other specialties such as oncology and nephrology, a low hemoglobin (commonly less than 9 g/dL) is an indicator of poor prognosis [38–42]. It is clearly not cause and effect, but rather the anemia is a disease marker. Mistaking disease markers for causes and treating them as such has usually been found to be frustrating, and there is no reason it should be different in the critically ill.

The debate now swings between caution and the suggestion that even lower might be even better [21, 33, 43, 44]. If outcome is the only meaningful end point, then a restrictive practice is important in this group of patients.

Burns

In burns the same conditions apply as in the critically ill with one large exception. The operative interventions cause massive bleeding, and cell salvage is often contraindicated because of infected eschars. There is some evidence that blood transfusion in burns is associated with outcome and may, unsurprisingly, be detrimental [26, 30, 45]. The subject is well recognized as being a significant issue [45]. The restrictive transfusion approach works equally well in this population and is gaining ground, although with no firm guidelines [46, 47]. A range of methods for managing burns so as to reduce surgical blood loss are being assessed as methods of predicting blood loss, all of which may help deciding how much to transfuse [48, 51]. An integrated approach with hemostasis-conscious surgical technique, conservation methods, and a restrictive approach has been shown to reduce blood usage, specifically in burns of less than 20% body surface, although it seems reasonable to extend this approach to bigger burns [52–54]. All the considerations regarding the CP still apply in this vulnerable population. The more chronic use of blood for "top ups" in the burns unit is very similar to that in the ICU, both in cause and in practice, and a similar approach should be adopted.

Acute coronary syndrome

Transfusion in acute coronary syndrome has been shown to be associated with increased mortality [55]. Yet, in the elderly it has been shown to reduce mortality if the hematocrit is less than 30% [56]. However, this is complicated by evidence that transfusion for those with a hemoglobin concentration less than 12 g/dL is good in ST-segment elevation myocardial infarction, but not so good in non-ST-segment elevation myocardial infarction. To confound matters further, there is excess mortality with both very high and very low hemoglobin concentrations [57]. The only conclusion would appear to be that a hemoglobin level between 10 g/dL and 14 g/dL is best left alone.

Chronic anemia

There are two areas of chronic anemia that exemplify the issues involved. They are renal impairment and palliative care.

Renal impairment

Renal impairment is associated with anemia that is often secondary to the condition, is perceived to cause functional problems and is associated with a poor outcome. It has also been investigated very extensively. More than 60% of renal patients have anemia. Previous studies indicated that correction of anemia was beneficial [58–60]. More recent studies emphasize that a hemoglobin level of around 10 g/dL is acceptable, while higher values are associated with increased morbidity and mortality, in particular seizures and hypertension [61–63]. Transfusion should not be indicated here, as other means, especially erythropoiesis-stimulating agents, are as effective.

Palliative care

In palliative care, anemia is clearly a problem, and quality-of-life indices are correlated with hemoglobin values in 15 out of 16 studies [64]. Transfusion has been used to provide symptom relief and a general improvement. In particular, weakness and dyspnea seem to be helped [65, 66]. The area is difficult to assess with relatively nonspecific and unpredictable responses in terms of pre- and postvalues, yet with a high perceived benefit rate [67, 68]. Whether these benefits could be achieved without transfusion needs elucidating and is controversial [69].

Sickle cell disease (Table 7.5)

There are specific emergency indications for transfusion in sickle cell disease (the decision to transfuse should always be made in consultation with a hematologist). As with other areas of transfusion, there is a trend away from its use because there are clearly defined problems with transfusion, especially chronically used transfusion in patients with

Table 7.5 Indications for transfusion in sickle cell disease.

Pulmonary (infection, fat emboli, infarction)	Transfusion if PaO_2 falling <8 kPa
Splenic sequestration [78, 79]	Rapid fall in Hb (may need splenectomy) [80]
CNS vascular damage/stroke [77, 81–84]	Early exchange transfusion for neurological deficit
Ophthalmic (retinal artery occlusion) [80]	Transfusion
Multiorgan failure [85, 86]	Often necessary
Heart failure if anemic	
Aplastic marrow	
Heart kidney transplantation [87]	
Preoperative transfusion	See *Preoperative transfusion*
Pain (acute or chronic)	Avoid. Transfusion could make it worse
Pulmonary hypertension	Promising but unproven
Priapism	Only if persistent >24 hours
Pregnancy	See Pregnancy

CNS, central nervous system; Hb, hemoglobin concentration.

sickle cell disease. The risk/benefit analysis is difficult except in extremis [70].

Transfusion therapy reduces the percentage of sickle cells and, at low levels of hemoglobin, improves oxygen transport. Reducing the number of cells helps to reduce blood viscosity, which in its own right causes significant problems, but also reduces sickling [71]. This is best achieved by exchange transfusion, although far more blood is involved than in a simple transfusion. Anemia may benefit from a standard transfusion; the literature suggests a threshold hemoglobin level of 8 or 9 g/dL, but this will almost certainly be reviewed as transfusion should be avoided where possible and exchange is at least iron neutral [72–74]. Too much blood—and certainly a hemoglobin level greater than 11 g/dL—is associated with increased viscosity and inherent problems [75–77].

Preoperative transfusion

There is a clear association between general anesthesia and sickling; preoperative transfusion reduces the incidence of complications [88, 89]. There is debate about whether exchange or simple transfusion is better as the results are similar. The United States National Institutes of Health recommend aiming for 10 g/dL but not greater for major surgery, as well as replacing blood loss. Previous recommendations for transfusion prior to eye surgery have been modified in order to mirror those for surgery under anesthesia [88, 90–92].

Pregnancy

There is no place for prophylactic transfusion in normal pregnancy, but in sickle cell disease the situation may be complicated [84, 93]. Opinions vary but complications in association with anemia may necessitate transfusion—simple transfusion if the hemoglobin is less than 5 g/dL, but exchange transfusion if it is higher [93, 94].

Pain

Pain has been used as an indication for transfusion, but it is generally agreed that transfusion should be avoided. Preventive therapy of sickle pain is best achieved with hydroxyurea, which was found to decrease the frequency of crises significantly, decrease the incidence of acute chest syndrome, and decrease the need for blood transfusion [95].

Other indications for transfusion in this condition lie as a specialty area within hematology and transfusion services. There is an excellent review by Josephson et al. [94].

Malaria

In severe malaria, exchange transfusion, in use since 1974, is an adjunctive measure [96]. Its mode of action is a combination of parasite and toxin removal and potentially improved rheology. The Centers for Disease Control and Prevention recommend that this treatment be considered in case of a parasitemia greater than 10% or the presence of major complications such as cerebral malaria, renal failure, or pulmonary edema [97, 98]. The only meta-analysis showed that there is inadequate controlled data and that no survival benefit for exchange transfusion could be seen, but the authors do comment that the populations may have been different [99].

Conclusion

Restrictive transfusion practice is not life-threatening and may even be beneficial where transfusion is clearly associated with increased morbidity. High hemoglobin targets in some populations increase morbidity and death. Blood transfusion should be avoided, and the evidence is compelling. Unfortunately, the situation is made more complex by other observations. Anemia is associated with morbidity, and acute anemia and hypovolemia have a strong association with major morbidity and death.

Probably less dramatic but of greater concern is that most human beings seem content with a hemoglobin level of 14 g/dL in men and 12 g/dL in women. Furthermore, most people subjected to sudden and unexpected anemia, albeit isovolemic, feel unwell, and fatigue easily. A physiological approach might be to ask why we have such high normal values when we do not need them or indeed if they are evolutionarily redundant. While that may be the case in those who are sitting in front of a computer desk, which in the modern age has replaced hunting and gathering, it can hardly be applied widely. Even if it were, acute critical illness and surgery have been shown to be physiologically challenging, and one might expect that physiological reserve would be important, if not in the acute phase then in the recovery. Few studies have addressed recovery from illness with low hemoglobins [100]. At least one study could find no evidence of problems, while another found higher hemoglobins to be better; so the evidence is sparse and unconvincing in either direction [101, 102].

Therefore, there are definite unknowns, and it would be foolish to accept the current evidence without reservation until the unknowns are known. The focus of research should address whether a normal hemoglobin confers recovery properties even if it is transfused blood and should define the actual mechanism by which transfusion does harm. With this knowledge, complacent acceptance of low hemoglobin values as being of no consequence is unlikely to result in embarrassment. More importantly, both authors wish to stress that if they are bleeding and are anywhere near their CP they would like to be transfused.

References

1. Kauvar DS, Holcomb JB, Norris GC, Hess JR. Fresh whole blood transfusion: a controversial military practice. J Trauma 2006;61:181–4.
2. Repine TB, Perkins JG, Kauvar DS, Blackborne L. The use of fresh whole blood in massive transfusion. J Trauma 2006;60(6 Suppl.):S59–69.
3. Spinella PC, Perkins JG, Grathwohl KW, et al. Risks associated with fresh whole blood and red blood cell transfusions in a combat support hospital. Crit Care Med 2007;35:2576–81.
4. Cain SM. Oxygen delivery and uptake in dogs during anemic and hypoxic hypoxia. J Appl Physiol 1977;42:228–34.
5. Suttner S, Piper SN, Kumle B, et al. The influence of allogeneic red blood cell transfusion compared with 100% oxygen ventilation on systemic oxygen transport and skeletal muscle oxygen tension after cardiac surgery. Anesth Analg 2004;99:2–11.
6. Kahn RC, Zaroulis C, Goetz W, Howland WS. Hemodynamic oxygen transport and 2,3-diphosphoglycerate changes after transfusion of patients in acute respiratory failure. Intensive Care Med 1986;12:22–5.
7. Woodson RD. Physiological significance of oxygen dissociation curve shifts. Crit Care Med 1979;7:368–73.

8. Dawson RB. Hemoglobin function in stored blood, XVII. Maintenance of red cell 2,3 DPG (function) and ATP (viability) for six weeks in ACD or CPD-adenine-inosine-methylene blue. Rev Fr Transfus Immunohematol 1976;19:527–38.
9. Smith MJ, Le Roux PD, Elliott JP, Winn HR. Blood transfusion and increased risk for vasospasm and poor outcome after subarachnoid hemorrhage. J Neurosurg 2004;101:1–7.
10. Wallis JP. Nitric oxide and blood: a review. Transfus Med 2005;15:1–11.
11. Almac E, Ince C. The impact of storage on red cell function in blood transfusion. Best Pract Res Clin Anaesthesiol 2007;21:195–208.
12. Mallett SV, Peachey TD, Sanehi O, Hazlehurst G, Mehta A. Reducing red blood cell transfusion in elective surgical patients: the role of audit and practice guidelines. Anaesthesia 2000;55:1013–19.
13. Carson JL, Duff A, Berlin JA, et al. Perioperative blood transfusion and postoperative mortality. JAMA 1998;279:199–205.
14. Dougenis D, Patrinou V, Filos KS, Theodori E, Vagianos K, Maniati A. Blood use in lung resection for carcinoma: perioperative elective anaemia does not compromise the early outcome. Eur J Cardiothorac Surg 2001;20:372–7.
15. Kulier A, Levin J, Moser R, et al. Impact of preoperative anemia on outcome in patients undergoing coronary artery bypass graft surgery. Circulation 2007;116:471–9.
16. Kreimeier U, Messmer K. Perioperative hemodilution. Transfus Apher Sci 2002;27:59–72.
17. Waggoner JR, 3rd, Wass CT, Polls TZ, et al. The effect of changing transfusion practice on rates of perioperative stroke and myocardial infarction in patients undergoing carotid endarterectomy: a retrospective analysis of 1114 Mayo Clinic patients. Mayo Perioperative Outcomes Group. Mayo Clin Proc 2001;76:376–83.
18. Carson JL, Chen AY. In search of the transfusion trigger. Clin Orthop Relat Res 1998;357:30–5.
19. Crosby ET. Perioperative haemotherapy: I. Indications for blood component transfusion. Can J Anaesth 1992;39:695–707.
20. Grover M, Talwalkar S, Casbard A, et al. Silent myocardial ischaemia and haemoglobin concentration: a randomized controlled trial of transfusion strategy in lower limb arthroplasty. Vox Sang 2006;90:105–12.
21. Fakhry SM, Fata P. How low is too low? Cardiac risks with anemia. Crit Care 2004;8(Suppl. 2):S11–14.
22. Hébert PC, Wells G, Blajchman MA, et al. A multicenter, randomized, controlled clinical trial of transfusion requirements in critical care. Transfusion Requirements in Critical Care Investigators, Canadian Critical Care Trials Group. N Engl J Med 1999;340:409–17.
23. Hardy JF. Should we reconsider triggers for red blood cell transfusion? Acta Anaesthesiol Belg 2003;54:287–95.
24. Van der Linden P, De Hert S, Bélisle S, et al. Comparative effects of red blood cell transfusion and increasing blood flow on tissue oxygenation in oxygen supply-dependent conditions. Am J Respir Crit Care Med 2001;163:1605–8.
25. Napolitano LM, Corwin HL. Efficacy of red blood cell transfusion in the critically ill. Crit Care Clin 2004;20:255–68.
26. Jeschke MG, Chinkes DL, Finnerty CC, et al. Blood transfusions are associated with increased risk for development of sepsis in severely burned pediatric patients. Crit Care Med 2007;35:579–83.
27. Corwin HL, Gettinger A, Pearl RG, et al. The CRIT Study: anemia and blood transfusion in the critically ill-current clinical practice in the United States. Crit Care Med 2004;32:39–52.
28. Koch CG, Li L, Duncan AI, et al. Morbidity and mortality risk associated with red blood cell and blood-component transfusion in isolated coronary artery bypass grafting. Crit Care Med 2006;34:1608–16.
29. Koch CG, Li L, Duncan AI, et al. Transfusion in coronary artery bypass grafting is associated with reduced long-term survival. Ann Thorac Surg 2006;81:1650–57.
30. Palmieri TL, Caruso DM, Foster KN, et al. Effect of blood transfusion on outcome after major burn injury: a multicenter study. Crit Care Med 2006;34:1602–7.
31. Shorr AF, Duh MS, Kelly KM, Kollef MH. Red blood cell transfusion and ventilator-associated pneumonia: a potential link? Crit Care Med 2004;32:666–74.
32. Silverboard H, Aisiku I, Martin GS, Adams M, Rozycki G, Moss M. The role of acute blood transfusion in the development of acute respiratory distress syndrome in patients with severe trauma. J Trauma 2005;59:717–23.
33. Corwin HL, Surgenor SD, Gettinger A. Transfusion practice in the critically ill. Crit Care Med 2003;31(12 Suppl.):S668–71.
34. Walsh TS, Lee RJ, Maciver CR, et al. Anemia during and at discharge from intensive care: the impact of

restrictive blood transfusion practice. Intensive Care Med 2006;32:100–109.
35. Carson JL, Poses RM, Spence RK, Bonavita G. Severity of anaemia and operative mortality and morbidity. Lancet 1988;1:727–9.
36. du Cheyron D, Parienti JJ, Fekih-Hassen M, Daubin C, Charbonneau P. Impact of anemia on outcome in critically ill patients with severe acute renal failure. Intensive Care Med 2005;31:1529–36.
37. Vincent JL, Baron JF, Reinhart K, et al. Anemia and blood transfusion in critically ill patients. JAMA 2002;288:1499–507.
38. Joynson CP, Sundar S, Symonds P. Anaemia is associated with poor overall survival but not with inferior local control in patients with muscle invasive bladder carcinoma treated by radical external beam radiotherapy. A retrospective study. Clin Oncol (R Coll Radial) 2006;18:728–34.
39. van de Pol SM, Doornaert P, de Bree R, Leemans C, Slotman B, Langendijk J. The significance of anemia in squamous cell head and neck cancer treated with surgery and postoperative radiotherapy. Oral Oncol 2006;42:131–8.
40. Citterio G, Bertuzzi A, Tresoldi M, et al. Prognostic factors for survival in metastatic renal cell carcinoma: retrospective analysis from 109 consecutive patients. Eur Urol 1997;31:286–91.
41. Kosiborod M, Smith GL, Radford MJ, Foody JM, Krumholz HM. The prognostic importance of anemia in patients with heart failure. Am J Med 2003; 114:112–19.
42. Mocroft A, Kirk O, Barton SE, et al. Anaemia is an independent predictive marker for clinical prognosis in HIV-infected patients from across Europe. EuroSIDA study group. Aids 1999;13:943–50.
43. Hébert PC, Yetisir E, Martin C, et al. Is a low transfusion threshold safe in critically ill patients with cardiovascular diseases? Crit Care Med 2001;29:227–34.
44. Lundsgaard-Hansen P. The 'critical hematocrit': a figure differing from patient to patient. Beitr Infusionsther 1992;30:208–15.
45. Palmieri TL, Greenhalgh DG. Blood transfusion in burns: what do we do? J Burn Care Rehabil 2004;25: 71–5.
46. Namias N. Advances in burn care. Curr Opin Crit Care 2007;13:405–10.
47. Kwan P, Gomez M, Cartotto R. Safe and successful restriction of transfusion in burn patients. J Burn Care Res 2006;27:826–34.
48. Criswell KK, Gamelli RL. Establishing transfusion needs in burn patients. Am J Surg 2005;189:324–6.
49. Hart D, Wolf S, Beauford R, Lai S, Chinkes D. Determinants of blood loss during primary burn excision. Surgery 2001;130:396–402.
50. Cartotto R, Musgrave MA, Beveridge M, Fish J, Gomez M. Minimizing blood loss in burn surgery. J Trauma 2000;49:1034–9.
51. Gomez M, Logsetty S, Fish JS. Reduced blood loss during burn surgery. J Bum Care Rehabil 2001;22: 111–17.
52. O'Mara MS, Hayetian F, Slater H, Goldfarb IW, Tolchin E, Caushaj PF. Results of a protocol of transfusion threshold and surgical technique on transfusion requirements in burn patients. Burns 2005; 31:558–61.
53. Sheridan R. Reducing blood loss in burn care. Crit Care Med 2007;35:665.
54. Jeschke MG, Herndon DN. Blood transfusion in burns: benefit or risk? Crit Care Med 2006;34:1822–3.
55. Rao SV, Jollis JG, Harrington RA, et al. Relationship of blood transfusion and clinical outcomes in patients with acute coronary syndromes. JAMA 2004; 292:1555–62.
56. Wu WC, Rathore SS, Wang Y, Radford MJ, Krumholz HM. Blood transfusion in elderly patients with acute myocardial infarction. N Engl J Med 2001;345:1230–36.
57. Sabatine MS, Morrow DA, Giugliano RP, et al. Association of hemoglobin levels with clinical outcomes in acute coronary syndromes. Circulation 2005;111: 2042–9.
58. Drueke TB, Eckardt KU, Frei U, et al. Does early anemia correction prevent complications of chronic renal failure? Clin Nephrol 1999;51:1–11.
59. McCullough PA, Lepor ME. The deadly triangle of anemia, renal insufficiency, and cardiovascular disease: implications for prognosis and treatment. Rev Cardiovasc Med 2005;6:1–10.
60. NKF/KDOQI. National Kidney Foundation. II. Clinical practice guidelines and clinical practice recommendations for anemia in chronic kidney disease in adults. Am J Kidney Dis 2006;47(Suppl. 3):SI6–85.
61. Strippoli GF, Manno C, Schena FP, Craig JC. Haemoglobin and haematocrit targets for the anaemia of chronic renal disease. Cochrane Database Syst Rev 2003;CD003967.
62. Drueke TB, Locatelli F, Clyne N, et al. Normalization of hemoglobin level in patients with chronic kidney disease and anemia. N Engl J Med 2006; 355:2071–84.

63. Singh AK, Szczech L, Tang KL, et al. Correction of anemia with epoetin alfa in chronic kidney disease. N Engl J Med 2006;355:2085–98.
64. Knight K, Wade S, Balducci L. Prevalence and outcomes of anemia in cancer: a systematic review of the literature. Am J Med 2004;116(Suppl. 7A):11S-26S.
65. Gleeson C, Spencer D. Blood transfusion and its benefits in palliative care. Palliat Med 1995;9:307–13.
66. Brown E, Bennett M. Survey of blood transfusion practice for palliative care patients in Yorkshire: implications for clinical care. J Palliat Med 2007;10: 919–22.
67. Monti M, Castellani L, Berlusconi A, Cunietti E. Use of red blood cell transfusions in terminally ill cancer patients admitted to a palliative care unit. J Pain Symptom Manage 1996;12:18–22.
68. Ripamonti C. Management of dyspnea in advanced cancer patients. Support Care Cancer 1999; 7:233–43.
69. Pohl GM, Ludwig H. Supportive treatment for anemic cancer patients. Wien Med Wochenschr 2004; 154:226–34.
70. Davies SC, Oni L. Management of patients with sickle cell disease. BMJ 1997;315:656–60.
71. Johnson CS. Arterial blood pressure and hyperviscosity in sickle cell disease. Hematol Oncol Clin North Am 2005;19:827–37.
72. Fung EB, Harmatz P, Milet M, et al. Morbidity and mortality in chronically transfused subjects with thalassemia and sickle cell disease: a report from the multi-center study of iron overload. Am J Hematol 2007;82:255–65.
73. Taher A. Iron overload in thalassemia and sickle cell disease. Semin Hematol 2005;42(Suppl. 1):S5–9.
74. Darbari DS, Kple-Faget P, Kwagyan J, Rana S, Gordeuk VR, Castro O. Circumstances of death in adult sickle cell disease patients. Am J Hematol 2006; 81:858–63.
75. Swerdlow PS. Red cell exchange in sickle cell disease. Hematology Am Soc Hematol Educ Program 2006; 48–53.
76. Riddington C, Wang W. Blood transfusion for preventing stroke in people with sickle cell disease. Cochrane Database Syst Rev 2002;CD003146.
77. Switzer JA, Hess DC, Nichols FT, Adams RJ. Pathophysiology and treatment of stroke in sickle-cell disease: present and future. Lancet Neural 2006; 5:501–12.
78. Okpala I. The management of crisis in sickle cell disease. Eur J Haematol 1998;60:1–6.
79. Koduri PR, Nathan S. Acute splenic sequestration crisis in adults with hemoglobin S-C disease: a report of nine cases. Ann Hematol 2006;85:239–43.
80. Claster S, Vichinsky EP. Managing sickle cell disease. BMJ 2003;327:1151–5.
81. Debaun MR, Field JJ. Limitations of clinical trials in sickle cell disease: a case study of the multi-center study of hydroxyurea (MSH) trial and the stroke prevention (STOP) trial. Hematology Am Soc Hematol Educ Program 2007;482–8.
82. Kirkham FJ, Lerner NB, Noetzel M, et al. Trials in sickle cell disease. Pediatr Neural 2006;34:450–8.
83. Adams RJ, McKie VC, Brambilla D, et al. Stroke prevention trial in sickle cell anemia. Control Clin Trials 1998;19:110–29.
84. Howard RJ. Management of sickling conditions in pregnancy. Br J Hasp Med 1996;56:7–10.
85. Khurshid I, Anderson L, Downie GH, Pape GS. Sickle cell disease, extreme hyperbilirubinemia, and pericardial tamponade: case report and review of the literature. Crit Care Med 2002;30:2363–7.
86. Hassell KL, Eckman JR, Lane PA. Acute multiorgan failure syndrome: a potentially catastrophic complication of severe sickle cell pain episodes. Am J Med 1994;96:155–62.
87. Audard V, Grimbert P, Kirsch M, et al. Successful combined heart and kidney transplantation in a patient with sickle-cell anemia. J Heart Lung Transplant 2006;25:993–6.
88. Vichinsky EP, Haberkern CM, Neumayr L, et al. A comparison of conservative and aggressive transfusion regimens in the perioperative management of sickle cell disease. The Preoperative Transfusion in Sickle Cell Disease Study Group. N Engl J Med 1995;333:206–13.
89. Haberkern CM, Neumayr LD, Orringer EP, et al. Cholecystectomy in sickle cell anemia patients: perioperative outcome of 364 cases from the National Preoperative Transfusion Study. Preoperative Transfusion in Sickle Cell Disease Study Group. Blood 1997;89:1533–42.
90. Firth PG, Head CA. Sickle cell disease and anesthesia. Anesthesiology 2004;101:766–85.
91. Neumayr L, Koshy M, Haberkern C, et al. Surgery in patients with hemoglobin SC disease. Preoperative Transfusion in Sickle Cell Disease Study Group. Am J Hematol 1998;57:101–8.
92. Riddington C, Williamson L. Preoperative blood transfusions for sickle cell disease. Cochrane Database Syst Rev 2001;CD003149.

93. Koshy M. Sickle cell disease and pregnancy. Blood Rev 1995;9:157–64.
94. Josephson CD, Su LL, Hillyer KL, Hillyer CD. Transfusion in the patient with sickle cell disease: a critical review of the literature and transfusion guidelines. Transfus Med Rev 2007;21:118–33.
95. Ballas SK. Management of sickle pain. Curr Opin Hematol 1997;4:104–11.
96. Griffith KS, Lewis LS, Mali S, Parise ME. Treatment of malaria in the United States: a systematic review. JAMA 2007;297:2264–77.
97. Powell VI, Grima K. Exchange transfusion for malaria and Babesia infection. Transfus Med Rev 2002;16:239–50.
98. Mehta SR, Das S. Management of malaria: recent trends. J Commun Dis 2006;38:130–38.
99. Riddle MS, Jackson JL, Sanders JW, Blazes DL. Exchange transfusion as an adjunct therapy in severe Plasmodium falciparum malaria: a meta-analysis. Clin Infect Dis 2002;34:1192–8.
100. Carson JL, Terrin ML, Jay M. Anemia and postoperative rehabilitation. Can J Anaesth 2003;50(6 Suppl.):S60–64.
101. Wallis JP, Wells AW, Whitehead S, Brewster N. Recovery from postoperative anaemia. Transfus Med 2005;15:413–18.
102. Lawrence VA, Silverstein JH, Cornell JE, Pederson T, Noveck H, Carson JL. Higher Hb level is associated with better early functional recovery after hip fracture repair. Transfusion 2003;43:1717–22.

PART 3
Volume Replacement

SECTION 1
Plasma and Albumin

CHAPTER 8
Plasma and Albumin

Philippe L. Baele
Department of Anesthesiology, Cliniques Universitaires Saint-Luc, Brussels, Belgium

Plasma

The composition of plasma reflects that of the extravascular extracellular space, the "milieu intérieur" of Claude Bernard, with some important differences. Indeed it also contains hormones, nutrients, and end products of metabolism transiting through the circulation; it contains clotting factors, components of the inflammatory and fibrinolytic pathways in various stages of activation, and immunoglobulins; the oncotic pressure generated by its soluble proteins—mainly albumin—plays a major role in the conservation of intravascular volume, allowing for adequate circulation. Extracellular viruses, bacteria, or parasites, and other infectious agents are conveyed through the bloodstream and can therefore be found in plasma, as can be toxins, drugs, chemicals, and environmental contaminants. Thus, the fluid bathing erythrocytes is by no means an inert medium and transfusing plasma has much more profound implications than perfusing a "physiologically balanced solution" to restore volemia.

Source

Human plasma has been obtained from various sources and is prepared in many ways [1]. The standard today is to obtain plasma from well-identified, medically examined, screened, and followed voluntary, unpaid donors, although the importance of the latter characteristic is still a matter of debate between nonprofit organizations and industrial companies involved in the field. Plasma can be centrifuged from whole blood donations or can be obtained by plasmapheresis. Apheresis yields larger volumes per donation and allows for more frequent donations, which favors the selection of a pool of stable regular donors. Collecting blood from placentas is still a matter of controversy [2]. In the past, plasma used for fractionation has also been collected from paid donors in developing countries, in prisons, or in impoverished areas of developed countries, all unacceptable practices by today's standards.

Alternatives to Blood Transfusion in Transfusion Medicine, 2nd edition. Edited by A. Maniatis, P. Van der Linden, J.-F. Hardy.

Testing

Every plasma unit must be tested for HIV, HBV (HBsAg, anti-Hbc antibodies), HCV, syphilis, and HTLV (where requested). Hepatic enzymes activities must be within normal limits in countries where this test is requested. All these tests must be carried out on individual donations. For pooled products, a second series of tests must be performed after pooling, and finally most countries request PCR testing for HCV on the final product.

Viro-inactivation

The AIDS epidemic prompted most countries to adopt viro-inactivation methods in the process of preparing plasma and derived products. It taught how pooled blood products could multiply the spread of an emerging, and yet undetectable, infectious agent, and how a single infected donation could possibly result in the contamination of all unitary doses made from an affected pool. It disclosed how vulnerable the transfusion system really is: no testing program will ever foresee emerging viruses or new forms of infectious agents. It also taught how the infectious risk concentrates on patients chronically depending on pooled products for their survival, such as hemophiliacs.

Two fundamentally different strategies have been developed to reduce the infectious risk of some blood products: single-unit versus pooled-unit viro-inactivation [3].

Pooled procedures are industrial processes applied to batches of thousand donations, involving several filtration, extraction, and viro-inactivating steps, resulting in highly standardized, purified, and predictable products. Dilution from pooling also considerably reduces those risks that are quantitatively related to the dose of some undesirable components such as drugs or specific anti-HLA immunoglobulins. All units produced from the same batch are identical. The potential danger of pooling comes from qualitative agents for which even the minutest dose carries the full risk, such as viruses. For such agents pooling initially multiplies the risk by the number of donations entering a batch, to eventually reduce it to zero during processing. As concerns these risks, the quality of the end product can only be as good as the efficiency of viro-inactivating methods.

By contrast, single-unit viro-inactivation applies to individual donations and obviates the need for pooling and industrial facilities. Another advantage is the simplicity of the process, which usually relies on adding small amounts of a photosensitizer to a leukofiltered plasma unit before exposing it to high intensity light of a wavelength chosen to optimally activate the photosensitizer. Initial variability among units is unaffected by the process: no two units are the same. Some sources of variation are systematic: group O donors have lower concentrations (0.75 IU/mL) of Factor VIII, for example Reference [1]. Other characteristics are specific to individuals, like the presence of specific immunoglobulins resulting from pregnancies or previous transfusions. Efficacy and side effects are therefore less predictable than with pooled products. On the contrary, if an (new) infectious agent escapes viro-inactivation, it will only affect the few units drawn from contaminated donors.

Currently, it can be said that advantages and disadvantages of both strategies balance out [3]. Both systems yield high-quality safe and effective products. As a reminder, plasma contains no cellular components; therefore, intracellular viruses (e.g., cytomegalovirus or CMV) or parasites (e.g., malaria) are not transmitted by fresh frozen plasma (FFP).

Single-unit viro-inactivation

Since 1992, minute amounts of the phenothiazine dye methylene blue (<100 μg) have been added to millions of units of FFP in Germany and Switzerland, and more recently in Spain and in the United Kingdom methylene blue has a high affinity for guanine in nucleic acids, but can also link to various proteins, including some viral core proteins. Activation by visible light yields highly reactive singlet oxygen, which will locally oxidate and inactivate nucleic acids or denaturate proteins. It influences minimally coagulation factors activity [4]. Most enveloped and many nonenveloped viruses are inactivated by methylene blue, but some are not. HIV-1 and -2, HBV, HCV, HSV, CMV, and many others are inactivated. Hepatitis A is not, and probably neither is Parvovirus B19 [3, 5]. Methylene blue has been used for decades in other fields of medicine in dosages hundred to several thousand times higher than the quantity contained in a 200 mL unit of FFP [6]. Side effects from this molecule should, therefore, not be a concern at least for adult recipients. Experience with neonates is still limited. One newborn has been reported with a photosensitivity reaction during phototherapy [7].

Psoralenes are another class of photosensitizers activated by UV light. They link strongly to nonadjacent DNA or RNA bases, preventing further replication of the involved segment. Their advantage is an easy penetration through cellular and nucleic membranes. They can thus be active in a dose-dependent way against all forms of life relying on nucleic acids to function and perpetuate. This includes viruses, bacteria, protozoa, but also leukocytes and intracellular forms of infectious agents. Future applications under investigation include inactivation of infectious agents and leukocytes in platelet or even red cell concentrates [8]. In the seventies, psoralens used in conjunction with UV therapy to treat psoriasis have been held responsible for provoking skin cancers. Psoralens are potentially mutagenic and oncogenic molecules. It is still unclear whether this should be a concern for the type and doses of psoralens proposed to viro-inactivate blood products. Their use in transfusion medicine is still experimental.

Viro-inactivation of pooled units

Plasma has been viro-inactivated with solvent and detergent since the mid-nineties, most often with tri(*n*-butyl)-phosphate and Tween 80. Tween must be from vegetal origin or certified from BSE-free bovine origin. Solvents and detergents effectively dissolve lipids and lipid membranes while minimally affecting proteins such as coagulation factors. Lipid-enveloped viruses like HBV, HCV, HIV, and HTLV are destroyed by solvents and detergents. By contrast, some small protein-encapsulated viruses remain unharmed, e.g., hepatitis A virus or Parovirus B19. Antibodies directed against HAV and present in the infected donor's plasma provide partial passive protection against the virus.

Quarantine

Plasma intended for fractionation is deep-frozen and stored for 50–120 days (depending on country and end product) before processing. This increases the chances to detect and exclude a donor in the early incubation phase of a viral illness, i.e., in its seronegative "window" period. Due to relative shortages of plasma the quarantine period for FFP distributed as such is shorter in most countries.

Fractionation

Many components of human plasma can be extracted from pools of up to 10,000 donations and prepared in concentrated, stable (mostly freeze-dried), purified, and viro-inactivated forms (see Table 8.1). Some can also be produced by genetic engineering. Whenever possible specific concentrated factors should be used to treat well-identified coagulation deficits.

Conservation

In order to prevent the alteration of coagulation factors, plasma must be frozen to −30°C within 6 hours of collection. The eutectic point of plasma is −23°C. Once cooling has started, complete freezing

Table 8.1 Available plasma fractions.

Albumin solutions
Stable plasma protein solutions
Cryoprecipitate, contains fibrinogen, factor VIIIc, von Willebrand factor, factor XIII, and fibronectin
Fibrinogen
Factor VI
Factor VII
von Willebrand Factor
Factor XI
Human prothrombin complex, contains concentrated vitamin K-dependent factors: factor II, factor VII, factor X, factor IX, protein C, + various proteins and heparin (5 μ/mL after reconstitution)
Antithrombin III
Protein C
Protein S
Fraction C1 of compliment esterase inhibitor
Immunoglobulins

- Polyvalent preparations (i.m. or i.v.)
- specific
  Anti-Rh(D)
  Anti-HBs, anti-herpes zoster, anti-CMV, anti-rubella, anti-tetanic, anti-pertussis, anti-rabies, etc.

Surgical glues

Table 8.2 European Council Specifications for FFP [9].

Volume	Specified within 10%	Standard = 200 mL + anticoagulant
Blood group*	ABO, Rh(D)	
Irregular erythrocyte antibodies	None	
Residual cells	Erythrocytes	$<0.6 \times 10^9$ per liter (about 0.05% vol)
	Leukocytes	$<0.1 \times 10^9$ per liter
	Platelets	$<50 \times 10^9$ per liter
Packing	No leaks	
Visual inspection	No abnormal color	
	No precipitates, no clot formation	
Viral tests (ELISA)*	HIV, HBV, HCV, HTLV	
Bacteriology	Sterility, negative tests for syphilis*	
Pyrogens	None	
Enzymes	Normal ALAT activity*	

*Tested on individual donations, before pooling.

to −30°C must be obtained rapidly to avoid factor VIII degradation by excessive concentration of salts: ideally the process must take less than 60 minutes and a maximum of 4 hours [1]. Plasma can be kept for 2 years at −30°C, for 6 months between −25 and −30°C, and for 3 months between −18 and −25°C. Such temperatures totally prevent bacterial replication. Deep-freezers containing derivates from human blood must be subjected to specific controls.

Product specifications

Table 8.2 details the Council of Europe standards for plasma prepared for transfusion [9] and Table 8.3 lists the expected concentrations of FFP constituents [10]. FFP from any source should contain near-normal concentrations of original plasma constituents; a slight dilution (1:4 for single donor plasma, 1:6 for pooled plasma) results from the presence of an anticoagulant, usually Citrate Phosphate Dextrose Adenine. Rapid transfusion of large volumes of FFP may therefore result in citrate toxicity requiring calcium administration. Albumin, fibrinogen, coagulation factors, and other plasma proteins are found in near-normal concentrations in FFP. This includes all kinds of immunoglobulins including antibodies directed against erythrocytes, occasionally against the recipient's. Some patients (with anti-IgA antibodies) may develop an anaphylactic reaction against any blood product containing normal IgA, including FFP.

Cryosupernatant plasma, i.e., plasma left after removal of cryoprecipitate has been in use in some countries. It has near-normal contents in albumin, immunoglobulins, and coagulation factors except for factor V and VIIIc, which are significantly decreased and for fibrinogen, which is almost entirely removed. The sole indication for this product is Thrombotic Thrombocytopenic Purpura [10].

Table 8.3 Expected concentrations of FFP constituents.

Factor VIIIc		>0.7	I U/mL
Fibrinogen		1.5–4	mg/mL
Other coagulation factors		>0.5	I U/mL
Total proteins		40–60	g/L
Osmolality		320–420	Mosmol/ kg
Electrolytes	Na^+	≤200	mEq/L
	K^+	≤5	mEq/L
	Ca^{+2}	≤5	mEq/L
	H^+	27–100	nEq/L
	pH	7.0–7.6	pH units
Citrate		15–25	mmol/L
Lactate		<5	mmol/L
Phosphate		3.5–7.5	mmol/L
Triton X-100		<5	μg/mL
Tri-(*n*-butyl)-phosphate		<2	μg/mL
Glycin		4–6	g/L
apt		30–45	Seconds

Adapted from United Kingdom Health Departments [10].

Labeling

Plasma is legally considered as a "labile" blood product; as such it is distributed by the blood bank, not the hospital pharmacy. Its label must contain the following information: name of product, its origin (whole blood vs apheresis), volume, anticoagulant, identification number of the donation or batch, ABO group, Rh(D) group (positive or negative), name, and address of the manufacturer, and whether the unit has been quarantined and viro-inactivated (and how). Labels may not mention donor's identity, except for autologous donations. Further information must be printed either on the label of the unit or on its outer packing: date of freezing, expiry date, temperature of storage, and instructions for storage, thawing, and administration.

Transfusion

Before transfusion, FFP must be thawed in a 37°C water bath or in specially designed microwave ovens. Exposure to higher temperatures can lead to protein denaturation with ensuing loss of transfusion efficiency or aspecific transfusion reactions. Every unit must be visually inspected after thawing; a unit in which insoluble matter can be seen may not be transfused. Once thawed plasma may not be refrozen for later use, but must be transfused within 2 hours to prevent decrease of coagulation factors concentrations, as well as bacteriological growth. Transfusion must occur through a 170–200 μm filter and its rate should be adapted to recipient's hemodynamic tolerance.

Pretransfusion check, traceability, and hemovigilance

Good clinical practice includes verifying every unit before connecting it to the patient's perfusion line, documenting every transfusion in the patient's file, and ensuring traceability for all transfused products. For FFP, documentation should include: identification of the patient, registration number of the donation or batch, patient's blood group, blood group of the unit, expiration date of the unit, hour and date of transfusion, type of blood product and quantity, reason for transfusing FFP (with laboratory results if relevant), name of prescribing physician, and name of the person executing the order. No proof of compatibility is required. Correct documentation of follow-up includes a mention in the patient's file of the occurrence or absence of any side effect, and a clinical or biological assessment of the transfusion efficacy. Side effects must be reported to the blood bank and this information included in hemovigilance data banks.

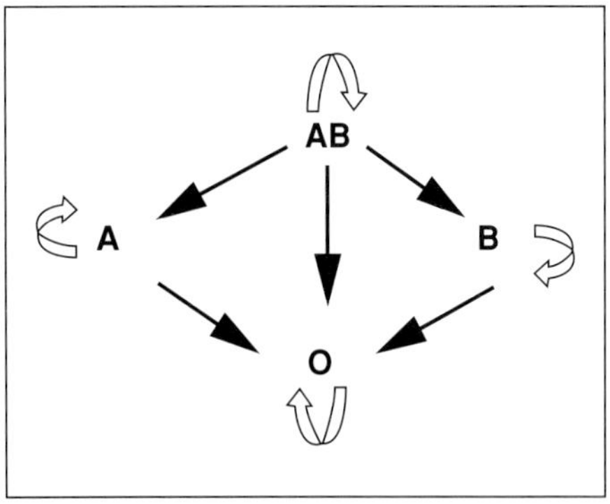

Figure 8.1 ABO transfusion rules for plasma.

Compatibility

Plasma contains antibodies against erythrocyte antigens. Concerning the ABO system, plasma compatibility transfusion rules must be followed to avoid hemolysis (Figure 8.1). Group O plasma is susceptible to contain antibodies against both A and B antigens, and can only be given to group O recipients. Conversely, group AB plasma cannot contain anti-A nor anti-B antibodies and can theoretically be used for recipients of any blood group. Unfortunately, AB donors only constitute 3% of the European population, which mandates to restrict the use of AB plasma for AB recipients, for the rare emergencies with unknown blood group, or for special indications such as neonatal exsanguino-transfusions.

Rh(D) compatibility is usually not requested. Rh(D) group is not always mentioned on pooled viro-inactivated plasma units because of the absence of residual erythrocytes. However, to avoid alloimmunization, it is advisable to transfuse only Rh(D) isogroup plasma to young females receiving single-donor units, since erythrocytes are not always filtered out during their preparation.

No compatibility tests are performed before transfusing plasma. Donors with the most frequent irregular antibodies are excluded. However, FFP may contain significant titers of antibodies unscreened for by standard testing panels: more or less severe immune reactions and hemolysis may ensue when large quantities of plasma are transfused in a short period of time [11, 12].

Passive transfusion of lymphocytotoxic, HLA, or granulocyte specific antibodies triggering complement activation and neutrophil sequestration in the lung microvasculature is evoked as a possible mechanism for transfusion-related acute lung injury (TRALI) [13–15]. This rare but severe complication has been associated with all plasma-containing products, including red cell concentrates and platelets [13–19]. Other authors have proposed that lipids from stored plasma might play a role [20]. It is unclear from published reports whether pooled viro-inactivated plasma has ever been implicated [18]; if not, the important dilution effect from pooling and the removal of lipids by detergents could both have a protective effect. TRALI presents initially like an adult respiratory distress syndrome, i.e., with low hydrostatic pressure pulmonary edema, but most patients recover without sequellae after a few days of adequate respiratory support; mortality is between 5 and 10%.

Acute and severe thrombocytopenia has also been reported within a few hours after transfusing single-donor FFP, due to passive transfer of antiplatelet antibody [21].

Table 8.4 Adverse effects of FFP transfusions.

- Anaphylactic or anaphylactoid reactions
- Hemolytic immunological reactions:
  - ☐ ABO incompatibility
  - ☐ Other anti-erythrocyte antibodies
- Nonhemolytic immunological reactions:
  - ☐ Fever, chills, and urticaria
  - ☐ Transfusion-related thrombocytopenia
  - ☐ Transfusion-related acute lung injury (TRALI)
  - ☐ Allo-immunization against residual erythrocytes
- Circulatory overload
- Bacterial contamination and septic shock
- Residual viral risk:
  - ☐ After viro-inactivation: hepatitis A and parovirus B19
  - ☐ Without viro-inactivation: same as whole blood or red cells
- Unknowns: transmission of prion diseases?

Indications for transfusing FFP

Coagulation disorders

Coagulation disorders become rarely obvious clinically until the concentration of a given factor has decreased substantially, usually below 30% of normal [22–26]. Therefore the effective initial dosage of FFP to correct coagulation disorders must be important: at least 10–15 mL/kg. By definition 1 mL of FFP contains about one unit of coagulation factor activity. Further dosage will depend on the expected ongoing losses (from the surgical field, for example) and on the half-life of the most depleted factor (Table 8.4).

It is now generally admitted that coagulation disorders only need correction if they result in clinical bleeding [27, 28]. FFP is sometimes prescribed in situations where bleeding is anticipated or could entail special risks, for example in patients with one or more depleted coagulation factors about to undergo a surgical or an invasive procedure such as central vein catheterization, liver biopsy, or thoracocentesis. The value of such prophylactic administration of FFP is controversial [29]. Limited clinical series, some of them retrospective, failed to support the use of FFP in such indications [30, 31]. However, prudence is required to correct coagulation abnormalities when performing invasive procedures.

Whenever possible, concentrated factors specific to the patient's needs should be used rather than FFP, which should only be used when specific factors are unavailable. Preparations of vitamin K-dependent factors, also called "Human Prothrombin Complex" (Prothrombin factor II, Proconvertin factor VII, Stuart factor X, and antihemophilic B factor IX) should be used preferentially to counteract *antivitamin K anticoagulants coumadin and warfarin* when urgent reversal is needed. Similarly, the von Willebrand moiety of factor VIII exists in purified preparations or can be expressed by platelets or endothelial cells after i.v. infusion of DDAVP, a vasopressin derivate devoid of

Table 8.5 Average half-lives of coagulation factors.

Factor	I	Fibrinogen	3–5 days
	II	Prothrombin	3–5 days
	V	Proaccelerin	15–24 hours
	VII	Proconvertin	4–6 hours
	VIII	Antihemophilic A factor	12–18 hours
	IX	Antihemophilic B factor	13–20 hours
	X	Stuart	48–72 hours
	XI	Thromboplastin antecedent	48–84 hours
	XII	Hageman	60 hours
	XIII	Fibrin stabilization factor	4 days
Antithrombin III			3 days

vasoconstrictive properties. The latter is a suitable first line therapy for patients with some form of mild to moderate congenital or acquired von Willebrand factor or factor VIII deficiency undergoing minor surgery. Advise of a coagulation specialist is required because DDAVP may be contra-indicated in other forms of these diseases [32] (Table 8.5).

Pediatrics

Newborns, especially prematures, have low concentrations of coagulation factors. Although, this should pose no direct clinical threat, any further hemodilution could bring these concentrations to dangerously low levels. Furthermore, albumin plays a critical role in the neonatal period due to its capacity to transport nonconjugated (toxic) bilirubin. For all these reasons, FFP is a commonly accepted therapy for volume replacement in neonatal care, especially for preterm babies [33]. However, its systematic use to treat hypovolemia in newborns, even preterm babies, has been challenged recently on the basis of a large randomized trial involving 776 babies from 21 hospitals, which compared on-demand therapy versus systematic aggressive volume loading with either FFP or gelatin. The end point was survival without major neurological deficit at 2 years; there were no differences between the three therapeutic regimens [34]. Another randomized controlled trial showed that crystalloids could be equally effective as colloids in treating hypotension in preterm babies [35]. In infants and children with meningococcal septicemia, 4.5% human albumin solution has been used in doses as large as 300 mL/kg within the first 12 hours and resulted in low mortalities [36]. As a consequence, routine use of FFP in the absence of coagulopathy is now discouraged in pediatrics [37].

Massive hemorrhage and dilution coagulopathy

Compensation of massive hemorrhage by transfusions of red cell concentrates eventually leads to multicomponent deficiency of hemostatic factors [22–24, 38]. Dilution and shock both play a role in the genesis of the resulting coagulopathy. Studies on massive transfusions have often been conducted with red cell concentrates, stored on CPD or ACD anticoagulants, and underlined the dangers of citrate toxicity. However, residual amounts of plasma in those preparations delay the advent of coagulation factor deficiencies. When using red cell concentrates resuspended in Sorbitol Adenine Glucose Mannitol solutions clinically significant coagulation factor deficiencies, especially fibrinogen, occur earlier and require treatment [39]. Studies on massive transfusions have repeatedly emphasized that there is no need to transfuse prophylactically FFP or platelets before clinical evidence of abnormal bleeding develops, which may not occur before replacement of one to two circulating blood volumes [10, 40]. Abnormal coagulation tests are effective in detecting situations where plasma is needed. However, these tests take time, as do thawing and transfusing FFP Transfusing FFP while waiting for laboratory results is therefore a reasonable attitude when confronted to microvascular bleeding during massive transfusion [27]: laboratory evidence will then help redirecting therapy if needed.

Dilution of coagulation factors during cardiopulmonary bypass does not justify replacement therapy in most instances [41]. Priming oxygenator and circuits with plasma has been abandoned without evidence of harm [42]. Consumption of platelets and coagulation factors does occur during bypass, but rarely results in clinical bleeding before numerous hours of bypass, and is encountered mostly during prolonged circulatory or respiratory assistance with Extra Corporeal Membrane Oxygenation.

Systematic FFP transfusions at the end of prolonged surgery is unwarranted in the absence of clinical bleeding and alteration of laboratory coagulation tests.

Other coagulopathies

Severe liver disease results in combined factor I, II, V, VII, VIII, IX, X, XIII, AT III, and plasminogen deficiencies. Transfusion of FFP is often required when these patients bleed clinically or must undergo surgical or invasive procedures.

In acute diffuse intravascular coagulopathy (DIC), therapy with FFP and platelets can only play a palliative role. Treating and reversing the cause of DIC is of paramount importance.

Under normal circumstances antithrombin III (AT III) deficiency can remain a silent feature. It prevents heparin-induced anticoagulation and can therefore be an unexpected intraoperative finding at the start of cardiac surgery, when activated clotting time fails to increase after repeated heparin doses. Under those circumstances, readily available FFP may be an acceptable substitute to AT III concentrates to restore heparin sensitivity and allow the start of extracorporeal circulation with minimal delay. AT III deficiency can also be acquired in critically ill patients. Normalizing its levels is possible by using high doses of AT III concentrates, but the effect of this therapy on survival is controversial [43].

Protein C and protein S preparations exist as do C1 esterase inhibitor concentrates, obviating the need to transfuse FFP for patients with such deficiencies.

Immunotherapy

Preparations of specific or aspecific immunoglobulins exist. FFP should therefore not be used to treat acquired or inherited immunodeficiencies.

Thrombotic thrombocytopenic purpura (TTP) remains an undisputed indication for FFP, preferentially during a plasma exchange program [44, 45]. It is advised to start plasma exchanges as soon as possible, once the diagnosis of TTP is established. Doses of 20 up to 60 mL/kg FFP during daily plasma exchanges have been proposed, to be continued 4–6 days after hemolysis and thrombopenia have disappeared. The highest doses will be required by patients suffering from nonfamilial TTP with high titers of inhibitor of von Willebrand factor cleaving protease [44]. Children affected by the milder type of thrombotic microangiopathy called hemolytic uremic syndrome usually respond to anti-infectious agents, FFP transfusions and supportive measures, but rarely need plasma exchanges.

Frequent misuses of plasma

Plasma is still too frequently prescribed for indications which rest on no scientific or clinical evidence [46–48]. The following are not indications to transfuse plasma. Plasma transfusion does not promote wound healing. Plasma should not be used as a volume expander, nor a nutritional source. Plasma should not be used to reconstitute whole blood when red cell concentrates are transfused. Plasma should not be used prophylactically or systematically because of the type of surgery or because of its duration.

Consensus conferences and guidelines for clinical practice

Guidelines about plasma transfusion have been published as early as 1985 [49], in response to evidence of widespread misuse of FFP [47]. Several other guidelines followed. A recent review of consensus conferences has been published by the Canadian Medical Association in 1997 [50, 51]. It refers to 17 guidelines and 42 review articles. Among the Guidelines, four focused on plasma and

Table 8.6 Indications and nonindications for FFP.

Definite indications for the use of FFP
1 □ Replacement of single coagulation factor deficiencies, where a specific or combined factor concentrate is unavailable.
2 □ Immediate reversal of warfarin effect.
3 □ Acute disseminated, intravascular coagulation (DIC).
Conditional uses: FFP only indicated in the presence of bleeding and disturbed coagulation
1 □ Massive transfusion.
2 □ Liver disease.
3 □ Cardiopulmonary bypass surgery.
4 □ Special pediatric indications.
No justification for the use of FFP
1 □ Hypovolemia.
2 □ Plasma exchange procedures.
3 □ "Formula" replacement to reconstitute whole blood with red cell concentrates.
4 □ Nutritional support.
5 □ Treatment of immunodeficiency states.

Adapted from Consensus Guidelines of the British Committee for Standards in Haematology [59].

eight concerned both plasma and red cell transfusions [27, 49, 52–60]. Other papers [48, 61, 62] delivered basically the same messages. Most refuted the concept of arbitrary transfusion triggers, but instead insisted on clinical judgment. For plasma transfusion, they repeatedly and invariably insisted on the need to combine a clinical assessment of bleeding and its risk, with a laboratory investigation of potential coagulation abnormalities. Most insisted also on transfusing concentrated products to correct specific deficits rather than transfusing FFP in a blind—and often less effective—way. Table 8.6 reproduces the conclusions of guidelines published in the UK in 1992, which also cite the most frequently invoked "wrong reasons" for transfusing plasma [59]. The Practice Guidelines, published in 1996 by the American Society of Anesthesiologists, differ from previous texts in their rating of the evidence on which is based every recommendation [28]. The authors emphasize how little of our transfusion practice has ever been build on randomized or even nonrandomized properly controlled trials.

Epidemiological surveys

Long after publication of the first guidelines, and despite the availability of fractionated products, plasma remained widely used, especially in surgery or intensive care. Various reasons may explain this: isolated deficits of one plasma fraction are rare in those settings, hypovolemia often accompanies coagulation deficits during hemorrhagic episodes, time is lacking to perform laboratory tests, fractionated products may be more expensive and more difficult to obtain than FFP in some hospitals. Despite the well-known capacity for plasma to convey pathogens, its use extended far beyond the accepted indications even before viro-inactivated FFP became available. Considerable variations could be demonstrated between centers for the same procedures, or even within the same hospital between teams performing procedures of similar importance.

A recent (1998) North-American multicentric survey [63] found large variations in the use of FFP in coronary surgery, ranging from 0 to 36% of operated patients, despite the existence of national guidelines specific to the field of cardiac revascularization surgery [54]. Similar findings had been made for orthopedic surgery [64].

The European Sanguis Study (1990–1991) [65, 66] revealed that 84% of patients receiving FFP had no laboratory test performed to assess coagulation on the day of plasma transfusion, that only 12% of recipients had evidence of abnormal coagulation, and that the average quantity of administered plasma was low, between 2 and 4 units depending on the type of surgery. In some places, plasma was still used in liquid form and given systematically for open-heart surgery. In other places, plasma was administered at the rate of one unit a day for up to five postoperative days after hemicolectomy [67]. These results strongly suggest that plasma was most often given for wrong indications: to restore volemia, to "reconstitute whole blood" during transfusion of red cell concentrates, or for nutritional purposes. Furthermore, it could be shown that teams transfusing much plasma also gave much human albumin and/or artificial colloids, probably reflecting their preference for active volemic expansion strategies over pharmacological alternatives, when facing clinical situations involving vasoplegia or third-sector formation. Six years after large diffusion of these results, a similar study conducted in Belgium [68] revealed a dramatic decrease in the proportion of operated patients receiving plasma, from 15.3 to 2.7% of operated patients. Plasma transfusions without coagulation tests virtually disappeared, decreasing from 36 to 1.3% of patients receiving FFP. Such reductions in FFP use have been reported elsewhere [69–72]. However, quantitative reductions do not necessarily mean improved practice. Indeed, in the Belgian study correlation between indications and objective needs remained very poor [68]. Only one out of seven patients with documented PTT values inferior to 15% of normal received a plasma transfusion, whereas 69 out of 79 patients who received plasma, had their lowest documented PTT value above 60% of normal. Finally autotransfusion was found to strongly influence the way plasma is prescribed: 45 out of 127 patients (35.4%) having predeposited autologous red cells and plasma, were transfused with their plasma, in contrast to 35 patients receiving allogeneic plasma among 1321 (2.6%) who also received allogeneic red cells.

Conclusions

Misuse and overuse of plasma have been prevalent in the field of surgery. Despite efforts to curb unwarranted use over the last 10 years, plasma is still seldom prescribed in its first indication, i.e., correction of coagulation deficiencies in situations where specific factor therapy is unsuitable or unavailable [73]. Furthermore, it cannot be excluded from existing surveys that patients who would benefit from plasma transfusions might not get it by lack of knowledge or surveillance. Finally, autotransfusion can introduce a strong bias in the way FFP is prescribed.

Teaching the indications of plasma transfusion should be part of basic specialty training in all specialties dealing with surgical procedures, intensive care, hematology, or transfusion in general (see Table 8.6).

Albumin

Physiology

Albumin is a hydrophilic protein with a molecular weight of 69,000 Da. The total body albumin content is about 4–5 g/kg. One third circulates in the intravascular space, and two thirds are located in the extravascular compartment. Half of the extravascular albumin is concentrated close to the skin, which explains the rapid and dramatic protein losses encountered after burns. Albumin is exchanged between intra- and extravascular compartments at a rate of about 5% per hour. This means that 90% of the extravascular pool can return to the circulation in 1 day, and also that 10% of infused albumin leaves the circulation within 2–3 hours [74]. Under normal circumstances albumin is the most abundant protein in the plasma and accounts for 70–80% of plasma oncotic pressure. This colloid osmotic pressure (COP) counteracts the exudation of water that would normally occur at the capillary level under the local hydrostatic pressure gradient [75]. Injury to the vascular endothelium can disrupt this equilibrium and allow albumin extravasation along its concentration gradient.

At pH = 7.40 albumin bears 17 negative charges and binds as many cations, which further increase its oncotic activity by the Donnan effect. One gram of albumin retains 15 mL of water. Albumin plays thus a major role in the water balance between intra- and extravascular fluid compartments [74].

Albumin synthesis takes place exclusively in hepatocytes and accounts for 10% of protein synthesis by the liver. Synthesis seems to respond to changes in plasma COP, but is also regulated by the nutritional status and by several hormones including insulin, glucagon, cortisol, and thyroid hormones. Cytokines liberated into the circulation following trauma or inflammation may also enhance its production. Albumin has a half-life of 2–3 weeks. It seems to be broken down primarily in the reticuloendothelial system.

Besides its oncotic power, albumin plays several other important physiological roles. Its abundance and its capacity to fix hydrogen ions make it an active buffer in the acid–base balance of blood. Capable to bind at different sites both cationic and anionic molecules, albumin transports (and neutralizes) a variety of active and sometimes toxic substances in the bloodstream, such as hormones, nonconjugated bilirubin, and many drugs. It has also been hypothesized that it may act as a free radical scavenger.

Rationale for using albumin infusions

Several pathological conditions interfering with albumin synthesis or with the glomerular capacity to retain it in the bloodstream can lead to severe hypoalbuminemia. This feature is a well-known marker of severity for many underlying conditions. It seemed therefore logical to believe that lack of albumin—and particularly circulating albumin—could be, at least, partially responsible for the poor outcome of severely hypoalbuminemic patients. The next logical step has been to try and restore lost albumin functions by albumin administration [76–78].

Manufacture and proposed clinical uses of albumin solutions

Albumin is usually extracted from human plasma through the cold alcohol fractionation technique invented by More and Harvey, Cohn, Kistler, and Nitschamnn, often referred to as the Cohn alcohol extraction method [79–82]. Coagulation factors and other enzymes are first removed by cryoprecipitation or chromatography. Contact with increasing alcohol concentrations then precipitates other proteic fractions such as immunoglobulins G, which must then be filtered out. Further phases using chromatography eliminate endotoxins, some salts and other undesirable contaminants. Aluminium and thermal stabilizers such as N-acetyl-tryptophane or sodium caprylate are added to the solution before heating, and must be removed later on. Their residual concentrations, as well as that of heme, are regulated by the U.S. and European Pharmacopoeias [83]. Albumin is then resuspended to obtain 4, 5, 20, or 25% solutions. A small proportion of molecules may differ slightly from native albumin in that some ligands may be lost in the process, and dimers or even polymeric forms can assemble.

In many countries, 5% stable plasma proteins solutions (SPPS) have been used abundantly. Such preparations contained predominantly albumin (4.5%), but also many other plasma proteins such as immunoglobulins, to which some recipients could develop anaphylactoid reactions. Release of activated kallikrein from its vector protein during the manufacturing process, has been incriminated as another cause for aspecific hypotensive episodes [84, 85]. SPPS has progressively been replaced by 4 or 5% solutions of purified albumin although some countries kept the original denomination "SPPS." The important point is that the quality of both purified albumin and SPPS have definitely improved over the last 10 years, which should be kept in mind when reviewing results of earlier trials.

The industrial process is applied to pools of up to ten thousand plasma donations, and is completed by pasteurization, i.e., 10 hours of heating at precisely 60°C, in the liquid phase; this ensures the destruction of all known viruses, bacteria or parasites. To date, there is no evidence that hepatitis A, B, or C; HIV; and HTLVI of CMV have ever been transmitted via transfusion of an albumin or SPPS solution [86]. One patient received, during a liver transplant a unit of albumin, to which a donor had contributed, who later developed Creutzfeldt Jakob disease (CJD); this recipient later developed CJD [87]. Coincidence, not causal relationship, is believed to link these two patients, because no other recipient of the same pool of albumin preparation developed CJD [88]. The way the AIDS epidemic spread via other pooled blood products such as coagulation factors, and the fear that someday new infectious agents might escape inactivation through pasteurization, have justified measures to better control the quality and origin of donations entering the plasma pools used to manufacture albumin. In December 1993, a major producer who used to manufacture albumin from placentas, rather than well-screened regular plasma donors, withdrew its product from the market. In 1998, the British government took the controversial decision to withdraw all blood products derived from plasma given by UK donors; theoretical concerns about the possible transmission of the new variant of CJD (actually the human form of Bovine Spongiform Encephalopathy) motivated this decision. The multiplying effect of pooling donations during the manufacturing processes was, again, at the heart of the debate. The decision also concerned human albumin, including its use as excipient for many vaccines.

The end products are ready-to-use sterile and pyrogen-free solutions, stable at room temperature if protected from light. Albumin represents at least 95% of their proteins. Their pH must be 7.0 ± 0.3. Sodium concentration should not exceed 160 mmol/L and potassium 0.05 mmol/ g of protein. Kallikrein and prekallikrein activator concentrations should be inferior to 15 IU/L and 20 IU/mL, respectively [9]. A 4–5% albumin solution is nearly isooncotic. More concentrated solutions are hyperoncotic; their infusion will result in fluid being drawn from the extravascular space into the circulation. Being a normal constituent of plasma, albumin is expected to be devoid of any toxic, oncogenic, mutagenic or teratogenic potential. Overdosage only comes from relative or absolute fluid overload of the circulation, and directly depends on the total dose administered and the speed of infusion. In Europe, albumin solutions are now considered medications and hence distributed by pharmacists, no longer by blood banks. Albumin solutions are labeled with a reference number, which must be reported in the patients' file at the time of transfusion to ensure traceability.

Clinical uses of albumin solutions

Albumin solutions were adopted with enthusiasm by the medical community with the hope that recipients would benefit from the many physiological roles of albumin, and because of the sense of security provided by pasteurization, and the perceived advantage of a human protein versus artificial colloids prone to provoke life-threatening allergic reactions [89–91]. In contrast to artificial colloids, albumin solutions have no maximal doses and have a sustained effect on volemia. Albumin solutions became used as the resuscitation fluids of choice and often as first-line infusions during surgery, in emergency situations, and in intensive care units. In some countries, albumin solutions led the list of in-hospital pharmaceutical expenses [92]. Profits from their sales compensated for losses endured to meet increasing testing costs for other blood products such as red cells. By the end of the 1980s, albumin solutions had turned into the driving force allowing national blood transfusion services to keep delivering high quality blood products in some countries, a role played by coagulation factors in other countries. This situation favored self-sufficiency in plasma at national and European levels, but was intrinsically unhealthy because it encouraged consumption beyond actual clinical needs, and tended to create artificial situations of unmet demand. As a result, 6- to 10-fold differences in albumin consumption could be documented between nations of the Council of Europe [93]. In most countries, the instructions accompanying albumin solutions featured a list of numerous and vaguely defined indications.

Albumin to treat hypoalbuminemia

Foley et al. [70] compared treatment with 25% human albumin in order to keep serum albumin concentrations above 25 g/L versus no treatment in 40 consecutive randomly assigned adult patients, referred to the nutrition support service in a major North American hospital. Albumin administration was effective in correcting hypoalbuminemia and maintaining serum albumin concentrations at target levels. However, no significant differences could be found in terms of mortality (7/18 treated patients vs 6/22 untreated) or major complications (16/18 treated vs 17/22 untreated). Lengths of hospital and ICU stay, and duration of artificial ventilation were shorter in the untreated group, but these differences failed to reach statistical significance. It is interesting to note that serum albumin levels rose spontaneously in the group of patients receiving no albumin, as their underlying condition improved.

The authors have been criticized for having used questionable allocation procedures (patients were randomized according to their medical record number). Nevertheless, their study has been instrumental in showing that, while hypoalbuminemia remains an ominous sign in many pathologies, correcting this symptom with albumin transfusions will not improve outcome.

Albumin to meet fluid demands in critically ill patients: the stockwell study

In this study, 475 consecutive adult patients admitted to an Intensive Care Unit were randomized to receive either a 4.5% human albumin solution or a synthetic colloid (polygelin), whenever volume replacement was considered, based on clinical status or invasive pressure measurements [78]. All patients received crystalloid solutions and enteral/parenteral nutrition to satisfy their basic fluid and nutritional requirements. Despite an older age (64 vs 60) and a slightly higher APACHE II score (14 vs 12) in the polygelin group, the mortality was exactly the same with both regimens (20%), and so was the length of ICU stay (3 days). Subpopulation analyses of patients starting with more severe clinical conditions (e.g., APACHE II >10) or staying longer than 5 days in the ICU yielded similar results. In an associated paper, the same authors focused on the influence of treatment allocation on serum albumin concentrations [94]. In the albumin group, nonsurvivors showed a tendency for serum albumin to decrease below 25 g/L. However, in the polygelin group serum albumin concentrations rapidly decreased below 22 g/L in all patients, survivors and nonsurvivors alike. These findings indicate that a low serum albumin concentration per se was not a direct cause of poor outcome, although failure to maintain near normal serum albumin concentrations despite albumin infusions heralded a poor outcome. Among patients who stayed more than 5 days in the ICU slightly more patients developed renal failure (10% vs 4%) pulmonary edema (15% vs 11%) or both (8% vs 6%) in the polygelin group, but these differences failed to reach statistical significance. Unfortunately, these issues are somewhat confounded because 4 patients in the albumin group and 13 in the polygelin group also received concentrated albumin to treat peripheral or pulmonary edema, mostly in association with dialysis. Besides confirmation of Foley's conclusions, the main value of this study for the clinician (and the manager) is its demonstration on a large scale that replacing expensive albumin solutions with polygelin solutions as first-line volume replacement in an ICU will not result in measurable changes in outcome.

Albumin to maintain COP

Grundmann and Heistermann [95] randomized 220 postoperative patients into two therapeutic strategies. One group received albumin whenever COP was lower than 29 cm H20 whereas the other group did no receive albumin until COP decreased below 24 cm H_2O; 77% of patients in the high COP group versus 65% in the low COP group required albumin. There were no differences in length of stay, recorded complications or need for artificial ventilation. Other studies have since shown the feasibility to manage patients at lower COP levels, sometimes below 15 mmHg [96].

Physiological effects of albumin and substitutes in trauma and sepsis

In 1996, Boldt et al. [97] reported on a carefully conducted study comparing over 5 days the physiological characteristics of adult patients treated for trauma or sepsis, randomized to receive either a 20% albumin solution or a 10% solution of hydroxyethyl starch (200,000 MW with a molar substitution ratio of 0.5). There were thus four groups of 15 patients each. Volemia was mainly adjusted according to pulmonary wedge pressure measurements. The most notable differences were that cardiac index, oxygen delivery index (Do21) and oxygen consumption index (Vo21) increased significantly over time in the groups treated with HES, but not in those receiving albumin. Sepsis patients receiving albumin therapy had significant decreases in gastric intramucosal pH (<7.20), which did not occur with HES. Five-day and late mortalities were comparable in the four groups. The principal value of this study is the prolonged and comprehensive scope of physiological observations. Its main finding is that HES solutions consistently improved cardiocirculatory and respiratory variables, while albumin did not. An unexpected additional finding is that albumin might actually contribute to deteriorate splanchnic circulation in some classes of critically ill patients.

Albumin for treatment of burns

Thermal injuries induce coagulation and dehydration of tissues. The resulting local hyperosmolarity and endothelial lesions provoke a rapid and massive fluid shift toward the affected zone; edema formation starts within minutes and culminates after 24 hours. The release of vasoactive (and cardiodepressive) substances by burned tissues disrupt endothelial permeability in the whole body, i.e., also in nonburned tissues, leading to generalized edema formation starting 4 hours after the initial injury and culminating around 12 hours after burn. The ensuing fluid and protein losses from the circulation quickly lead to acute hemoconcentration and hypoalbuminemia, requiring the administration of important quantities of intravenous fluids [98]. Since 1978, several consensus conferences have regularly updated guidelines concerning the treatment of postburn shock. Current guidelines favor the exclusive use of crystalloids during the first hour postburn and propose the introduction of artificial colloids and human albumin solutions after the eighth hour postburn [99–104]. At this stage, colloids could have a positive effect by reclaiming water from edematous nonburned tissues when they regain normal endothelial permeability. No attempt should be made to normalize serum albumin levels: it has been shown that concentrations as low as 15 g/L can be tolerated without deleterious consequences [105]. Furthermore, improving circulating volume may not improve renal function [106]. Therapy should be guided by the hemodynamic status as assessed by urine output, cardiac echography, or more invasive pressure and output measurements, rather than by serum albumin concentrations.

Albumin usage in infants and neonates

Neonates and infants present specific features regarding their circulating proteic and fluid balances [33] (see Table 8.7). First, their plasmatic volume is relatively large when compared to adults. Second, their endothelial permeability is greater than that of adults. Third, their serum albumin concentration varies over time: it is low at birth but increases with age. Albumin plays a vital role during the first days of life because it transports and neutralizes unconjugated bilirubin, preventing this toxic metabolite to reach the intracranial gray matter and protecting from the feared "kernicterus." Fourth, maternal immunoglobulins contribute to the COP. Their concentration is lower in prematures and decreases after the third month of life. For all these reasons, newborns, and especially premature babies, are at high risk of significant fluid shifts from the intravascular to the extravascular compartment with subsequent hypovolemia and circulatory failure. Mild to moderate hypovolemia can be treated with 0.9% normal saline or lactated Ringer solutions, but fluid resuscitation should quickly resort to human albumin solutions because of the specific transport capacity of this protein. Artificial colloids are therefore not recommended in infants. Because newborns, and especially prematures, have low concentrations of coagulation factors (especially factors II, VII, and fibrinogen) viro-inactivated FFP is a suitable alternative whenever hemostasis is a concern, e.g., in endotoxinic shock or during major surgery. A recent uncontrolled series [37] reported excellent results by using albumin solutions as first line therapy in meningococcemia, underlining the need for controlled, randomized studies to better define the indications of FFP and albumin solutions.

Other usages and the Erstad literature review

In 1991, Erstad and his group [77] reviewed the available literature concerning the use of albumin solutions in trauma patients, aortic surgery patients, patients undergoing cardiopulmonary bypass, patients with acute pulmonary insufficiency, sepsis, burns, hypovolemia, or other critical conditions. Historical comparisons, open or randomized trials consistently failed to document major significant differences in outcome between groups

Table 8.7 Pediatrics reference values.

	Blood volume (mL/ kg)	Total body water (%)	Extracellular volume (%)	Serum protein concentration (g/L)	Serum albumin concentration (g/L)
Preterm baby	90–100	80	45	43–75	30–42
Newborn	80–90	75	40	46–75	36–54
1–12 months	80	65	30	50–75	40–50
1–12 years	70–80	60	20–25	62–80	35–50
Adult	60–65	50–55	20–25	60–78	35–50

Data from Moulin [33].

receiving albumin versus crystalloids (occasionally other colloids).

Patients with cirrhosis undergoing repeated paracentesis had less renal dysfunction and less hyponatremia when given 20% albumin [107]. Similar benefits could occasionally be obtained by others with i.v. or oral sodium chloride supplements [108]. Whether albumin offers an advantage over other fluids in this indication remains, therefore, an open question.

A more recent study (posterior to Erstad's review) compared antibiotics alone with albumin supplements in patients with cirrhosis and spontaneous bacterial peritonitis and disclosed no difference in infection resolution but showed a threefold reduction in renal impairment and mortality in the group receiving albumin [126]. However, patients receiving antibiotics alone did not receive other fluids, let alone colloids, to compensate to paracenteses.

In young patients with severe nephrosis failing to respond adequately to diuretics a normal response to treatment could be restored after albumin infusion in at least two studies [109, 110].

Controversial data exist as to whether enteral feeding intolerance could be improved by albumin: a study in children reported encouraging results [111] while another reported no benefits in adults [70]. No definitive advantage seems to result from adding albumin to total parenteral nutrition [70, 112].

Prospective randomized controlled studies are lacking in the field of cerebral ischemia, renal transplantation, and partial hepatectomy comparing albumin, artificial colloids, and crystalloids.

Finally, albumin replacement is recommended and preferred to plasma transfusions during large plasma exchange procedures, except for Thrombotic Thrombocytopenic Purpura [59, 113–115].

The overall picture provided by this literature review was that, in many fields of medicine, albumin therapy had been adopted and was widely used without adequate scientific evidence on the basis of properly conducted prospective randomized trials.

The Cochrane meta-analysis

The Cochrane group is an Oxford-based international group of physicians and other scientists interested in reviewing the evidence underlying current medical interventions. Well known for its epidemiological work on perinatal medicine, it also includes subgroups studying other aspects of medicine. In 1998, the Cochrane Injuries Group published a meta-analysis of available randomized controlled trials comparing the administration of albumin solutions with standard therapies [116]. Thirty-two trials representing 1495 patients were included and were subdivided according to the main indication for albumin administration: hypovolemia (20 trials, 790 patients), burns (3 trials, 163 patients), and hypoalbuminemia (9 trials, 542 patients). Some trials concerned only neonatology, while others concerned perioperative or intensive care adult populations. They had been published between 1975 and 1997. Rather strict criteria determined the inclusion or exclusion of trials including

Table 8.8 The Cochrane meta-analysis—main results [116].

	Trials (*n*)	Trials with deaths (*n*)	*n* deaths/n cases*		Relative risk trials with deaths (95% CI)
			Albumin	Controls	
Hypovolemia	20	13	38/256	26/278	1.46 (0.97–2.22)
Burns	3	3	19/81	8/82	2.40 (1.11–5.19)
Hypovolemia	9	8	41/259	24/248	1.69 (1.07–2.67)
Total	32	24	98/596	58/608	1.68 (1.26–2.23)

*Trials with zero mortality being excluded from analysis.

random allocation of patients between the albumin and control groups, clear definitions of treated conditions, and availability of mortality figures. A few trials comparing low with high dosage albumin regimens were included, along with a majority of trials comparing albumin with crystalloid administration. Neither Stockwell's [78, 94] nor Boldt's [97] studies comparing albumin to other colloid solutions were included in the meta-analysis (Table 8.8).

For all three main indications, the Cochrane analysis found an excess mortality in the albumin (or high-albumin) patients. The relative risk of dying when allocated to receive albumin was 1.46 when the indication was hypovolemia, 1.69 for hypoalbuminemia, and 2.40 for burns. The overall excess mortality was 6.8%, or about six additional deaths for every 100 patients treated with albumin. The conclusion of the study was that "[...] *the use of human albumin in the management of critically ill patients should be reviewed. A strong argument could be made that human albumin should not be used outside the context of a properly concealed and otherwise rigorously conducted randomized controlled trial with mortality as the endpoint.*"

Many critics have been voiced concerning the selection of trials, the pooling of neonatal and adult populations, or the inclusion of studies conducted with old solutions of albumin prepared before the advent of modern purification techniques. It is indeed possible that some of the oldest trials bore heavily on the reported excess mortality. Reconsidering the data to answer such critics could reduce the calculated excess mortality, but never reverse it. The major conclusion of the Cochrane analysis remains therefore unchallenged, namely that the administration of albumin solutions to a wide variety of acutely ill patients provides no proven benefit over crystalloids [117, 118]. Its main shortcoming is that it did not address the comparison between albumin and artificial colloids.

Epidemiological surveys

The European Sanguis Study conducted in 1990 and 1991 in 43 teaching hospitals across the European Union, confirmed extreme variations in the use of human albumin solutions between countries [65, 66]. Schematically, northern countries, which produced most albumin solutions, used them more often and in larger quantities than southern countries such as Greece, Italy, Spain, and Portugal. Belgium, where 15% of studied patients had been enrolled, had used about 50% of the total amount of human albumin administered during the study [67]. In several countries, surgical teams could be divided according to their near-exclusive usage of one type of colloid solution versus any other. Such choices were not consistent for a given surgical procedure, nor did they affect outcome as far as could be judged from in-hospital mortality or length of hospital stay.

A study using the same methodology was conducted 6 years later in Belgium, under the aegis of the European BIOMED program [68]. At least, two surgical procedures allowed meaningful comparison between surveys. A dramatic decrease in the use of human albumin was noted for both operations: the overall consumption was reduced by 85% for hemicolectomy and 81% for total hip replacement. Several factors may have contributed to the decrease in albumin consumption during the nineties: lack of scientific evidence, publication of the mentioned surveys allowing for international and inter-hospital comparisons, new reimbursement regulations obliging to justify its use, and new guidelines issued after consensus conferences.

Consensus conferences

Consensus conferences were held about the use of albumin in Australia [119], Belgium [120], and France [86, 121–123]. Their main conclusions are similar: there is no scientifically documented minimal albumin plasma concentration above which a specific treatment must be instituted; there is no obvious indication for using human albumin solutions to treat hypovolemia in emergency or intensive care situations; human albumin solutions are not first line treatments for perioperative hypovolemia; human albumin is justified only when artificial colloids are contraindicated in case of severe hypoproteinemia (<35 g/L) unrelated to dilution during resuscitation. Several guidelines also reemphasized that FFP should not be used to correct hypovolemia, nor as a mere source of albumin. The impact of these consensus conferences has been questioned [92].

Conclusion and moral

The story of therapeutic use of albumin has gone a full circle and is exemplative of how missing some logical steps to jump to "obvious" conclusions can lead to widespread adoption of a questionable therapy. Since hypoalbuminemia and poor outcome were so strongly associated, it has been assumed they were linked by a cause-to-effect relationship. In the process of thought, two questions were skipped: (1) what is the mechanism by which lack of albumin increases mortality in hypoalbuminemic patients? and (2) does restoration of normal serum (and tissue) albumin concentration improve outcome?

As the story goes, albumin could be isolated, purified, and produced at industrial scale. With hindsight, the Cohn alcohol extraction method and pasteurization constituted exceptionally efficient safety measures against infectious agents. With time, infrequent hypotensive reactions disappeared with improved fractionation methods. Without maximal dose and no direct effect on hemostasis, albumin solutions achieved an unchallenged leadership among colloid solutions. Technically, it undoubtedly has been a success story.

Quality improvement of albumin production and the crystalloid versus colloid resuscitation controversy generated much scientific work, but comparatively few prospective randomized controlled trials assessed the two forgotten questions. Ironically, the ever enlarging usage of albumin therapy created the conditions for reaction: perceived shortages or excessive dependence of whole transfusion systems on albumin sales led to reconsider the scientific evidence underlying clinical use. Despite the unmatched safety record of albumin solutions, the AIDS epidemic also contributed to revisit indications for transfusing albumin, like those of any other pooled blood product.

A few consensus conferences later, very little is left of the once accepted uses of albumin [124,125]. Residual indications concern mainly neonatology, end-stage medical conditions, adjuvant therapy for infrequent techniques such as plasma exchange, some transplantation surgeries, and burns (with some controversy). Almost nothing remains from its main usage as ideal volume replacement for the operated or critically ill patient. Many questions remain unanswered concerning, for example, the pharmacological interactions of albumin transfusions. The place in modern pharmacopoeia of this colloid featuring both a long intravascular half-life and a remarkable absence of toxicity remains to be defined. Despite so many years of clinical use, there is still a definite need for properly conducted prospective randomized trials.

References

1. Myllylä G. Factors determining quality of plasma. Vox Sang 1998;74(Suppl. 2):507–11.
2. Annas GJ. Waste and longing – the legal status of placental blood banking. N Engl J Med 1999;340:1471–5.
3. Mohr H. Virus inactivation of fresh plasma. Vox Sang 1998;74(Suppl. 2):171–2.
4. Zeiler T, Riess H, Wittmann G, et al. The effect of methylene blue phototreatment on plasma proteins

and in vitro coagulation capability of single-donor fresh-frozen plasma. Transfusion 1994;34:685–9.
5. Lambrecht B, Mohr H, Knuver-Hopf J, Schmitt H. Photoinactivation of viruses in human fresh plasma by phenothiazine dyes in combination with visible light. Vox Sang 1991;60:207–13.
6. Martindale. *The Extra Pharmacopoeia*, 30th edn. The Pharmaceutical Press, London, 1993, pp. 684–5.
7. Porat R, Gilbert S, Magilner D. Methylene Blue-induced phototoxicity: an unrecognized complication. Pediatrics 1996;97:717–21.
8. Corash L. Inactivation of viruses, bacteria, protozoa, and leukocytes in platelet concentrates. Vox Sang 1998;74(Suppl. 2):173–6.
9. Conseil de l'Europe. *Guide pour la préparation, l'utilisation et l'assurance de qualité des composants sanguins*, 5e édition. Editions du Conseil de l'Europe, 1999.
10. United Kingdom Health Departments. *Handbook of Transfusion Medicine*. Her Majesty's Stationery Office, London, 1996.
11. Wells JV, King MA. Adverse reactions to human plasma proteins. Anaesth Intensive Care 1980;8:139–44.
12. Carlson SA, Kosinski KS, Akins CW, Buckley MJ, Lowenstein E. Vasodilator effect of fresh frozen plasma (FFP). Anesthesiology 1983;59(3):A19.
13. Bux J, Becker F, Seeger W, Kilpatrick D, Chapman J, Waters A. Transfusion-related acute lung injury due to HLA-A2-specific antibodies in recipient and NB1-specific antibodies in donor blood. Br J Haematol 1996;93:707–13.
14. Cailleux N, Levesque H, Bastit D, Cuvelier A, Muir JF, Courtois H. An uncommon cause of alveolar hemorrhage: transfusion-related acute lung injury caused by granulocyte-specific antibody. Rev Med Interne 1998;19:434–7.
15. Davenport RD, Polak TJ, Kunkel SL. White cell-associated procoagulant activity induced by ABO incompatibility. Transfusion 1994;34:943–9.
16. Densmore TL, Goodnough IT, Ali S, Dynis M, Chaplin H. Prevalence of HLA sensitization in female apheresis donors. Transfusion 1999;39:103–6.
17. Santamaria A, Moya F, Martinez C, Martino R, Martinez-Perez J, MunizDiaz E. Transfusion-related acute lung injury associated with an NI1-specific antigranulocyte antibody. Haematologica 1998;83:951–2.
18. Popovsky MA, Saidman SL, Shepard JO, Colvin RB, Mark EJ, A 49-year-old woman with thrombotic thrombocytopenic purpura and severe dyspnea during plasmapheresis and transfusion. N Engl J Med 1998;339(27):2005–12.
19. Ramanathan RK, Triulzi DJ, Logan TF. Transfusion-related acute lung injury following random donor platelet transfusion: a report of two cases. Vox Sang 1997;73:43–5.
20. Silliman CC, Voelkel NF, Allard JD, et al. Plasma and lipids from stored packed red blood cells cause acute lung injury in animal model. J Clin Invest 1998;101:1458–67.
21. Brunner-Bolliger S, Kiefel V, Horber FF, Nydegger UE, Berchtold P. Antibody studies in a patient with acute thrombocytopenia following infusion of plasma containing anti PIA1. Am J Hematol 1997;56(2):119–21.
22. Myllylä G. New transfusion practice and haemostasis. Acta Anaesthesiol Scand 1988;89(Suppl. 32):76–80.
23. Murray, DJ, Olson JD, Strauss R, Tinker JH. Coagulation changes during packed red cell replacement of major blood loss. Anesthesiology 1988;69:839–45.
24. Murray DJ, Pennel BJ, Weinstein SL, Olson JD. Packed red cell in acute blood loss: dilutional coagulopathy as a cause of surgical bleeding. Anesth Analg 1995;80:336–42.
25. Ciavarella D, Reed RL, Counts RB, et al. Clotting factor levels and the risk of microvascular bleeding in the massively transfused patient. Br J Haematol 1987;67:365–8.
26. Reed RL, Heimbach DM, Counts RB, et al. Prophylactic platelet administration during massive transfusion. Ann Surg 1986;203:40–48.
27. American Society of Anesthesiologists. Practice guidelines for blood component therapy: a report by the American Society of Anesthesiologists Task Force on Blood Component Therapy. Anesthesiology 1996;84:732–47.
28. American Society of Anesthesiologists. *Questions and Answers About Transfusion Practices*, 3rd edn. American Society of Anesthesiologists, Illinois, 1998.
29. Ewe K. Bleeding after liver biopsy does not correlate with indices of peripheral coagulation. Dig Dis Sci 1981;26:388–93.
30. Foster PF, Moore LR, Sankary HN, Hart ME, Ashmann MK, Williams JW. Central venous catheterization in patients with coagulopathy. Arch Surg 1992;127:273–5.
31. Mc Vay PA, Toy PT. Lack of increased bleeding after paracentesis and thoracocentesis in patients with mild coagulation abnormalities. Transfusion 1991;31:164–71.

32. Rodeghiero F, Castaman G, Mannucci PM. Clinical indications for desmopressin (DDAVP) in congenital and acquired von Willebrand disease. Blood Rev 1991;5:155–61.
33. Moulin D. Human albumin and substitutes in pediatric intensive care and neonatalogy. Arch Public Health 1994;52:417–23.
34. Northern Neonatal Nursing Initiative Trial Group. Randomised trial of prophylactic early fresh-frozen plasma or gelatin or glucose in preterm babies: outcome at 2 years. Lancet 1996;348:229–32.
35. Nadel S, De Munter C, Britto J, Levin M, Habib P. Albumin: saint or sinner? Arch Dis Child 1998;79:384–5.
36. So KW, Fok TF, Ng PC, Wong WW, Cheung KL. Randomised controlled trial of colloid or crystalloid in hypotensive preterm infants. Arch Dis Child 1997;76:F43–6.
37. Hope P. Pump up the volume? The routine early use of colloid in very preterm infants. Arch Dis Child 1998;78:F163–5.
38. Leslie SD, Toy PTCY. Laboratory hemostatic abnormalities in massively transfused patients given red-blood cells and crystalloids. Am J Pathol 1991;96:770–73.
39. Hiippala, ST, Myllylä GJ, Vahtera EM. Hemostatic factors and replacement of major blood loss with plasma-poor red cell concentrates. Anesth Analg 1995;81(2):360–65.
40. O'Connor MF, Roth S, Roizen MF. Blood transfusion therapy for vascular surgery. In: Roizen MF (ed.) *Anesthesia For Vascular Surgery*. 1990, pp. 441–62.
41. Martinowitz U, Goor DA, Ramot B, Mohr R. Is transfusion of fresh plasma after cardiac operations indicated? J Thorac Cardiovasc Surg 1990;100: 92–8.
42. Roy RC, Stafford MA, Hudspeth AS, Meredith JW. Failure of prophylaxis with fresh frozen plasma after cardiopulmonary bypass. Anesthesiology 1988;69:254–7.
43. Van Beek EJ, von der Mohlen MA, ten Cate JW, Brandjes DP, Buller HR. Antithrombin III concentrate in the treatment of DIC: a retrospective follow-up study. Neth J Med 1994;45:206–10.
44. Furlan M, et al. von Willebrand factor-cleaving protease in Thrombotic Thrombocytopenic Purpura and the Hemolytic-Uremic Syndrome. N Engl J Med 1998;339:1578–84.
45. Rochant H, Gordjani N, Hénon P, Rondeau E, Hermine O. Purpuras thrombotiques thrombocytopéniques, Syndromes hémolytiques et urémiques, microangiopathies thrombotiques: Forum. Hématologie 1998;1:75–87.
46. McClelland DBL. Fresh frozen plasma – opinion and evidence. Transfus Med 1992;2:97–8.
47. Blumberg N, Laczin J, McMican A, Heal J, Arvan D. A critical survey of fresh-frozen plasma use. Transfusion 1986;26:511–13.
48. Thomson A, Napier JAF, Wood JK. Use and abuse of fresh frozen plasma (Editorial). Br J Anaesth 1992;237–8.
49. Consensus Conference, Office of Medical Applications of Research, National Institutes of Health, Bethesda. Fresh-frozen plasma: indications and risks. JAMA 1985;253(4):551–3.
50. Calder L, Hebert PC, Carter AO, Graham ID. Review of published recommendations and guidelines for the transfusion of allogeneic red blood cells and plasma. Can Med Assoc J 1997;156(Suppl. 11): S1–8.
51. Hume HA, Kronick JB, Blanchette VS. Review of the literature on allogeneic red blood cell and plasma transfusions in children. Can Med Assoc J 1997;156(Suppl. 11):S41–9.
52. ACOG technical bulletin. Blood component therapy. Int J Gynaecol Obstet 1995;48:233–8.
53. Petz LD, Tomasulo PA. Red cell transfusion. In: Kolins J, McCarthy LJ (eds) *Contemporary Transfusion Practice*. American Association of Blood Banks, Arlington, VA, 1987, pp. 1–26.
54. Goodnough LT, Johnston MFM, Ramsey G, et al. Guidelines for transfusion support in patients undergoing coronary artery bypass grafting. Ann Thorac Surg 1990;50:675–83.
55. Bested AC, Francombe W, Freedman J, Herst R, Norman C. *Medical Advisory Council of Canadian Red Cross Toronto Centre*. Criteria for transfusion of blood components. Canadian Red Cross Society, Toronto, 1992.
56. Description of blood components and plasma fractions. In: *Canadian Red Cross Society Clinical Guide to Transfusion*, 3rd edn. Canadian Red Cross Society, Ottawa, 1993.
57. Silberstein LE, Kruskall MS, Stehling LC, Johnston MFM, Rutman RC, Samia CT, et al. Strategies for the review of transfusion practices. JAMA 1989;262:1993–7.
58. Ali AM, VanderGliessen B, Blajchman MA. Hospital blood transfusion audit systems. In: Smit Sibinga CT, Das PC, Heiniger HJ (eds) *Good Manufacturing Practice in Transfusion Medicine: Proceedings of the 18th International Symposium on Blood Transfusion*. Kluwer

Academic Publishers, Dordrecht, the Netherlands, 1994, pp. 269–79.
59. Contreras M, Ala FA, Greaves M, et al. Guidelines for the use of fresh frozen plasma. British Committee for Standards in Haematology, Working Party of the Blood Transfusion Task Force. Transfusion Med 1992;2:57–63.
60. Development Task Force of the College of American Pathologists. Practice parameters for the use of fresh-frozen plasma, cryoprecipitate, and platelets: fresh-frozen plasma, cryoprecipitate, and platelets administration practice guidelines. JAMA 1994;271:777–81.
61. Crosby ET. Preoperative haemotherapy: I. Indications for blood component transfusion. Can J Anaesth 1992;39:695–707.
62. Medical Directors Advisory Committee, National Blood Transfusion Council. Guideline for the use of fresh-frozen plasma. S Afr Med J 1998;88: 1344–7.
63. Stover EP, Siegel LC, Parks R, et al. Variability in transfusion practice for coronary artery bypass surgery persists despite national consensus guidelines: a 24-institution study. Anesthesiology 1998;88:327–33.
64. Surgenor DM, Churchill WH, Wallace EL, Rizzo RJ, et al. Determinants of red cell platelet, plasma, and cryoprecipitate transfusions during coronary artery bypass graft surgery: the collaborative hospital transfusion study. Transfusion 1996;36:521–32.
65. Sirchia G, Giovanetti AM, McClelland DBL, Fracchia GN. Safe and good use of blood in surgery (SANGUIS). In: *Use of Blood Products and Artificial Colloids in 43 European Hospitals*. European Commission, Brussels, 1994.
66. SANGUIS Study Group (the). Use of blood products for elective surgery in 43 European hospitals. Transfus Med 1994;4:251–68.
67. Baele P, De Bruyère M, Deneys V, et al. Results of the SANGUIS study in Belgium. A concerted action of the Commission of the European Communities IVth Medical and Health Research Programme. Acta Chir Belg 1994;94(Suppl.).
68. Baele P, Beguin C, Waterloos H, et al. Results, of the Belgian biomed study about transfusion for surgery. Acta Anaesthesiol Belg 1998;49:243–303.
69. Ayoub MM, Clarck JA. Reduction of fresh frozen plasma use with a simple education program. Am Surg 1989;55:563–5.
70. Barnette RE, Fish DJ, Eisenstaedt RS. Modifications of fresh frozen plasma transfusion practices through educational intervention. Transfusion 1990;30:253–7.
71. Giovanetti AM, Paraviccini A, Baroni L, et al. Quality assessment of transfusion practice in elective surgery. Transfusion 1988;28:166–9.
72. Shanberge JN. Reduction of fresh frozen plasma use through a daily survey and education program. Transfusion 1987;27:226–7.
73. Ellison N, Silberstein LE. A commentary on three consensus development conferences on transfusion medicine. Anesthesiol Clin North Am 1990;8:609–25.
74. Salmon JB, Mythen MG. Pharmacology and physiology of colloids. Blood Rev 1993;114–20.
75. Starling EH. On the absorption of fluids from the connective tissue spaces. J Physiol 1896;19:312–26.
76. Foley EF, Borlase BC, Dzik WH, Bistrian BR, Benotti PN. Albumin supplementation in the critically ill. Arch Surg 1990;125:739–42.
77. Erstad BL, Gales BJ, Rappaport WD. The use of albumin in clinical practice. Arch Intern Med 1991;151:901–11.
78. Stockwell MA, Soni N, Riley B. Colloid solutions in the critically ill: a randomised comparison of albumin and polygeline. 1. Outcome and duration of stay in the intensive care unit. Anaesthesia 1992;47:3–6.
79. Burnouf T, Huart JJ. Human albumin: toxicological and viral safety. Arch Public Health 1994;52:331–45.
80. More JE, Harvey MJ. Purification technologies for human plasma albumin. In: *Blood Separation and Plasma Fractionation*. Wiley-Liss Inc, 1991, pp. 261–306.
81. Cohn EJ, Strong LE, Hughes WL, et al. Preparation and properties of serum and plasma proteins. IV A system for the separation into fractions of the protein and lipoprotein components of biological tissues and fluids. J Am Chem Soc 1946;68:459–75.
82. Kistler P, Nitschmann HS. Large-scale production of human plasma fractions. Vox Sang 1962;7:414–24.
83. European Pharmacopoeia. *Albumin Solution*. Human Press, 1998.
84. Bland JM, Laver MB, Lowenstein E. Vasodilator effect of commercial 5% plasma protein fraction solutions. JAMA 1973;224:1721–4.
85. Isbistet JP, Fisher MM. Adverse effects of plasma volume expanders. Anaesth Intensive Care 1980;8:145–51.
86. Conference de consensus. Utilisation des solutions d'albumine humaine en anesthésie-réanimation chirurgicale de l'adulte. Ann Fr Anesth Reanim 1996;15:405–568.

87. Créange A, Gray F, Cesaro P, et al. Creutzfeldt-Jakob disease after liver transplantation. Ann Neurol 1995;38:269–72. See also from the same team: Pooled plasma derivatives and Creutzfeldt-Jakob disease. Letters in Lancet, 1996;347:482; and Lancet, 1996;347:967.
88. Turner ML, Ironside J. New-variant Creutzfeldt-Jakob disease: the risk of transmission by blood transfusion. Blood Rev 1998;12:255–68.
89. Ring J, Messmer K. Incidence and severity of anaphylactoid reactions to colloid volume substitutes. Lancet 1977;466–9.
90. Messmer K. What is new in the therapy of hemorrhagic shock? Curr Opin Anaesthesiol 1990;3: 265–8.
91. Laxenaire MC, Charpentier C, Feldman L. Anaphylactoid reactions to colloid plasma substitutes: incidence, risk factors, mechanisms. A French multicenter prospective study. Ann Fr Anesth Reanim 1994;13:301–10.
92. Audibert G, Charpentier C, Savoye E, Laxenaire MC. Outcome of the use of albumin and colloid plasma substitutes from 1989 to 1993 in a French University Hospital Center. Ann Fr Anesth Reanim 1995;14:517–22.
93. Leikola J, Van Aken WG, Högman C, Lee D, Muglia M, Schmitt H, for the Committee of Experts on Blood Transfusion and Immunohaematology. *Plasma Products and European Self-Sufficiency: Collection, Preparation and Use*. Council of Europe, Publishing and Documentation Service, Strasbourg, 1992.
94. Stockwell MA, Scott A, Day A, Riley B, Soni N. Colloid solutions in the critically ill. A randomised comparison of albumin and polygenine 2. Serum albumin concentration and incidences of pulmonary oedema and acute renal failure. Anaesthesia 1992;47:7–9.
95. Grundmann R, Heistermann S. Postoperative albumin infusion therapy based on colloid osmotic pressure. Arch Surg 1985;120:911–15.
96. Grootendorst AF, van Wilgenburg M, de Laat PH, van der Hoven B. Albumin abuse in intensive care medicine. Intensive Care Med 1988;14:554–7.
97. Boldt J, Heesen M, Müller M, Pabsdorf M, Hempelmann G. The effects of albumin versus hydroxyethyl starch solution on cardiorespiratory and circulatory variables in critically ill patients. Anesth Analg 1996;83:254–61.
98. Kramer GC, Nguyen TT. Pathophysiology of burn shock and burn edema. Total Burn Care 1996;44–52.
99. Warden GD. Fluid resuscitation and early management. Total Burn Care 1996;53–60.
100. Vanderkelen A, Reper P, Duinslaeger L. Human albumin and substitutes: effectiveness in the treatment of burn shock. Arch Public Health 1994;52:391–404.
101. Monafo WW. Initial management of burns. N Engl J Med 1996;335:1581–6.
102. Goodwin CW, Dorethy J, Lam V, Pruit BA, Jr. Resuscitation trial of efficacy of cristalloid and colloid resuscitation on hemodynamic response and lung water following thermal injury. Ann Surg 1983;197:520–29.
103. Greenhalgh DG, Housinger TA, Kagan RJ, et al. Maintenance of serum albumin levels in pediatric burn patients: a prospective, randomized trial. J Trauma 1995;39:67–73.
104. Jelenko C, III, Williams JB, Wheeler ML, et al. Studies in shock and resuscitation, I: use of a hypertonic, albumin-containing, fluid demand regimen (HALFD) in resuscitation. Crit Care Med 1979;7:157–67.
105. Schlagintweit S, Snelling CGT, German E, et al. Major burns managed without blood or blood products. J Burn Care Rehabil 1990;11:214.
106. Gore DC, Dalton JM, Gehr TW. Colloid infusions reduce glomerular filtration in resuscitated burn victims. J Trauma 1996;40:356–60.
107. Gines P, Tito L, Arroyo V. Randomized comparative study of therapeutic paracentesis with and without intravenous albumin in cirrhosis. Gastroenterology 1988;94:1493–1502.
108. Nelson WP, Rosenbaum JD, Strauss MB. Hyponatremia in hepatic cirrhosis following paracentesis. J Clin Invest 1951;30:738–44.
109. Davison AM, Lambie AT, Verth AH, Cash JD. Salt-poor albumin in management of nephrotic syndrome. Br Med J 1974;1:481–4.
110. Weiss RA, Schoenemann M, Greifer I. Treatment of severe nephrotic edema with albumin and furosemide. New York State J Med 1984;84:384–6.
111. Ford EG, Tennings M, Andrassy RJ. Serum albumin (oncotic pressure) correlates with enteral feeding tolerance in the pediatric surgical patient. J Pediatr Surg 1987;22:597–9.
112. Brown RO, Bradley JE, Bekemeyer WB, Luther RW. Effect of albumin supplementation during parenteral nutrition on hospital morbidity. Crit Care Med 1998;16:1177–82.
113. Osselaer JC, Bosly A. Human albumin and synthetic substitutes in therapeutic plasma exchange

and in the treatment of hypoproteinemia. Arch Public Health 1994;52:383–90.

114. Leblond PF, Rock G, Herbert CA. The use of plasma as a replacement fluid. in plasma exchange. Canadian Apheresis Group. Transfusion 1998;38:834–8.

115. Raphael JC, Chevret S, Gajdos P. Plasma exchange in neurological diseases. Transfus Sci 1996;17:267–82.

116. Cochrane Injuries Group Albumin Reviewers. Human albumin administration in critically ill patients: systematic review of randomised controlled trials. Br Med J 1998;317:235–39.

117. McClelland DBL. Albumin: don't confuse us with the facts. Br Med J 1998;317:829–30 (Editorial).

118. Offringa M. Excess mortality after human albumin administration in critically ill patients. Br Med J 1998;317:223–4.

119. Subcommittee of the Victorian Drug Usage Advisory Committee. Human albumin solutions: consensus statements for use in selected clinical situations. Med J Aust 1992;157(5):340–43.

120. Consensus text. In: Conference de consensus – Corcsensusconferentie "Les perfusions d'albumine humaine et les produits de substitution/Perfusie van menselijke albumine en vervangoplossingen", Vol. 52. Arch Public Health, 1994,301–6 and 307–12.

121. Perret C, Bedock B, Boles JM, Bussel A, Laxenaire MC, Paillard M, Petit P, Schlemmer B. Choix des produits de remplissage vasculaire pour le traitement des hypovolémies chez l'adulte: IV, Conférence de Consensus en réanimation et en médecine d'urgence. Réan Soins Intens Méd Urg 1989;5(5):295–304.

122. Agence pour le Développement de l'Evaluation Médicale; ad hoc task force. *Recommandations pour la pratique clinique: remplissage vasculaire au cours des hypovolémies relatives ou absolues.* Paris, January 1997. See also: Réan Urg; 1997;6:special issue.

123. Conférence de consensus. Choix du produit de remplissage vasculaire pour le traitement des hypovolémies chez l'adulte. Réan Soins Intens Méd Urg 1989;5:295–304.

124. Nilsson E, Lamke O, Liljedahl SO, Elfstrom K. Is albumin therapy worth-while in surgery for colorectal cancer? Acta Chir Scand 1980;146:619–22.

125. Durant-Zaleski I, Bonnet F, Rochant H, Bierling P, Lemaire F. Usefulness of consensus conferences: the case of albumin. Lancet 1992;340:1388–90.

126. Sort P, et al. Effects of intravenous albumin on renal impairment and mortality in patients with cirrhosis and spontaneous bacterial peritonitis. N Engl J Med 1999;341:403–9.

SECTION 2
Crystalloids and Synthetic Colloids

CHAPTER 9
Pharmacology of Intravenous Fluids

Michael F.M. James
Department of Anaesthesia, University of Cape Town Faculty of Health Sciences, Cape Town, Western Cape, South Africa

Intravenous fluids can be broadly categorized into crystalloids and colloids. As the colloids are suspended in a crystalloid solution, there is some overlap in the pharmacology of these preparations, but this categorization will be used for convenience in this discussion.

Crystalloids

Crystalloids are aqueous solutions of mineral salts that pass readily through biological membranes. The term "crystalloid" is derived from the fact that when these solutions are evaporated to dryness all that remains are pure crystals of the dissolved salts. Crystalloids are true solutions with all the associated physical characteristics of such solutions, including depression of freezing point.

Crystalloid solutions expand the extracellular fluid (ECF) space and are redistributed between the intravascular and extracellular compartments in a ratio of 1:4 in proportion to the normal distribution of fluid between these two spaces. Consequently, full volume expansion after blood loss requires 3–4 times the volume lost to be replaced with crystalloids alone to replenish the intravascular losses. In the initial resuscitation phase, crystalloids may be deceptively effective, but once the capillary perfusion is re-established, the crystalloid will rapidly move out of the vascular space. Crystalloids will result in a reduction plasma oncotic pressure and excessive quantities of crystalloids used for resuscitation may have adverse effects, particularly in terms of abdominal compartment syndrome [1].

None of the currently available crystalloid solutions completely resembles the electrolyte content of plasma. The most widely used crystalloids, 0.9% saline and balanced salt solutions such as Ringer's lactate, fall well short of the desired composition.

(Ab)normal saline

"Normal" saline is a simple solution of sodium chloride containing 154 mmol/L (0.9%) sodium chloride salt. It is significantly hypertonic (osmolarity 308 mOsm/L) and has a very high chloride content (154 mmol/L; normal plasma range, 95–105 mmol/L). Infusions of as little as 2 L 0.9% saline during surgical procedures will produce a significant, measurable metabolic acidosis due to the chloride load [2, 3]. Hyperchloremia has been shown to be one of the main causes of progressive metabolic acidosis in critically ill patients [4]. The clinical significance of this metabolic acidosis has not yet been established, but a number of adverse effects have been ascribed to excessive chloride administration, including decreased survival in animals, abdominal discomfort, impaired cerebral function, and delayed renal clearance of fluid loads [5]. Chloride regulates renal vascular resistance markedly within the clinical range [6] and hyperchloremia produces dose-dependent renal vasoconstriction and reductions in glomerular filtration rate [7]. Diminished renal function has been demonstrated in patients receiving saline-based fluids perioperatively and decreased water clearance and greater fluid retention with saline as opposed to Ringer's lactate shown in volunteers [3].

Alternatives to Blood Transfusion in Transfusion Medicine, 2nd edition. Edited by A. Maniatis, P. Van der Linden, J.-F. Hardy.

There is substantial evidence that chloride loading may impair renal function and may interfere with coagulation. However, there are no human outcome data suggesting that this may lead to decreased survival. There is a common misconception that 0.9% saline is a safer intravenous fluid to use than Ringer's lactate in patients with renal dysfunction and an elevated serum potassium. However, the acidosis associated with saline administration may cause extracellular migration of potassium from the intracellular space, leading to a paradoxical rise in plasma potassium concentrations, despite the administered fluid containing no potassium itself. A recent study has shown that, in patients undergoing renal transplantation, potassium concentrations were better controlled with Ringer's lactate than with saline [8]. Similar considerations apply to the recommendation to use 0.9% saline in the management of the ketoacidosis of diabetes mellitus. The policy frequently advocated is to use saline until such time as renal function is established and then to switch to a more balanced salt. Again, this ignores the effect of the hyperchloremic acidosis on potassium release. There is no scientific basis for this recommendation.

Balanced salt solutions

The composition of a variety of electrolyte solutions is shown in Table 9.1. Ringer's lactate (or acetate), like 0.9% saline, is not an ideal solution. The Cl^- content is substantially higher than plasma chloride (111 mmol/L), the Na^+ content is lower (131 mmol/L), and the osmolarity of the solution is 274 mOsm/L. This may be of some relevance in critically ill patients in whom antidiuretic hormone production results in water retention in excess of sodium, and may be clinically important in patients with head injury. Several studies have demonstrated that reduced plasma osmolality is associated with increased cerebral edema where the blood–brain barrier has been disrupted [9–11], but these have not been translated into clinical outcome studies. Nevertheless, most authorities recommend limited use of Ringer's lactate in patients at risk of cerebral edema.

Lactate is rapidly metabolized to CO_2 and water, resulting in a positive strong ion difference, which may lead to metabolic alkalosis, despite the fact that the pH of Ringer's lactate is 6.5. The conversion of lactate to glucose may impair glucose control in diabetics, but Ringer's lactate has been widely used without problems in these patients and there is no evidence that the lactate substantially disturbs glucose metabolism. However, it should probably be avoided in patients taking metformin where lactate metabolism may be impaired. A further problem with the use of lactated solutions is that they may interfere with the use of lactate as a marker of adequate tissue perfusion in critically ill patients.

Alternative solutions have used different anions to replace the lactate in an attempt to avoid the theoretical considerations mentioned above. The most popular anion for this purpose has been acetate. Arguments in favor of acetate include the fact that it can be metabolized by peripheral tissues, requires less oxygen for its metabolism, and is not solely dependent on the liver for its breakdown. However, the fact that it is rapidly metabolized may actually worsen the alkalosis problem as the strong ion difference will increase more rapidly. Gluconate has also been used as an alternative anion in some solutions. Currently, there are no

Table 9.1 Approximate constituents of some common electrolyte solutions (vary from country to country).

Solution	Na	K	Ca	Mg	Cl	Lac	Bic	Acet	Gluc	Osm
0.9% Saline	154	154	—	—	—	—		—	—	308
RL	131	5	1.8	—	111	27		—	—	274
Plas B	131	5	1.8	1.5	111		29			276
Plas A	140	5		1.5	98			27	23	294

RL, Ringer's lactate; Plas B, plasmalyte-B; Plas A, plasmalyte-A; Lac, lactate; Bic, bicarbonate; Acet, acetate; Gluc, gluconate (all in mmol/L); Osm, approximate osmolarity (mOsm/L).

clinical comparative studies demonstrating any benefit of one anion over another.

A near-ideal crystalloid solution exists in the form of plasmalyte-A. This solution contains 140 mmol/L of sodium and appropriate concentrations of the other cations. However, the anion component is made up of a mixture of gluconate and acetate. Despite the obvious theoretical benefits of this solution, it has not gained any widespread acceptance and there are no studies demonstrating its clinical advantages (or disadvantages).

In summary, an ideal crystalloid solution currently does not exist. Ringer's lactate (acetate) is moderately hypo-osmolar, while 0.9% saline may have substantial adverse effects due to the chloride load. At present, the best compromise, other than plasmalyte-A, is probably a combination of Ringer's lactate and 0.9% saline to achieve a balance between hyperchloremia and adequate sodium administration.

There is growing evidence of a substantial problem associated with excessive crystalloid use, including acid-based disturbances, osmolality problems, and increased risks of fluid overload [12]. A more rational approach to perioperative fluid therapy would suggest that crystalloids should be limited in volume, blood loss replaced largely with colloid and red blood cells using balanced salt solutions [13].

Hypertonic solutions

Hypertonic solutions, both crystalloid and colloid, will draw ECF into the vascular compartment, resulting in a greater expansion of the vascular space than the volume infused, but at the price of a further depletion of ECF and intracellular fluid (ICF). This may be valuable in prehospital resuscitation, but has limited application and requires subsequent re-expansion of the ECF. Hypertonic saline (7.5%) allows initial resuscitation with relatively small volumes of fluid and is theoretically indicated in patients with head injury. However, the duration of benefit is limited and no overall survival benefit has been demonstrated [14]. There is some evidence that hypertonic saline may improve the immune status of traumatized patients [15].

Colloids

The term "colloid" is derived from the Greek word for glutinous and is described as the residue left when a colloid suspension is evaporated to dryness. It defines a substance comprising very small, insoluble particles, usually 1–1000 nm in diameter, that are uniformly dispersed or suspended in a finely divided state throughout a continuous dispersion medium. If all particles in a colloidal system are of approximately the same size, the system is called *monodisperse*; where there is a substantial range of molecular size, the system is referred to as *polydisperse*. The average size of the particles in the suspension is critical as this will determine the extent to which the colloid is retained within the circulation. The determination of the effective molecular size depends on the dispersity of the system.

Albumin is a uniform size molecule and so an albumin suspension is a monodisperse system for which the molecular mass is easily established. The synthetic colloids (gelatins, dextrans, and hydroxyethyl starches) are all, to a greater or lesser extent, polydisperse systems. In polydisperse systems the determination of particle mass or relative molecular mass gives averages, which depend on the method used. The molecular weight (MW) can be described in one of the two ways: weight-averaged MW (MW_W) and number-averaged MW (MW_N).

Number-averaged molecular weight is calculated as:

$$MW_N = \frac{\sum n_i M(i)}{\sum n_i}$$

The weight-averaged (or mass-averaged) molecular weight is calculated as:

$$MW_N = \frac{\sum n_i \{M(i)\}^2}{\sum n_i M(i)}$$

where n_i and $M(i)$ are the amount of substance and the relative molecular mass of the species i respectively.

The weight-averaged molecular weight is more influenced by the larger molecules in the system and gives a larger value for the averaged MW than the number-averaged MW. The ratio MW_W/MW_N

gives an index of the degree of polydispersity in the system. When a polydisperse colloid is infused into the circulation, small molecules below the renal threshold (approximately 65 kDa) are rapidly excreted, while the larger molecules are retained for varying periods of time depending on their size and ease of breakdown. However, since osmotic effectiveness depends on the number of particles, and not the molecular size, the excretion of the smaller particles continuously reduces the osmotic effectiveness of the infused solution, and the retained larger particles have less osmotic action.

None of the currently unavailable colloids is ideal. Albumin has recently been criticized as leading to a higher mortality in critically ill patients [16]. The gelatins pose a considerable risk of anaphylaxis, which is significantly greater than that posed by the other colloid solutions [17]. The dextrans also represent a significant anaphylaxis risk, although the use of Dextran 1 may significantly reduce this risk, while hydroxyethyl starch (HES) solutions have the lowest risk of allergic reactions among colloids. Both the dextrans and the HES solutions significantly interfere with coagulation to varying degrees. All colloids carry some risk of inducing hyperosmolar renal failure if they are infused without adequate accompanying crystalloid, or if the hyperosmolar particles are allowed to accumulate in the circulation. This problem has been most widely described with the dextrans and HES, particularly when hyperoncotic solutions are administered.

Gelatins

The gelatins are the oldest of the synthetic colloids available and are derived from the degradation of bovine collagen with alkali. Two types of gelatins are available, the urea-linked form as typified by Haemaccel® and the succinylated form as typified by Gelofusin®.

Urea-linked gelatin consists of polypeptides linked through a urea bond giving an average MW of 35 kDa. It is suspended in a saline-based solution containing additional potassium and calcium. The high calcium concentration (approximately 6 mmol/L) makes it inadvisable to mix citrated blood in the same giving set as urea-linked gelatin as this may lead to the formation of clots in the fluid line or filter. The low MW means that it is fairly rapidly filtered through the kidneys and consequently the duration of the plasma expansion is quite limited.

The succinylated gelatins have the NH_3 groups replaced with COO^-, which gives the molecule a negative charge. This changes the shape of the molecule, opening up the coiled structure, resulting in an effectively larger molecule for the same MW [18]. Together with the negative charge, this enhances intravascular retention, despite MW of only 30 kDa. However, there is currently no published evidence that the succinylated gelatins have a longer duration of action than the older gelatins. The electrolyte content of Gelofusin® is similar to 0.9% saline, although the osmolarity is slightly lower than that of plasma, and the chloride content is lower than that of normal saline, with part of the cation content being made up of the negatively charged gelofusin particles.

The polydispersity of the gelatins results in a large number of small molecules with an intense, but short lived, plasma volume expansion lasting for 1–3 hours [18]. Consequently, the gelatins are useful plasma expanders in circumstances where a short-term increase in volume is desirable, such as during neuraxial blockade, or as an interim measure while waiting for red cell infusions to become available. The gelatins are fully cleared from the body through the kidney.

The gelatins exert little effect on coagulation, although they may impair clot strength, mainly on a dilution basis. The succinylated gelatins may have a greater effect on the von Willebrand (vWF) factor than the urea-linked type [19], but no coagulation disturbances are recognized and no volume limitation applies. The main adverse effect attributable to the gelatins is that of anaphylaxis. The risk is significantly greater for the urea-linked gelatins than the fluid gelatins, but both appear to have a higher risk of allergic reactions than other colloids. It is possible that the gelatins may be preferable to some of the starches in patients with impaired renal function, particularly in association with renal transplantation.

Dextrans

The dextrans are glucose polymers derived from the action of leuconostoc bacteria growing in sucrose-containing media. The parent, natural polymer has a mean MW of 450 kDa, and this molecule is then hydrolyzed to various smaller units. They are polydisperse colloids with a wide range of molecular sizes. There is some in vivo metabolism, but the main route of elimination is through the kidney.

There are various dextran preparations, defined by the average MW, ranging from Dextran 1 (MW 1 kDa) to the, now obsolete, Dextran 110. The dextrans generally enhance tissue plasma flow by reducing blood viscosity and by diminishing red cell aggregation and enhancing endothelial integrity. From a purely pharmacokinetic point of view, Dextran 70 may be regarded as a near-ideal volume expander because it has a long dwell time, is biodegradable, and is a good volume expander.

Dextran 40 (generally available in a 10%, hyperoncotic preparation) produces greater volume expansion than Dextran 70, but has a shorter duration of action due to the smaller mean molecular size. The smaller dextran molecules are readily filtered in the kidney where they have significant osmotic effects. The most noted adverse effect of dextrans is their ability to interfere with coagulation, largely through binding to the vWF, thus inhibiting platelet adhesion. They also impair the action of thrombin, resulting in reduced clot strength and enhanced plasmin activity. Dextrans have been used for the prevention of thromboembolism, where they are as effective as low-dose heparin [20, 21]. In addition, Dextran 40 may be beneficial in decreasing the incidence of cerebral embolism and improving the cerebral blood flow following carotid endarterectomy [22]. However, no benefit has been shown in other forms of vascular surgery.

For simple volume replacement, and for the prevention of thromboembolism, Dextran 70 is the dextran of choice, whereas Dextran 40 is used to enhance the microcirculation, particularly in free-flap surgery. Recent research has suggested that the combination of hypertonic saline and dextran may have advantages in resuscitation, particularly in patients with brain injury [23].

The dextrans have numerous adverse effects. The osmotic diuresis associated with Dextran 40, may lead to hyperosmotic renal failure. Rarely, adverse reactions including the dextran syndrome (which consists of a combination of hypotension, acute respiratory distress syndrome, anemia, and coagulopathy) and anaphylaxis may occur. Dextran anaphylaxis is a true immunoglobulin-mediated reaction for which no prior exposure is necessary, since dextrans occur in very low concentrations in the gut. However, the risk of anaphylaxis with the dextrans can be almost completely eliminated by pretreatment with the low-MW hapten compound Dextran 1. Its use is now standard practice in many European countries as a pretreatment where dextran is to be used.

Hydroxyethyl starches

The starches are a group of compounds characterized by hydroxyethyl substitution of plant-derived starch molecules. Hydroxyethylation increases the water solubility of the starch and inhibits breakdown of the starch molecule by amylase. Starches used in the manufacture of these products are derived either from waxy corn or from potato, producing compounds with somewhat different properties. Hydroxyethyl groups attach to the glucose subunits at the C2, C3, and C6 positions on the molecule. Substitution in the C2 position is the most important in terms of preventing the action of amylase and substitution seldom occurs in the C3 position. The extent of substitution may be described either by the degree of substitution, which is the ratio of glucose units containing hydroxyethyl groups to the total number of glucose units, or by the molar substitution (MS), which is the average number of hydroxyethyl groups per glucose molecule. The latter is the term that is generally used as it is easier to characterize, but in practice, the two are not greatly different.

A variety of different HES products exist with considerable differences in their pharmacological properties. HES solutions are classified according to the average in vitro MW into high MW (450–700 kDa), medium MW (100–200 kDa), and low MW (70 kDa). However, further classification is necessary as the starches undergo some metabolism in the plasma which results in changes in the MW. The rate of metabolism is determined by the extent of hydroxyethyl substitution (MS) ranging from 0.4 to 0.7 and the ratio of the carbon atom position at which the substitution occurs (C2/C6). High values for MW, MS, and C2/C6 ratio all result in a reduction in metabolic rate with a long-lasting volume effect and extended persistence within the body. Large molecules increase the incidence of bleeding complications and may be associated with an increased risk of pruritis. Since the degree of in vivo metabolism is critical, it is now more common to classify the starches by their MS ratios. The current classification is as follows:

MS ratio	Generic name	Commercial products
0.7	Hetastarch	Hespan®, Plasmasteril®, Hextend®
0.6	Hexastarch	Elohes®
0.5	Pentastarch	HAES-Steril®, Pentaspan®, Hemohes®
0.4	Tetrastarch	Voluven®, Venofundin®, Tetraspan®

The starches, therefore, are characterized by both the MW and the MS, and typical nomenclature gives both of these values; hence, Hespan® is characterized as 450/0.7 while Voluven® is characterized as 130/0.4 and Venofundin® as 130/0.42.

The lower MS of the newer HES products results in more rapid breakdown of the starch in the plasma, resulting in lower in vivo MW in the order of 70 kDa. This has resulted in substantial decreases in the major adverse effects of the HES products including impaired coagulation [24], tissue accumulation, and potential for renal dysfunction [25]. However, as the in vivo MW remains above the crucial value of 65 kDa there is minimal loss of efficacy, and tetrastarch has been shown to be as effective and to have similar duration of action as the older HES products [26].

In clinical terms, starches are characterized by effective plasma expansion that is usually more than 100% of the volume infused, a relatively long duration of action of 4–8 hours, and a possible protective effect of the endothelium. Adverse effects include interference with coagulation as a result of binding and inactivation of the factor VIII/vWF complex, tissue persistence that may result in skin itching and possible renal dysfunction that is probably the result of hyperosmolar states, rather than a direct toxic effect of the starch molecules. All of these effects appear to be related to the higher levels of MS and are of minimal importance with the tetrastarches.

Recently, potato-derived starches have been introduced that are substantially different from the waxy cornstarch product. Waxy cornstarch is almost pure amylopectin, whereas the potato starch contains a significant proportion of amylase. The potato starch also has a significant phosphate content that is not present in the waxy cornstarch product. The physical characteristics of the two starch products are different and the pharmacokinetic profiles are similar but not truly bioequivalent. Older potato starch (200/0.5) was associated with a greater bleeding risk than the equivalent cornstarch in one comparative study [27]. In another study, clinical use of potato starch 200/0.5 and 130/0.42 was associated with a postoperative increase in bilirubin in both groups [28]. A recent analysis of the cornstarch and potato starch HES preparations has demonstrated substantial differences between the products in terms of in vitro MW, MS, amylose content, and phosphate content [29]. Whether these differences are clinically important remains to be established, but at present, these HES preparations should not be regarded as being interchangeable.

HES as a group have the lowest incidence of allergic reactions of all the colloid preparations, including albumin.

Most starch products are suspended in saline, with the potential for hyperchloremic acidosis referred to above. Recently, starch solutions containing balanced salts have been introduced. These include an HES 650/0.7 available in the United States (Hextend®), and two products that have recently entered the market containing HES 130/0.4 or HES 130/0.42. The latter two products should be available internationally in the near future and may go some way to resolving the problem of hyperchloremic acidosis where large volumes of resuscitation fluid are used.

Conclusions

The crystalloid–colloid controversy is far from being resolved, and absolute recommendations regarding the choice of intravenous fluid cannot be made at this time. However, the general consensus appears to be that a balanced approach using a rational mix of crystalloid and colloid based on the condition of the patient is the best choice. In order to make such a rational choice, the pharmacological properties of each of the crystalloid and colloid solutions must be understood and considered when making clinical decisions.

References

1. Balogh Z, McKinley BA, Cocanour CS, et al. Supranormal trauma resuscitation causes more cases of abdominal compartment syndrome. Arch Surg 2003;138:637–42.
2. Ho AM, Karmakar MK, Contardi LH, Ng SS, Hewson JR. Excessive use of normal saline in managing traumatized patients in shock: a preventable contributor to acidosis. J Trauma 2001;51:173–7.
3. Reid F, Lobo DN, Williams RN, Rowlands BJ, Allison SP. (Ab)normal saline and physiological Hartmann's solution: a randomized double-blind crossover study. Clin Sci (Lond) 2003;104:17–24.
4. Leblanc M. Acid–base balance in acute renal failure and renal replacement therapy. Best Pract Res Clin Anaesthesiol 2004;18:113–22.
5. Williams EL, Hildebrand KL, McCormick SA, Bedel MJ. The effect of intravenous lactated Ringer's solution versus 0.9% sodium chloride solution on serum osmolality in human volunteers. Anesth Analg 1999;88:999–1003.
6. Hansen PB, Jensen BL, Skott O. Chloride regulates afferent arteriolar contraction in response to depolarization. Hypertension 1998;32:1066–70.
7. Lobo DN. Fluid, electrolytes and nutrition: physiological and clinical aspects. Proc Nutr Soc 2004;63: 453–66.
8. O'Malley CM, Frumento RJ, Hardy MA, et al. A randomized, double-blind comparison of lactated Ringer's solution and 0.9% NaCl during renal transplantation. Anesth Analg 2005;100:1518–24.
9. Drummond JC, Patel PM, Cole DJ, Kelly PJ. The effect of the reduction of colloid oncotic pressure, with and without reduction of osmolality, on post-traumatic cerebral edema. Anesthesiology 1998;88:993–1002.
10. Tommasino C, Moore S, Todd MM. Cerebral effects of isovolemic hemodilution with crystalloid or colloid solutions. Crit Care Med 1988;16:862–8.
11. Zornow MH, Scheller MS, Todd MM, Moore SS. Acute cerebral effects of isotonic crystalloid and colloid solutions following cryogenic brain injury in the rabbit. Anesthesiology 1988;69:180–84.
12. Brandstrup B, Tonnesen H, Beier-Holgersen R, et al. Effects of intravenous fluid restriction on postoperative complications: comparison of two perioperative fluid regimens: a randomized assessor-blinded multicenter trial. Ann Surg 2003;238:641–8.
13. Joshi GP. Intraoperative fluid restriction improves outcome after major elective gastrointestinal surgery. Anesth Analg 2005;101:601–5.
14. Cooper DJ, Myles PS, McDermott FT, et al. Prehospital hypertonic saline resuscitation of patients with hypotension and severe traumatic brain injury: a randomized controlled trial. JAMA 2004;291: 1350–57.
15. Coimbra R, Junger WG, Hoyt DB, Liu FC, Loomis WH, Evers MF. Hypertonic saline resuscitation restores hemorrhage-induced immunosuppression by decreasing prostaglandin E2 and interleukin-4 production. J Surg Res 1996;64:203–9.
16. Alderson P, Bunn F, Lefebvre C, et al. Human albumin solution for resuscitation and volume expansion in critically ill patients. Cochrane Database Syst Rev 2002;CD001208.
17. Laxenaire MC, Charpentier C, Feldman L. Anaphylactoid reactions to colloid plasma substitutes: incidence, risk factors, mechanisms. A French multicenter prospective study. Ann Fr Anesth Reanim 1994;13: 301–10.
18. Salmon JB, Mythen MG. Pharmacology and physiology of colloids. Blood Rev 1993;7:114–20.
19. de Jonge E, Levi M. Effects of different plasma substitutes on blood coagulation: a comparative review. Crit Care Med 2001;29:1261–7.
20. Bergman A, Andreen M, Blomback M. Plasma substitution with 3% dextran-60 in orthopaedic surgery: influence on plasma colloid osmotic pressure, coagulation parameters, immunoglobulins and other plasma constituents. Acta Anaesthesiol Scand 1990;34:21–9.

21. Randell T, Lindgren L, Yli HA, Hekali R, Orko R, Lalla M. The effect of dextran infusion on antithrombin III concentrations and on platelet function during minor surgery. Ann Chir Gynaecol 1996;85:17–21.
22. Lennard N, Smith J, Dumville J, et al. Prevention of postoperative thrombotic stroke after carotid endarterectomy: the role of transcranial Doppler ultrasound. J Vasc Surg 1997;26:579–84.
23. Wade CE, Grady JJ, Kramer GC. Efficacy of hypertonic saline dextran fluid resuscitation for patients with hypotension from penetrating trauma. J Trauma 2003;54:S144–8.
24. Kozek-Langenecker SA. Effects of hydroxyethyl starch solutions on hemostasis. Anesthesiology 2005;103:654–60.
25. Jungheinrich C, Neff TA. Pharmacokinetics of hydroxyethyl starch. Clin Pharmacokinet 2005;44:681–99.
26. James MF, Latoo MY, Mythen MG, et al. Plasma volume changes associated with two hydroxyethyl starch colloids following acute hypovolaemia in volunteers. Anaesthesia 2004;59:738–42.
27. Jamnicki M, Zollinger A, Seifert B, Popovic D, Pasch T, Spahn DR. The effect of potato starch derived and corn starch derived hydroxyethyl starch on in vitro blood coagulation. Anaesthesia 1998;53:638–44.
28. Sander O, Reinhart K, Meier-Hellmann A. Equivalence of hydroxyethyl starch HES 130/0.4 and HES 200/0.5 for perioperative volume replacement in major gynaecological surgery. Acta Anaesthesiol Scand 2003;47:1151–8.
29. Sommermeyer K, Cech F, Schossow R. Differences in chemical structures between waxy maize- and potato starch-based hydroxyethyl starch volume therapeutics. Transfus Altern Transfus Med 2007;9:1–7.

CHAPTER 10

Crystalloids versus Colloids: The Controversy

Hengo Haljamäe
Department of Anaesthesiology and Intensive Care, Sahlgrenska University Hospital, Göteborg, Sweden

Introduction

Fluid therapy with water and salts was first given in the 1830s for treatment of dying cholera patients and dramatic responses to the treatment were noted [1]. In spite of remarkable immediate effects of the fluid resuscitation on vital signs, the effects on outcome were less impressive at that time due to problems with electrolyte composition, tonicity, and sterility of the solutions. The importance of the electrolyte composition of crystalloids used for plasma volume support was shown by Sydney Ringer in the 1880s [2]. Further improvements of the composition of Ringer's solution were achieved in the 1920s when Alexis Hartmann could demonstrate that by the inclusion of lactate it was possible to reduce the chloride load and thereby the risk of hyperchloremic acidosis. At the same time a buffering capacity was achieved since bicarbonate is produced at the metabolic breakdown of lactate [2]. It is interesting to note that Ringer worked quite a lot with frog tissue, which explains the sodium level of about 130 mmol/L of the Ringer's solution. Today, more than 100 years later, we are still treating our patients with hyponatremic Ringer's/Harmann's type of solutions more suitable for frogs than for humans.

The use of saline fluid resuscitation in shock was initially described by the turn of the century while colloids were introduced much later [1]. Gelatin, the first artificial plasma substitute to be used clinically for shock treatment, was introduced in 1915 [3] and it was used rather extensively during World War I [4]. Gelatin was in the 1940s and 1950s followed by dextrans and later also by different hydroxyethyl starch preparations.

Increasing knowledge about disturbances in fluid homeostasis induced by trauma and blood losses was gained during the First and Second World Wars. It was, however, not until the 1940s and 1950s when, by the use of standardized animal models, the pathophysiology of hypovolemia and the physiological importance of fluid resuscitation were understood more in detail [5]. At that time it was claimed that pronounced acute internal fluid fluxes between the different compartments of the body constituted an important endogenous physiological response to trauma and hypovolemia [6–12]. It was also suggested that these internal fluid derangements had to be compensated for in order to reestablish fluid homeostasis in the posttraumatic period. Since extravascular fluids were primarily involved, infusion of crystalloids rather than of colloids was suggested by Shires and coworkers [13, 14]. The existence and importance of these so-called *third space fluid losses* advocated by Shires and coworkers have recently been questioned [15]. The evidence supporting the idea that hemorrhage or operation will cause a contraction of the extracellular volume (ECV) was considered weak, and probably a result of flawed methodology [15].

A superior relative effectiveness of colloids in comparison with crystalloids for support of plasma volume and thereby for normalization of the

Alternatives to Blood Transfusion in Transfusion Medicine, 2nd edition. Edited by A. Maniatis, P. Van der Linden, J.-F. Hardy.

hemodynamics in emergency resuscitation has, however, been acknowledged for years [16–18]. Therefore, a colloid-based fluid regimen has often been suggested as a better alternative than infusion of crystalloids in many clinical situations [16–18]. The optimal fluid regimen has, however, remained a matter of controversy and a crystalloid versus colloid debate has been going on for years and is still not satisfactorily settled.

It is obvious that intravenous infusion of an electrolyte solution results in a rather poor plasma volume supporting effect because of rapid redistribution of the solution throughout the whole extracellular fluid space [19]. This implies that for restitution of a plasma volume deficit there is a volume requirement of crystalloid far in excess of the actual intravascular volume deficit. At the fluid resuscitation a major part of the infused crystalloid is deposited in extravascular tissues whereby interstitial hydration is markedly increased [17, 18]. When more extensive volume deficits are substituted with crystalloid this interstitial deposition of fluid may include a risk of tissue edema formation, compressing capillaries and impairing microvascular blood flow. Therefore, it is not surprising that the rationale for choosing crystalloid in the clinical treatment of more extensive plasma volume deficits or perioperative blood losses may be questioned.

About 20 years ago *"An end of the crystalloid era"* was suggested by Twigley and Hillman [20]. Toward the end of 1980s as well as 1990s, however, some rather alarming reports, based on meta-analyses of published randomized studies, were published [21–23]. These meta-analyses indicated an increased risk of mortality for critically ill patients resuscitated with colloids. Although albumin was suggested the possible main cause of negative colloid-associated influences on outcome, at least in critically ill patients [23], still the discussions induced by these publications [21–23] caused a major push for increased use of crystalloids, both in the perioperative period and in the intensive care surroundings. The clinical relevance of these meta-analyses were, however, questioned and within short several papers appeared showing no difference in mortality, pulmonary edema, or hospital stay between crystalloid- and colloid-based resuscitation [24] or presence of albumin-associated outcome hazards [25].

It should be obvious, however, that the type of fluid required to correct fluid deficits and derangements will to a considerable extent depend on which fluid compartment is depleted and if more than one fluid compartment is affected [1]. Since the optimal fluid regimen in different clinical conditions has remained a matter of controversy, this survey will summarize the basic physiological concepts of crystalloid and colloid resuscitation, including the present status of the ongoing crystalloid versus colloid debate.

Fluid spaces and internal fluid fluxes in response to trauma

Fluid spaces

The fluid spaces of the body are schematically presented in Figure 10.1. Total body water in the adult usually ranges from about 50 to 65% of body weight, somewhat lower in females than in males, and there is a general decrease in body water with increasing age in the elderly. About 2/3 of the body water is found within the intracellular space, i.e., approximately 28 L in a 70 kg adult male. Most of the remaining body fluid (about 14 L) is distributed within the interstitial and intravascular spaces. The relationship between the fluid content of the intravascular and interstitial spaces is in the range of 1/4 to 1/5. The capillary membrane is freely permeable to water. Therefore, the fluid movements between the intravascular and interstitial spaces are primarily influenced by the osmotic gradients of solutes. At fluid homeostasis the osmolality of both these extracellular compartments is approximately equivalent.

The total fluid fluxes between the intra- and extravascular compartments are influenced by hydrostatic and colloid osmotic gradients as predicted by the Starling transcapillary fluid equilibrium equation. A near-equilibrium situation usually exists between several forces tending to move fluid out through the capillary membrane (mean capillary hydrostatic pressure, negative interstitial free fluid pressure, interstitial fluid colloid osmotic pressure

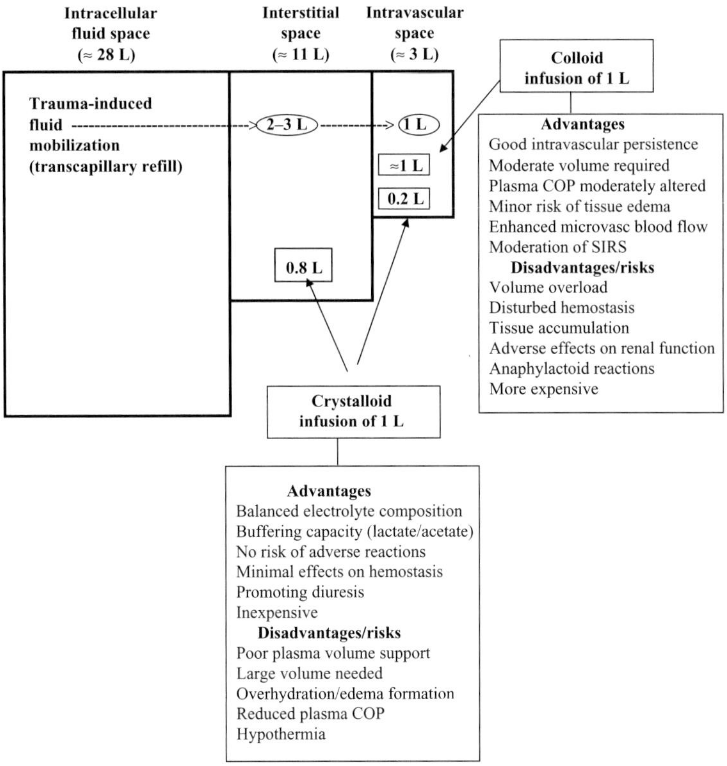

Figure 10.1 Fluid spaces, trauma induced fluid fluxes, and the effects and advantages/disadvantages of colloid- and crystalloid-based fluid resuscitation.

[COP]), and one major force tending to move fluid back into the capillary bed (plasma COP). At near-equilibrium there is a slight imbalance in favor of outward filtration, which is balanced by return of the fluid via the lymphatics. Alterations in any of these variables, including changes in capillary permeability, will change the overall balance of the fluid exchange process across the capillary membrane.

Fluid fluxes in response to surgery and trauma

The general response of the body to trauma and blood loss is a pronounced neuroendocrine activation whereby different major compensatory defense mechanisms are set into action in order to secure the perfusion and substrate availability of central vital organs [26]. In this process major internal changes of the fluid homeostasis between the different fluid spaces of the body are induced [11, 12]. In response to the neuroendocrine activation induced by trauma and/or hemorrhage about 1.0 L of fluid can be transferred in the adult individual from the intracellular and interstitial spaces into the intravascular compartment (Figure 10.1). The main components of this endogenous plasma volume supporting defense mechanism are:

• A glucose-osmotic transcapillary refill process [11, 12].

In response to the hyperglycemia induced by the trauma, plasma osmolality will increase and about 2–3 L of fluid can be mobilized along the osmotic gradient from the intracellular compartment into the interstitial fluid space. Of this fluid about 0.5 L will reach the intravascular compartment and support blood volume. Trauma-induced insulin resistance will contribute to the maintenance of the hyperglycemia and thereby increase the efficacy and duration of this glucose-osmotic transcapillary refill process.

• A resetting of the pre- to postcapillary resistance ratio [11, 12].

The capillary hydrostatic pressure is reduced due to precapillary vascular constriction in response to the neuroendocrine activation induced by trauma and/or hemorrhage. Thereby, the equilibrium of the Starling transcapillary exchange process is changed so that fluid reabsorption from extravascular sources is favored. In the adult individual about 0.5 L of fluid can be mobilized by this compensatory mechanism from the interstitial fluid space into the intravascular compartment.

In addition to direct losses of blood and plasma in connection with surgical procedures or following trauma, there is an increased overall transcapillary fluid loss resultant from increased trauma-induced activation of the cascade systems evoking a systemic inflammatory response syndrome (SIRS) influencing endothelial cell barrier function and thereby capillary permeability [27]. This more generalized increase of capillary permeability in response to trauma will further enhance the hypovolemia and jeopardize tissue perfusion [28].

Shires and coworkers [6, 7] have suggested a reduction of the extracellular fluid volume during major surgery and following trauma due to internal redistribution of fluid into traumatized tissues (wound edema) and into organs, the function of which is disturbed (e.g., paralytic intestine). Such fluid movements were considered to constitute so-called *third space losses*. The occurrence and clinical significance of possible internal *third space losses* has remained unclear [1]. Trauma is often considered associated with a relative increase rather than a reduction in extracellular fluid content. A relative increase in the interstitial fluid content is explained by stress-induced salt and water retention, as well as the above-discussed mobilization of intracellular fluid into the extracellular fluid space. Recently the existence and importance of these so-called *third space fluid losses* advocated by Shires and coworkers have been seriously questioned by Brandstrup and coworkers [15]. On the basis of a systematic review of original trials measuring ECV changes during hemorrhage or operation it was considered that the evidence supporting the idea that these conditions will cause a contraction of the ECV was weak, and probably a result of flawed methodology [15]. It seems obvious, however, that in order to achieve normovolemia and hemodynamic stability and reestablish fluid homeostasis in surgical patients or trauma victims, it is necessary at the fluid resuscitation not only to consider direct blood losses but also to take the internal compensatory fluid fluxes into consideration [12, 17, 18].

Distribution of infused resuscitation fluids

The relative distribution of crystalloids and colloids between the different fluid spaces of the body and the advantages and disadvantages of crystalloid- versus colloid-based fluid resuscitation regimes are summarized in Figure 10.1. As indicated in the figure, the plasma volume support achieved at the infusion of a colloid is usually good while the more prolonged plasma volume-supporting efficacy of crystalloids is poor [17, 18].

Crystalloids

General aspects

Crystalloid resuscitation fluids usually have a balanced electrolyte composition since infusion of a rather large volume is needed for restoration of hemodynamic stability in hypovolemic patients (Figure 10.1). Infusion of large volume of saline (154 mmol/L of sodium and chloride) will include a risk of hyperchloremic acidosis negatively affecting acid–base status, hemostasis, and renal perfusion [29–32]. Predominant use of 0.9% saline solution in major surgery may have little impact on outcome as assessed by duration of mechanical ventilation, intensive care unit stay, hospital stay, and postoperative complications, but it does appear to be associated with increased perioperative blood loss [32]. Although hyperchloremic metabolic acidosis and a hypocoagulable state may not necessarily harm the patient, still metabolic acidosis is not observed after administration of lactated Ringer's type of solutions [30, 32]. The use of fluids with a balanced electrolyte composition and "buffering capacity", i.e., Ringer's type of solutions containing either lactate or acetate therefore seems advantageous [18]. When the lactate or acetate ions are metabolized by tissue cells, bicarbonate ions will be produced and a buffer effect is achieved. Acetate-containing Ringer's solutions seem even more advantageous than lactate containing ones since the capacity of the body to metabolize lactate may be reduced in case of disturbed organ perfusion, as seen in the connection with shock and trauma [18, 33, 34]. Therefore, a lactate containing solution may even aggravate an already existing lactic acidosis since the metabolic capacity of the two main lactate-clearing organs, i.e., the liver and the kidney, is disturbed in severe shock. Acetate, on the other hand, can be metabolized by most tissue cells of the body and therefore includes advantages in case of compromised liver function [35].

Additional advantages of Ringer's type of crystalloids are: absence of adverse anaphylactoid reactions, minimal influences on hemostasis other than those caused by the hemodilution per se, and diuresis promoting effects (Figure 10.1). Thromboelastographic studies indicate mild hypercoagulability induced by crystalloids but the effect is similar for saline as for Ringer's solution [36, 37]. The low cost of crystalloids as compared to colloids is often also considered advantageous.

Distribution between the different fluid spaces

Balanced salt solutions will freely cross capillary membranes and equilibrate within the whole extracellular fluid space. The intravascular retention of a crystalloid is consequently poor and it is usually considered that in connection with blood losses a large volume, i.e., 4–5 times the actual intravascular volume deficit, has to be infused in order to achieve normovolemia [17–19]. In surgical patients it has been shown by Lamke and Liljedahl [19] that infusion of 1 L of crystalloid in the postoperative period will result in a remaining plasma volume expansion of only about 0.2 L after an equilibration period of 90 minutes. Cervera and Moss [38] have also pointed out that crystalloid resuscitation of hemorrhage for reexpansion of the lost plasma volume may require much larger volumes than appreciated by most clinicians.

It has been claimed by Riddez and coworkers [39], however, that for optimal volume substitution following acute hypovolemia, infusion of a much smaller volume of Ringer's solution may be sufficient. In their study young volunteers were subjected to acute moderate venesection, i.e., withdrawal of 900 mL of blood. It was noted that these young individuals were able to restore up to 50% of the blood loss by internal shift of fluid from extravascular sources into the intravascular compartment, as expected on the basis of the above-considered transcapillary refill process. On the basis of these observations it was suggested that infusion of Ringer's solution corresponding to about twice the lost volume was sufficient for restitution of central and regional hemodynamics. Young individuals subjected only to withdrawal of blood and not exposed to any tissue injury and/or anesthesia may not be representative for the average surgical or trauma patient population seen in the clinics. However, the SAFE (Saline vs Albumin Fluid Evaluation) study [40] showed that on an average only 1.4 times more saline than 4% albumin was needed to cope with the fluid requirements of intensive care patients. It should be noted, however, that the initial fluid resuscitation of the ICU patients was not included so the fluid administered was for satisfaction of the basal fluid requirements and the maintenance of hemodynamic stability during the ICU stay. Still, the observations of the SAFE study seem to favor a more restrictive administration of crystalloids than the traditional concept of infusion of 3–5 times the estimated plasma volume deficit. A perioperative intravenous fluid restriction was by Brandstrup et al. [41, 42] suggested to reduce complications after elective colorectal resection and such a more restrictive fluid therapy concept has recently been supported by others [43, 44]. Consequently it seems justified, on the basis of current best clinical evidence suggestions, to recommend the principle of a more "restricted intravenous fluid therapy." The concept basically means that fluid losses should be replaced but crystalloid fluid overload should be avoided.

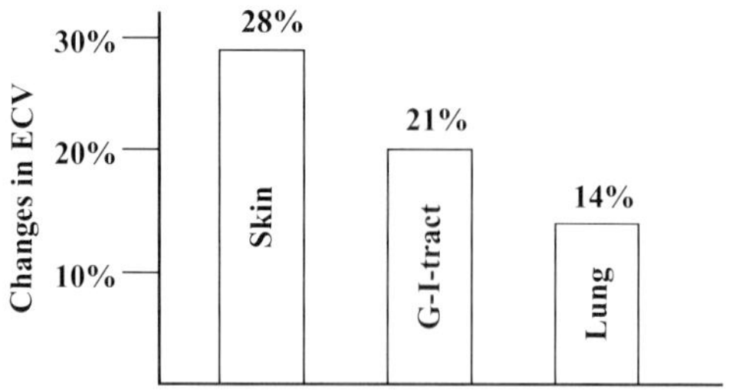

Figure 10.2 An experimental study of the effects of a massive intravenous isotonic fluid load (5% of body weight; corresponding to infusion of 3.5 L in a 70 kg man) on the extravascular fluid content of different tissues. Data from Larsson and Ware [46].

Crystalloid-associated disadvantages/risks

After a rather short time period 75–80% of the infused volume of a crystalloid will lodge in the extravascular compartments [17, 18, 45]. Therefore, it is obvious that crystalloid resuscitation includes a risk of increased tissue hydration and edema formation (Figure 10.1). Quite often it is thought that the edema formation caused by excessive crystalloid infusion is mainly a cosmetic problem affecting peripheral tissues. An experimental study of the effects of a massive intravenous isotonic fluid load (5% of body weight; corresponding to infusion of 3.5 L in a 70 kg man) on the extravascular fluid content of different tissues has also verified that fluid will accumulate mainly in tissues with a high compliance such as skin and connective tissue [46]. However, the crystalloid load was found also to increase the fluid content of more vital organs, e.g., the lungs and the intestine (Figure 10.2).

Extravascular lung water: In the lungs a reduction of the COP in response to crystalloid resuscitation will influence the threshold hydrostatic capillary pressure at which pulmonary fluid overload will occur [17, 47]. The hydrostatic gradient (difference between the pulmonary capillary and the tissue fluid pressures) tends to push fluid out of the vasculature. However, it is counteracted by the high COP gradient between plasma and tissue fluid favoring retention of fluid within the vascular compartment. This oncotic gradient, however, is dependent on the ability of the capillary membrane to reflect substances that are colloid-osmotically active, i.e., to prevent leakage of colloidal substances out of the vascular compartment into the interstitial fluid space.

Major causes for increased extravascular lung water are increases in the hydrostatic gradient across the pulmonary capillary during fluid resuscitation and increases in the protein permeability of the capillary membrane due to systemic activation of the cascade systems influencing endothelial cell barrier function. The maintenance of a gradient of 7–9 mmHg between plasma COP and cardiac filling pressure has been suggested to be of importance for prevention of pulmonary edema [48]. However, there are several important antiedema safety factors, which will prevent moderate changes in capillary hydrostatic pressure from influencing the extravascular fluid content of the lung [49]. One component of this physiological defense mechanism is the increase in interstitial pressure that is initially created by an increased fluid filtration. Thereby the hydrostatic pressure gradient across the pulmonary capillary is shifted back toward the normal level and further fluid movement is prevented. Increased fluid filtration will also influence the COP gradient by diluting the protein content of the extravascular fluid. Such a reduction of the interstitial COP will oppose fluid-flux by widening the colloid osmotic gradient across the pulmonary capillary bed.

Although the above-considered antiedema safety factors are of importance in the early phase of increased pulmonary capillary hydrostatic pressure, the most important edema preventive factor is the capacity of the lung to increase its lymph flow. From basal levels lung lymph flow can increase several fold, up to 7–10 times [50]. Therefore, as long as the lymph drainage of the lung can clear the amount of fluid that is filtered across the pulmonary capillary, no manifest clinical pulmonary edema will occur. This may explain why crystalloid treatment of hypovolemia in many situations does not seem to increase extravascular lung water to any significant extent [51–55]. Still, infusion of 40 mL/kg body weight over a 3-hour period in healthy volunteers has been shown to result in a significant decrease in pulmonary function and a body weight increase persisting 24 hours after the infusion [56]. The occurrence of hypoxemic episodes of patients in a postanesthesia care unit also seems associated with intraoperative infusion of greater volumes (>1500 mL) of intravenous fluid [57]. Excessive perioperative fluid administration resulting in major net fluid retension has been shown to include even a risk of fatal postoperative pulmonary edema [58]. Furthermore, resuscitation with crystalloids has been suggested to predispose for pulmonary dysfunction in case of later major challenges of the homeostatic balance [59]. Especially in elderly patients with reduced functional capacity of vital organs, including the cardiovascular and respiratory systems, crystalloid fluid overload may disturb the recovery process after surgery and trauma. Late adverse effects after an initial resuscitation with large quantities of fluid, seen as a "third-day" transient circulatory overload, may in addition occur due to the subsequent redistribution of the tissue edema [60]. Therefore, it seems likely that in several clinical situations the functional respiratory capacity may be disturbed by infusion of a large volume of crystalloid resuscitation fluids. The risk seems more pronounced in connection with lung surgery than other types of surgical procedures [61].

Peripheral tissue edema: A crystalloid-based treatment regime of profound hypovolemia may initially restore cardiac output during the fluid resuscitation but, due to rapid leakage of fluid out into the extravascular tissues, may be insufficient for the maintenance of an adequate intravascular volume support [62]. Laser doppler flowmetric studies have demonstrated a persistent depression of the microvascular blood flow following hemorrhage in spite of infusion of Ringer's lactate up to four times the volume of maximal bleeding [63]. It seems obvious that crystalloid fluid resuscitation includes a risk of edema formation in peripheral tissues, which by compression of capillaries, may jeopardize microvascular blood flow and thereby also tissue oxygenation [64–67]. Generalized edema may consequently disturb the transport of oxygen and nutrients to tissue cells and thereby contribute to the development of multiple organ failure.

Iatrogenic tissue edema caused by crystalloid resuscitation is reflected by a significant weight gain and has been considered to result in prolonged need of respirator treatment, impaired wound healing, and prolonged ICU-stay [66, 67]. Also regain of gastrointestinal function following surgery or trauma resuscitation seems influenced by the fluid treatment strategy chosen. A postoperative increase in body weight of more than 3 kg has been shown to delay regain of gastrointestinal function (passage of flatus and feces) and thereby also prolonging hospital stay and cost of surgery [68]. Studies of liberal versus restrictive perioperative infusion of crystalloid indicate that the main cause for delayed regain of gastrointestinal function and prolonged hospital stay is liberal administration of fluid [43]. Liberal fluid strategies in gastrointestinal surgery have repeatedly been suggested to impair clinical outcome [41, 43, 44].

The association between excessive crystalloid fluid resuscitation and major problems within the gastrointestinal tract is also obvious from the experiences at the management of trauma patients. The pressure within the abdominal cavity is normally little more than atmospheric pressure but even small increases in intra-abdominal pressure can induce adverse effects on renal function, cardiac output, hepatic blood flow, respiratory mechanics, splanchnic perfusion, and intracranial pressure [69–71]. Massive fluid resuscitation may consequently not only induce hypothermia leading to coagulopathy but also include a risk of abdominal hypertension and abdominal compartment syndrome [72]. An association between massive fluid resuscitation and abdominal compartment syndrome seems obvious [72, 73] and excessive use of crystalloids seems to be the primary determinant [74]. Consequently, supranormal trauma resuscitation requiring more Ringer's solution infusion seems associated with decreased intestinal perfusion (higher GAP CO_2), and increased incidence of intra-abdominal hypertension, abdominal compartment syndrome, multiple organ failure, and death [75].

Most of the extravasating crystalloid will distribute within the interstitial space but some will probably leak into hypoxic or traumatized cells in connection with surgery or trauma, i.e., into cells with a reduced functional capacity to regulate their membrane electrolyte balance and hence their volume [28]. Therefore, the problem of extravascular fluid accumulation after crystalloid volume loading seems even more critical for trauma patients suffering head injuries [76] and edema formation may occur even in the heart following massive crystalloid resuscitation [77].

It seems evident that nowadays there is an increased awareness of the clinical problems caused by fluid overload and, as stated by Lowell et al. [78] almost 20 years ago, "fluid overload is not a benign problem." Fluid administration routines resulting in negative fluid balance in septic shock patients has been claimed to predict good outcome prognosis and survival [79].

Colloids

General aspects

The advantages and disadvantages of colloid-based fluid resuscitation are summarized in Figure 10.1. Colloid solutions contain, to varying degrees, larger, oncotically active molecules, which do not easily cross the capillary membrane. The greater capacity of colloids to remain within the intravascular space includes not only a more efficient expansion of the intravascular plasma volume but also a better maintenance of plasma COP. Therefore, the addition of colloid, even in low concentrations, will markedly reduce the overall fluid volume requirements for achievement of hemodynamic stability in the treatment of hypovolemia [80–82]. Infusion of only a rather moderate volume is usually needed and therefore the risk of fluid overload of extravascular tissues, as seen in connection with only crystalloid-based fluid resuscitation, is reduced.

Plasma volume supporting efficacy

The overall plasma volume-expanding efficacy of a colloid solution is dependent on the size and concentration of its colloid-osmotically active molecules and their intravascular persistence [82]. The COP of a colloid is the major factor influencing its initial plasma volume expanding capacity. Intravenous infusion of colloids with a COP lower than or equal to that of plasma will even at high infusion rates result in a mainly isovolemic initial plasma volume expansion. Colloids with a high COP, on the other hand, will mobilize fluid from extravascular sources into the vascular compartment along the created COP gradient. Rapid infusion of colloids with a high COP may consequently include a risk of acute intravascular volume overload [82].

The more prolonged plasma volume supporting capacity of a colloid is determined by the numbers, sizes, and configurations of the molecules in the suspension and the breakdown and elimination characteristics for the substance [82]. It has repeatedly been claimed that infusion of colloid will improve the oxygen transport to tissues and thereby favor aerobic tissue metabolism better than crystalloid fluid resuscitation [67, 82, 83]. This may be explained by favorable hemorheological effects of colloids. In patients undergoing major abdominal surgery a colloid-based volume replacement regimen has been shown to increase tissue oxygen tension while crystalloids were found to impair tissue oxygenation [84].

Hemorheological effects

The rheological behavior of blood is altered in many clinical situations and hemorheological aspects are important to consider at the choice of resuscitation fluid. The hemorheological effectiveness of a colloid is determined by its hemodilutional capacity in combination with its inherent specific pharmacological effects on red cell aggregation, platelet function, plasma viscosity, and blood corpuscle–endothelial cell interactions [82].

The reduction of the hematocrit level of the blood at the hemodilution seems to be the most important determinant for the rheologic effects and thereby for enhancement of tissue perfusion and oxygenation. Vascular resistance is reduced by lowered whole blood viscosity, which will enhance venous return and increase cardiac output [85–87]. In comparison with the dominating role played by the hemodilution per se changes in plasma viscosity seem to be of minor importance for alterations of tissue perfusion [88, 89]. Colloid-associated reduction of red blood cell aggregation and leukocyte–endothelium interactions may be additional factors of importance for the enhancement of blood flow in the microvasculature [82,90,91]. Thereby the potential activation of a SIRS by surgery or trauma will be moderated and the risk of multiple organ dysfunction syndrome may be reduced (Figure 10.1).

Colloid-associated disadvantages/risks

In addition to the risk of volume overload at extensive fluid resuscitation with colloids, several of the available artificial colloids will influence the hemostatic competence of the body [29,92]. The effects on hemostasis are partly due to hemodilution, resulting in decreased concentrations of coagulation factors, and partly to colloid-specific effects on the clotting of blood. Dextrans seem to reduce the hemostatic competence more than hydroxyethyl starch preparations and gelatins [29, 82]. As recently pointed out by Van der Linden and Ickx [93] the clinical consequences of the biological effects of colloids on hemostasis are limited, provided that safety considerations are observed (maximum daily dosage, duration of treatment, patient's hemostatic status, clinical conditions). The implications may be different in patients with hemostatic disorders, either inherited or related to preoperative antiplatelet or anticoagulant treatment. The total volume of fluid infused, crystalloid as well as colloid, also seems to be a factor of importance. Barak et al. [94] reported that administration of more than 3 L of crystalloids or 500 mL of colloids during abdominal surgery correlated with postoperative coagulopathy.

Colloid-associated factors such as tissue accumulation, potential adverse effects on renal function, and risk of anaphylactoid reactions are also of importance, as is the cost factor (Figure 10.1)[29]. Considering the above-mentioned pros and cons of colloid-based fluid resuscitation, it seems obvious that at the choice of colloid the following aspects should be considered:

- Plasma volume supporting capacity
  - size, concentration, and elimination characteristics of the macromolecules
- Clinical safety
  - minimal effects on hemostasis
  - complete elimination/no tissue accumulation
  - absence of adverse effects on organ function
  - no risk of allergic/anaphylactoid reactions

Therapeutic goals of clinical fluid resuscitation

It is obvious that colloids and crystalloids, due to their specific fluid characteristics, are distributed differently within the fluid spaces of the body. Since colloids are distributed mainly to the intravascular space and crystalloids to the interstitial space, the decision to use colloid or crystalloid solution should depend to a considerable extent on whether the intravascular or the interstitial space is depleted [1]. The intravascular space is the more accessible one to clinical estimation of its fluid status. Cardiac output, arterial blood pressure, pulse rate, central venous pressure, pulmonary artery wedge pressure, peripheral tissue perfusion, and urine output are all indicators contributing to the assessment of the adequacy of the intravascular blood volume. The response of these variables may also be considered to be of value in conjunction with a fluid challenge. A challenge with colloid, mainly staying in the circulation, is much easier to interpret than a challenge with crystalloid, which to a considerable extent relatively rapidly is redistributed to the extravascular space [1].

Appropriate goals for the fluid resuscitation in connection with surgical procedures or in the treatment of critically ill patients and the optimal choice of fluid to reach the goals can be summarized as follows [18,82]:

- Provide daily basal fluid requirements (crystalloid)
- Rehydrate fluid deficient patients (crystalloid)
- Maintain normovolemia and hemodynamic stability (colloid)
- Enhance microvascular blood flow (colloid)
- Maintain adequate plasma COP (colloid)
- Avoid tissue edema formation (colloid)
- Prevent/moderate trauma-induced activation of cascade systems and enhancement of coagulation (colloid)
- Prevent reperfusion type of cell injury caused by generation of free radicals (colloid)

- Guarantee adequate transport of oxygen to tissue cells (colloid + RBCs)
- Promote diuresis (colloid + crystalloid)

In order to achieve all these clinical goals of fluid resuscitation the use of both crystalloids and colloids seems indicated. However, as indicated in the above summary, colloids seem to play a more important role in not only the maintenance of central hemodynamic stability and microvascular blood flow but also the moderation of trauma induced inflammatory reactions [82]. In spite of quite a bit of evidence in favor of colloids, a crystalloid versus colloid controversy has continued and, as discussed below, presently there does not seem to exist any generally accepted consensus on the optimal fluid therapy in different clinical situations [20–25, 40, 44, 95–97].

Choice of fluid regimen and clinical outcome

Major surgery

In most situations about 60–80% of infused crystalloids will leave the intravascular compartment before the end of the infusion, i.e., within a rather limited time period [18–20]. The correction of the intravascular hypovolemia with a moderate volume of crystalloid is in most cases therefore rather insufficient. Even minor remaining degrees of hypovolemia can predispose to insufficient organ perfusion. The splanchnic circulation may be critically affected and a decrease in splanchnic blood flow may occur even after a brief episode of normotensive hypovolemia [98, 99]. Infusion of too large volumes of crystalloid solution, on the other hand, will lead to interstitial sequestration of fluid and tissue edema that will impair tissue oxygenation and organ function. It has been suggested on the basis of systematic reviews (meta-analyses) of randomized controlled studies that colloid administration, at least for critical ill patients, may rather increase than reduce mortality [21–23]. However, data related to major surgery included in these meta-analyses were rather in favor of colloid-based perioperative fluid regimes [21–23].

The studies by Lobo et al. [68] and Nisanevich et al. [43] clearly indicate that perioperative increase in body weight due to excessive infusion of fluid will delay regain of postoperative gastrointestinal function and thereby prolong hospital stay and the cost of the surgical care. Preoperative as well as intraoperative expansion of plasma volume with colloid has been shown to reduce mucosal hypoperfusion and improve outcome [99, 100]. In the study of Moretti et al. [101] it was found that postoperative nausea and emesis was much more common in patients receiving only crystalloid as compared with patients given a balanced fluid resuscitation also including colloid. Still, the difference in total amount of fluid infused was only about 1.5 L. A reasonable explanation for the difference in the occurrence of nausea and emesis could be increased fluid content (edema) of the GI tract influencing GI function in the patients not getting colloid. Furthermore, the inclusion of colloid also reduced postoperative pain experiences, tissue edema, and incidence of dubble vision [101]. The findings clearly indicate that the choice of fluid therapy will influence "the quality of care" for the surgical patient. On the basis of the above-considered studies in Figure 10.3, suggested intraoperative fluid treatment strategy seems advantageous [44, 102].

The main arguments in favor of the concepts presented in Figure 10.3 are:

1 Prior to surgery the patient is usually subjected to a period of fluid restriction and the basal fluid requirements of the patient have to be satisfied. Therefore, start with a crystalloid (1 L) since compensation of the dehydration may improve symptoms related to preoperative dehydration [103]. Prefer balanced (Ringer's type) crystalloid to avoid effects on acid–base balance (hyperchloremic metabolic acidosis), hemostasis, and renal perfusion [29, 30, 32].

2 In case of epidural anesthesia (EDA) or spinal anesthesia (SPA) do not volume preload with crystalloid but rather use vasoconstrictors to prevent hypotension caused by venous pooling [44, 102]. For volume loading with crystalloid large volume is needed which may include a risk of tissue edema impairing nutritional blood flow. Furthermore, fluid (water) overload may occur once the

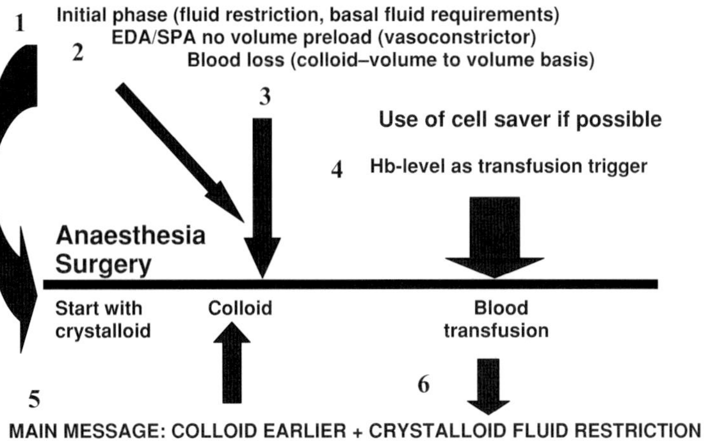

Figure 10.3 Suggested best strategy for fluid resuscitation in major surgery [44, 102]. For details see text.

sympathetic block has regressed. If volume support for some reasons is considered a better choice for the patient than vasoconstrictors—choose colloid [44, 102].

3 Do not substitute blood loss with crystalloid but use colloid on a volume-to-volume basis. For blood salvage use cell saver whenever possible.

4 The optimal hemoglobin trigger level for blood transfusion has to be determined individually for each surgical patient. The lowest safe limit or "transfusion trigger" for surgical patients approximates hemoglobin and hematocrit levels of 7.0 g/dL and 21%, respectively. Some patient subsets, such as elderly patients suffering from complicating medical disorders, appear to have better outcomes when a hematocrit level of 30–33% and hemoglobin of about 10 g/dL are aimed at [104].

5 The main message for fluid therapy is *use colloid earlier*. . .and . . . .

6 *Restrict the infusion of crystalloid* so that perioperative weight increase can be maintained at level <4% of body weight [41, 44, 68].

The above aspects have in a recent survey been supported by Joshi [44] suggesting the following clinically useful guidelines:

• Avoid deep general anesthesia
• Eliminate preload for EDA patients
• Use balanced approach to fluid management with colloids to provide hemodynamic stability and maintain urine output of 0.5 mL $\times$ kg^{-1} $\times$ h^{-1}
• Crystalloids only for maintenance
• Blood loss replaced with colloid on a volume-to-volume basis
• Replacements of *third space losses* and losses through diuresis are unnecessary.

An all too restrictive ("dry") perioperative fluid therapy, as suggested by Brandstrup et al. [41, 42], however, has been questioned. Although the basic concept is that fluid lost should be replaced and fluid overload should be avoided [42], still a somewhat more liberal but balanced strategy, including crystalloid as well colloid, has by Holte et al. [105, 106], been considered more advantageous. Fluid optimization by proper monitoring of the physiological effects of the fluid therapy given may be more important than the choice of fluid for the clinical outcome [97]. Goal-directed intraoperative fluid administration has been reported to result in earlier return to bowel function, lower incidence of postoperative nausea and vomiting, and decrease in length of postoperative hospital stay [107]. Proper intraoperative monitoring and fluid challenge has been shown as advantageous also for patients with hip fracture by shortening the duration of hospital stay [108]. Postoperative restriction of fluid and sodium may not have a similar impact as intraoperative moderation of fluid therapy on postoperative recovery and hospital stay [109].

Recent reviews, often including meta-analytic data assessments, do not provide any conclusive evidence of the most optimal strategy for perioperative fluid management of patients undergoing major surgical procedures [24, 97, 105, 106, 110]. As recently commented by Boldt [111] the ongoing debate on fluid management of surgical patients may arise more questions than answers. Conclusive data on definite advantages of a "dry approach" to fluid management of surgical patients are not available but still the advantages of "a more restrictive intravenous fluid therapy policy" are often stressed [42, 112]. The concept of an optimal fluid therapy approach in major surgery seems to be avoidance of fluid overload by replacing only the fluids lost during surgery and by early inclusion of colloid for plasma volume support. At the choice of colloid the advantages and disadvantages of the different available colloids should be taken into account [29, 82]. Furthermore, in case of major surgery the perioperative fluid administration should be monitored and individualized goals for the fluid administration should be set [97, 107, 108, 113].

Intensive care

Crystalloids or colloids

Clinical outcome data on mortality of different meta-analytic comparisons published in the late 1990s [21–23] suggested that crystalloids may be the superior alternative in the treatment of critically ill patients with increased capillary permeability. Original publications included in these meta-analyses [19–22] cover a time period of about 25 years. During this long time period many basic clinical therapeutic procedures, in addition to the choice of fluid regimen, have changed considerably and do not reflect present practice. Subsequent meta-analyses [24, 25] taking such aspects into consideration and the extensive clinical SAFE studies [40], including almost 7000 intensive care patients, could not verify critical differences in clinical outcome between colloid and crystalloid-based fluid resuscitation regimes. However, colloids are in general more effective than crystalloids for optimizing physiological variables related to flow in critically ill patients and for maintaining an adequate delivery of oxygen to tissue cells. The clinical experience reported by Rackow et al. [114] almost 25 years ago was that by colloid-based fluid resuscitation hemodynamic stability was obtained at infusion of much less fluid than if crystalloid was chosen. The larger crystalloid fluid load was at the same time found to increase the incidence of pulmonary edema considerably. The association between crystalloid fluid load and increased pulmonary edema is obvious in many studies but may not necessarily affect long-term outcome (survival) [115–117].

Questionnaire-based assessments of the routines of fluid resuscitation used in the ICUs have indicated that there are major national [118] as well as international differences [119, 120]. The data of the CRYCO Study Group [120] indicate that in Europa a combination of colloid and crystalloid is most commonly used for critically ill patients and that starches are the most widely used colloids while the use of albumin is declining. Although decreased survival in acutely ill patients given albumin has been suggested in subgroups of acutely ill patients [121], still the clinical value of albumin in the treatment of ICU patients is being reevaluated [122–124]. Alderson et al. [125] still claims that for patients with hypovolemia there is no evidence that albumin reduces mortality when compared with cheaper alternatives, but at the same time it is commented that there is a possibility that for highly selected populations of critically ill patients albumin may be indicated. Data showing that albumin administration may improve organ function in hypoalbuminemic critically ill patients have recently been presented [126]. Furthermore, long-term albumin infusion seems to improve survival of patients with cirrhosis and ascites [127]. Use of albumin in resuscitation of burn patients may even reduce the likelihood of mortality [128]. Therefore, considering the above-commented more recent studies it seems obvious that the use of albumin in different ICU settings is beneficial in influencing morbidity as well as mortality. However, it is becoming more and more obvious considering rational use of colloids that synthetic colloids may be superior to albumin especially in patients with increased capillary permeability [129–133].

Fluid resuscitation practice in the ICU

Important factors to consider at fluid resuscitation of critically ill patients are:

- Timing of fluid resuscitation—tissue hypoperfusion should be avoided by fluid administration whenever hypovolemia is suspected.
- Choice of fluid—avoid saline excess (risk of hyperchloremic metabolic acidosis) by using balanced (Ringer's type of solutions) and avoid crystalloid fluid overload (tissue edema) by addition of colloid at an early phase of the resuscitation efforts.
- Rate of fluid administration and monitoring of the response to the infusion—the response to the fluid administration should be monitored as closely as possible, preferably by evaluation of the stroke volume response to the fluid infusion, and when in doubt—use fluid challenge (colloid bolus) to evaluate optimal cardiac response to the fluid resuscitation.
- Endpoints for the resuscitation—for optimal safety individualized endpoints for the resuscitation should be defined.
- Assessment of tissue perfusion—monitoring of blood (base excess, lactate levels) or direct tissue variables (tissue oxygen tension, tonometry, CO_2 gap, microdialysis) to be able to optimize the fluid resuscitation.

Conclusions

The crystalloid versus colloid controversy in the treatment of surgical and critically ill patients seems in favor of a balanced fluid therapy strategy on the basis of administration of crystalloid as well as colloid. The following aspects should be considered:

- Fluid therapy should be based on the specific needs of each individual patient.
- Crystalloids are needed to satisfy basal fluid requirements and for correction of extravasacular fluid derangements.
- At the choice of crystalloid use balanced (Ringer's type of solutions) rather than saline.
- Infusion of large volume of crystalloids for correction of major intravascular volume deficit includes a risk of tissue edema and organ dysfunction.
- Colloids are in most situations to be preferred when the main indication is to increase intravascular volume.
- At the choice of colloid consider the plasma volume supporting capacity, and the hemorheological effects, the anti-inflammatory potential, the elimination characteristics, and the clinical safety of the colloid.
- Favor a balanced fluid treatment strategy including crystalloids and colloids for surgical as well as for intensive care patients.
- Use well-defined individual endpoints for the monitoring of the fluid therapy.

References

1. Hillman K, Bishop G, Bristow P. The crystalloid versus colloid controversy: present status. Baillière's Clin Anaestesiol 1997;11:1.
2. Lee JA. Sydney Ringer (1834–1910) and Alexis Hartmann (1898–1964). Anaesthesia 1981;36:1115.
3. Hogan JJ. The intravenous use of colloidal (gelatin) solutions in shock. JAMA 1915;64:721.
4. Richter W, Hedin H. Solutions and emulsions used for intravenous infusions. Handbook Exp Pharmacol 1983;63:581.
5. Wiggers CJ. *Physiology of Shock*. The Commonwealth Fund, New York 1950.
6. Shires GT, Brown FT, Canizaro PC, Sommerville N. Distributional changes in extracellular fluid during acute hemorrhagic shock. Surg Forum 1960;11:115.
7. Shires GT, Williams J, Brown F. Acute changes in extracellular fluids associated with major surgical procedures. Ann Surg 1961;154:803.
8. Gutelius JR, Shizgal HM, Lopez G. The effect of trauma on extracellular water volume. Arch Surg 1968;97:206.
9. Reid DJ. Intracellular and extracellular fluid volume during surgery. Br J Surg 1968;55:594.
10. Järhult J. Osmotic fluid transfer from tissue to blood during hemorrhagic hypotension. Acta Physiol Scand 1973;89:213.
11. Drucker WR, Chadwick CDJ, Gann DS. Transcapillary refill in hemorrhage and shock. Arch Surg 1981;116:1344.
12. Haljamäe H. Interstitial fluid response. Clin Surg Internat 1984;9:44.
13. Shires GT, Canizaro PC. Fluid resuscitation in the severly injured. Surg Clin N Am 1973;53:1341.

14. Shires GT. Pathophysiology and fluid replacement in hypovolaemic shock. Ann Clin Res 1977;9:144.
15. Brandstrup B, Svensen C, Engquist A. Hemorrhage and operation cause a contraction of the extracellular space needing replacement- evidence and implications? A systematic review. Surgery 2006;139:419.
16. Shoemaker WC, Schluchter M, Hopkins JA, Appel PL, Schwartz S, Chang PC. Comparison of the relative effectiveness of colloids and crystalloids in emergency resuscitation. Am J Surg 1981; 142:73.
17. Haljamäe H. Rational for the use of colloids in the treatment of shock and hypovolemia. Acta Physiol Scand 1985;29(Suppl. 82): 48.
18. Haljamäe H. Use of fluids in trauma. Int J Intensive Care 1999;6:20.
19. Lamke LO, Liljedahl SO. Plasma volume changes after infusion of various plasma expanders. Resuscitation 1976;5:93.
20. Twigley AJ, Hillman KM. The end of the crystalloid era? A new approach to perioperative fluid administration. Anaesthesia 1985;40:860.
21. Velanovich V. Crystalloid versus colloid fluid resuscitation: a meta-analysis of mortality. Surgery 1989;105:65.
22. Schierhout G, Roberts I. Fluid resuscitation with colloid or crystalloid solutions in critically ill patients: a systematic review of randomised trials. BMJ 1998;316:961.
23. Cochrane Injuries Group Albumin Reviewers. Human albumin administration in critically ill patients: systemic review of randomised controlled trials. BMJ 1998;317:235.
24. Choi PT, Yip G, Quinonez LG, Cook DJ. Crystalloids vs. colloids in fluid resuscitation: a systematic review. Crit Care Med 1999;27:200.
25. Wilkes MM, Navickis RJ. Patient survival after human albumin administration. A meta-analysis of randomized, controlled trials. Ann Intern Med 2001;135:149.
26. Haljamäe H. Metabolic consequences of trauma. In: Aasen AO, Risberg B (eds) *Surgical Pathophysiology*. Harwood Academic Publishers, Chur, 1990, pp. 47–67.
27. Baue AE. Multiple organ failure, multiple organ dysfunction syndrome, and the systemic inflammatory response syndrome – where do we stand? Shock 1994;6:385.
28. Haljamäe H. Cellular metabolic consequences of altered perfusion. In: Gutierrez G, Vincent JL (eds) *Tissue Oxygen Utilization*. Springer-Verlag, Berlin Heidelberg. 1991, pp. 71–86.
29. Haljamäe H. Adverse reactions to infusion fluids. In: Hahn RG, Prough DS, Svensen CH (eds) *Perioperative Fluid Therapy*. Informa Healthcare USA, Inc., New York, 2006, pp. 459–75.
30. Scheingraber S, Rehm M, Sehmisch C, Finsterer U. Rapid saline infusion produces hyperchloremic acidosis in patients undergoing gynecologic surgery. Anesthesiology 1999;90:1265.
31. Stephens R, Mythen M. Optimizing intraoperative fluid therapy. Curr Opin Anaesthesiol 2003;16:385.
32. Waters JH, Gottlieb A, Schoenwald P, Popovich MJ, Sprung J, Nelson DR. Normal saline versus lactated Ringer's solution for intraoperative fluid management in patients undergoing abdominal aortic aneurysm repair: an outcome study. Anesth Analg 2001;93:817.
33. Haljamäe H. Lactate metabolism. Int Care World 1987;4:118.
34. Eldridge FL. Relationship between lactate turnover rate and blood concentration in hemorrhagic shock. J Appl Physiol 1974;37:321–3.
35. Nakayama M, Kawana S, Yamauchi M, Tsuchida H, Iwasaki H, Namiki A. Utility of acetated Ringer solution as intraoperative fluids during hepatectomy. Masui 1995;44:1654.
36. Ruttmann TG, James MF, Viljoen JF. Haemodilution induces a hypercoagulable state. Br J Anaesth 1996;76:412.
37. Boldt J, Haisch G, Suttner S, Kumle B, Schellhase F. Are lactated Ringer's solution and normal saline solution equal with regard to coagulation? Anesth Analg 2002;94:378.
38. Cervera AL, Moss G. Crystalloid requirements and distribution when resuscitating with RBC's and noncolloid solutions during hemorrhage. Circ Shock 1978;5:357.
39. Riddez L, Hahn RG, Brismar B, Strandberg A, Svensen C, Hedenstierna G. Central and regional hemodynamics during acute hypovolemia and volume substitution in volunteers. Crit Care Med 1997;25:635.
40. Finfer S, Bellomo R, Boyce N, French J, Myburgh J, Norton R. SAFE Study Investigators. A comparison of albumin and saline for fluid resuscitation in the intensive care unit. N Engl J Med 2004;350:2247.
41. Brandstrup B, Tonnesen H, Beier-Holgersen R, et al. Danish Study Group on Perioperative Fluid Therapy. Effects of intravenous fluid restriction on postoperative complications: comparison of two

perioperative fluid regimens: a randomized assessor-blinded multicenter trial. Ann Surg 2003;238:641.
42. Brandstrup B. Fluid therapy for the surgical patient. Best Pract Res Clin Anaesthesiol 2006;20:265.
43. Nisanevich V, Felsenstein I, Almogy G, Weissman C, Einav S, Matot I. Effect of intraoperative fluid management on outcome after intraabdominal surgery. Anesthesiology 2005;103:25.
44. Joshi GP. Intraoperative fluid restriction improves outcome after major elective gastrointestinal surgery. Anesth Analg 2005;101:601.
45. Shoemaker WC. Comparison of the relative effectiveness of whole blood transfusions and various types of fluid therapy in resuscitation. Crit Care Med 1976;4:71.
46. Larsson M, Ware J. Effects of isotonic fluid load on plasma water and extracellular fluid volumes in the rat. Eur Surg Res 1983;15:262.
47. Guyton AC, Lindsey AW. Effect of left atrial pressure and decreased plasma protein concentration on the development of pulmonary edema. Circ Res 1959;7:649.
48. da Luz PL, Shubin H, Weil MH, et al. Pulmonary edema related to changes in colloid osmotic pressure and pulmonary artery wedge pressure in patients after myocardial infarction. Circulation 1975;51:350.
49. Haljamäe H. Lung water in the ICU. Refresher course lecture. *10th World Congress of Anaesthesiologists*, Hague, 1992; B 304.
50. Zarins CK, Rice CL, Peters RM, Virgilio RW. Lymph and pulmonary response to isobaric reduction in plasma oncotic pressure. Circ Res 1978;43:925.
51. Virgilio RW, Rice Cl, Smith DE, et al. Crystalloid vs. colloid resuscitation: is one better? Surgery 1979;85:129.
52. Shires III GT, Peitzman AB, Albert SA, et al. Response of extravascular lung water to intraoperative fluids. Ann Surg 1983;197:515.
53. Boldt J, Bormann BV, Kling D, Scheld H, Hempelmann G. Influence of acute normovolemic hemodilution on extravascular lung water in cardiac surgery. Crit Care Med 1988;16:336.
54. Zadrobilek E, Hackl W, Sporn P, Steinbereithner K. Effect of large volume replacement with balanced electrolyte solutions on extravascular lung water in surgical patients with sepsis syndrome. Intensive Care Med 1989;15:505.
55. Bickell WH, Barrett SM, Romine-Jenkins M, Hull SS Jr, Kinasewitz GT. Resuscitation of canine hemorrhagic hypotension with large-volume isotonic crystalloid: impact on lung water, venous admixture, and systemic arterial oxygen tension. Am J Emerg Med 1984;12:36.
56. Holte K, Jensen P, Kehlet H. Physiologic effects of intravenous fluid administration in healthy volunteers. Anesth Analg 2003;96:1504.
57. Russell GB, Graybeal JM. Hypoxemic episodes of patients in a postanesthesia care unit. Chest 1993;104:899.
58. Arieff AI. Fatal postoperative pulmonary edema: pathogenesis and literature review. Chest 1999;115:1371.
59. Demling RH, Manohar M, Will JA. Response of the pulmonary microcirculation to fluid loading after hemorrhagic shock and resuscitation. Surgery 1980;87:552.
60. Lucas CE, Ledgerwood AM, Shier RM, et al. The renal factor in the post-traumatic "fluid overload" syndrome. Trauma 1977;17:667.
61. Jordan S, Mitchell JA, Quinlan GJ, Goldstraw P, Evans TW. The pathogenesis of lung injury following pulmonary resection. Eur Respir J 2000;15:790.
62. Wang P, Chaudry IH. Crystalloid resuscitation restores but does not maintain cardiac output following severe hemorrhage. J Surg Res 1991;50:163.
63. Wang P, Hauptman JG, Chaudry IH. Hemorrhage produces depression in microvascular blood flow which persists despite fluid resuscitation. Circ Shock 1990;32:307.
64. Schött U, Lindbom LO, Sjöstrand U. Hemodynamic effects of colloid concentration in experimental hemorrhage: a comparison of Ringer's acetate, 3% dextran-60, and 6% dextran 70. Crit Care Med 1988;16:346.
65. Amundson B, Jennische E, Haljamäe H. Skeletal muscle microcirculatory and cellular metabolic effects of whole blood, Ringer's acetate, and dextran 70 infusions in hemorrhagic shock. Circ Shock 1980;7:111.
66. Heughan C, Ninikoski J, Hunt TK. Effect of excessive infusion of saline solution on tissue oxygen transport. Surg Gynecol Obstet 1972;135:257.
67. Hauser CJ, Shoemaker WC, Turpin I, Goldberg SJ. Oxygen transport responses to colloids and crystalloids in critically ill surgical patients. Surg Gynecol Obstet 1980;150:811.
68. Lobo DN, Bostock KA, Neal KR, et al. Effect of salt and water balance on recovery of gastrointestinal function after elective colonic resection: a randomised controlled trial. Lancet 2002;359:1812.

69. Bailey J, Shapiro MJ. Abdominal compartment syndrome. Crit Care 2000;4:23.
70. Hunter JD, Damani Z. Intra-abdominal hypertension and the abdominal compartment syndrome. Anaesthesia 2004;59:899.
71. Sugrue M. Abdominal compartment syndrome. Curr Opin Crit Care 2005;11:333.
72. Shafi S, Kauder DR. Fluid resuscitation and blood replacement in patients with polytrauma. Clin Orthop Relat Res 2004;422:37.
73. Rodas EB, Malhotra AK, Chhitwal R, et al. Hyperacute abdominal compartment syndrome: an unrecognized complication of massive intraoperative resuscitation for extra-abdominal injuries. Am Surg 2005;71:977.
74. Cotton BA, Guy JS, Morris JA Jr, Abumrad NN. The cellular, metabolic, and systemic consequences of aggressive fluid resuscitation strategies. Shock 2006;26:115.
75. Balogh Z, McKinley BA, Cocanour CS, et al. Supranormal trauma resuscitation causes more cases of abdominal compartment syndrome. Arch Surg 2003;138:637.
76. Fein IA, Rackow EC, Sprung CL, et al. Relation of COP to arterial hypoxemia and cerebral edema during crystalloid volume loading of patients. Ann Intern Med 1982;96:570.
77. Moon PF, Hollyfield MA, Myers TL, Kramer GC. Effects of isotonic crystalloid resuscitation on fluid compartments in hemorrhaged rats. Shock 1994;2:355.
78. Lowell JA, Schifferdecker C, Driscoll DF, Benotti PN, Bistrian BR. Postoperative fluid overload: not a benign problem. Crit Care Med 1990;18:728.
79. Alsous F, Khamiees M, DeGirolamo A, Amoateng-Adjepong Y, Manthous CA. Negative fluid balance predicts survival in patients with septic shock: a retrospective pilot study. Chest 2000;117:1749.
80. Dawidson I, Ottoson J, Eriksson B, Hedman L, Söderberg R. Relation of colloid concentration to volume expansion for resuscitation of rats subjected to intestinal ischemic shock. Crit Care Med 1982;10:597.
81. Dawidson I, Eriksson B. Statistical evaluation of plasma substitutes based on 10 variables. Crit Care Med 1982;10:653.
82. Haljamäe H, Dahlqvist M, Walentin F. Artificial colloids in clinical practice: pros and cons. Baillière's Clin Anaesthesiol 1997;11:49.
83. Shoemaker WC. Hemodynamic and oxygen transport effects of crystalloids and colloids in critically ill patients. Curr Stud Hematol Blood Transfus 1986;53:155.
84. Lang K, Boldt J, Suttner S, Haisch G. Colloids versus crystalloids and tissue oxygen tension in patients undergoing major abdominal surgery. Anesth Analg 2001;93:405.
85. Brückner UB, Messmer K. Organ perfusion and tissue oxygenation after moderate isovolemic hemodilution with HES 200/0.62 and dextran-70. Anaesthetist 1991;40:434.
86. Le Veen HH, Ip M, Ahmed N, Mascardo T, Guinto RB, Falk G, D'Ovidio N. Lowering blood viscosity to overcome vascular resistance. Surg Gynecol Obstet 1980;150:139.
87. Kouraklis G, Sechas M, Skalkeas G. Effects of hemodilution on peripheral circulation. Vasc Surg 1989;23:20.
88. Krieter H, Brückner UB, Kefalianakis F, Messmer K. Does colloid-induced hyperviscosity in haemodilution jeopardize perfusion and oxygenation in vital organs? Acta Aneasthesiol Scand 1995;39:236.
89. Brückner UB, Messmer K. Blood rheology and systemic oxygen transport. Biorheology 1990;27:903.
90. Lang K, Suttner S, Boldt J, Kumle B, Nagel D. Volume replacement with HES 130/0.4 may reduce the inflammatory response in patients undergoing major abdominal surgery. Can J Anaesth 2003;50:1009.
91. Boldt J, Ducke M, Kumle B, Papsdorf M, Zurmeyer EL. Influence of different volume replacement strategies on inflammation and endothelial activation in the elderly undergoing major abdominal surgery. Intensive Care Med 2004;30:416.
92. Strauss RG. Volume replacement and coagulation: a comparative review. J Cardiothorac Anesth 1988;2(Suppl. 1): 24.
93. Van der Linden P, Ickx BE. The effects of colloid solutions on hemostasis. Can J Anaesth 2006;53(6 Suppl): S30.
94. Barak M, Rudin M, Vofsi O, Droyan A, Katz Y. Fluid administration during abdominal surgery influences on coagulation in the postoperative period. Curr Surg 2004;61:459.
95. Bunn F, Alderson P, Hawkins V. Colloid solutions for fluid resuscitation. Cochrane Database Syst Rev 2003; (1): CD001319.
96. Roberts I, Alderson P, Bunn F, Chinnock P, Ker K, Schierhout G. Colloids versus crystalloids for fluid resuscitation in critically ill patients. Cochrane Database Syst Rev 2004; (4): CD000567.

97. Grocott MP, Mythen MG, Gan TJ. Perioperative fluid management and clinical outcomes in adults. Anesth Analg 2005;100:1093.
98. Price HL, Deutsch S, Marshal BNE, Stephen GW, Behar MG, Neufeld GR. Hemodynamic and metabolic effects of hemorrhage in man, with particular reference to the splanchnic circulation. Circ Res 1966;18:469.
99. Mythen MG, Webb AR. Intra-operative gut mucosal hypoperfusion is associated with.increased postoperative complications and cost. Intensive Care Med 1994;20:99.
100. Mythen MG, Webb AR. Perioperative plasma volume expansion reduces the incidence of gut mucosal hypoperfusion during cardiac surgery. Arch Surg 1995;130:423.
101. Moretti EW, Robertson KM, El-Moalem H, Gan TJ. Intraoperative colloid administration reduces postoperative nausea and vomiting and improves postoperative outcomes compared with crystalloid administration. Anesth Analg 2003;96:611.
102. Haljamäe H. Intraoperative fluid therapy and postoperative gastrointenstinal (GI) function – possible impact on early enteral nutrition. ROSPEN. In press.
103. Holte K, Kehlet H. Compensatory fluid administration for preoperative dehydration – does it improve outcome? Acta Anaesthesiol Scand 2002;46:1089.
104. Carson JL, Hill S, Carless P, et al. Transfusion triggers: a systematic review of the literature. Transfus Med Rev 2002;16:187.
105. Holte K, Sharrock NE, Kehlet H. Pathophysiology and clinical implications of perioperative fluid excess. Br J Anaesth 2002;89:622.
106. Holte K, Hahn RG, Ravn L, Bertelsen KG, Hansen S, Kehlet H. Influence of "liberal" versus "restrictive" intraoperative fluid administration on elimination of a postoperative fluid load. Anesthesiology 2007;106:75.
107. Gan TJ, Soppitt A, Maroof M, et al. Goal-directed intraoperative fluid administration reduces length of hospital stay after major surgery. Anesthesiology 2002;97:820.
108. Venn R, Steele A, Richardson P, Poloniecki J, Grounds M, Newman P. Randomized controlled trial to investigate influence of the fluid challenge on duration of hospital stay and perioperative morbidity in patients with hip fractures. Br J Anaesth 2002;88:65.
109. MacKay G, Fearon K, McConnachie A, Serpell MG, Molloy RG, O'Dwyer PJ. Randomized clinical trial of the effect of postoperative intravenous fluid restriction on recovery after elective colorectal surgery. Br J Surg 2006;93:1469.
110. Stephens R, Mythen M. Optimizing intraoperative fluid therapy. Curr Opin Anaesthesiol 2003;16:385.
111. Boldt J. Fluid management of patients undergoing abdominal surgery–more questions than answers. Eur J Anaesthesiol 2006;23:631.
112. Lobo DN, Macafee DA, Allison SP. How perioperative fluid balance influences postoperative outcomes. Best Pract Res Clin Anaesthesiol 2006;20:439.
113. Bundgaard-Nielsen M, Holte K, Secher NH, Kehlet H. Monitoring of peri-operative fluid administration by individualized goal-directed therapy. Acta Anaesthesiol Scand 2007;51:331.
114. Rackow EC, Falk JL, Fein IA, Siegel JS, Packman MI, Haupt MT, Kaufman BS, Putnam D. Fluid resuscitation in circulatory shock: a comparison of the cardiorespiratory effects of albumin, hetastarch, and saline solutions in patients with hypovolemic and septic shock. Crit Care Med 1983;11:839.
115. Haupt MT, Teerapong P, Green D, Schaeffer RC Jr, Carlson RW. Increased pulmonary edema with crystalloid compared to colloid resuscitation of shock associated with increased vascular permeability. Circ Shock 1984;12:213.
116. Wiedemann HP, Wheeler AP, Bernard GR, et al., for National Heart, Lung, and Blood Institute Acute Respiratory Distress Syndrome (ARDS) Clinical Trials Network, Comparison of two fluid-management strategies in acute lung injury. N Engl J Med 2006;354:2564.
117. Su F, Wang Z, Cai Y, Rogiers P, Vincent JL. Fluid resuscitation in severe sepsis and septic shock: albumin, hydroxyethyl starch, gelatin or ringer's lactate-does it really make a difference? Shock 2007;27:520.
118. Boldt J, Lenz M, Kumle B, Papsdorf M. Volume replacement strategies on intensive care units: results from a postal survey. Intensive Care Med 1998;24:147.
119. Boldt J. Fluid choice for resuscitation of the trauma patient: a review of the physiological, pharmacological, and clinical evidence. Can J Anaesth. 2004;51:500.
120. Schortgen F, Deye N, Brochard L, for CRYCO Study Group. Preferred plasma volume expanders for critically ill patients: results of an international survey. Intensive Care Med 2004;30:2222.
121. Vincent JL, Sakr Y, Reinhart K, Sprung CL, Gerlach H, Ranieri VM. 'Sepsis Occurrence in Acutely Ill

Patients' Investigators. Is albumin administration in the acutely ill associated with increased mortality? Results of the SOAP study. Crit Care 2005;9: R745.
122. Groeneveld AB. Albumin and artificial colloids in fluid management: where does the clinical evidence of their utility stand? Crit Care 2000;4(Suppl. 2): S16.
123. Haynes GR, Navickis RJ, Wilkes MM. Albumin administration–what is the evidence of clinical benefit? A systematic review of randomized controlled trials. Eur J Anaesthesiol 2003;20:771.
124. Vincent JL, Navickis RJ, Wilkes MM. Morbidity in hospitalized patients receiving human albumin: a meta-analysis of randomized, controlled trials. Crit Care Med 2004;32:2029.
125. Alderson P, Bunn F, Lefebvre C, et al., for Albumin Reviewers. Human albumin solution for resuscitation and volume expansion in critically ill patients. Cochrane Database Syst Rev 2004; (4):CD001208.
126. Dubois MJ, Orellana-Jimenez C, et al. Albumin administration improves organ function in critically ill hypoalbuminemic patients: a prospective, randomized, controlled, pilot study. Crit Care Med 2006;34:2536.
127. Romanelli RG, La Villa G, Barletta G, et al. Long-term albumin infusion improves survival in patients with cirrhosis and ascites: an unblinded randomized trial. World J Gastroenterol 2006;12:1403.
128. Cochran A, Morris SE, Edelman LS, Saffle JR. Burn patient characteristics and outcomes following resuscitation with albumin. Burns 2007;33: 25.
129. Mythen MG, Salmon JB, Webb AR. The rational administration of colloids. Blood Rev 1993;7:223.
130. Hoffmann JN, Vollmar B, Laschke MW, Inthorn D, Schildberg FW, Menger MD. Hydroxyethyl starch (130 kD), but not crystalloid volume support, improves microcirculation during normotensive endotoxemia. Anesthesiology 2002;97: 460.
131. Tian J, Lin X, Guan R, Xu JG. The effects of hydroxyethyl starch on lung capillary permeability in endotoxic rats and possible mechanisms. Anesth Analg 2004;98:768.
132. Marx G, Pedder S, Smith L, et al. Resuscitation from septic shock with capillary leakage: hydroxyethyl starch (130 KD), but not Ringer's solution maintains plasma volume and systemic oxygenation. Shock 2004;21:336.
133. Marx G, Pedder S, Smith L, et al. Attenuation of capillary leakage by hydroxyethyl starch (130/0.42) in a porcine model of septic shock. Crit Care Med 2006;34:3005.

CHAPTER 11
Effects of Synthetic Colloids on Hemostasis

Sibylle A. Kozek-Langenecker & Gisela Scharbert
Department of Anesthesiology and Pain Management, Medical University of Vienna, Vienna, Austria

Introduction

Synthetic colloids are frequently used plasma expanders, which are indicated to restore and maintain intravascular volume, to stabilize hemodynamic conditions, and to improve tissue perfusion. Among them, hydroxyethyl starch (HES) solutions are most widely used. Developments of HES preparations since their introduction into clinical practice centered on designing starch molecules with an increased oncotic pressure and hemodynamic efficacy while minimizing the risk of adverse reactions such as plasma and tissue accumulation and anticoagulant effects. Hemostatic alterations associated with the use of plasma expanders are related to both nonspecific dilutional effects and specific effects. This chapter will extend the focus of previous reviews on specific anticoagulant side effects of various HES generations, including hetastarch, pentastarch, and tetrastarch [1–4] and compares HES to gelatin and dextran.

Chemistry

Adverse effects on hemostasis are determined by the in vivo degradation of a particular HES preparation. HES solutions are classified:

1 According to the molar substitution (mol hydroxyethyl residues per mol glucose subunit) into hetastarch (highly substituted: 0.62–0.75), pentastarch (medium substituted: 0.5), and tetrastarch (low substituted: 0.4);

2 According to the C2/C6 ratio (pattern of hydroxyethylation at the carbon position C2 and C6) into solutions with a high C2/C6 ratio (>1:8) and low C2/C6 ratio (<1:8); and

3 According to the manufactured mean molecular weight into high molecular weight (450–670 kDa), medium molecular weight (130 and 200 kDa), and low molecular weight solutions (<70 kDa).

Especially molar substitution and C2/C6-ratio determine the in vivo behavior of specific HES types and the rate of HES degradation. Hetastarch and pentastarch are slowly degradable, whereas tetrastarch is rapidly degradable. The development of HES over the past decades has been characterized by a concomitant reduction in molecular weight and molar substitution (from HES 450/0.7 to HES 200/0.5 to HES 130/0.4). Molecular design of HES products differ between the continents: in Europe medium molecular weight HES solutions with low substitution are predominant. The standard solutions in the United States are relatively high molecular weight HES (450 or 670 kDa) with a high substitution (0.7 or 0.75). In the light of the importance of pharmacokinetic parameters on coagulation, future papers need to clearly indicate molar substitution, C2/C6 ratio, molecular weight, and the concentration in the carrier solution in order to permit precise interpretation of the results.

Linkage of carboxymethyl rather than hydroxyethyl groups to the starch backbone

Alternatives to Blood Transfusion in Transfusion Medicine, 2nd edition. Edited by A. Maniatis, P. Van der Linden, J.-F. Hardy.

results in polyanionic, negatively charged and more hydrophilic starches. Carboxymethyl starches may therefore exert a more pronounced volume expansion effect compared with conventional HES.

Gelatins are polypeptides produced from collagen by hydrolysis. Although prepared from bovine origin, gelatins are sterile, pyrogen free, and contain no preservatives. Chemical conformation is modified by addition of succinic acid anhydride in fluid-modified gelatins. Urea-linked gelatins are prepared by cross-linking polypeptides by addition of hexamethyl di-isocyanate. The third type of modified gelatin products available is oxypolygelatin. Molecular weight of gelatins ranges from 5 to 50 kDa.

Dextran molecules are chain-like polymers with a low degree of branching. Dextrans are prepared from glucose by enzymatic degradation and partial acid hydrolysis. High molecular weight dextrans have a molecular weight of 60–70 kDa; the commercially available 6% solution is hyperoncotic. Low molecular weight dextrans have a molecular weight of 40 kDa; the commercially available 3.5% solution is isooncotic, whereas 10% solution is hyperoncotic.

Decrease in coagulation factor VIII and von Willebrand factor

Acquired von Willebrand syndrome and the decreasing effect on factor VIII of slowly degradable HES have repeatedly been observed since the introduction of slowly degradable HES solutions into clinical practice (Figure 11.1). Treib et al. systematically investigated differences of HES preparations with regard to coagulation [5–7]. Physicochemical differences have been shown to be important for the factor VIII/von Willebrand factor (vWF)-lowering properties of particular HES preparation: Slowly degradable HES solutions have been consistently shown to decrease circulating plasma levels of coagulation factor VIII and vWF by up to 80% in healthy volunteers [8–10] and in patients [11, 12] even when used below the recommended daily amounts of 25–50 mL/kg. Hemostatic dysfunction after HES administration has been intensively investigated in vitro [13–19] and in vivo [20–23]. The pathophysiological consequence of the decrease in factor VIII and vWF antigen is an impairment of functional parameters such as ristocetin cofactor activity or activated partial thromboplastin time, or thrombelastographic parameters. Patients with type 0 blood may have increased coagulation compromise after acute hemodilution with HES owing to lower baseline values of vWF (and factor VIII:c) [24]. VWF is a high molecular weight glycoprotein (GP) that plays an important role in hemostasis by interacting with platelet membrane receptors. The defect in vWF activity can be estimated by ristocetin cofactor activity (vWF:RCo), collagen binding activity (vWF:CBA). The degree of vWF synthesis, degradation, consumption, or nonspecific binding can be detected by the measurements of vWF:antigen (Ag).

In contrast to slowly degradable HES, rapidly degradable tetrastarch had negligible effects in orthopedic patients, in patients with cerebrovascular disease after chronic administration, and in volunteers [9, 25]. Recent trials reported the use of high tetrastarch doses of up to 50–70 mL/kg without deterioration of VIII [26, 27]. In parallel to the lower in vivo molecular weight of tetrastarch, factor VIII and vWF returned to almost normal up to 5 hours postoperatively, but not in hetastarch-treated orthopedic patients [25]. There is a physiologic increase in acute phase parameters such as coagulation factor VIII and vWF in the postoperative period starting upon the arrival at the recovery room, which plays a role in the postoperative hypercoagulability. Slowly degradable HES [28], but not rapidly degradable HES diminished the postoperative increase in factor VIII and vWF [29–32].

Gelatins and dextrans share the same factor VIII/vWF-lowering potency. This effect appears to be proportional to the molecular weight of the dextran molecules [33]. Gelatin decreases factor VIII and vWF more than tetrastarch [34]. In this study, however, prothrombin time, fibrinogen concentration (despite substitution), and factor VII decreased more from preoperative baseline in the gelatin group than in the tetrastarch group.

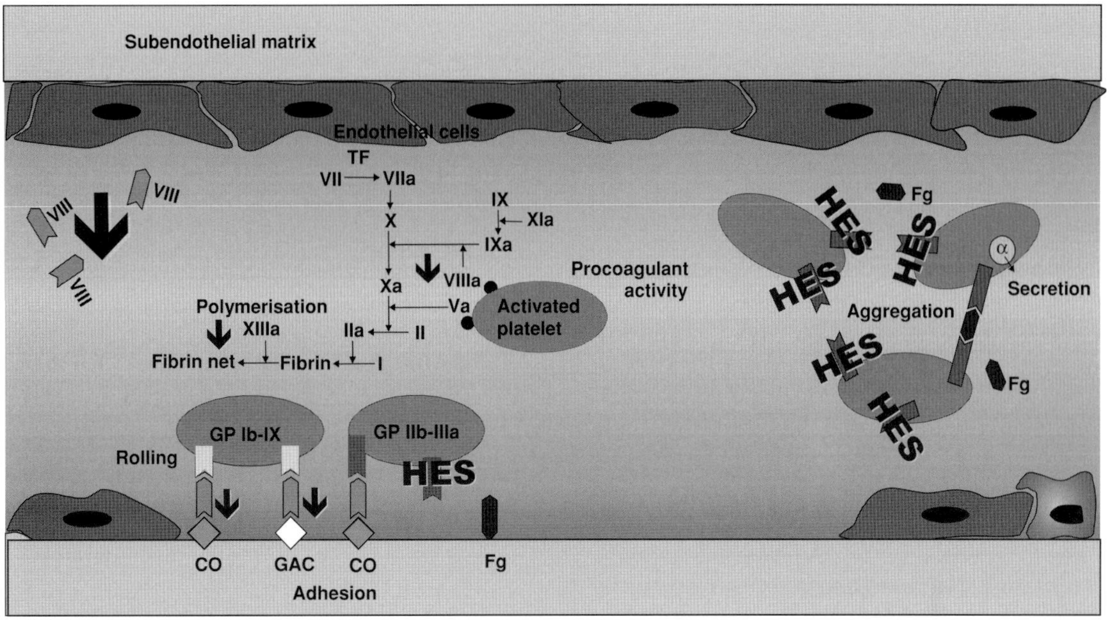

↓ Decrease in the plasma concentration of coagulation factor VIII

von Willebrand factor (vWF)

Platelet GP Ib-IX and GP IIb-IIIa

HES HES macromolecules

● Phospholipids

Figure 11.1 Effect of hydroxyethyl starch (HES) molecules on hemostasis. Slowly degradable HES solutions decrease the plasma concentration of coagulation factor VIII and its carrier glycoprotein (GP) von Willebrand factor (vWF). Consequently, vWF-mediated rolling and adhesion of platelets to subendothelial collagen (CO) and heparin-like glycosaminoglycanes (GAC) involving platelet GP Ib-IX and GP IIb-IIIa is impaired in the presence of HES. Reduced availability of activated GP IIb-IIIa by platelets surface coating of HES macromolecules impairs adhesion to surface-bound fibrinogen (Fg) and, most important, soluble fibrinogen (Fg) ligand binding between neighboring platelets causing platelet aggregation. Activated platelets expose negatively charged phospholipids on their surface, which bind constituents of the prothrombinase (Va) and tenase complex (VIIIa; procoagulant activity). Consequently, reduced availability of the accelerator VIIIa results in diminished activation of factor X in the intrinsic coagulation pathway. HES impairs fibrin polymerization required for stable clot formation. The in vivo pharmacokinetic behavior of HES types, especially the in vivo molecular weight and HES plasma concentration, determine side effects on hemostasis: Rapidly degradable HES (tetrastarch) has fewer effects when compared with slowly degradable HES (hetastarch and pentastarch). Modified from [1].

Pathophysiology: coagulation factor VIII and vWF

The pathogenetic mechanism responsible for the adverse effects on plasmatic coagulation is not yet understood. While passive hemodilutional effects are observed immediately after infusion (such as the decrease in hemoglobin, fibrinogen concentration, and platelet count), vWF reaches its minimum 1–2 hours afterward, and exceeds the degree of decrease (20% vs 47%) indicating additional mechanisms responsible for the decrease beyond the dilutional effect [9]. Nondilutional mechanisms, however, remain hypothetical. While each in vivo study found a decrease in factor VIII (although the decrease did not reach statistical significance in some studies [28, 35]) in vitro studies failed to reproduce the lowering effect of HES on factor VIII (except for one experimental study [17]). This result may suggest the absence or blockade of the pathogenic mechanism in the in vitro testing milieu.

A decreased release is unlikely considering the half-life of vWF of 8 hours. Antibody-mediated mechanisms also seem to be unlikely because of the very rare occurrence of preformed HES antibodies [36]. Increased proteolytic degradation is unlikely because both small and large vWF multimers decrease similarly after HES infusion [5, 37]. Association of vWF with collagen has been suggested to regulate glycoprotein Ib binding function. Similarly, association with larger colloid molecules may occur [37, 38] and accelerated elimination after complexing has been considered as a pathogenic mechanism responsible for the adverse effect on factor VIII/vWF-complex. In this context it remains to be determined whether its nonspecific binding to colloid molecules reduces vWF levels, modulates vWF function, and whether the interaction of vWF with platelet receptors blocked by colloid molecules modulates vWF-cleaving protease secretion or activity.

Decrease in platelet function

The introduction of near-patient coagulation monitoring such as Platelet Function Analyzer PFA-100 and thrombelastography, and novel platelet testing techniques such as whole blood flow cytometry advanced our understanding of HES-dependent platelet effects. Similar to the plasmatic coagulation changes, physicochemical differences were found to be important for the platelet-inhibiting properties of particular HES preparations: Slowly degradable HES solutions have been found to prolong PFA-100 closure times significantly [39, 40], while rapidly degradable HES had minimal specific effects, if any, in healthy volunteers [40]. PFA-100 measures global platelet function that is dependent upon the interaction of GP IIb-IIIa and GP Ib with their ligands such as fibrinogen and vWF. HES-induced prolongations in PFA-100 closure times have been confirmed in the majority of studies [8, 40, 41] except in a single study in which surgery per se may have counteracted the effect of HES on platelet function [29]. Fitting into the above elaborated picture, rapidly degradable HES did not decrease platelet aggregation [29], while slowly degradable HES impaired platelet aggregation [42].

Platelet inhibition by HES molecules has been further investigated at the cellular level using flow cytometry, which permits evaluation of surface receptor expression and intracellular messenger status on individual platelets [39]. The interaction of GP Ib-IX with vWF is essential for platelet adhesion. Platelet activation transforms the extracellular portion of platelet membrane GP IIb-IIIa complex into a conformational state that is competent for binding its ligands such as soluble fibrinogen and vWF. This reaction is a prerequisite for platelet aggregation and irreversible adhesion to the subendothelium. P-selectin is present in internal α-granules and translocates to the cell surface upon platelet activation and secretion. Our own recent experiments suggest that not only their physicochemical differences but also the composition of the solvent determines side effects of HES preparations on platelet function: The novel high molecular weight HES (670 kDa, molar substitution 0.75) exerts platelet-stimulating effects, which may be, at least partly, due to the high calcium concentration in the solvent [43]. While 10 mL/kg HES 130/0.4 had no platelet inhibiting effects [40], 20 mL/kg inhibited the expression of platelet membrane GP Ib-IX (CD42b), GP IIb-IIIa (CD41/61), and P-selectin (CD62P) on ADP-stimulated platelets [44]. Platelet function recovered within 6 hours after infusions of HES 130/0.4 but not after HES 200/0.5 [44].

Dextrans share platelet inhibiting effects [3]. Chemical characteristics of gelatin solutions modulate their influence on platelet reactivity. The extent of antiplatelet effects of oxypolygelatin is minimal and comparable to tetrastarch [45]. Both fluid-modified gelatin and urea-linked gelatin have been shown to impair aggregability [45] resulting in increased bleeding times [46, 47].

Pathophysiology: platelet inhibition

Slowly degradable HES induces cellular abnormalities with a decreased agonist-induced expression and activation of platelet surface GP IIb-IIIa [39, 40]. Reduced activated GP IIb-IIIa availability in turn leads to impaired platelet adhesion and aggregation, and prolongs PFA-100 closure times. Slowly degradable HES molecules appear not to exert their inhibitory effect on platelet function by interfering with intracellular signal transduction because the agonist-induced increase in cytoplasmic calcium, the key second messenger in platelets, was unchanged in the presence of HES [48]. Platelet secretion is a downstream platelet function dependent on intracellular calcium. Supporting the independence of platelet-inhibiting HES effects on intracellular signal transduction, platelet secretion assessed by the expression of P-selectin, was not [40] or only slightly decreased [49] by slowly degradable HES. Further in vitro experiments investigated unspecific binding of fluorochrome-coupled HES molecules to the platelet surface as another potential mechanism of HES-induced platelet inhibition [50]. These flow cytometric experiments visualized extracellular coating of human platelets by HES macromolecules as proposed by early studies. HES may inhibit platelet reactivity by blocking the access of ligands to surface receptors or by an unspecific modification of cytoplasmic membrane structures, and a consecutive inhibition of the conformational change of GP IIb-IIIa. It remains to be determined whether extracellular coating impairs platelet procoagulant activity by modifying the binding of constituents of the prothrombinase and tenase complex to the negatively charged phospholipids exposed on activated platelets.

Dextrans [3] and gelatins [45] have also been accused to induce extracellular coating.

Thrombelastography and thrombelastometry reveal hypocoagulability

Blood coagulation is increasingly compromised by HES hemodilution toward hypocoagulability characterized by an increase in the time to thrombelastographic clot initiation, a decrease in the speed of clot propagation, or a decrease in clot strength. By employing either conventional or platelet inhibitor-modified thrombelastography, hypocoagulability has been documented extensively with slowly degradable HES having the most pronounced effect [9, 21, 23, 28, 35, 51–54]. In line, HES 650/0.42 had a significantly greater impact on routine coagulation and thrombelastographic parameters than HES 130/0.42 [55]. However, effects were similar when observed antihemostatic effects were related to the measured HES plasma concentration. Plasma concentration in g/L, integrating both number and size of circulating molecules, determined the effect on blood coagulation [56]. This study also showed that HES 650/0.42 has a lower efficacy in immediate plasma expansion [56]. Another study by Spahn's group systematically investigated the isolated effect of molar substitution and C2/C6 ratio of HES molecules. Although the dynamic of in vivo molecular weight measurements was unlikely (increase starting from 30 kDa), Madjdpour et al. [53] reported lower in vivo molecular weight in pigs after infusion of HES 130 compared with HES 500 and HES 900 at the same low degree of molar substitution (0.42), while coagulation tests revealed no differences between these HES infusions. The authors thus questioned the in vivo molecular weight as the key factor compromising blood coagulation in tetrastarch. Less accumulation of HES 130 may be considered.

High molecular weight HES (700 kDa) with a low molar substitution of 0.42 and a low C2/C6 ratio of 2.7 had the lowest effect on in vitro coagulation [52]. Spahn's group recently described the effect of novel carboxymethyl starches on hemostatis: carboxymethyl starches impaired thrombelastographic variables more than HES [56].

The antihemostatic effect of dextran in viscoelastic parameters is more pronounced than that of other colloids [17, 57–60]. Clot firmness in thrombelastometric assays was more deteriorated after tetrastarch infusion compared with gelatin [34, 61].

Decrease in thrombin–fibrinogen interaction and fibrin polymerization

HES impairs thrombin–fibrinogen interactions and fibrin clot formation [62]. HES solutions diminish the profile of the propagation phase of citrated whole blood exposed to 55% in vitro hemodilution [63]. Polymerization of fibrin monomers is impaired in the presence of HES macromolecules [16, 34, 35, 61]. Using pooled human plasma samples subjected to factor-supplemented TEG analyses and frozen plasma samples stored from previous hemodilution studies in rabbits, Nielsen explored the pathomechanism of decreased clot propagation [18, 64, 65]: Thrombin-mediated polymerization of fibrin and activation of factor XIII with consequent fibrin polymer cross-linking are inhibited by HES molecules. A higher C2/C6 ratio of two tetrastarch solutions only showed a trend toward a more pronounced decreasing effect on shear elastic modulus, maximum and total thrombus generation 1 hour after test infusion (possibly due to low statistical power or counteracting lower molar substitution).

Combinations of drugs are likely to exert additive effects. Recent experiments showed that HES dilution increase the time to clot initiation, decrease the velocity of clot propagation, and clot strength in one lot of pooled citrated control plasma incubated with argatroban [65].

Dextrans share the diminishing effect on clot propagation [63]. Gelatins also reduce the quality of the clot but the inhibiting effect on thrombin–fibrinogen interactions and fibrin clot formation is less pronounced when compared with HES [34, 35, 66].

Fibrinolysis

The effect of colloids on fibrinolysis has been discussed controversially. Some studies showed increased fibrinolysis in vivo and in vitro in the presence of HES [11, 20–22, 51], whereas others found no effect [10, 12, 42]. HES could favor fibrinolysis by incorporation of HES macromolecules in the clot [20] or increased plasminogen activator activity [67]. HES enhanced tissue plasminogen activator-induced fibrinolysis in plasma secondary to decreased factor XIII-mediated clot strength [22]. Hence, HES modulates the response of plasma to fibrinolytic stress and decreases clot resistance to fibrinolytic disintegration. A definite conclusion on the clinical importance of the effect of HES on fibrinolysis cannot be drawn from the available (experimental) data.

Dextrans accelerate fibrinolysis by increasing fibrinolysis activators and altering polymerization of fibrin monomers [68].

Suspension medium

Both the molecular design of HES and the suspension medium may alter blood coagulation. Most HES compounds are prepared in normal saline or plasma adapted, balanced solutions (6 or 10%). The higher the HES concentration the more anticoagulant effects may be observed. Hetastarch prepared in balanced solution containing lactate buffer, calcium chloride, and glucose resulted in a better coagulation status in vivo than the same HES prepared in saline [69]. Hyperchloremic metabolic acidosis may be caused by large volumes of saline-based fluid administration, which per se may impair coagulation [70]. Balanced salt solutions caused fewer coagulation abnormalities in vitro than similar HES types dissolved in saline [43, 71–73]. However, the content of calcium, magnesium, and buffer per se may enhance aggregation and overall coagulation in the test cuvette at high degrees of hemodilution. Hence, the clinical relevance of these in vitro experiments remains to be determined.

Clinical aspects—perioperative blood loss

Side effects of HES on the coagulation system have been accused to worsen clinical outcome [74]. A meta-analysis involving 16 trials and 653 randomized patients showed a significant higher postoperative bleeding in cardiopulmonary bypass patients exposed to slowly degradable hetastarch and pentastarch than albumin [75]. The authors reported increased costs of care since excessive bleeding triggers blood transfusion, prolonged mechanical ventilation, or reexploration for bleeding in many centers.

A recent pooled analysis included 449 patients undergoing major surgical procedures prospectively randomized in 7 studies having compared HES 130/0.4 ($n = 228$) or HES 200/0.5 ($n = 221$) [76]. The use of HES 130/0.4 was associated with a significant reduction in perioperative blood loss, resulting in a decrease in allogeneic blood transfusion by about 140 mL RBC unit per patient. Differences between HES 130/0.4 and 200/0.5 appear larger then those reported in a previous meta-analysis comparing slowly degradable starches (HES 450 and 200 kDa) and albumin [75]. Decreased interaction of tetrastarch with factor VIII, vWF, and platelet function might translate to a smaller blood loss. Even after repetitive large-dose infusion up to 70 mL/kg/day for up to 28 days, blood loss and transfusion of packed red blood cells were lower in patients treated with tetrastarch [26]. The increased therapeutic safety index of the tetrastarch HES 130/0.4 has recently been acknowledged by the European regulatory authorities by increasing the maximum daily dose to 50 mL/kg bodyweight per day.

Dextran acts as an anticoagulant and is not recommended as a volume expander in patients at risk for bleeding.

Gelatins have been suggested not to increase perioperative blood loss in human [77]. However, gelatin increased blood loss compared to albumin in several clinical setting, e.g., cardiac surgery [78]. In contrast to slowly degradable hetastarch and pentastarch, patients receiving rapidly degradable tetrastarch were not different in respect to blood loss and transfusion requirements after cardiac, major abdominal, and orthopedic surgery when compared with albumin or gelatin [27, 29–31, 79–81]. A recent study indicated that gelatin increases blood loss and blood product requirements compared to tetrastarch in orthopedic surgery [34]. The relationship between bleeding and laboratory coagulation parameters (e.g., clot polymerization) in the presence of synthetic colloids need to be determined in humans.

Clinical aspects—hypercoagulability

Colloid-induced hemostatic changes may be either beneficial or unwanted depending on the status of a given patient. Hypercoagulability remains a major source of morbidity and mortality in trauma patients, the manifestations of which include deep vein thrombosis and multiple organ failure. Attenuation of the postoperative hypercoagulability as a physiologic component of the acute phase reaction after surgery by hetastarch and pentastarch solutions may be beneficial in patients at risk for thrombotic episodes. Long-term repeated infusion of slowly degradable HES, e.g., in patients with cerebral perfusion disorders who are at an increased risk for thrombosis may benefit from the HES-induced antithrombotic and platelet-inhibiting effects. High molecular weight hetastarches attenuate hypercoagulability when compared with crystalloids and albumin [58, 82].

Mild to moderate hemodilution with HES has been reported to accelerate the onset of clotting [9, 35]. This phenomenon may either be an in vitro artifact or HES may indeed serve as an additional surface able to activate coagulation factors, thus accelerating the conversion of fibrinogen to fibrin. In contrast to crystalloid-induced hypercoagulability an imbalance between thrombin generation and antithrombin concentration is not suggested to be involved in HES-induced hypercoagulability [35]. Decreased endogenous heparinoid release has been suspected as a cause of increased clot initiation in the presence of HES 450/0.75 [83]. Mild to moderate hemodilution with gelatin has been reported to accelerate the onset of clotting [84].

Reversing strategies

The administration of desmopressin has been reported to reverse the lowering effect of slowly degradable HES as well as dextan and gelatin on factor VIII and vWF, as well as to shorten bleeding times [12,85]. Other therapeutic approaches for acquired vWS by colloids may involve the administration of factor VIII/vWF-concentrates [38]. Symptomatic treatment is typically complicated by the short half-life of endogenous and exogenous vWF.

Platelet transfusion may correct platelet alterations induced by slowly degradable HES by distributing HES macromolecules to an increased pool of platelets. Sorensen's group [63, 86] investigated possible approaches to reverse HES-induced decreased dynamic whole blood clotting profile. While platelets, factor VIII, and recombinant activated factor VII failed to restore whole blood thrombin generation capacity and clot strength, fibrinogen substitution was effective. Fries et al. [87] confirmed these findings in a porcine model. Fibrinogen supplementation also partially improved clot strength in plasma samples hemodiluted with various colloids [64]. Factor XIII addition partially restored clot propagation in samples diluted with HES 450/0.7, HES 200/0.45, or albumin [64]. Tranexamic acid failed to reverse HES-associated impairment of clot strength [88]. Prospective clinical studies have to evaluate indications for reversing strategies, as well as efficacy and safety issues. Prothrombotic complications and side effects of the reversing agents per se have to be considered before their administration.

Practical considerations

Judging by currently available evidence, adverse hemostasis effects appear to be inherent to dextran, gelatin, and HES molecules, although hetastarch and pentastarch definitely have a more pronounced impact than tetrastarch. Tetrastarch HES 130/0.4 appears to be a suitable volume expander in the routine perioperative setting owing to adequate volume efficacy and the minimal risk for hemostatic derangements. Contraindications such as anuria and maximum daily doses (50 mL/kg for HES 130/0.4) need to be acknowledged.

Dextran has its clinical indication in the prevention and treatment of deep vein thrombosis [3] but not as a volume expander in patients at risk for bleeding due to its multifold side effects (antihemostatic, allergic, and renal) [89,90]. These side effects of dextran (70 kDa 6%) are also present in novel hypertonic preparations for low volume resuscitation with additional antihemostatic effects of hypertonic saline per se [91–93]. Maximum daily doses are 1.5 g/kg/day for conventional dextran solutions and 4 mL/kg for hypertonic, hyperoncotic dextran solutions.

Volume efficacy of gelatin is lower compared with tetrastarch [2, 3]. Accordingly, repeated infusions of gelatin are necessary to maintain adequate intravascular volume. This disadvantage is balanced by the absence of maximum daily dose limitations and lack of accumulation. Gelatin is frequently used as a second-line colloid in Europe after maximum daily doses of HES have been administered, while it is no longer approved in the United States for fluid therapy.

Limitations of study designs

Mixing defined doses of colloids to blood stored in the cuvette may allow for studying selected biological effects [17, 22, 57, 64, 65, 94]. However extrapolations from such experimental study designs to clinical practice are not feasible because the in vitro model only shows what happens in this particular model not necessarily representing reality. The increasing understanding of the crucial importance of the in vivo molecular weight and the specific in vivo pharmacokinetic behavior of a particular HES preparation suggest that some experimental in vitro study designs may be inadequate to detect HES-dependent hemostatic side effects due to the absence of endothelium, metabolic degradation, and compensatory mechanisms such as buffering, control of pH, and electrolyte environment.

Limitations of the thrombelastography and thrombelastometry must be considered such as it is not a satisfactory surrogate parameter for plasma levels of factor VIII, vWF, platelet function, or antithrombin levels. Small differences in percent change of clot strength between HES preparations do not necessarily translate into clinically relevant phenomena.

The use of plasma instead of whole blood for thrombelastography employs a nonphysiological test milieu despite our understanding of a cell-based model of hemostasis. Although the use of plasma may allow for simplifying the complex interactions during hemostasis, and the use of factor-deficient plasma or factor-supplemented plasma devoid of platelets, red and white blood cells may isolate the effect of HES on individual steps of the plasmatic cascade reactions, this methodology remains highly artificial. Studies employing whole blood instead of plasma-modified artificial study designs appear to give a closer picture of reality [63, 86, 95].

Subgroup analysis revealed a significant difference in mortality in trauma patients in favor of crystalloid resuscitation versus hetastarch and pentastarch [96]. Although these analyses contributed to our understanding, the crystalloid versus colloid debate is not answered until clinical studies employing tetrastarch are available.

We need adequately powered in vivo studies in humans to assess the clinical consequences of the administration of novel tetrastarch preparations and (oxypoly-)gelatin on coagulation, perioperative blood loss, and transfusion requirements in the relevant clinical situation of procedures with high volume shifts and imminent bleeding. However methodology of some in vivo studies may also be questioned because intravenous infusion of 20 mL/kg within 10 minutes does not necessarily represent common practice [18, 22]. Furthermore, blood substitution strategy and individual circumstances, like comorbidities and co-medication, individual anatomy, as well as operative sites influences blood loss sometimes to a larger extent than coagulopathy. Fluid volume regimens need to be adjusted to the different volume effects of the test solutions.

References

1. Kozek-Langenecker S. Effects of hydroxyethyl starch solutions on hemostasis. Anesthesiology 2005;103:654–60.
2. Van der Linden P, Ickx B. The effects of colloid solutions on hemostasis. Can J Anaesth 2006;53:S30–39.
3. deJonge E, Levi M. Effects of different plasma substitutes on blood coagulation: a comparative review. Crit Care Med 2001;29:1261–7.
4. Boldt J, Suttner S. Plasma substitutes. Minerva Anestesiol 2005;71:741–58.
5. Treib J, Haass A, Pindur G, et al. HES 200/0.5 is not HES 200/0.5: influence of the C2/C6 hydroxyethylation ratio of hydroxyethyl starch (HES) on hemorheology, coagulation and elimination kinetics. Thromb Haemost 1995;74:1452–6.
6. Treib J, Haass A, Pindur G, et al. All medium starches are not the same: influence of the degree of hydroxyethyl substitution of hydroxyethyl starch on plasma volume, hemorrheologic conditions, and coagulation. Transfusion 1996;36:450–55.
7. Treib J, Haass A, Pindur G, et al. Influence of intravascular molecular weight of hydroxyethyl starch on platelets. Eur J Haematol 1996;56:168–72.
8. deJonge E, Levi M, Buller R, Berends F, Kesecioglu J. Decreased circulating levels of von Willebrand factor after intravenous administration of a rapidly degradable hydroxyethyl starch (HES 200/0.5/6) in healthy human subjects. Intensive Care Med 2001;27: 1825–9.
9. Jamnicki M, Bombeli T, Seifert B, et al. Low- and medium-molecular-weight hydroxyethyl starches: comparison of their effect on blood coagulation. Anesthesiology 2000;93:1231–7.
10. Kapiotis S, Quehenberger P, Eichler H, et al. Effect of hydroxyethyl starch on the activity of blood coagulation and fibrinolysis in healthy volunteers: comparison with albumin. Crit Care Med 1994;22:606–12.
11. Strauss R, Stansfield C, Henriksen R, Villhauer P. Pentastarch may cause fewer effects on coagulation than hetastarch. Transfusion 1988;28:257–60.
12. Conroy J, Fishman R, Reeves S, Pinosky M, Lazarchick J. The effects of desmopressin and 6% hydroxyethyl starch on factor VIII:C. Anesth Analg 1996;83:804–7.

13. Niemi T, Kuittunen A. Hydroxyethyl starch impairs in vitro coagulation. Acta Anaesth Scand 1998;42:1104–9.
14. Tobias M, Wambold D, Pilla M, Greer F. Differential effects of serial hemodilution with hydroxyethyl starch, albumin, and 0.9% saline on whole blood coagulation. J Clin Anesth 1998;10:366–71.
15. Entholzer E, Mielke L, Calatzis A, et al. Coagulation effects of a recently developed hydroxyethyl starch (HES 130/0.4) compared to hydroxyethyl starches with higher molecular weight. Acta Anaesth Scand 2000;44:1116–21.
16. Fries D, Innerhofer P, Klingler A, et al. The effects of the combined administration of colloids and lactated Ringer's solution on the coagulation system: an in vitro study using thrombelastograph coagulation analysis (ROTEG). Anesth Analg 2002;94:1280–87.
17. Petroianu G, Maleck W, Koetter K, Liu J, Schmitt A. Effect of in vitro hemodilution with hydroxyethyl starch and dextran on the activity of plasma clotting factors. Crit Care Med 2003;31:250–54.
18. Nielsen V. Effects of PentaLyte and Voluven hemodilution on plasma coagulation kinetics in the rabbit: role of thrombin-fibrinogen and factor XIII-fibrin polymer interactions. Acta Anaesthesiol Scand 2005;49:1263–71.
19. McCammon A, Wright J, Figueroa M, Nielsen V. Hemodilution with Albumin, but not Hextend®, results in hypercoagulability as assessed by thrombelastography® in rabbits:Role of Heparin-dependent Serpins and Factor VIII complex. Anesth Analg 2002;95:844–50.
20. Strauss R, Pennell B, Stump D. A randomized controlled trial comparing the hemostatic effects of pentastarch versus hetastarch. Transfusion 2002;42:27–36.
21. Boldt J, Haisch G, Suttner S, Kumle B, Schellhaass A. Effects of a new modified, balanced hydroxyethyl starch preparation (Hextend) on measures of coagulation. Br J Anaesth 2002;89:722–8.
22. Nielsen V. Hemodilution modulates the time of onset and rate of fibrinolysis in human and rabbit plasma. J Heart Lung Transplant 2006;25:1344–52.
23. Niemi T, Kuitunen A. Artificial colloids impair haemostasis. An in vitro study using thromboelastometry coagulation analysis. Acta Anaesthesiol Scand 2005;49:373–8.
24. Kang J, Ahn H, Kim S, et al. The hemostatic profiles of patients with type 0 and non-0 blood after acute normovolemic hemodilution with 6% hydroxyethyl starch (130/0.4). Anesth Analg 2006;103:1543–8.
25. Jungheinrich C, Sauermann W, Bepperling F, Vogt N. Volume efficacy and reduced influence on measures of coagulation using hydroxyethyl starch 130/0.4 (6%) with an optimised in vivo molecular weight in orthopedic surgery: a randomised, double-blind study. Drugs R D 2004;5:1–9.
26. Neff T, Doelberg M, Jungheinrich C, et al. Repetitive large-dose infusion of the novel hydroxyethyl starch 130/0.4 in patients with severe head injury. Anesth Analg 2003;96:1453–9.
27. Kasper S, Meinert P, Kampe S, et al. Large-dose hydroxyethyl starch 130/0.4 does not increase blood loss and transfusion requirements in coronary artery bypass surgery compared with hydroxyethyl starch 200/0.5 at recommended doses. Anesthesiology 2003;99:42–7.
28. Kuitunen A, Hynynen M, Vahtera E, Salmenpera M. Hydroxyethyl starch as a priming solution for cardiopulmonary bypass impairs hemostasis after cardiac surgery. Anesth Analg 2004;98:291–7.
29. Huttner I, Boldt J, Haisch G, et al. Influence of different colloids on molecular markers of haemostasis and platelet function in patients undergoing major abdominal surgery. Br J Anaesth 2000;85:417–23.
30. Gallandat-Huet R, Siemons A, Baus D, et al. A novel hydroxyethyl starch (Voluven) for effective perioperative plasma volume substitution in cardiac surgery. Can J Anaesth 2000;47:1207–15.
31. Langeron O, Doelberg M, Ang E, et al. Voluven, a lower substituted novel hydroxyethyl starch (HES 130/0.4), causes fewer effects on coagulation in major orthopedic surgery than HES 200/0.5. Anesth Analg 2001;92:855–62.
32. Ellger B, Freyhoff J, van Aken H, Booke M, Marcus M. High-dose volume replacement using HES 130/0.4 during major surgery. Ned Tijdschr Anesthesiol 2006;19:63–8.
33. Battle J, del Rio F, Lopez Fernandez M, Martin R, Lopez BA. Effect of dextran on factor VIII/von Willebrand factor structure and function. Thromb Haemost 1985;54:697–9.
34. Mittermayr M, Streif W, Haas T, et al. Haemostatic changes after crystalloid or colloid fluid administration during orthopedic surgery: the role of fibrinogen administration. Anesth Analg 2007;105:905–17.
35. Innerhofer P, Fries D, Margreiter J, et al. The effects of perioperatively administered colloids and crystalloids on primary platelet-mediated hemostasis and clot formation. Anesth Analg 2002;95:858–65.

36. Dietrich H, Kraft D, Sirtl C, et al. Hydroxyethyl starch antibodies in humans: incidence and clinical relevance. Anesth Analg 1998;86:1123–6.
37. Dalrymple-Hay M, Aitchison R, Collins R, et al. Hydroxyethyl starch induced acquired von Willebrand's disease. Clin Lab Haematol 1992;14:209–11.
38. Mohri H. Acquired von Willebrand syndrome: features and management. Am J Hematol 2006;81:616–23.
39. Stögermüller B, Stark J, Willschke H, et al. The effects of hydroxyethyl starch 200 kD on platelet function. Anesth Analg 2000;91:823–7.
40. Franz A, Bräunlich P, Gamsjäger T, et al. The effects of hydroxyethyl starches of varying molecular weight on platelet function. Anesth Analg 2001;92: 1402–7.
41. Scharbert G, Deusch E, Kress H, et al. Inhibition of platelet function by hydroxyethyl starch solutions in chronic pain patients undergoing peridural anesthesia. Anesth Analg 2004;99:823–7.
42. Omar M, Shouk T, Khaleq M. Activity of blood coagulation and fibrinolysis during and after hydroxyethyl starch (HES) colloidal volume replacement. Clin Biochem 1999;32:269–74.
43. Deusch E, Thaler U, Kozek-Langenecker S. The effects of high molecular weight hydroxyethyl starch solutions on platelets. Anesth Analg 2004;99:665–8.
44. Chen G, Yan M, Lu Q, Gong M. Effects of two different hydroxyethyl starch solutions (HES200/0.5 vs. HES130/0.4) on the expression of platelet membrane glycoprotein. Acta Anaesthesiol Scand 2006;50:1089–94.
45. Thaler U, Deusch E, Kozek-Langenecker S. In vitro effects of various gelatin solutions on platelet function and their comparison to hydroxyethyl starch solutions. Anaesthesia 2005;60:554–9.
46. deJonge E, Levi M, Berends F, et al. Impaired haemostasis by intravenous administration of a gelatin-based plasma expander in human subjects. Thromb Haemost 1998;79:286–90.
47. Evans P, Glenn J, Heptinstall S, Madira W. Effects of gelatin-based resuscitation fluids on platelet aggregation. Br J Anaesth 1998;80:204–7.
48. Gamsjäger T, Gustorff B, Kozek-Langenecker S. The effects of hydroxyethyl starches on intracellular calcium in platelets. Anesth Analg 2002;95:866–9.
49. Jüttner B, Kuse E, Elsner H, et al. Differential platelet receptor expression following hydroxyethyl starch infusion in thrombocytopaenic orthotopic liver transplantation recipients. Eur J Anaesthesiol 2004;21:309–13.
50. Deusch E, Gamsjäger T, Kress H, Kozek-Langenecker S. Binding of hydroxyethyl starch molecules to the platelet surface. Anesth Analg 2003;97:680–83.
51. Jamnicki M, Zollinger A, Seifert B, et al. Compromised blood coagulation: an in vitro comparison of hydroxyethyl starch 130/0.4 and hydroxyethyl starch 200/0.5 using thrombelastography. Anesth Analg 1998;87:989–93.
52. von Roten I, Madjdpour C, Frascarolo P, et al. Molar substitution and C2/C6 ratio of hydroxyethyl starch: influence on blood coagulation. Br J Anaesth 2006;96:455–63.
53. Madjdpour C, Dettori N, Frascarolo P, et al. Molecular weight of hydroxyethyl starch: is there an effect on blood coagulation and pharmacokinetics? Br J Anaesth 2005;94:569–76.
54. Butwick A, Carvalho B. The effect of colloid and crystalloid preloading on thromboelastography prior to Cesarean delivery. Can J Anaesth 2007;54:190–95.
55. Thyes C, Madjdpour C, Frascarolo P, et al. Effect of high- and low-molecular-weight low-substituted hydroxyethyl starch on blood coagulation during acute normovolemic hemodilution in pigs. Anesthesiology 2006;105:1228–37.
56. Madjdpour C, Thyes C, Buclin T, et al. Novel starches. Anesthesiology 2007;106:132–43.
57. Coats T, Brazil E, Heron M. The effects of commonly used resuscitation fluids on whole blood coagulation. Emerg Med J 2006;23:546–9.
58. Jones S, Whitten C, Despotis G, Monk T. The influence of crystalloid and colloid replacement solutions in acute normovolemic hemodilution: a preliminary survey of hemostatic markers. Anesth Analg 2003;96:363–8.
59. Mortier E, Ongenae M, De Baerdemaeker L, et al. In vitro evaluation of the effect of profound haemodilution with hydroxyethyl starch 6%, modified fluid gelatin 4% and dextran 40 10% on coagulation profile measured by thrombelastography. Anaesthesia 1997;52:1061–4.
60. Petroianu G, Liu J, Maleck W, Mattinger C, Bergler W. The effect of in vitro hemodilution with gelatin, dextran, hydroxyethyl starch, or ringer's solution on thrombelastogramm. Anesth Analg 2000;90: 795–800.
61. Haas T, Preinreich A, Oswald E, et al. Effects of albumin 5% and artificial colloids on clot formation in small infants. Anaesthesia 2007;62:1000–1007.
62. Strauss R, Stump D, Henriksen R, Saunders R. Effects of hydroxyethyl starch on fibrinogen, fibrin clot formation and fibrinolysis. Transfusion 1985;25:230–34.

63. Fenger-Eriksen C, Heslop J, Anker-Moller E, Ingerslev J, Sorensen B. Thrombelastographic whole blood clot formation following ex vivo addition of plasma substitutes: improvements of the induced coagulopathy with fibrinogen concentrate. Br J Anaesth 2005;94:324–9.
64. Nielsen V. Colloids decrease clot propagation and strength: role of factor XIII-fibrin polymer and thrombin-fibrinogen interactions. Acta Anaesthesiol Scand 2005;49:1163–71.
65. Nielsen V, Kirklin J. Hydroxyethyl starch enhances argatroban-mediated decrease in clot propagation and strength by diminishing thrombin-fibrinogen interactions. Blood Coagul Fibrinolysis 2007;18:49–54.
66. Konrad C, Markl T, Schuepfer G, Gerber H, Tschopp M. The effects of in vitro hemodilution with gelatin, hydroxyethyl starch, and lactated ringer's solution on markers of coagulation: an analysis using Sonoclot™. Anesth Analg 1999;88:483–8.
67. Ickx B, Van der Linden P. Interactions entre les solutes colloides et l'hemostase. STV 2002;14:408–16.
68. Eriksson M, Saldeen T. Effect of dextran on plasma tissue plasminogen activator (t-PA) and plasminogen activator inhibitor-1 (PAI-1) during surgery. Acta Anaesthesiol Scand 1995;39:163–6.
69. Gan T J, Bennett-Guerrero E, Phillips-Bute B, et al. Hextend, a physiologically balanced plasma expander for large volume use in major surgery: a randomized phase III clinical trial. Anaesth Analg 1999;88: 992–8.
70. Waters J, Gottlieb A, Schoenwald P, et al. Normal saline versus lactated Ringer's solution for intraoperative fluid management in patients undergoing abdominal aortic aneurysma repair: an outcome study. Anesth Analg 2001;93:817–22.
71. Roche AM, James MF, Bennett-Guerrero E, Mythen MG. A head-to-head comparison of the in vitro coagulation effects of saline-based and balanced electrolyte crystalloid and colloid intravenous fluids. Anesth Analg 2006;102:1274–9.
72. Roche AM, James MF, Bennett-Guerrero E, Mythen MG. Calcium supplementation of saline-based colloids does not produce equivalent coagulation profiles to similarly balanced salt preparations. J Cardiothorac Vasc Anesth 2006;20:807–11.
73. Boldt J, Wolf M, Mengistu A. A new plasma-adapted hydroxyethylstarch preparation: in vitro coagulation studies using thrombelastography and whole blood aggregometry. Anesth Analg 2007;104:425–30.
74. Roberts J, Evans P, Bunn F, Kwan I, Crowhurst E. Is the normalisation of blood pressure in bleeding trauma patients harmful? (review). Lancet 2001;357:385–7.
75. Wilkes M, Navickis R, Sibbald W. Albumin versus hydroxyethyl starch in cardiopulmonary bypass surgery: a meta-analysis of postoperative bleeding. Ann Thorac Surg 2001;72:527–37.
76. Kozek-Langenecker S, Jungheinrich C, Sauermann W, Van der Linden P. Hydroxyethyl starch 130/0.4 reduces blood loss in major surgery. Intensive Care Med 2006;32 (Suppl. 1): A-0836.
77. Hobisch-Hagan P, Wirleitner B, Mair J. Consequences of acute normovolaemic haemodilution on haemostasis during major orthopaedic surgery. Br J Anaesth 1999;82:503–9.
78. Tabuchi N, de Haan J, Gallandat-Huet R, Boonstra P, van Oeveren W. Gelatin use impairs platelet adhesion during cardiac surgery. Thromb Haemost 1995;74:1447–51.
79. Haisch G, Boldt J, Krebs C, et al. The influence of intravascular volume therapy with a new hydroxyethyl starch preparation (6% HES 130/0.4) on coagulation in patients undergoing major abdominal surgery. Anesth Analg 2001;92:565–71.
80. Boldt J, Knothe C, Zickmann B, et al. Influence of different intravascular volume therapies on platelet function in patients undergoing cardiopulmonary bypass. Anesth Analg 1993;76:1185–90.
81. Gandhi S, Weiskopf R, Jungheinrich C, et al. Volume replacement therapy during major orthopedic surgery using Voluven (hydroxyethyl starch 130/0.4) or hetastarch. Anesthesiology 2007;106:1120–27.
82. Todd S, Malinoski D, Muller P, Schreiber M. Hextend attenuates hypercoagulability after severe liver injury in swine. J Trauma 2005;59:589–94.
83. Nielsen V. Resuscitation with Hextend decreases endogenous circulating heparin activity and accelerates clot initiation after hemorrhage in the rabbit. Anesth Analg 2001;93:1106–10.
84. Karoutsos S, Nathan N, Lahrimi A, et al. Thrombelastogram reveals hypercoagulability after administration of gelatin solution. Br J Anaesth 1999;82: 175–7.
85. Fordal P, Svensson J, Ljungstrom K. Effects of desmopressin and dextran on coagulation and fibrinolysis in healthy volunteers. Thromb Res 1991;62:355–64.
86. Sorensen B, Fenger-Eriksen C, Ingerslev J. Recombinant factor VIIa fails to correct coagulopathy induced by haemodilution with colloids. Br J Anaesth 2006.
87. Fries D, Krismer A, Klingler A, et al. Effect of fibrinogen on reversal of dilutional coagulopathy: a porcine model. Br J Anaesth 2005;94:862–3.

88. Kuitunen A, Suojaranta-Ylinen R, Kukkonen S, Niemi T. Tranexamic acid does not correct the haemostatic impairment caused by hydroxyethyl starch (200 kDa/0.5) after cardiac surgery. Blood Coagul Fibrinolysis 2006;17:639–45.
89. Wills B, Nguyen M, Ha T, et al. Comparison of three fluid solutions for resuscitation in dengue shock syndrome. N Engl J Med 2005;353:877–89.
90. Ellingson T, Aboulafia D. Dextran syndrome. Acute hypotension, noncardiogenic pulmonary edema, anemia, and coagulopathy following hysteroscopic surgery using 32% dextran 70. Chest 1997;111:513–8.
91. Watters J, Tieu B, Differding J, Muller P, Schreiber M. A single bolus of 3% hypertonic saline with 6% dextran provides optimal initial resuscitation after uncontrolled hemorrhagic shock. J Trauma 2006;61:75–81.
92. Wiedermann I, Scharbert G, Schöchl H, Kozek-Langenecker S. Hydroxyethyl starch in hypertonic saline and platelet function [abstract]. Anesthesiology 2007.
93. Brummel-Ziedins K, Whelihan M, Ziedins E, Mann K. The resuscitation fluid you choose may potentiate bleeding. J Trauma 2006;61:1350–58.
94. Nielsen V. High-molecular-weight hydroxyethyl starch accelerates kallikrein-dependent clot initiation. J Trauma 2007;62:1491–4.
95. De Lorenzo C, Calatzis A, Welsch U, Heindl B. Fibrinogen concentrate reverses dilutional coagulopathy induced in vitro by saline but not by hydroxyethyl starch 6%. Anesth Analg 2006;102:1194–200.
96. Choi P, Yip G, Quinonez L, Cook D. Crystalloids vs. colloids in fluid resuscitation: a systematic review. Crit Care Med 1999;27:200–210.

CHAPTER 12
Hydroxyethyl Starch and Renal Dysfunction

Laurent Jacob[1], *Nicholas Heming*[1] *& Bertrand Guidet*[2]
[1]Department of Anesthesiology and Intensive Care, Saint-Louis Hospital, Assistance Publique-Hôpitaux de Paris, Paris, France
[2]UMR-S 707, Pierre-et-Marie-Curie University (Paris 6), Department of Intensive Care, Saint-Antoine Hospital, Assistance Publique-Hôpitaux de Paris, Paris, France

Introduction

Beyond the controversy regarding the role of colloids and crystalloids in fluid therapy, another debate—just as impassioned—concerns hydroxyethyl starch (HES) solutions and their effect on renal function. When assessing the evidence, the type of HES used should be considered. Studies performed with "old" high-molecular-weight and high-substitution-ratio HES solutions are probably not applicable to newly marketed HES. The data regarding the nephrotoxicity of HES solutions should also be analyzed with consideration to the clinical circumstances in which these solutions are prescribed [1]. Given the wide heterogeneity of the published material, it would be inappropriate to compare an organ donation, which is a model of ischemia-reperfusion, to a septic shock, where a multiple organ dysfunction syndrome is associated with an alteration of glomerular perfusion and filtration even before fluid resuscitation, or to intraoperative compensation of blood loss. In all these circumstances, the volume and duration of fluid administration are different.

The difficulties in addressing intraoperative renal protection because of the lack of understanding of its complex physiology were underlined by the consensus conference sponsored by the French Society of Anesthesiology and Intensive Care in 2004 [2]. However, in patients at risk of renal failure, rapid restoration of perfusion pressure to the kidney is probably just as important for the prognosis of renal function as the choice of the fluid replacement solution [3].

Nephrotoxicity associated with fluid replacement solutions

Part of the nephrotoxicity ascribed to HES falls within the scope of colloid-induced lesions during fluid resuscitation or immunotherapy with intravenous immunoglobulin [4, 5]. These fluids can alter renal function by increasing oncotic pressure in the glomerular capillaries, thereby opposing glomerular filtration. This happens when large quantities of colloids are administered to dehydrated patients without administration of crystalloids. Moreover, filtration of low-molecular-weight (<50 to 60 kD) colloid substances, increase of viscosity of tubular urine, and colloid deposit in the tubular lumen could all contribute to altering renal function.

Osmotic-nephrosis lesions have been described after administration of HES in kidney transplantation [6]. We have known about osmotic-nephrosis lesions for a long time and they are reported after administration of sugar, mannitol, radiocontrast dyes, gelatins, and dextrans. The most probable

Alternatives to Blood Transfusion in Transfusion Medicine, 2nd edition. Edited by A. Maniatis, P. Van der Linden, J.-F. Hardy.

mechanism is based on resorption of filtered molecules by tubular epithelial cells through pinocytosis. These cells lack the enzymes capable of degrading internalized molecules, leading to intracellular accumulation. The proximal and distal distribution of osmotic-nephrosis lesions and their persistence are arguments in favor of HES-induced nephrotoxicity. On the other hand, these lesions are not associated with clinically significant modifications of renal function, neither has the presence of molecules of HES in cytoplasmic vacuoles ever been demonstrated, which pleads against induced nephrotoxicity and suggests that the modifications of renal function observed in these clinical circumstances are generated by multiple factors such as ischemia-reperfusion and/or inflammation of the kidney.

However, long-lasting deposition of HES in typical vacuoles can be found in other organs such as the liver, the spleen, and the reticuloendothelial system. In 2001, Stander et al. [7] elegantly proved by antibody studies that such vacuoles in endothelial and nerve cells contained HES and were responsible for HES-induced pruritus. Pillebout et al. [8] found osmotic-nephrotis lesions characteristic for HES toxicity which persisted up to 10 years in 16 out of 29 patients (61%) who previously had received orthotopic liver transplantation and developed chronic renal failure. The authors, who did not expect this finding, called it "chronic HES nephrotoxicity" and concluded that this chronic renal failure "can be attributed to four associated primary lesions: (i) specific chronic CsA/FK506 arteriolopathy; (ii) typical diabetic nephropathy; (iii) acute or chronic thrombotic microangiopathy attributed to CsA/FK506 or α-IFN; and (iv) tubular changes related to administration of hydroxyethylstarch" [8]. Patients receiving large amounts of HES, in particular after several plasma exchanges, were found to have widespread HES deposition resembling acquired lysosomal storage disease [9–11].

Considering the accumulation of material in tubular cells, possibly related to starches, large amounts of HES should be avoided and basic intravenous hydration with crystalloids should be performed in parallel.

HES solutions and kidney transplantation

In a letter published by *The Lancet* in 1993, Legendre et al. [6] underlined the increased incidence of osmotic-nephrosis lesions observed on biopsies of kidneys transplanted in 1992, compared with the period preceding the introduction of HES 200/0.62 in organ-donor resuscitation protocols. This study found 80% of osmotic-nephrosis lesions after introduction of HES 200/0.62, compared with 14% previously. Of note, these osmotic-nephrosis lesions had no impact on transplanted kidney function; there was no delay in graft function nor any difference in terms of plasmatic creatinine 3 months or 6 months after transplantation. From the start, osmotic-nephrosis lesions were described as persistent as they were found on routine biopsies at 3 months in three patients. This study concluded with the absence of impact on renal function but underlined the added difficulty of interpretation of histological findings concerning grafted kidneys.

These results led Marie-Laure Cittanova's team to undertake an open prospective study on the impact of the use of HES 200/0.62 on renal function in kidney-transplant recipients [12]. This study was interrupted after an intermediate analysis showed a negative effect on graft function. The criteria of renal function alteration were an increased need for renal replacement therapy (33% versus 5%) in the HES group and a slower decrease of plasma creatinine. The following factors, although not significant, may have contributed to these results:

- The total volume of fluid administered to the donor was 1000 mL higher in the gelatin group.
- Early administration of cyclosporine was more fre quent in the HES group (33% versus 25%).
- The need for vasopressor support was more frequent (40% versus 33%) in the HES group.
- The use of Euro-Collins as kidney graft preservation liquid was twice as important in the HES group.
- The distribution of the kidneys across the transplan tation sites was not specified. Care of the kidney-transplant recipient varies from one hospital to another, in particular with regard to fluid replace ment therapy before release of vascular

clamps, and can have an impact on the frequency of early graft function.

• The indications of renal replacement therapy—the primary outcome—were not specified, particularly with regard to the presence of urine output.

In this context, acute tubular necrosis after ischemia and delayed graft function might be caused by multiple factors. The impact of this study was considerable and resulted in abandoning the use of HES with high in vivo molecular weight for fluid resuscitation of brain-death patients. Long-term followup of the patients included in this study did not show a significant difference in renal function after 5–6 years [13].

During the same period, the above-mentioned studies were contradicted by three papers [14–16]. Coronel et al. [14] reported that the frequency of osmotic-nephrosis lesions (20%) was not influenced by the use of HES, that these lesions had no impact on graft function and that hemo-dynamic status of the donor could affect the incidence of these lesions just as much as the type of fluid replacement solution used. This letter confirmed the data from a 1994 study [15] reporting that administration of HES 200/0.62 to the donors of 26 transplanted kidneys was associated with no use of renal replacement therapy nor any difference in plasmatic creatinine or oliguria during the first week. During this study, four biopsies were performed in the HES group, showing osmotic-nephrosis lesions in all four cases, with no relation to the HES volume administered or graft function. In 1999, Deman et al. [16] reported a retrospective study comparing administration of HES 200/0.5, HES 450/0.7, and albumin associated with gelatin. A delay in graft function was found in 15, 31, and 19% of patients, respectively, but the differences did not reach statistical significance. The delay in graft function observed with HES 450/0.7 was associated with donor hemodynamic instability. Of note, preservation liquids containing HES (U Wisconsin) offer better results on graft function than Euro-Collins [17].

In summary, high-molecular-weight, high-substitution-ratio HES solutions with a prolonged half-life should not be used for fluid therapy in organ donors. The use of medium-molecular-weight HES solutions has been shown to increase the frequency of osmotic-nephrosis lesions, without any demonstrated correlation with the prognosis of graft function. As suggested by the French Society of Anesthesiology and Intensive Care expert recommendations for the management of organ donors [2], restrictions on the use of HES 200/0.62 do not concern HES solutions with a low molecular weight and a low substitution ratio.

HES solutions and perioperative renal function

The use of HES for compensation of perioperative blood loss is equally controversial with regard to the effects on renal function. On one hand, a number of studies covering multiple surgical situations and involving large patient populations did not demonstrate any increase in postoperative renal dysfunction [18–26]. On the other hand, case reports have blamed HES for causing renal dysfunction [27]. In this context, where a number of factors related to the patient, the surgical procedure, and the perioperative events are associated with an increased risk of acute renal failure, it is difficult to isolate HES administration from all the other potential causative factors.

It must be noted that studies reporting an impact on renal function use different specific markers of renal tubular function, such as N-acetyl-β-D-glucosaminidase (NAG), α1-microglobulin, or π and λ, glutathione transferase, without demonstrating any alteration in glomerular filtration, requirements for renal replacement therapy or vital prognosis [19, 28]. These markers of tubular function are extremely sensitive to ischemia-reperfusion damage, which occurs frequently in these patients. The association with HES administration remains unclear. For example, during cardiac surgery on 40 patients over 70 years of age, who already combined two major risk factors for developing postoperative acute renal failure, the use of low-molecular-weight and low-substitution-ratio HES was not associated with a significant increase of renal function markers, compared with a group receiving gelatin [18]. None of the patients developed acute renal failure in the first 48 hours after surgery. Mortality was not modified and the increased level of renal function markers was identical in both groups, underlining the impact of the type of surgery rather than the fluid replacement solution. These results confirmed the study by Kumle et al. [23] comparing two HES solutions (with medium and low molecular weights) and gelatin during major abdominal surgery.

The use of large volumes of HES during major urologic surgery [25] or orthopedic surgery [26] is not associated with changes in renal function during the first 24 hours, compared with a control group receiving albumin. During thoracic and thoracoabdominal surgery of the aorta [22], significant alterations of renal function were noted in 25% of the 475 patients studied. HES (200/0.62) was used in 217 patients, 25% of whom developed acute renal failure, whereas 26% of the 258 remaining patients developed acute renal failure. The multivariate analysis did not find the use of medium-molecular-weight HES to be an independent risk factor. These results were confirmed when using HES 130/0.4 in abdominal aortic surgery [29]. The peak plasma creatinine level and the minimum postoperative creatinine clearance did not differ between HES and gelatin patients. A randomly conducted comparison of HES 200/0.62, HES 130/0.4, and gelatin administration in 62 patients undergoing abdominal aortic aneurysm surgery showed a lower creatinine level in the HES 130/0.4 patients at days 1, 2, and 5 after surgery [30]. The use of large volumes (up to 70 mL/kg/day) of HES (130/0.4) during 1–5 days in head injury patients is not associated with an altered renal function when these patients are compared with a group receiving another HES (200/0.5) solution at a 33 mL/kg/day dose, associated with albumin [24].

A deleterious effect on the evolution of renal function after coronary artery bypass has been reported [31]. This study showed a decrease of the glomerular filtration rate by approximately 10 mL/min at days 3 and 5 after surgery. The glomerular filtration rate was evaluated using the Cockroft formula, which has only been validated in stable patients, a situation very different from the perioperative period. The creatinine values were not reported. The multivariate analysis found an association between HES administration and renal dysfunction, without demonstrating a causality link. The HES used in small volumes (650 mL) was a high-molecular-weight and high-substitution-ratio HES. It is not easy to determine the specific role of HES in the genesis of the observed lesions.

Finally, an evaluation of the effects of fluid therapy on renal function in 60 ears, nose, and throat (ENT) patients receiving either Ringer's lactate or one of three different HES solutions (200/0.5; 200/0.62; 450/0.7) at a dose of 15 mL/kg at induction of anesthesia found no modification of renal function [21]. These results are observed during the first 2 days following the operation. The markers studied were urea, creatinine, and urine output, as well as more sophisticated markers of renal function such as renal plasmatic flow, p-aminohippurate clearance, glomerular filtration rate (inuline clearance), or biochemical markers of tubular injury (α-1-microglobulin, NAG, Tamm-Horsfall protein).

In conclusion, administration of moderate volumes of HES to patients without renal dysfunction is not associated with alterations of renal function.

HES solutions and fluid therapy in intensive care

Severe sepsis, i.e., sepsis associated with acute organ dysfunction, is a major problem in intensive care, accounting for 10–20% of intensive care unit (ICU) stays longer than 24 hours [32]. Adequate fluid resuscitation is a major step in the management of severe sepsis or septic shock [33]. The objective of fluid resuscitation is to improve regional, local, and general circulation in order to prevent tissue damage. The rapidity and quality of fluid resuscitation are important factors for the prevention of secondary multiorgan failure. The time devoted to correcting hypovolemia is a decisive element in the prognosis of severe sepsis. In the study by Rivers et al. [34], optimization of the management of severe sepsis in the first 6 hours was shown to significantly reduce mortality. During sepsis, fluid therapy is administered to compensate fluid losses and to restore a normal hemodynamic status characterized by a decrease in systemic vascular resistance and capillary leak syndrome. The choice of the fluid replacement regimen is debated between partisans of albumin, crystalloids, and gelatins, or starches [28].

Early restoration of intravascular volume requires a strategy of aggressive filling. Isoosmotic crystalloids (0.9% NaCl, Ringer's lactate) are distributed to all extracellular compartments; therefore, larger volumes are needed than with colloids to obtain the same intravascular volume expansion. Colloids have a longer volume effect than crystalloids. However, this property has not been shown to have an impact on mortality. A meta-analysis comparing albumin and crystalloids showed no difference between the two groups [35]. In the only randomized, prospective study with a large number of patients, no effect on 28-day mortality was found with intensive treatment consisting of 4% albumin compared with 0.9% NaCl [36]. A subgroup analysis showed a trend toward reduced mortality in patients with severe sepsis resuscitated with albumin versus patients treated with crystalloids (30.7% versus 35.3%; $P = 0.06$). Further studies evaluating colloid administration in this patient group are needed.

Beyond the alteration of renal function associated with the type of fluid replacement solution used, the interaction between the fluid replacement strategy, and injury to the vascular endothelium should be considered [37–39]. Moreover, in these situations, alterations of renal perfusion caused by changes in cardiac output or systemic blood pressure play a role, just as alterations of intrarenal circulation. Intrarenal circulation is compromised because of an imbalance between renal vasoconstrictor and vasodilatator mediators.

A prospective randomized study assessed renal function in patients with severe sepsis or septic shock receiving either HES (200/0.62), at a total dose of 31 mL/kg for up to 4 days, or gelatin [40]. This study concluded that there was an increased risk of acute renal failure (defined as a twofold increase of plasmatic creatinine, irrespective of the baseline value). However, the two patient groups differed with regard to baseline renal function (plasmatic creatinine: 143 (μmol/L in the HES group versus 114 (μmol/L in the gelatin group). The difference in plasmatic creatinine levels recorded from day 0 to day 8 only reached significant levels at days 6 and 7, with relatively minor differences considering the clinical context. Most importantly, these alterations of renal function had no effect on patient outcomes (overall mortality, need for renal replacement therapy, or length of hospital stay). In most analyses of ICU registries, development of acute renal failure is predictive of an increase in mortality and length of hospital stay [41]. The clinical significance of these modifications of plasmatic creatinine remains unclear.

In a recent observational study [42], 1075 of 3147 critically ill patients admitted to 198 ICUs received HES. Administration of HES had no influence on renal function or the need for renal replacement therapy in the ICU.

The results of the VISEP (Efficacy of Volume Substitution and Insulin Therapy in Severe Sepsis) study were presented in 2006 [43]. Administration of HES 200/0.5 was compared with Ringer's lactate infusion to achieve the Surviving Sepsis Campaign hemodynamic goals in septic patients. Although neither the 28-day mortality nor the mean SOFA score reached any significant differences, the study was suspended because of a significant increase in the frequency of acute renal failure and need for renal replacement therapy in the HES group. These data have yet to be published and special attention should be paid to the type of HES used, the duration of HES administration, and the results should be interpreted cautiously. It should be emphasized that the dose of HES was not tapered when acute renal failure appeared, basic hydration was not adequately performed, and acute renal failure was not diagnosed before the fifth ICU day.

In trauma patients, administration of HES (250/0.45) resulted in significantly lower capillary leak syndrome and higher PaO_2/FiO_2 ratio than gelatin [44]. Finally, no difference in plasma creatinine or urine output was reported. Administration of large volumes of HES, compared with albumin, is associated with no increase of acute renal failure in the high-risk population of patients suffering from toxic hepatitis after ingestion of paracetamol.

The 2004 consensus statement of the American Thoracic Society stated that "HES administration may increase the risk of acute renal failure in patients with sepsis (II-A)" and that "hydroxyethyl starch solutions should be used with caution in cardiopulmonary bypass (meta-analysis) and in patients with sepsis (II-A)" [45].

Conclusion

HES-induced renal dysfunction is at the center of a major debate between advocates of crystalloids, those who prefer gelatins, those who consider that albumin would be more appropriate, and finally those who believe in the renal toxicity of HES. HES incrimination in renal alterations is based on a limited number of studies to which the following arguments—both methodological and pathophysiological—can be opposed:

• The use of medium-molecular-weight and low-substitution-ratio HES for patients with risk factors for acute renal failure is associated with no changes in renal function modification, whatever marker is used. The use of large volumes of this type of HES does not have any undesirable effect on renal function. Accumulation of solutions with a longer half-life imposes limitations on both the duration of administration and the volume administered.

• In cases of preexisting alterations of renal function, the use of low-molecular-weight and low-substitution-ratio HES is not associated with a decline of renal function.

• The use of low- or medium-molecular-weight and low-substitution-ratio HES is not associated with a degradation renal function in high-risk perioperative situations such as cardiac, vascular, orthopedic, and ENT surgery or neurosurgery. Most published studies support this observation.

• In organ donors and ICU patients, administration of HES has been associated with transient increases of serum creatinine levels which did not affect mortality, the need for renal replacement therapy in septic patients, or the prognosis of kidney graft function in organ donors. Considering that osmotic-nephrosis lesions do not contain any HES and that they remain in place even after renal function returns to normal, the link between the use of HES and renal dysfunction remains to be demonstrated.

References

1. Jungheinrich C, Scharpf R, Wargenau M, Bepperling F, Baron JF. The pharmacokinetics and tolerability of an intravenous infusion of the new hydroxyethyl starch 130/0.4 (6%, 500 mL) in mild-to-severe renal impairment. Anesth Analg 2002;95:544–51.
2. French Society of Anesthesiology and Intensive Care. Consensus Conference on Perioperative Renal Protection, September 14, 2004. Accessed at http://www.sfar.org.
3. Mehta RL, Clark WC, Schetz M. Techniques for assessing and achieving fluid balance in acute renal failure. Curr Opin Crit Care 2002;8:535–43.
4. Davidson IJ. Renal impact of fluid management with colloids: a comparative review. Eur J Anaesthesiol 2006;23:721–38.
5. Perazella MA. Drug-induced renal failure: update on new medications and unique mechanisms of nephrotoxicity. Am J Med Sci 2003;325:349–62.
6. Legendre C, Thervet E, Page B, et al. Hydroxyethylstarch and osmotic-nephrosis-like lesions in kidney transplantation. Lancet 1993;342:248–9.
7. Slander S, Szepfalusi Z, Bohle B, et al. Differential storage of hydroxyethyl starch (HES) in the skin: an immunoelectron-microscopical long-term study. Cell Tissue Res 2001;304:261–9.
8. Pillebout E, Nochy D, Hill G, et al. Renal histopathological lesions after orthotopic liver transplantation (OLT). Am J Transplant 2005;5:1120–29.
9. Auwerda JJ, Leebeek FW, Wilson JH, et al. Acquired lysosomal storage caused by frequent plasmapheresis procedures with hydroxyethyl starch. Transfusion 2006;46:1705–11.
10. Ginz HF, Gottschall V, Schwarzkopf G, Walter K. [Excessive tissue storage of colloids in the reticuloendothelial system]. Anaesthesist 1998;47:330–34.
11. Schmidt-Hieber M, Loddenkemper C, Schwartz S, et al. Hydrops lysosomalis generalisatus – an underestimated side effect of hydroxyethyl starch therapy? Eur J Haematol 2006;77:83–5.
12. Cittanova ML, Leblanc I, Legendre C, et al. Effect of hydroxyethylstarch in brain-dead kidney donors on renal function in kidney-transplant recipients. Lancet 1996;348:1620–22.

13. Cittanova ML, Mavre J, Riou B, Coriat P. Long-term follow-up of transplanted kidneys according to plasma volume expander of kidney donors. Intensive Care Med 2001;27:1830.
14. Coronel B, Mercatello A, Martin X, Lefrancois N. Hydroxyethylstarch and renal function in kidney transplant recipients. Lancet 1997;349:884.
15. Coronel B, Laurent V, Mercatello A, et al. [Can hydroxyethylstarch be used during intensive care of brain-dead organ donors?] Ann Fr Anesth Reanim 1994;13:10–16.
16. Deman A, Peelers P, Sennesael J. Hydroxyethyl starch does not impair immediate renal function in kidney transplant recipients: a retrospective, multicentre analysis. Nephrol Dial Transplant 1999;14:1517–20.
17. de Boer J, De Meester J, Smits JM, et al. Euro transplant randomized multicenter kidney graft preservation study comparing HTK with UW and Euro-Collins. Transpl Int 1999;12:447–53.
18. Boldt J, Brenner T, Lang J, Kumle B, Isgro F. Kidney-specific proteins in elderly patients undergoing cardiac surgery with cardiopulmonary bypass. Anesth Analg 2003;97:1582–9.
19. Boldt J, Brenner T, Lehmann A, et al. Influence of two different volume replacement regimens on renal function in elderly patients undergoing cardiac surgery: comparison of a new starch preparation with gelatin. Intensive Care Med 2003;29:763–9.
20. Boldt J, Priebe HJ. Intravascular volume replacement therapy with synthetic colloids: is there an influence on renal function? Anesth Analg 2003;96:376–82.
21. Dehne MG, Muhling J, Sablotzki A, et al. Hydroxyethyl starch (HES) does not directly affect renal function in patients with no prior renal impairment. J Clin Anesth 2001;13:103–11.
22. Godet G, Fleron MH, Vicaut E, et al. Risk factors for acute postoperative renal failure in thoracic or thoracoabdominal aortic surgery: a prospective study. Anesth Analg 1997;85:1227–32.
23. Kumle B, Boldt J, Piper S, et al. The influence of different intravascular volume replacement regimens on renal function in the elderly. Anesth Analg 1999;89:1124–30.
24. Neff TA, Doelberg M, Jungheinrich C, et al. Repetitive large-dose infusion of the novel hydroxyethyl starch 130/0.4 in patients with severe head injury. Anesth Analg 2003;96:1453–9.
25. Vogt N, Bothner U, Brinkmann A, de Petriconi R, Georgieff M. Peri-operative tolerance to large-dose 6% HES 200/0.5 in major urological procedures compared with 5% human albumin. Anaesthesia 1999;54:121–7.
26. Vogt NH, Bothner U, Lerch G, Lindner KH, Georgieff M. Large-dose administration of 6% hydroxyethyl starch 200/0.5 total hip arthroplasty: plasma homeostasis, hemostasis, and renal function compared to use of 5% human albumin. Anesth Analg 1996;83:262–8.
27. De Labarthe A, Jacobs F, Blot F, Glotz D. Acute renal failure secondary to hydroxyethylstarch administration in a surgical patient. Am J Med 2001;111:417–8.
28. Celik I. Renal dysfunction after hydroxyethyl starch. Anesth Analg 2004;99:309–10.
29. Godet G, Lehot J, Janvier G, et al. Does volume substitution with HES 130/0.4 affect renal safety in abdominal aortic surgery? Crit Care 2006;10(Suppl. 1):173.
30. Mahmood A, Gosling P, Vohra RK. Randomized clinical trial comparing the effects on renal function of hydroxyethyl starch or gelatine during aortic aneurysm surgery. Br J Surg 2007;94:427–33.
31. Winkelmayer WC, Glynn RJ, Levin R, Avorn J. Hydroxyethyl starch and change in renal function in patients undergoing coronary artery bypass graft surgery. Kidney Int 2003;64:1046–9.
32. Guidet B, Aegerter P, Gauzit R, Meshaka P, Dreyfuss D. Incidence and impact of organ dysfunctions associated with sepsis. Chest 2005;127:942–51.
33. Dellinger RP, Carlet JM, Masur H, et al. Surviving Sepsis Campaign guidelines for management of severe sepsis and septic shock. Intensive Care Med 2004;30:536–55.
34. Rivers E, Nguyen B, Havstad S, et al. Early goal-directed therapy in the treatment of severe sepsis and septic shock. N Engl J Med 2001;345:1368–77.
35. Wilkes MM, Navickis RJ. Patient survival after human albumin administration. A meta-analysis of randomized, controlled trials. Ann Intern Med 2001;135:149–64.
36. Finfer S, Bellomo R, Boyce N, et al. A comparison of albumin and saline for fluid resuscitation in the intensive care unit. N Engl J Med 2004;350:2247–56.
37. Hoffmann JN, Vollmar B, Laschke MW, et al. Hydroxyethyl starch (130 kD), but not crystalloid volume support, improves microcirculation during normotensive endotoxemia. Anesthesiology 2002;97:460–70.
38. Lang JD Jr, Figueroa M, Chumley P, et al. Albumin and hydroxyethyl starch modulate oxidative inflammatory injury to vascular endothelium. Anesthesiology 2004;100:51–8.

39. Tian J, Lin X, Guan R, Xu JG. The effects of hydroxyethyl starch on lung capillary permeability in endotoxic rats and possible mechanisms. Anesth Analg 2004;98:768–74.
40. Schortgen F, Lacherade JC, Bruneel F, et al. Effects of hydroxyethylstarch and gelatin on renal function in severe sepsis: a multicentre randomised study. Lancet 2001;357:911–16.
41. Druml W. Acute renal failure is not a 'cute' renal failure!. Intensive Care Med 2004;30:1886–90.
42. Sakr Y, Payen D, Reinhart K, et al. Effects of hydroxyethyl starch administration on renal function in critically ill patients. Br J Anaesth 2007;98:216–24.
43. Reinhart K, Bloos F, Engel C, for the German Competence Network Sepsis. Hydroxyethyl starch and Ringer's lactate for fluid resuscitation in patients with severe sepsis: result from the VISEP study (abstract). Intensive Care Med 2006;32:S213.
44. Allison KP, Gosling P, Jones S, Pallister I, Porter KM. Randomized trial of hydroxyethyl starch versus gelatine for trauma resuscitation. J Trauma 1999;47:1114–21.
45. Evidence-based colloid use in the critically ill: american Thoracic Society Consensus Statement. Am J Respir Crit Care Med 2004;170:1247–59.

CHAPTER 13
Choice of a Synthetic Colloid for Surgery

Joachim Boldt
Department of Anesthesiology and Intensive Care Medicine, Klinikum der Stadt Ludwigshafen, Ludwigshafen, Germany

Introduction

During surgery, absolute or relative blood volume deficits often occur. Absolute volume deficits are secondary to bleeding, relative volume deficit may result from vasodilation mediated by vasodilating substances (e.g., anesthetics) or rewarming of the patient. Fluid deficits can also occur in the absence of obvious fluid loss due to generalized alterations of the endothelial barrier resulting in diffuse capillary leak. This situation is characterized by a panendothelial injury with subsequent development of increased endothelial permeability, leading to a loss of proteins and a fluid shift from the intravascular to the interstitial compartment resulting in interstitial edema.

Concern about the risk of allogenic blood supply has forced us to reduce the use of allogenic blood and blood products. Even severe reduction in hemoglobin is not deleterious since compensating mechanisms (e.g., increase in cardiac output) are able to guarantee tissue oxygenation and systemic oxygen transport [1]. However, the "safe" hemoglobin level is still not definitely known and it is unlikely that any level of hemoglobin can be used as a universal threshold for transfusion. Myocardial oxygen supply is determined by coronary blood flow and its oxygen content. Especially in the critically ill patient showing cardiovascular diseases augmentation of coronary blood flow may not provide adequate myocardial oxygenation when arterial blood oxygen content is decreased by reducing hemoglobin to critical levels owing to extreme hemodilution.

Alternatives to Blood Transfusion in Transfusion Medicine, 2nd edition. Edited by A. Maniatis, P. Van der Linden, J.-F. Hardy.

Consequences of surgery and hypovolemia

Current evidence suggests that hypovolemia is associated with flow alterations that are inadequate to fulfill the nutritive role of the circulation. The hypovolemic patient is at risk of experiencing significant organ hypoperfusion with subsequent development of (multiple) organ failure [2, 3]. Shoemaker et al. [4] demonstrated the importance to maintain VO_2 (oxygen consumption) and DO_2 (oxygen delivery) to reduce the incidence of MOF (multiple organ failure) and overall mortality in high-risk surgical patients. Thus, in patients undergoing complex, long-lasting surgery, maintenance of an adequate circulating volume appear to be a prerequisite to avoid postoperative organ dysfunction.

During hypovolemia, the organism tries to compensate perfusion deficits by redistribution of flow to vital organs (e.g., heart and brain) resulting in an underperfusion of other organs such as splanchnic bed, kidneys, muscles, and skin. Release of inflammatory mediators and vasoactive substances are of particular importance for impaired perfusion in this situation. Activation of the sympathetic nervous system (SNS) and the renin–angiotensin–aldosteron system (RAAS) are compensatory mechanisms to maintain peripheral perfusion. This compensatory neurohumoral activation is beneficial at first, but becomes deleterious and may be involved in the bad outcome of the critically ill surgical patient. Thus an adequate restoration of intravascular volume in the perioperative period is an important therapeutic maneuver. The controversy in this area focuses on the ideal kind of volume therapy [5–11]. This controversy does not only refer to the crystalloid–colloid debate, but has been widened in recent years to include a colloid–colloid debate since synthetic colloids have proven to be of benefit for volume therapy in this situation [12].

Principles of volume therapy in the surgical patient

The administered fluid may stay in the intravascular compartment or equilibrate with the interstitial/intracellular fluid compartments. The antidiuretic system (ADH), the RAAS, and the SNS are involved in the control of volume and composition of each body compartment. The principal action of these systems is to retain water in order to restore water or intravascular volume deficits, to retain sodium in order to restore the intravascular volume, and to increase the hydrostatic perfusion pressure through vasoconstriction. The control of ADH secretion depends on plasmatic osmolality, whereas the most important stimulus for activation of the RAAS is depletion of the intravascular volume. Enhanced activity of ADH, RAAS, and SNS is known to occur in stress situations, e.g., during surgery. Although the normal response to surgery and starvation results in increased metabolic activity, it can be expected that a preexisting deficit of water or intravascular volume further may increase this activity. If water or intravascular volume deficits and the stress-related stimulus of ADH, RAAS, and SNS are additive, fluid management could inhibit this process through counterregulatory mechanisms. Several attempts to inhibit or attenuate the activity of ADH and RAAS by administering different volumes of isotonic crystalloid solutions were made. It is known that the ADH production is dependent on the maintenance of the extracellular volume and, in particular, the intravascular compartment. Administration of a restricted volume of crystalloids could possibly replace a previous deficit of water, but the replacement of a previous intravascular volume deficit would require much more volume in order to inhibit the secretory stimulus of all the hormones committed to maintain it. It can be expected that the replacement of crystalloids alone will not inhibit the normal response of ADH and RAAS, whereas administration of a combination of crystalloid and colloid solutions (replacement of water deficit simultaneous with improvement of the effective intravascular volume) may achieve this goal.

Practical strategies of volume replacement in the surgical patient

The primary goal of volume administration is to guarantee stable systemic hemodynamics, whereas overloading of the circulation and extreme hemodilution should be avoided [7, 13].

Large volumes of crystalloids are necessary for effectively increasing plasma volume and may subsequently result in severe hemodilution with subsequent reduction in colloid oncotic pressure (COP) followed by the risk of increased interstitial edema and an impaired organ function. For these reasons, colloids have been established for rapid restoration of the circulating plasma volume, thus avoiding excessive fluid accumulation, particularly in the interstitial tissue. Several different colloids are available varying with regard to their physicochemical properties and efficacy.

Human Albumin (HA)

HA is the naturally occurring colloid. The molecular weight of albumin is approximately 69,000 Da. Owing to its preparation procedures it is free of risk of transmitting infections and thus generally held to be safe. Four percent of albumin is slightly hypooncotic, 5% albumin is isooncotic, whereas

20 and 25% solutions are hyperoncotic expanding plasma volume by fluid shift from the interstitial to the intravascular compartment. The effects of 5% HA are not well predictable—infusion of 500 mL of albumin expanded plasma volume by 490 or 750 mL [13]. The retention of the infused albumin in the intravascular compartment and therefore its hemodynamic efficacy greatly vary with regard to the patient's disease. In patients with altered vascular endothelial integrity, albumin may pass into the interstitial space, by which fluid shift from the intravascular compartment is promoted. The importance of albumin is also related to its transport function for various drugs and endogenous substances (e.g., bilirubin, free fatty acids)—the clinical relevance of administration of HA in surgical patients for this purpose, however, have never been shown.

The worth of using HA in surgical appears to be very uncertain. In a study in elderly patients (>70 years) undergoing major abdominal surgery, it has been shown that although total protein concentration was kept normal by administering HA, these patients did not profit from the use of HA compared to a much cheaper nonprotein modern hydroxyethyl starch (HES) preparation [14]. Inflammatory response and endothelial activation/injury was even more beneficially influenced by HES 130/0.4 than by HA. When considering the effects on hemodynamics, organ function (renal), coagulation, inflammatory response or endothelial activation/integrity, and finally costs, HA cannot be recommended in this patient population and the use of a modern HES preparation should be favored to correct hypovolemia.

Synthetic colloids

Due to the high costs of albumin, less extensive synthetic colloids are widely used as cheap alternatives. The term "synthetic colloids" is somewhat misleading because all of them are from biological origin. Thus "nonprotein" colloids sound not as negative as synthetic colloids. In contrast to albumin, which is a monomer (i.e., all molecules have the same size and weight), synthetic colloids are polydispersed, i.e., they are a combination of many differently sized molecules. Large molecules only contribute minimally to the volume expansion effects; they reflect viscosity and persistence in the circulation. Smaller molecules are quickly lost by renal filtration or diffusion into the interstitial space.

Dextrans

Dextrans are a polydispersed mixture of glucose polymers. The two available dextran preparations are 6% Dextran 70 (average molecular weight 70,000 Da) and 10% Dextran 40 (average molecular weight 40,000 Da). The two solutions mainly differ with regard to their influence on microcirculation. Infusion of Dextran 40 increases microcirculatory flow because of a reduced red cell and platelet sludging, volume expansion, and hemodilution-induced reduction in whole blood viscosity. Dextrans are associated with anaphylactic reactions, coagulation abnormalities (e.g., interference with platelet adhesion and a von Willebrand-like syndrome), and impaired blood crossmatching. They have been replaced by other plasma substitutes in several countries and cannot any longer be recommended for correcting hypovolemia in the surgical patient.

Gelatins

Gelatins are modified beef collagens. Gelatin solution was introduced in 1915 for shock treatment and was used extensively during World War I. Gelatin is listed by the World Health Organization as an essential drug. In the USA, however, gelatins were abandoned in 1978 owing to its high incidence of hypersensitivity reactions [15, 16]. Gelatins exist in three different modifications: cross-linked gelatin (e.g., Gelofundiol®), urea-linked gelatin (e.g., Haemaccel®), and succinylated gelatin (e.g., Gelofusine®). The only major difference between these preparations is the different electrolyte concentrations: urea-linked gelatin includes high calcium and potassium contents, succinylated preparations have low calcium and potassium contents. Due to the very low molecular weight average (approximately 35,000 Da), plasma half-life is only short. Subsequently repeated doses are necessary to maintain adequate blood volume. Because of their poor volume-supporting capacity, their low intravascular persistence, and their high incidence of severe anaphylactic reactions, gelatins are not ideal for replacement of volume deficits in the surgical patient [7].

Hydroxyethyl starch

Hydroxyethyl starch is a high polymeric glucose compound that is manufactured through hydrolysis and hydroxyethylation from the highly branched starch amylopectin. Polymerized D-glucose units are joined primarily by 1–4 linkages with occasional 1–6 branching linkages. Natural starches cannot be used as plasma substitutes because they are unstable and rapidly hydrolyzed by circulating amylase. HES preparations are characterized by [17, 18]:

- concentration (low: 3%; medium: 6%; high: 10%),
- molar substitution (MS [low: 0.4 or 0.42; medium: 0.5; high: 0.62 and 0.7]),
- mean molecular weight (MW [low molecular weight [LMW]–HES: 70 kDa; medium molecular weight [MMW]–HES: from 130 to 260 kDa; high molecular weight [HMW]–HES: >450 kDa),
- the ratio of the C2:C6 hydroxyethylation,
- the solvent (nonbalanced HES are solved in saline solution; balanced HES are solved in a plasma-adapted solution).

The extent and duration of plasma expansion are extremely dependent on the physicochemical characteristics of the HES solution. The different HES preparations cause different effects on hemodynamics, rheology, coagulation, oncotic pressure, and intravascular half-lives. Comparison of the different studies on HES solutions is difficult because they vary widely concerning the subjects that were studied, rate and amount of infused volume, and end point of fluid therapy.

The beneficial hemodynamic effects of HES by effectively restoring hypovolemia have been showing by several studies in all kind of surgery. Aside from adequately restoring hypovolemia, certain HES preparations beneficially influenced tissue oxygenation. In patients undergoing major abdominal surgery, the influence of 6% HES 130/0.4 on tissue pO_2 was compared to patients who received saline solution for volume replacement [19]. Skeletal muscle tissue pO_2 ($ptiO_2$) was monitored for 24 hours after surgery using flexible minimal-invasive microsensoric pO_2 catheters. Although systemic hemodynamics and oxygenation data were kept unchanged from baseline and were similar in both groups, $ptiO_2$ increased significantly in the HES-treated patients (59%), but decreased in the RL group (−23%). This was confirmed by a study in volunteers undergoing acute normovolemic hemodilution, in whom three HES preparations were used to replace withdrawn blood [20]: HES 130/0.4 showed the significantly highest increase in skeletal muscle $ptiO_2$ in comparison to prehemodilution values. In patients undergoing abdominal aortic aneurysm repair, 6% HES 450/0.7 (hetastarch) -treated patients showed higher gastric mucosal pH than a RL group indicating improved splanchnic blood flow and tissue oxygenation by HES [21]. In patients undergoing major surgery with large blood loss, volume resuscitation with a MMW-HES (MW 200 kDa) also improved splanchnic blood flow and tissue oxygenation [22].

Finally, there is increasing evidence that some HES preparations possess additional effects on organ perfusion, microcirculation, tissue oxygenation, inflammation, endothelial activation, capillary leakage, and tissue edema that are beyond their volume replacing properties. In normal aged as well as elderly patients undergoing major abdominal surgery, inflammation (IL-6 and IL-8 plasma levels) and endothelial injury/activation (plasma levels of adhesion molecules [sICAM-1, sELAM-1]) were significantly higher in crystalloid-treated patients than in patients in whom 6% HES 130/0.4 was given indicating attenuated inflammatory response with this HES preparation [23, 24].

A new concept: the balanced volume replacement strategy

Almost all colloids (dextrans, albumin, HES, gelatins) are prepared in unphysiologic solutions—most of them are solved in saline solution containing unphysiologically high concentrations of sodium and chloride and thus can be can be defined as "unbalanced colloids." In the beginning of the nineties, substantial alterations in acid–base status have been described in patients in whom large amounts of saline solution were infused—this phenomenon has been defined as "hyperchloremic acidosis" [25]. Subsequently, use of considerable amounts of unbalanced colloids may be associated with unwanted electrolyte disturbances or acid–base derangements (acidosis). Avoidance of acid–base alterations by the choice of volume replacement regimen is a widely accepted policy, because base excess (BE) may serve as an important marker to identify patients with malperfused tissues. Producing hyperchloremic acidosis by administering large amounts of unbalanced fluids may mask diagnosis of perfusion deficits or may result in inappropriate clinical interventions due to the erroneous presumption of ongoing tissue hypoxia secondary to hypovolemia. In a study in intensive care unit (ICU) patients, the BE was shown to predict outcome, the BE may also be utilized to identify patients who have a high risk for mortality and thus should be administered to the ICU [26]. In patients undergoing cardiac surgery with cardiopulmonary bypass, the BE measured during the first hour after surgery was correlated with the length of stay on the ICU [27].

Aside from substance-specific beneficial effects on hemodynamics and substance-related unwanted adverse effects of certain colloids (e.g., on coagulation kidneys), a total balanced fluid resuscitation concept including balanced colloids may add another piece in the puzzle of finding the ideal fluid therapy in the hypovolemic surgical patient. Embedded in a total balanced, plasma-adapted volume replacement strategy (balanced crystalloid plus balanced 6% HES 130/0.42) and given in moderate doses (approximately 2.500 mL of HES within 24 hours), this concept showed favorable effects in electrolyte concentrations and BE in patients undergoing complex abdominal surgery [28]: the unbalanced volume replacement concept was associated with significantly more patients showing a BE of less than −5 mmol/L (maximum: −11.5 mmol/L) and a Cl^- plasma levels of >115 mmol/L (maximum: 128 mmol/L) than the balanced concept.

A balanced volume replacement regimen appears to show other beneficial effects aside from less acid–base disturbances. In a prospective, randomized, double-blinded clinical trial in elderly patients (>60 years) undergoing elective open surgical procedures, either a conventional high-MW HES with a high MS (hetastarch, $n = 24$) or a similar high MW, highly substituted HES prepared in a balanced electrolyte formulation (Hextend®, $n = 23$) was used [29]. Only patients treated with the unbalanced hetastarch developed acidosis (postoperative BE: −3.8 mmol/L in the hetastarch group versus −0.2 mmol/L in the Hextend® patients). Gastric tonometry indicated improved gastric mucosal perfusion with the balanced HES when compared to the patients treated with saline-based HES.

Finally, balanced starched have been shown to be associated with significantly less alterations in coagulation—especially when a high degree of dilution reached [14, 30]. In an in vitro study, whole blood from 20 healthy volunteers was hemodiluted either with a low-MW HES (130 kDa) with a low MS (0.42) dissolved in a balanced solution, a conventional 6% HES 130/0.4 (dissolved in saline solution) or RL [14]. Modified thrombelastography was used to measure influence on coagulation and whole blood aggregometry was used for assessing platelet function. Induction of platelet aggregation was performed with ADP (ADPTest), collagen (COLTest), or thrombin-receptor-activating protein (TRAPTest). Fifty percent dilution with nonbalanced HES resulted in significantly more altered platelet aggregation than in the balanced HES group. These beneficial influence on coagulation may be of interest especially in those surgical patients that are at risk of extensive bleeding problems.

Volume replacement strategies in surgical patients in the mirror of literature analysis

There exists some meta-analyses or evidence-based analyses dealing with different volume

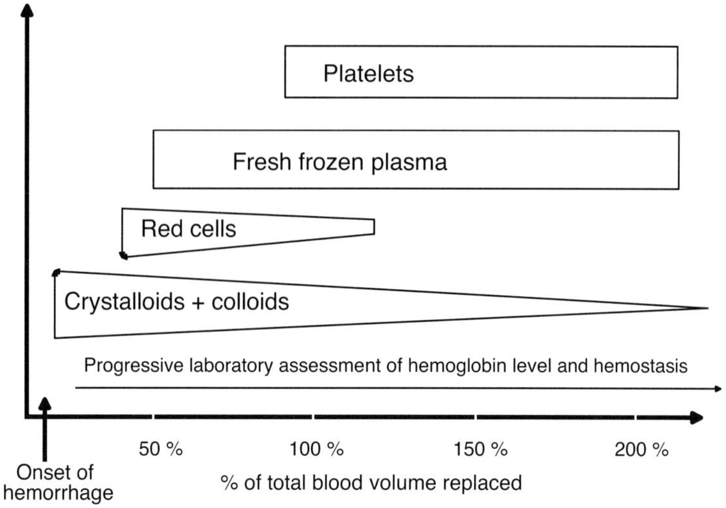

Figure 13.1 Volume resuscitation in the bleeding patient including crystalloids, nonprotein colloids, and blood/blood products.

replacement strategies in the surgical patient [31–34]. These analyses are far from being conclusive. Mostly, all kind of patients (e.g., burns, trauma, cardiac surgery patients) comparing all kinds of volume (e.g., "colloids" vs "crystalloids" without distinguishing the different "colloids") were included, the study population differ widely ranging from 5 to 247 patients in each volume group, the amount of infused volume ranged from 500 mL up to 3000 mL of the particular solution, and either fixed doses of the different solutions were administered or the amount of fluid replacement was adjusted with regard to defined hemodynamic variables (e.g., MAP, HR, CVP). Some studies tailored volume therapy only according to "clinical estimation," to "maintain hemodynamics," or "according to blood loss." Moreover, several of the included studies in these analyses have been published 20 years or more ago. Several innovative strategies have been developed in the past 10–15 years including improved surgical/anesthetic techniques, monitoring, ventilation strategies, and postoperative critical care management. Thus data from these analyses are more confusing than they are helping to solve current problem on the ideal volume replacement strategy in the surgical patient. The more it is astonishingly that guidelines of volume replacement therapy have been published recommending crystalloids as first choice in the surgical patient [35]. The American College of Surgeons Classes of Acute Hemorrhage specified four classes of acute hemorrhage classifying blood loss from up to 750 mL to >2000 mL and using some additional variables such as blood pressure and urine [36]. Fluid replacement is recommended to be performed with crystalloids (3:1 rule). There is no place for colloids in this recommendation. By contrast, in a study comparing the effects of crystalloids with two colloids (albumin and 10% HES 200/0.5) in patients undergoing abdominal surgery, the significantly largest intestinal edema was demonstrated with the use of crystalloids [37]. Others also reported on negative effects of crystalloid volume replacement on the gut in comparison to colloids [21]. Thus it has to be questioned on what results these recommendations refer to. More reliable recommendations for volume therapy in this situation are based on an individualized approach including crystalloids, nonprotein colloids, and blood/blood products (Figure 13.1).

Changes in hemostasis was the target of several studies. The majority of studies compared different HES preparations with albumin. Use of modern HES preparations was never associated with differences in the hemostatic competence or increased bleeding tendency in comparison with the natural colloid albumin. By contrast, use of dextran was shown to result in higher bleeding and use of more packed red blood cells than use of albumin [38]. Hemodynamic efficacy was another target of some studies. There were no differences in hemodynamic efficacy of albumin versus nonprotein colloids particularly HES. Some studies were only safety studies looking at possible negative side effects of nonprotein colloids (e.g., on kidney function, itching). Several studies showed that renal function was not negatively influenced by HES during surgery even in the elderly patient who is at risk to develop kidney dysfunction [15, 39–41].

A much-debated issue is which end points should be used to assess the benefit of volume replacement regimens—patients' outcome (morbidity or mortality?), length of stay in the hospital, physician's satisfaction? Mortality does not seem to be an appropriate end point when comparing different volume replacement regimens in surgery as outcome was not shown in most studies. Thus the influence of different volume replacement strategies on outcome in surgery cannot be determined today.

Conclusions

The "optimal" way of volume replacement in the surgical patient still represents a challenge. An extensive search is currently in progress to define which solution is best for which patient. What did we learn from past on the issue of volume therapy in the surgical patient?

- Extensive and complex surgical procedures may be associated with considerable perioperative hemodynamic alterations and organ complications [42, 43]. Fluid administration restores plasma volume and increases venous return to the heart, thus increasing cardiac output and improving systemic hemodynamics and organ perfusion. A substantial body of evidence supports the concept that deterioration in systemic and regional may be of particular importance for postoperative complications. An adequate volume therapy is accepted as the mainstay of managing perfusion deficits in this situation. The efficacy of different fluid preparations is still discussed controversially. The "ideal" solution should not only stabilize systemic hemodynamics but organ perfusion and microcirculation should also be guaranteed or even improved without being associated with side effects (Table 13.1).

Table 13.1 Important issues for an ideal volume therapy in surgery.

Hemodynamic efficacy
Influence on interstitial fluid
Influence on coagulation
Side effects (e.g., kidney, liver)
Availability
Costs

- Several studies have revisited the crystalloid–colloid or colloid–colloid controversies. Meta-analyses, however, must be viewed with some skepticism. Mortality does not seem to be an appropriate end point when comparing different volume replacement strategies, because mortality was never an end point of any of the studies [44]. The influence of the different colloids on organ function, endothelial inflammation, or perfusion should also be focused on.
- Blood volume can be definitely restored more rapidly with synthetic colloids rather than with crystalloids. Even excessive amounts of crystalloids do not always guarantee circulating blood volume and sufficient hemodynamics.
- When comparing albumin and nonprotein ("synthetic") colloids, several studies demonstrated no differences between these colloids and subsequently use of albumin for volume therapy cannot be justified. In today's climate of cost consciousness and cost containment, financial considerations may come into play. The major advantage of nonprotein colloids is in their relative economy. Although cost considerations are very difficult because of different medical systems of the countries, treatment with albumin cannot be recommended also from the economic point of view.
- Balanced colloids offer a promising approach and may add an important piece in the puzzle of finding an ideal volume replacement strategy in the surgical patient.

• We should always remember when caring for our patients "*Quidquid agis prudenter agas et respice finem.*"

Key points

• Adequate volume replacement is important in all surgical procedures.
• Volume replacement should be aimed at restoring systemic hemodynamics and tissue perfusion.
• Colloids are superior to crystalloids for restoration of the intravascular volume.
• Synthetic colloids should be better termed "non-protein colloids"
• Synthetic colloids appear to be equal to natural colloid albumin.
• Synthetic colloids can be recommended for volume therapy in surgery.
• Albumin cannot anymore recommended for correcting hypovolemia in the surgical patient.
• Dextran has the most pronounced side effects (e.g., negative influence on hemostasis, induction of anaphylactic reactions).
• The different hydroxyethyl starch preparations widely differ with regard to efficacy and side effects.
• Modern HES preparations with a moderate mean molecular weight (MW) and a low molar substitution (MS) should be preferred for volume therapy in surgery.
• Current available meta-analyses are not helpful to identify the "ideal" solution for volume replacement in surgery.

References

1. Spence RK, Carson JA, Poses R, et al. Elective surgery without transfusion: influence of preoperative hemoglobin level and blood loss on mortality. Am J Surg 1990;159:320–24.
2. Mythen MG, Webb AR. The role of gut mucosal hypoperfusion in the pathogenesis of post-operative organ dysfunction. Intensive Care Med 1994;20: 203–9.
3. Fiddian-Green RG. Association between intramucosal acidosis in the gut and organ failure. Crit Care Med 1993;21:S103–7.
4. Shoemaker WC, Appel PL, Kram HB. Prospective trial of supranormal values of survivors as therapeutic goals in high-risk surgical patients. Chest 1988;94:1176–86.
5. Prough DS, Johnston WE. Fluid restoration in septic shock: no solution yet. Anesth Analga 1898;69: 699–704.
6. Davidson I. Fluid resuscitation of shock: current controversies. Crit Care Med 1989;17:1078–80.
7. Haljamäe H. Volume substitution in shock. Acta Anaesthesiol Scand 1993;37(Suppl. 98): 25–8.
8. Stockwell MA, Scott A, Day A, Riley B, Soni N. Colloid solutions in the critically ill. Anaesthesia 1992;47:3–9.
9. Beards SC, Watt T, Edwards JD, Nightingale P, Farragher EB. Comparison of the hemodynamic and oxygen transport responses to modified fluid gelatin and hetastarch in critically ill patients: a prospective, randomized trial. Crit Care Med 1994;22: 600–605.
10. Kreimeier U, Peter K. Strategies of volume therapy in sepsis and systemic inflammatory response syndrome. Kidney Int 1998;53(Suppl. 64):75–9.
11. Zornow MH, Prough DS. Fluid management in patients with traumatic brain injury. New Horizons 1995;3:488–98.
12. Edwards JD. A new debate: colloid versus colloid? In: Vincent JL (ed.) *Yearbook of Intensive Care and Emergency Medicine*. Springer, Berlin; Heidelberg, New York, 1994, pp. 152–64.
13. London MJ, Ho SJ, Triedman JK, et al. A randomized clinical trial of 10% pentastarch (low molecular weight hydroxyethyl starch) versus 5% albumin for plasma volume expansion after cardiac operations. J Thorac Cardiovasc Surg 1989;97:785–97.
14. Boldt J, Wolf M, Mengistu A. A new plasma-adapted hydroxyethylstarch preparation: in vitro coagulation studies using thrombelastography and whole blood aggregometry. Anesth Analg 2007;104: 425–30.
15. Nearman HS, Herman ML. Toxic effects of colloids in the intensive care unit. Crit Care Med 1991;7: 713–23.
16. Watkins J. Reactions to gelatin plasma expanders. Lancet 1994;344:328–9.
17. Warren BB, Durieux ME. Hydroxyethylstarch: safe or not? Anesth Analg 1996;84:206–12.
18. Jungheinrich C, Neff TA. Pharmacokinetics of hydroxyethyl starch. Clin Pharmacokinet 2005;44: 681–99.

19. Lang K, Boldt J, Suttner S, Haisch G. Colloids versus crystalloids and tissue oxygen tension in patients undergoing major abdominal surgery. Anesth Analg 2001;93:405–9.
20. Standl T, Burmeister MA, Schroeder F, Currlin E, Freitag M, Schulte am Esch J. Hydroxyethyl starch (HES) 130/0.4 provides larger and faster increases in tissue oxygen tension in comparison with prehemodilution values than HES 70/0.5 or HES 200/0.5 in volunteers undergoing acute normovolemic hemodilution. Anesth Analg 2003;96:936–43.
21. Marik PE, Iglesias J, Marini B. Gastric intramucosal pH changes after volume replacement with hydroxyethyl starch or crystalloid in patients undergoing elective abdominal aortic aneurysm repair. J Crit Care 1997;12:51–5.
22. Guo X, Xu Z, Ren H, Luo A, Huang Y, Ye T. Effect of volume replacement with hydroxyethyl starch solution on splanchnic oxygenation in patients undergoing cytoreductive surgery for ovarian cancer. Chin Med J 2003;116:996–1000.
23. Lang K, Suttner S, Boldt J, Kumle B, Nagel D. Volume replacement with HES 130/0.4 may reduce the inflammatory response in patients undergoing major abdominal surgery. Can J Anaesth 2003;50: 1009–16.
24. Boldt J, Ducke M, Kumle B, Papsdorf M, Zurmeyer E. Influence of different volume replacement strategies on inflammation and endothelial activation in the elderly undergoing major abdominal surgery. Intensive Care Med 2004;30:416–22.
25. McFarlane C, Lee A. A comparison of Plasmalyte 148 and 0.9% saline for intra-operative fluid replacement. Anaesthesia 1994;49:779–81.
26. Smith I, Kumar P, Molloy S, et al. Base excess and lactate as prognostic indicators for patients admitted to intensive care. Intensive Care Med 2001;27: 74–83.
27. Hugot P, Sicsic JC, Schaffuser A, et al. Base deficit in immediate postoperative period of coronary surgery with cardiopulmonary bypass and length of stay in intensive care unit. Intensive Care Med 2003;29:257–61.
28. Boldt J, Schöllhorn T, Schulte G, Pabsdorf M. Volume replacement with a new balanced hydroxyethylstarch preparation (HES 130/0.42) in patients undergoing major abdominal surgery. Eur J Anaesthesiol 2007;24:267–75.
29. Wilkes NJ, Woolf R, Mutch M, et al. The effects of balanced versus saline-based hetastarch and crystalloid solutions on acid-base and electrolyte status and gastric mucosal perfusion in elderly surgical patients. Anesth Analg 2001;93:811–6.
30. Roche AM, James MF, Grocott MP, Mythen MG. Coagulation effects of in vitro serial haemodilution with a balanced electrolyte hetastarch solution compared with a saline-based hetastarch solution and lactated Ringer's solution. Anaesthesia 2002;57: 950–55.
31. Choi P, Yip G, Quinonez L, Cook D. Crystalloids versus colloids in fluid resuscitation: a systematic review. Crit Care Med 1999;27:200–210.
32. Velanovich V, Crystalloid versus colloid fluid resuscitation: a meta-analysis of mortality. Surgery 1989;105:65–71.
33. Schierhout G, Roberts I. Fluid resuscitation with colloids or crystalloids in critically ill patients: a systematic review of randomised trials. Br Med J 1998;316:961–4.
34. Cochrane Injuries Group Albumin Reviewers. Human albumin administration in critically ill patients: systematic review of randomised controlled trials. Br Med J 1998;317:235–9.
35. Vermeulen LC, Ratko MA, Estad BL. A paradigm for consensus – the university hospital consortium guidelines for the use of albumin, nonprotein colloids, and crystalloid solutions. Arch Int Med 1995;55:373–9.
36. Miller RD. Update on blood transfusions and blood substitutes. Anesth Analg 1999;88(Suppl. IARS): 71–8.
37. Prien T, Backhaus N, Pelster F, Pircher W, Bünte H, Lawin P. Effect of intraoperative fluid administration and colloid osmotic pressure on the formation of intestinal edema during gastrointestinal surgery. J Clin Anesth 1990;2:317–23.
38. Lisander B, Jacobsson SA, Ivarsson I, Vegfors M, Engdahl O. Giving both enoxaparin and dextran increases the need for transfusion in revison hip arthroplasty. Eur J Surg 1996;162:861–6.
39. Hiippala S, Linko K, Myllylä G, Lalla M, Heckali R, Makelainen A. Replacement of major surgical blood loss by hypo-oncotic or conventional plasma substitutes. Acta Anaesthesiol Scand 1995;39: 228–35.
40. Vogt NH, Bothner U, Lerch G, Lindner KH, Georgieff M. Large-dose administration of 6% hydroxyethyl starch 200/0.5 for total hip arthroplasty: plasma homeostasis, hemostasis, and renal function compared to use of 5% human albumin. Anesth Analg 1996;83:262–8.

41. Beyer R, Harmening U, Rittmeyer O, et al. Use of modified gelatin and hydroxyethyl starch for volume replacement in major orthopaedic surgery. Brit J Anaesth 1997;78:44–50.
42. Wade TP, elGhazzawy AG, Virgo KS, Jonson FE. The Whipple resection for cancer in U.S. Department of Veterans Affair Hospitals. Ann Surg 1995;221:241–6.
43. Boyd O, Grounds R, Bennett ED. A randomized clinical trial of the effect of deliberate perioperative increase of oxygen delivery on mortality in high-risk surgical patients. J Am Med Assoc 1993;270:2699–707.
44. Astiz ME, Rackow EC. Crystalloid-colloid controversy revisited. Crit Care Med 1999;27:34–5.

CHAPTER 14
Choice of Colloid for Intensive Care Patients

Yasser Sakr & Yalcin Inel
Department of Anesthesiology and Intensive Care, Friedrich-Schiller-University Hospital, Jena, Germany

Introduction

The never-ending crystalloid/colloid debate is still unresolved. In addition, recent years have brought another issue to the frontline, namely the colloid/colloid debate. Indeed, a recent multicenter observational study [1] showed a marked variation in the use of colloids among European countries (Figure 14.1). Hypovolemia is common in the intensive care unit (ICU). Whatever the cause of hypovolemia, a well-defined approach is needed to correct this condition because failure in treating it appropriately may lead to the development or worsening of organ dysfunction and subsequent worse outcome. In order to deal with hypovolemia and to restore an adequate intravascular volume, a physician needs to have a profound knowledge of the underlying pathophysiology of hypovolemia in various ICU settings and the properties of the fluids and drugs at his/her disposal. Furthermore, the ability to evaluate a patient's macro- and microcirculatory status and to act according to these parameters is probably the most essential aspect of volume therapy, since the definition of a clear volume replacement strategy remains elusive.

In this chapter, we will concisely review the factors influencing the choice between various colloids and their potential application in different case scenarios in critically ill patients.

Alternatives to Blood Transfusion in Transfusion Medicine, 2nd edition. Edited by A. Maniatis, P. Van der Linden, J.-F. Hardy.

Colloids: the bright side

The ideal colloid should have a rapid and sustained volume effect with a low risk profile. It should also be cost-effective and easy to use, ideally with no dose limitations. Isooncotic, plasma isotonic fluids, preferably with low viscosity, are favored in this context [2]. Colloid administration offers several advantages over other fluid types, which vary from one colloid to another (Table 14.1).

Albumin is a naturally occurring protein in humans and is synthesized in hepatocytes. In a healthy person, albumin accounts for 70–80% of the total plasma oncotic pressure [3]. About 5% of the albumin leaks from the circulation per hour in healthy subjects, with 90% of this extravascular pool of albumin returning to the circulation each day. This movement of albumin is also known as the transcapillary escape rate and can be increased threefold in sepsis [3]. Albumin solution has long been regarded as the gold standard solution for treatment of hypovolemia [3]. Since more than 95% of its particles are of uniform molecular size with a molecular weight (MW) of 69 kDa, albumin solutions are the only known monodisperse colloid. The high safety profile of albumin solutions and low costs in some countries were the major advantages of its use in ICU patients. Recently, the saline versus albumin fluid evaluation (SAFE) study provided evidence of the safety of using albumin solution for volume resuscitation [4]. Vincent et al. [5] have also recently reported that albumin administration may improve organ function in hypoalbuminemic critically ill patients,

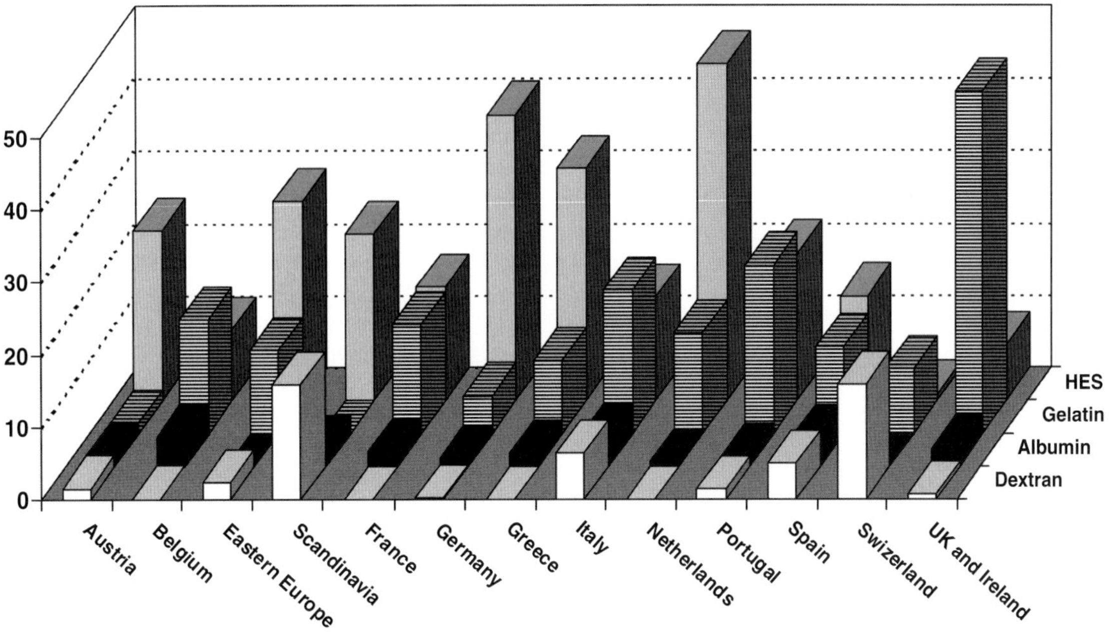

Figure 14.1 Bar chart demonstrating the use of various colloids in European countries. Reproduced from Sakr et al. [36], with permission from Oxford University Press.

Table 14.1 Overview of some advantages of colloids.

Colloid	Advantages
Albumin	• Since it is a natural colloid, it has the lowest incidence of adverse effects among colloid solutions
Gelatin	• Rapid effect • No accumulation in the body • Osmotic diuretic effect if given rapidly
Dextran	• Useful in reducing ischemia-reperfusion injury • Improves peripheral blood flow
HES	• HES solutions, especially those with a high MW, remain longer in the intravascular space, resulting not only in a rapid volume substitution, but also in a sustained effect • Fewer allergic reactions than many semisynthetic colloids • Improves microcirculation, albeit without an effect on tissue oxygenation • Lowers the circulating levels of adhesion molecules in sepsis • May have useful effects on the microvascular coagulation cascade by elevating levels of protein C and protein S

HES, hydroxyethyl starch solutions.

being associated with a less positive fluid balance and better tolerance to enteral feeding. Nevertheless, the high costs of albumin solutions in some countries and the high efficacy of semisynthetic colloid solutions as plasma substitutes have led many clinicians to switch to alternative volume expanding methods.

Semisynthetic colloids that are commonly used in clinical practice include gelatins, dextrans, and hydroxyethyl starch (HES) solutions. These solutions differ considerably in composition and physical properties (Table 14.2). Gelatin solutions are polydispersed polypeptides derived from bovine gelatin, a derivative of collagen. Since 1915, gelatin solutions have been used in the treatment of hypovolemia. Nowadays, there are three types of gelatin available: cross-linked or oxypolygelatins, urea cross-linked, and succinylated fluid gelatins. The MW is around 30 kDa, which is the renal threshold. The large number of small molecules make a rapid initial osmotic effect possible, but they are then cleared from the intravascular space (half-life: 3.5–4 hours) [6]. This clearance may be even more rapid in sepsis because of the endothelial capillary leak. After filtration, gelatin solutions may act as osmotic diuretics in the glomeruli, since 60% of the given volume appears in the urine within the first 24 hours [7]. Gelatin solutions are, therefore, rapidly acting without tissue accumulation and may have an osmotic diuretic effect if given rapidly.

Dextrans are a group of branched polysaccharides derived from the bacteria *Leuconostoc mesenteroides*. Currently available formulations of dextran are 10% dextran with a MW of 40 kDa, and 6% dextran with a MW of 70 kDa [8]. Being a polydisperse solution, 90% of Dextran 40 has a MW between 10 and 80 kDa. Since the renal threshold for dextran is between 50 and 55 kDa, about 70% of the given dose will be observed in the urine within the first 24 hours [3]. A smaller fraction enters the interstitial space and returns to the bloodstream via lymphatic drainage or is metabolized by certain organs. Small amounts may also be eliminated by the gastrointestinal tract. The effects of dextran solutions depend on their MW. Molecules having MW smaller than 60 kDa promote peripheral blood flow by disaggregating red blood cells and reducing blood viscosity. Both vessel endothelium and the cellular components of blood are coated by dextrans resulting in fewer interactions between the two components. This aspect may prove

Table 14.2 Overview of properties of semisynthetic colloid solutions.

	Concentration (%)	Volume efficacy (%)	Volume effect (hours)	Mean molecular weight (kDa)	Maximum daily dose	Osmolarity (mosmol/L)	Molar substance	C2/C6 ratio
Urea-cross-linked gelatins	3.5	80	1–3	35	No limitations	301	NA	NA
Cross-linked gelatins	5.5	80	1–3	30	No limitations	296	NA	NA
Succinylated gelatins	4.0	80	1–3	30	No limitations	274	NA	NA
6% Dextran 70	6	100	5	70	1.5 g/kg	—	NA	NA
10% Dextran 40	10	175–200	3–4	40	1.5 g/kg	—	NA	NA
HES 70/0.5	6	100	1–2	70	20 mL/kg	290	0.5	4:1
HES 130/0.4	6	100	2–3	130	50 mL/kg	308	0.4	9:1
HES 200/0.5	6	100	3–4	200	20 mL/kg	308	0.5	6:1
HES 200/0.5	10	130	3–4	200	20 mL/kg	308	0.5	6:1
HES 200/0.62	6	100	5–6	200	20 mL/kg	308	0.62	9:1
HES 450/0.7	6	100	5–6	450	20 mL/kg	308	0.4	4.6:1

Table 14.3 Classification of hydroxyethyl solutions according to their physical properties.

Criteria	Available options
Concentration	3, 6, and 10%
Molecular weight	
Low	70 kDa
Medium	130–270 kDa
High	>450 kDa
Molar substitution*	
Low	0.4 and 0.5
High	0.62 and 0.7

*The ratio of the total number of hydroxyethyl groups to the total number of glucose molecules. High molar substitution leads to slower degradation.

useful especially in ischemia-reperfusion injury, where leukocyte adherence plays an important role [9]. Dextrans also impair factor VIII activity by inhibiting the formation of FVIII/vWF complex [3]. Therefore, Dextran 40 is used mainly to improve peripheral blood flow, but it is not advisable to use it in ICU patients because of its adverse effects on coagulation. On the other hand, Dextran 70 could be used for volume expansion in hypovolemic patients but it is not commonly used for this purpose in many countries due to its adverse effects.

Hydroxyethyl starch solutions are synthetic colloid solutions containing glycogen-like modified natural polysaccharides [10]. HES solutions can be classified by their molecular properties according to their MW, concentration, and degree of substitution (Table 14.3). HES solutions, especially those with a high MW, remain longer in the intravascular space than other colloids, resulting not only in rapid volume substitution, but also in a sustained effect. Fewer allergic reactions have been reported with HES solutions compared to other semisynthetic colloids [11]. HES solutions have been reported to improve the microcirculation, albeit without an effect on tissue oxygenation [12]. Favorable effects of these solutions in sepsis include reducing circulating levels of adhesion molecules [13] and increasing levels of protein C and S [13].

The downside: adverse effects

Colloid use is associated with various adverse effects (Table 14.4) that must be taken into consideration when selecting a colloid in specific groups of ICU patients. Serious adverse effects include anaphylactic reactions, tissue accumulation with subsequent organ dysfunction, pulmonary edema, and adverse effects on coagulation. The choice of colloid requires a risk-benefit assessment in view of these adverse events (Figure 14.2).

Anaphylactic or anaphylactoid reactions may occur with naturally occurring and semisynthetic colloids. Histamine release commonly occurs after administration of gelatin solutions [3]. Cardiorespiratory arrest has been reported with urea-linked gelatin (Haemaccel), which has also been associated with more anaphylactoid reactions than succinylated gelatins. High MW dextrans have also been linked to anaphylactoid reactions, probably because of their multiple side branches, and all dextrans may cause true anaphylaxis. This effect is thought to result from previous cross-immunization against commensal gut bacterial antigens, causing a type III immune complex

Table 14.4 Risks associated with colloid administration.

	Albumin	Dextrans	Gelatins	Hydroxyethyl starches (low MW)	Hydroxyethyl starches (high MW)
Anaphylactoid reactions	+	++	+++++	+++	+++
Pruritus	–	–	–	+	++
Tissue accumulation	–	–	–	+	++
Coagulopathy	+	+++	++	++	++
Renal failure	+	++	+	+	++

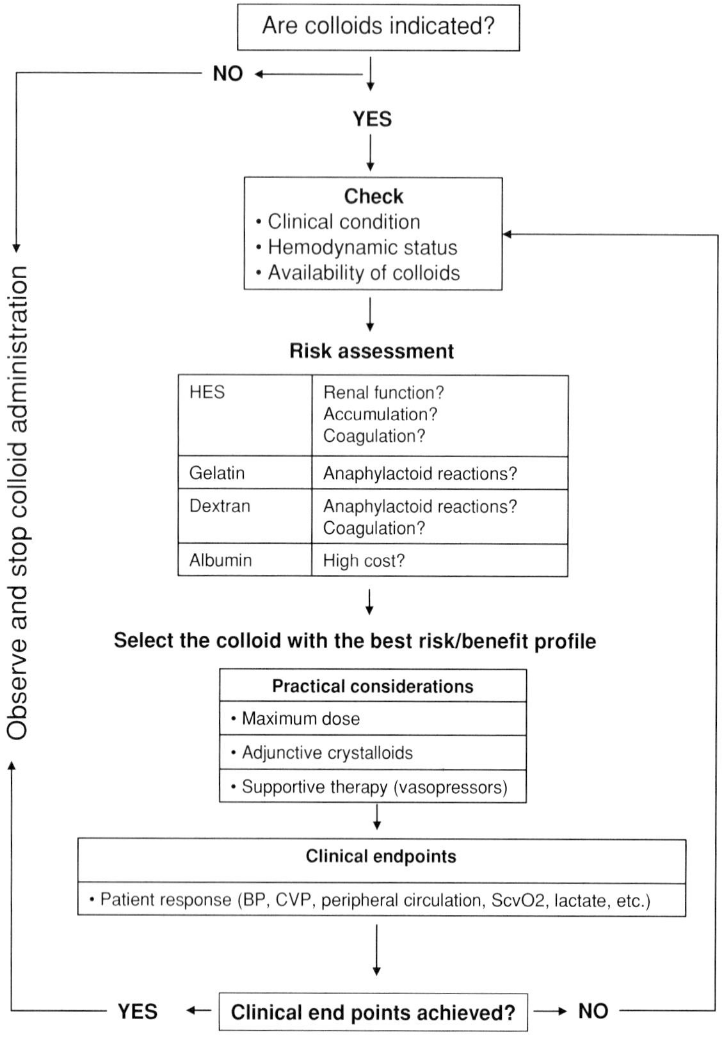

Figure 14.2 Practical approach to selecting a colloid for intensive care patients. BP, blood pressure; CVP, central venous pressure; $ScvO_2$, central venous oxygen saturation; HES, hydroxyethyl starch.

anaphylaxis. These antibodies are found in 70% of humans, and their titers correlate with the severity of the reaction. The incidence of anaphylaxis is quoted at 1:4500, but can be reduced to 1:84,000, after pretreatment with 3 g Dextran 1 (MW 1 kDa). Anaphylactoid reactions after HES infusions may be related to complement-mediated hypersensitivity [3]. Human albumin is known to have the lowest incidence of anaphylaxis among the colloids. The pooled incidence of anaphylactoid reactions after albumin infusion is about 9.4 in 100,000 [11]. The pooled incidence rate ratios of anaphylactoid reactions for gelatin, HES, and dextran solutions are 12.4, 4.5, and 2.3% when compared to albumin solutions [11].

Tissue deposits and accumulation occur after administration of some plasma substitutes, most commonly with HES solutions. After administration of HES, deposition in the cells of the monocyte–macrophage system of various organs has been demonstrated, slowing elimination [14]. Tissue deposition is thought to be transitory and dose- and MW-dependent, with differences in severity and duration among subjects [14].

However, in some patients, storage of HES can be shown by immunohistochemistry and immunoelectron microscopy more than 2 years after administration. Pruritus may occur due to tissue accumulation of HES and may last for years [14]. In some patients suffering from pruritus, additional deposition was observed in cutaneous nerves [9, 15]. Pruritus mostly occurs in patients who receive large amounts of HES (e.g., 20 L) over a long period of time (10–20 days). In a study that included 700 critically ill patients, the incidence of pruritus was similar after low and medium MW HES compared with lactated Ringer's solution [16].

Gelatins do not accumulate in the body [17]. Tissue deposition of albumin has not been observed in necroscopic studies [11].

Pulmonary edema is a serious adverse effect of fluid resuscitation. There are considerable interindividual differences in the development of pulmonary edema in response to volume substitution. A balance should be maintained between optimizing cardiac performance and ensuring adequate gas exchange. The status of the alveolocapillary membrane plays a role in the contribution of colloid osmotic pressure (COP) to this problem [18]. In an intact alveolocapillary membrane, lymphatic drainage and COP may protect the lung from pulmonary edema. Lymphatic drainage can increase 20-fold, thus maintaining the transcapillary COP gradient and restoring protein content into the vascular compartment. This is the case with pulmonary artery occlusion pressure (PAOP) levels up to 25 mmHg; but when PAOP increases and, at the same time, COP decreases, the PAOP threshold for pulmonary edema also decreases from 25 mmHg to 11 mmHg [19]. Alveolocapillary membrane permeability may be altered after insults such as sepsis, trauma, burns, and toxic agents. In an impaired alveolocapillary membrane, the COP gradient is nearly negligible. Experimental animal models of fluid resuscitation in previously damaged lungs showed that albumin infusions given to increase COP by 5 mmHg, failed to reduce pulmonary edema, whereas a reduction in PAOP by 5 mmHg decreased the extravascular fluid volume by 50% [20]. In other similar models, where the pulmonary effects of crystalloids and colloids were measured, there were no significant changes between groups [20–23]. These studies, along with a recent study on the effect of fluid loading with saline or colloids on pulmonary permeability, edema, and lung injury score after cardiac and major vascular surgery, demonstrate that the type of fluid used does not affect pulmonary permeability and edema [24].

Disturbances in renal function: Since 1970, dextrans have been known to cause acute renal failure associated with the vacuolization of the proximal tubular cells, osmotic nephrosis-like lesions [25]. Many hypotheses have been formulated to explain the renal failure and the most recent, albeit still relatively old, suggests that the administration of hyperoncotic colloid solutions may increase the viscosity of the urine causing stasis in renal tubular flow. Concerns about the adverse effects of HES on renal function were first raised by Legendre and colleagues [26], who reported an association between organ donors exposure to HES and osmotic nephrosis-like lesions in the transplant recipients. The first randomized trial exploring possible deleterious effects of HES administration on renal function was conducted by Cittanova and coworkers [27], who compared HES (200 kDa/0.60) with gelatin and revealed that the use of HES solutions in brain-dead kidney donors was followed by immediate impairment in renal function in the recipients with an increased rate of hemodialysis and higher serum creatinine concentrations. However, subsequent studies yielded conflicting results [28–32]. The debate regarding HES solutions was fuelled when a multicenter randomized study by Schortgen and colleagues [30], comparing the effects of 6% HES (200/0.62) and fluid modified gelatin on renal function in 129 patients with severe sepsis, found that the frequencies of acute renal failure, oliguria, and raised serum creatinine concentrations were higher in the HES group than in the gelatin group. A limiting factor in that study was the better renal function at baseline in the gelatin group [33–35]. A recent retrospective analysis of a large European database showed that HES had no influence on renal function or on the need for subsequent renal replacement therapy. The presence of sepsis, hematological cancer, or cardiovascular failure, and the baseline renal function were more important risk factors for development of subsequent renal dysfunction [36].

Coagulopathy: All the semisynthetic colloid solutions have a negative effect on coagulation. One of the main reasons for this is the hemodilutionary effects of colloids. Although some studies have shown that clot strength can be reduced after administration of gelatins in large volumes [37], thromboelastographic studies in patients undergoing surgery revealed a tendency to hypercoagulopathy after gelatin infusions for substitution of blood loss, compared with controls and with patients receiving albumin or HES [38]. Dextrans on the other hand have more significant effects on hemorheology and coagulation. As mentioned earlier, Dextran 40 can reduce blood viscosity, reduce Factor VIII activity, and increase plasminogen activation and fibrinolysis. The net effect is that clot strength is reduced and thrombocyte activity is impaired [3]. The more rapidly eliminated members of the HES family, such as HES 200/0.5 and HES 130/0.4, seem not to have a significant effect on hemostasis [39]. However, there are also data from a randomized controlled trial in 69 cardiac surgery patients, which suggest that bleeding is increased by HES with medium and high MW compared to albumin [40].

Other reported adverse effects of colloids include acute fetal distress because of uterine hypertonia when dextrans are administered during delivery [41] and elevation of alpha amylase levels in blood after HES administration [42].

Choice of colloids in specific subgroups of critically ill patients

Severe sepsis and septic shock

Animal studies suggest that the type of fluid used in severe sepsis and septic shock has little influence on outcome. Timely resuscitation to rapidly restore hemodynamic parameters can be achieved independent of the type of fluid used [43]. Although albumin and HES solutions were more efficient in improving cardiac output and oxygen delivery, and in lowering blood lactate levels than gelatin and Ringer's lactate, the type of intravenous fluid used for initial fluid resuscitation has limited effects on outcome [44]. In another animal study, HES solutions were shown to have a protective in vivo effect on endotoxin-induced microcirculatory disorders. HES 130 kDa is effective in preventing LPS-induced leukocyte adherence, improving capillary perfusion, and reducing macromolecular leakage. Because there were no signs of in vivo HES 130 kDa toxicity or bleeding diathesis, HES 130 kDa may offer an anti-inflammatory potential when used during experimental sepsis [45], whereas modified fluid gelatin did not show anti-inflammatory properties in a rat model of polymicrobial sepsis [46]. A porcine septic shock model also demonstrated a protective effect of HES solutions on sepsis-induced capillary leakage and showed that the 130 kDa variant was significantly more effective than the 200 kDa variant [47]. Similarly, the formation of platelet-derived microvesicles was increased significantly by volume replacement with Ringer's solution compared to colloid solutions [48]. However, renal and liver failure, coagulation defects and pruritus may represent a potential risk of using HES solutions in patients with severe sepsis and septic shock, especially those with borderline renal function or those requiring high doses over a long period of time with the risk of tissue accumulation.

Despite the fact that the SAFE study failed to demonstrate differences in outcome in critically ill patients requiring fluid repletion who were treated with 4% albumin compared to those treated with saline, albumin may not be harmless in all ICU patients. In subgroup analyses of the SAFE study [4], discordant results were reported for patients with severe sepsis and those admitted because of traumatic injuries. In a recent observational multicenter study [1], albumin administration was found to be associated with decreased survival in acutely ill patients admitted to European ICUs. Although this study was not designed primarily to investigate this issue, it may cast some doubts on the presence of a differential effect of albumin solutions on outcome in various subgroups of critically ill patients. Nevertheless, until further study results are available, human albumin may be used when considered appropriate, notably in hypoalbuminemic patients [49].

Recently, the guidelines of the Surviving Sepsis Campaign did not support the use of one type of fluid over another in the resuscitation of patients with severe sepsis [50]. The resuscitation of a patient with severe sepsis or sepsis-induced tissue hypoperfusion (hypotension or lactic acidosis) should begin as soon as the syndrome is recognized and should not be delayed pending ICU admission. In a key randomized controlled study by Rivers et al. [51], early goal-directed therapy in emergency department patients with septic shock was shown to improve survival. During the first 6 hours of resuscitation, the goals of initial resuscitation of sepsis-induced hypoperfusion included mean arterial pressure (>65 mmHg), central venous pressure (8–12 mmHg), urine output (>0.5 mL/kg/h), and central venous oxygen saturation (>70%). Resuscitation directed toward these goals was able to reduce 28-day mortality rates. Therefore, optimal resuscitation of patients with sepsis requires early volume substitution with either crystalloids or colloids. Vasopressor therapy should be initiated when volume resuscitation is not able to rapidly restore an acceptable hemodynamic profile [50].

Fluid challenge is a term used to describe the initial fluid resuscitation period where the response of the patient to fluid infusion is carefully evaluated. In this process, large amounts of fluids may be used over a short period of time, so there must be close monitoring to evaluate the patient's response and to avoid pulmonary edema. The severity of intravascular volume deficit in patients with severe sepsis is variable. Because of vasodilation and increased capillary permeability, most patients require aggressive fluid resuscitation during the first 24 hours of treatment [49]. Fluid challenge in patients with suspected hypovolemia may be given at a rate of 500–1000 mL of crystalloids or 300–500 mL of colloids over 30 minutes and repeated based on response (increase in blood pressure and urine output) and tolerance [49].

Acute lung injury and acute respiratory distress syndrome

Sepsis is the most frequent cause of death in the ICU and the most common cause of acute lung injury (ALI) and acute respiratory distress syndrome (ARDS), occurring in 30–40% of patients. The reason for the pulmonary edema that develops in ALI/ARDS is alveolocapillary barrier dysfunction. Reduced COP may also play a role in the generation and persistence of pulmonary edema [52]. Reduced COP, particularly if hydrostatic pressures rise above normal, contributes to an exaggerated pulmonary edema. However, COP is less important in preventing pulmonary edema than the efficiency of the lymphatic system in the lung. This is particularly important when capillary permeability is impaired, like in sepsis or ALI/ARDS, where the protein reflection coefficient is reduced and hydrostatic pressure is more important in affecting the accumulation of fluid in the extravascular region, which causes edema [53].

In ALI/ARDS patients, there is no evidence that a given fluid improves clinical outcomes, just as in sepsis. In patients with established pulmonary insufficiency, albumin infusion significantly improved the intrapulmonary shunt [53]. Combined use of albumin and furosemide in hypoproteinemic patients with ALI created significant diuresis and weight loss with around 40% improvement in oxygenation and long lasting amelioration of hemodynamic stability [53]. One study suggests that positive fluid balance per se is at least partially responsible for poor outcome in patients with pulmonary edema. The authors defend the strategy of attempting to achieve a negative fluid balance if tolerated hemodynamically [54]. Which colloid—if at all—to use in ALI/ARDS is still debatable, since there is no study comparing the effects of different colloids in these patients. Moreover, patients may benefit from a conservative fluid strategy. Although this strategy does not achieve any significant improvements in mortality, it improves lung function and shortens the duration of mechanical ventilation and intensive care without increasing nonpulmonary organ failures [55]. A risk-benefit assessment, considering the underlying etiology and associated conditions seems to be the most appropriate strategy in this population.

Trauma and hemorrhagic shock

Severe trauma may cause hemorrhagic shock, resulting in mortality rates exceeding 50%. Early fluid resuscitation has traditionally been used to avoid shock and its complications, but clinical data suggest that definitive bleeding control is imperative before aggressive fluid resuscitation [56]. The clinical trajectory of patients who develop multiple organ failure is set early in the resuscitation process (i.e., within 6 hours of injury). Many patients at high risk require emergency surgery or interventional radiology and arrive in the ICU after this time window [57, 58]. Primary resuscitation using colloids requires one quarter to one half of the infusion volume of crystalloids and may reduce resuscitation time by up to 75%, depending on illness severity. However, colloids have only inconsistently been shown to reduce subsequent organ dysfunction, such as ALI/ARDS. Studies of relevant pulmonary function are inconclusive [53]. On the basis of a prospectively defined subset in the SAFE trial, crystalloids are the best choice for general resuscitation of trauma patients (relative risk for death with colloids, 1.36; 95% confidence interval, 0.99–1.86). This is particularly true among these patients when associated with traumatic brain injuries (colloid relative risk, 1.62; 95% confidence interval, 1.12–2.34) [43]. Secondary insults after major trauma may incite an inflammatory reaction with altered capillary permeability; intravenous fluid resuscitation in this phase should be guided by the same principles as in sepsis.

Conclusion

The choice of a colloid in critically ill patients requires an integration of clinical data with the properties and risk profile of the available solutions. There are few large randomized clinical studies comparing various colloids and the current evidence does not support the use of one specific colloid over any of the others. A risk-benefit approach should be considered when colloid administration is indicated and predefined clinical end points should be set to guide fluid therapy. Careful attention should be paid to dose limitations and contraindications of some colloid solutions, especially HES solutions. Careful observation is required to identify and adequately manage side effects, whenever they occur. Due to the potential risks of colloid solutions, their use as an alternative to crystalloids in stable critically ill patients without urgent need for rapid volume expansion, should be discouraged.

References

1. Vincent JL, Sakr Y, Reinhart K, et al. Is albumin administration in the acutely ill associated with increased mortality? Results of the SOAP study. Crit Care 2005;9:R745–54.
2. Suttner S, Boldt J. Volume replacement with hydroxyethyl starch: is there an influence on kidney function?. Anasthesiol Intensivmed Notfallmed Schmerzther 2004;39:71–7.
3. Vercueil A, Grocott MP, Mythen MG. Physiology, pharmacology, and rationale for colloid administration for the maintenance of effective hemodynamic stability in critically ill patients. Transfus Med Rev 2005;19:93–109.
4. Finfer S, Bellomo R, McEvoy S, et al. Effect of baseline serum albumin concentration on outcome of resuscitation with albumin or saline in patients in intensive care units: analysis of data from the saline versus albumin fluid evaluation (SAFE) study. BMJ 2006; 333:1044.
5. Dubois MJ, Orellana-Jimenez C, Melot C, et al. Albumin administration improves organ function in critically ill hypoalbuminemic patients: a prospective, randomized, controlled, pilot study. Crit Care Med 2006; 34:2536–40.
6. Saddler JM, Horsey PJ. The new generation gelatins. A review of their history, manufacture and properties. Anaesthesia 1987;42:998–1004.
7. Mishler JM. Synthetic plasma volume expanders–their pharmacology, safety and clinical efficacy. Clin Haematol 1984;13:75–92.
8. Salmon JB, Mythen MG. Pharmacology and physiology of colloids. Blood Rev 1993;7:114–20.
9. Boldt J, Suttner S. Plasma substitutes. Minerva Anestesiol 2005;71:741–58.
10. Treib J, Baron JF, Grauer MT, et al. An international view of hydroxyethyl starches. Intensive Care Med 1999;25:258–68.
11. Barron ME, Wilkes MM, Navickis RJ. A systematic review of the comparative safety of colloids. Arch Surg 2004;139:552–63.
12. Schaper J, Ahmed R, Schafer T, et al. Volume therapy with colloid solutions preserves intestinal microvascular perfusion in endotoxaemia. Resuscitation 2008; 76:120–28.

13. Schortgen F, Brochard L, Burnham E, et al. Pro/con clinical debate: hydroxyethylstarches should be avoided in septic patients. Crit Care 2003;7:279–81.
14. Sirtl C, Laubenthal H, Zumtobel V, et al. Tissue deposits of hydroxyethyl starch (HES): dose-dependent and time-related. Br J Anaesth 1999;82:510–15.
15. Metze D, Reimann S, Szepfalusi Z, et al. Persistent pruritus after hydroxyethyl starch infusion therapy: a result of long-term storage in cutaneous nerves. Br J Dermatol 1997;136:553–9.
16. Bothner U, Georgieff M, Vogt NH. Assessment of the safety and tolerance of 6% hydroxyethyl starch (200/0.5) solution: a randomized, controlled epidemiology study. Anesth Analg 1998;86:850–55.
17. Muchmore E, Bonhard K, Kothe N. Distribution and clearance from the body of an oxypolygelatin plasma substitute determined by radioactive tracer study in chimpanzees. Arzneimittelforschung 1983;33: 1552–4.
18. Humphrey H, Hall J, Sznajder I, et al. Improved survival in ARDS patients associated with a reduction in pulmonary capillary wedge pressure. Chest 1990; 97:1176–80.
19. Guyton AC, Lindsey AW. Effect of elevated left atrial pressure and decreased plasma protein concentration on the development of pulmonary edema. Circ Res 1959;7:649–57.
20. Harms BA, Pahl AC, Radosevich DG, et al. The effects of hypoproteinemia and volume expansion on lung and soft tissue transvascular fluid filtration. Surgery 1989;105:605–14.
21. Pearl RG, Halperin BD, Mihm FG, et al. Pulmonary effects of crystalloid and colloid resuscitation from hemorrhagic shock in the presence of oleic acid-induced pulmonary capillary injury in the dog. Anesthesiology 1988;68:12–20.
22. Prewitt RM, McCarthy J, Wood LD. Treatment of acute low pressure pulmonary edema in dogs: relative effects of hydrostatic and oncotic pressure, nitroprusside, and positive end-expiratory pressure. J Clin Invest 1981;67:409–18.
23. Haupt MT, Teerapong P, Green D, et al. Increased pulmonary edema with crystalloid compared to colloid resuscitation of shock associated with increased vascular permeability. Circ Shock 1984;12:213–24.
24. Verheij J, van Lingen A, Raijmakers PG, et al. Effect of fluid loading with saline or colloids on pulmonary permeability, oedema and lung injury score after cardiac and major vascular surgery. Br J Anaesth 2006; 96:21–30.
25. Diomi P, Ericsson JL, Matheson NA. Effects of dextran 40 on urine flow and composition during renal hypoperfusion in dogs with osmotic nephrosis. Ann Surg 1970;172:813–24.
26. Legendre C, Thervet E, Page B, et al. Hydroxyethylstarch and osmotic-nephrosis-like lesions in kidney transplantation. Lancet 1993;342:248–9.
27. Cittanova ML, Leblanc I, Legendre C, et al. Effect of hydroxyethylstarch in brain-dead kidney donors on renal function in kidney-transplant recipients. Lancet 1996;348:1620–22.
28. Deman A, Peeters P, Sennesael J. Hydroxyethyl starch does not impair immediate renal function in kidney transplant recipients: a retrospective, multicentre analysis. Nephrol Dial Transplant 1999;14:1517–20.
29. Kumle B, Boldt J, Piper S, et al. The influence of different intravascular volume replacement regimens on renal function in the elderly. Anesth Analg 1999;89: 1124–30.
30. Schortgen F, Lacherade JC, Bruneel F, et al. Effects of hydroxyethylstarch and gelatin on renal function in severe sepsis: a multicentre randomised study. Lancet 2001;357:911–6.
31. Boldt J, Brenner T, Lehmann A, et al. Influence of two different volume replacement regimens on renal function in elderly patients undergoing cardiac surgery: comparison of a new starch preparation with gelatin. Intensive Care Med 2003;29:763–9.
32. Neff TA, Doelberg M, Jungheinrich C, et al. Repetitive large-dose infusion of the novel hydroxyethyl starch 130/0.4 in patients with severe head injury. Anesth Analg 2003;96:1453–9.
33. Gosling P, Rittoo D, Manji M, et al. Hydroxyethylstarch as a risk factor for acute renal failure in severe sepsis. Lancet 2001;358:581.
34. Godet G. Hydroxyethylstarch as a risk factor for acute renal failure in severe sepsis. Lancet 2001;358:581.
35. Boldt J. Hydroxyethylstarch as a risk factor for acute renal failure in severe sepsis. Lancet 2001;358:581–3.
36. Sakr Y, Payen D, Reinhart K, et al. Effects of hydroxyethyl starch administration on renal function in critically ill patients. Br J Anaesth 2007;98:216–4.
37. Mardel SN, Saunders FM, Allen H, et al. Reduced quality of clot formation with gelatin-based plasma substitutes. Br J Anaesth 1998;80:204–7.
38. Karoutsos S, Nathan N, Lahrimi A, et al. Thrombelastogram reveals hypercoagulability after administration of gelatin solution. Br J Anaesth 1999;82: 175–7.

39. Dieterich HJ. Recent developments in European colloid solutions. J Trauma 2003;54:S26–30.
40. Wilkes MM, Navickis RJ, Sibbald WJ. Albumin versus hydroxyethyl starch in cardiopulmonary bypass surgery: a meta-analysis of postoperative bleeding. Ann Thorac Surg 2001;72:527–33.
41. Barbier P, Jonville AP, Autret E, et al. Fetal risks with dextrans during delivery. Drug Saf 1992;7:71–3.
42. Baron JF. Plasma, albumin and synthetic colloids: pharmacology of crystalloids and colloids. In: *Transfusion Medicine and Alternatives to Blood Transfusion.* R&J Editions Médicales, Paris, 2000, pp. 123–137.
43. Finfer S, Bellomo R, Boyce N, et al. A comparison of albumin and saline for fluid resuscitation in the intensive care unit. N Engl J Med 2004;350:2247–56.
44. Su F, Wang Z, Cai Y, et al. Fluid resuscitation in severe sepsis and septic shock: albumin, hydroxyethyl starch, gelatin or ringer's lactate-does it really make a difference? Shock 2007;27:520–26.
45. Hoffmann JN, Vollmar B, Laschke MW, et al. Hydroxyethyl starch (130 kD), but not crystalloid volume support, improves microcirculation during normotensive endotoxemia. Anesthesiology 2002;97: 460–70.
46. Feng X, Yan W, Wang Z, et al. Hydroxyethyl starch, but not modified fluid gelatin, affects inflammatory response in a rat model of polymicrobial sepsis with capillary leakage. Anesth Analg 2007;104:624–30.
47. Marx G, Pedder S, Smith L, et al. Attenuation of capillary leakage by hydroxyethyl starch (130/0.42) in a porcine model of septic shock. Crit Care Med 2006;34: 3005–10.
48. Schuerholz T, Sumpelmann R, Piepenbrock S, et al. Ringer's solution but not hydroxyethyl starch or modified fluid gelatin enhances platelet microvesicle formation in a porcine model of septic shock. Br J Anaesth 2004;92:716–21.
49. Vincent JL, Gerlach H. Fluid resuscitation in severe sepsis and septic shock: an evidence-based review. Crit Care Med 2004;32:S451–4.
50. Dellinger RP, Carlet JM, Masur H, et al. Surviving Sepsis Campaign guidelines for management of severe sepsis and septic shock. Intensive Care Med 2004;30:536–55.
51. Rivers E, Nguyen B, Havstad S, et al. Early goal-directed therapy in the treatment of severe sepsis and septic shock. N Engl J Med 2001;345:1368–77.
52. Mangialardi RJ, Martin GS, Bernard GR, et al. Hypoproteinemia predicts acute respiratory distress syndrome development, weight gain, and death in patients with sepsis. Ibuprofen in Sepsis Study Group. Crit Care Med 2000;28:3137–45.
53. American Thoracic Society. Evidence-based colloid use in the critically ill: American Thoracic Society Consensus Statement. Am J Respir Crit Care Med 2004;170:1247–59.
54. Schuller D, Mitchell JP, Calandrino FS, et al. Fluid balance during pulmonary edema. Is fluid gain a marker or a cause of poor outcome? Chest 1991;100: 1068–75.
55. Wiedemann HP, Wheeler AP, Bernard GR, et al. Comparison of two fluid-management strategies in acute lung injury. N Engl J Med 2006;354:2564–75.
56. Bickell WH, Wall MJ, Jr, Pepe PE, et al. Immediate versus delayed fluid resuscitation for hypotensive patients with penetrating torso injuries. N Engl J Med 1994;331:1105–9.
57. Botha AJ, Moore FA, Moore EE, et al. Postinjury neutrophil priming and activation: an early vulnerable window. Surgery 1995;118:358–64.
58. Balogh Z, McKinley BA, Holcomb JB, et al. Both primary and secondary abdominal compartment syndrome can be predicted early and are harbingers of multiple organ failure. J Trauma 2003;54:848–59.

CHAPTER 15

Hypertonic Saline Solutions for the Initial Treatment of Patients with Traumatic Injuries

Charles E. Wade & Michael A. Dubick
US Army Institute of Surgical Research, San Antonio, TX, USA

Initial fluid resuscitation of the patient, who is hypotensive, with traumatic injuries impacts survival as well as other measures of outcome, such as days on ventilator support and intensive care unit (ICU), and length of hospital stay. Yet, of the standard of care (SOC) fluids presently used, none has been required to demonstrate an improvement in the primary outcomes of survival, morbidity, or avoidance of allogeneic blood transfusions. Trauma is a major cause of death in the first 40 years of life in developed countries and is increasing worldwide [1,2]. The primary cause of death in this population is hemorrhage, which also contributes to morbidity. Early control of bleeding, restoration of blood volume, and reestablishment of adequate tissue perfusion to vital organ are essential to improved outcomes. Early and aggressive fluid resuscitation to treat blood loss due to hemorrhage, while being recommended for many decades, remains controversial.

This review focuses on investigations into the use of hypertonic (~2400 mOsm/kg) fluids as resuscitation for the initial care of victims of trauma. Hypertonic solutions usually consist of 7.5% sodium chloride (NaCl), though other salts have been used, often combined with hyperoncotic colloids, such as 6% Dextran 70 or hetastarch. Clinical interest in these fluid formulations has been stimulated by an extensive basic science literature elucidating a number of mechanisms of action and an expanding positive clinical experience.

The issues that must be considered while evaluating the efficacy of a resuscitation fluid are the effects on the relationship of oxygen delivery and demand, possible aggravation of bleeding resulting in additional loss of blood, and the time delay in gaining vascular access before initiation of definitive interventions.

Any asanguinous fluid used for resuscitation may expand the blood volume and therefore improve cardiac output, but it may also dilute the concentration of hemoglobin and thus, reduce oxygen carrying capacity. The net result could be a decrease in oxygen delivery. The balance of the cost of increasing flow at the expense of oxygen content must be considered in the evaluation of a resuscitation fluid.

The aggravation of bleeding by fluid administration may occur by two means. The first is by an increase in blood pressure in the presence of uncontrolled bleeding. This has led some to advocate hypotensive or permissive resuscitation [3,4]. The second is by the dilution of clotting factors. When evaluating the benefit of a resuscitation fluid the effects on clotting and blood pressure must be considered in light of the possibility of increasing blood loss.

Safety and ease of administration must also be considered in use of a resuscitation fluid in an

Alternatives to Blood Transfusion in Transfusion Medicine, 2nd edition. Edited by A. Maniatis, P. Van der Linden, J.-F. Hardy.

emergent situation. The fluid should have a well-defined safety profile of which any side effects can be corrected easily. Administration should be rapid to attain early efficacy to mitigate or attenuate the consequences of hemorrhagic hypotension.

Thus, the ideal resuscitation fluid to treat the emergent patient with traumatic injuries who is hypotensive should be safe, expand blood volume, be able to improve oxygen delivery, and possibly reduce oxygen demand, not increase bleeding, and be easy to administer. Currently, none of the fluids considered as SOC meets all of these criteria. Furthermore, of the presently available fluids for the replacement of blood loss due to traumatic injuries, none has undergone extensive clinical and regulatory investigations. Recently, questions have been raised about the use of these SOC fluids as information on efficacy and safety has accumulated [5]. These issues have stimulated an effort to develop new resuscitation solutions such as the hypertonic fluids discussed here.

Physiological properties

The initial incentive for clinical evaluation of hypertonic saline (HS) fluids came from early work in a number of animal models on survival after major hemorrhage. Velasco et al. [6] reported that dogs who were lightly anesthetized and hemorrhaged to a blood pressure of 40 mmHg for 30 minutes survived if infused with 4 mL/kg (10% of the blood volume lost) of 7.5% HS. Upon administration there was a rapid improvement in blood pressure and cardiac output. None of the control animals survived while 100% of the treatment animals were alive at 7 hours. In a study in conscious pigs that were hemorrhaged 70% of their estimated blood volume, Maningas and Bellamy [7] reported that none of the control animals survived while 50% of animals administered 11 mL/kg of HS survived; when given an equal volume of hypertonic saline dextran (HSD) 100% survived. These finding were reiterated in numerous other studies employing a wide range of species and hemorrhage models.

Expansion of blood volume

The increased survival noted with administration of hypertonic fluids in animal studies was associated with the expansion of blood volume as fluid moves from the extravascular space into the vascular compartment as a result of the osmotic gradient. The expansion of blood volume and retention was greater when the fluids contained colloids [8]. Studies of these solutions in human experimental subjects have contrasted hypertonic solutions with SOC crystalloid fluids such as Lactated Ringer's (LR) and normal saline [9–11]. In subjects who were hypovolemic there was a greater expansion of central blood volume with hypertonic fluids that persisted longer than SOC (Figure 15.1).

In the presence of hypotension, the increase in blood volume with hypertonic fluid administration is accompanied by an increase in blood pressure and cardiac output [12–15]. A reduction in total peripheral resistance also occurs. These changes improve blood flow to vital organs. Of note is that the administration of HS results in a greater increase in cardiac output for a given increase in blood volume. This improvement in cardiac output with HS could be related to increases in left ventricular contractile force associated with the increase in plasma osmolality as well as the greater preload because of expansion of blood volume. The reduction in total peripheral resistance may also contribute to the reduction in afterload. Hypertonic fluids cause hemodilution resulting in a reduction in oxygen carrying capacity; however, the increase in cardiac output proportionally exceeds this reduction resulting in a net increase in oxygen delivery [12–15].

Immune function

Studies of the hemodynamic aspects of HS or HSD for the treatment of hemorrhagic hypotension revealed a marked increase in flow in the microvasculature compared to conventional crystalloid fluids. It has been well documented that in response to hypoperfusion and subsequent rapid reperfusion, adherent leukocytes activate which release cytotoxic substances and reactive oxygen species damaging the endothelial barrier. With this damage comes leakage of fluid and

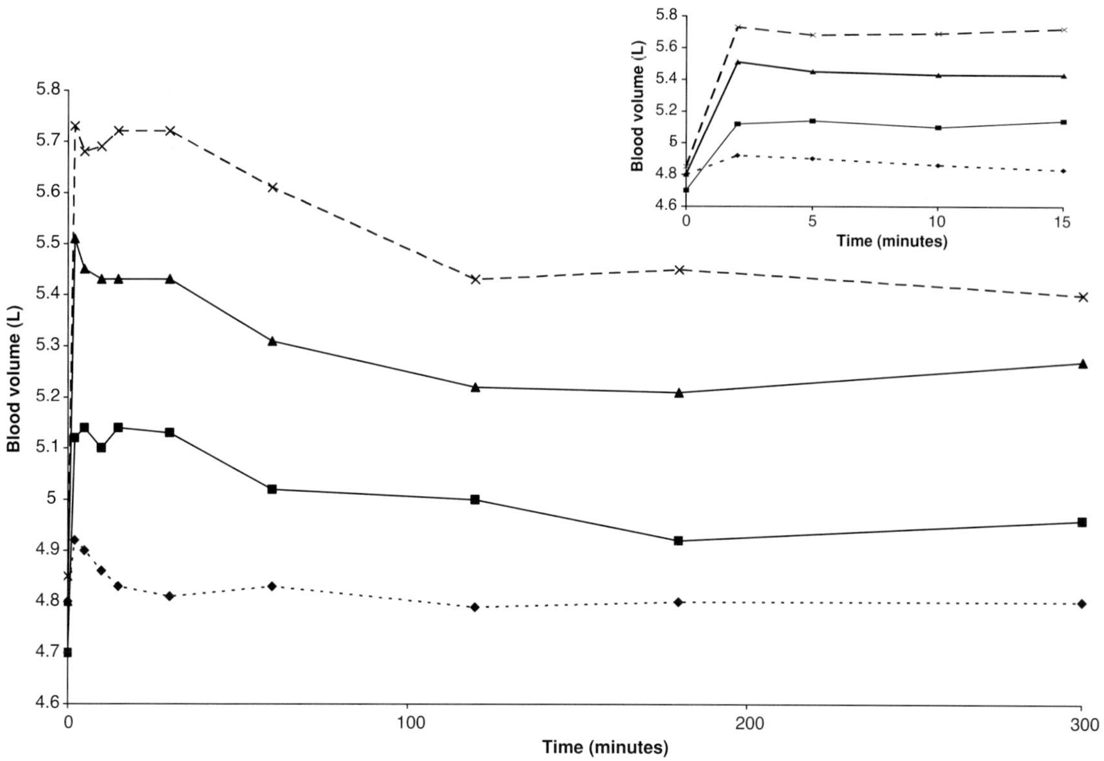

Figure 15.1 Central blood volume after the administration of 250 mL of isotonic saline. (♦···♦), 6% Dextran (■—■), 7.5% hypertonic saline (▲---▲) or hypertonic saline 6% Dextran (×- - -×) in human subjects. Inset graph represents first 15 minutes after infusion.

macromolecules into the extravascular space and development of tissue or organ injury. Subsequent to improved microcirculatory flow, use of hypertonic fluids has been associated with a reduction of neutrophils rolling and sticking to the endothelial cells of blood vessels [16–26]. Hypertonicity has been shown to inhibit leukocyte adherence and activation [16–20, 25]. Furthermore, HS reduced L-selectin shedding in isolated polymorphonuclear neutrophils (PMNs). This was also observed with choline chloride, but not with hypertonic mannitol or sucrose [27]. In addition, in isolated PMNs from healthy human volunteers, it was observed that HS decreased β_2-integrin expression, superoxide production, and elastase release, but only if HS was added before PMNs became primed or activated [28, 29]. Others have also found that incubation of human PMNs with HS or HSD inhibited their respiratory burst [30, 31]. However, if HS was added after PMN priming or activation, superoxide production and elastase release were actually enhanced. This observation further supports the use of HS as the first resuscitation fluid in the treatment of hemorrhage [32, 33].

These observations have led to the notion that hypertonic fluids may actually inhibit the immune suppression associated with hemorrhagic shock, supported by numerous studies in isolated blood cells, animal hemorrhage studies, and recent human clinical trials. In an early study, incubation of HS with human and rabbit monocytes resulted in enhanced monocyte function and T-cell proliferation [18]. This effect was also seen with HSD [34].

Other studies have evaluated the protective effects of HS on immune cells. Using murine thiocholate-elicited peritoneal exudative macrophages to model the effects of HS on Kupffer cells, it was observed that HS increased IL-10 mRNA levels and enhanced the increase in IL-10 induced by lipopolysaccharides (LPS) [35].

Recent studies have also identified a number of immune pathways which appear mediated by hypertonicity [16–20, 25]. For example, Junger et al. demonstrated that HS-mediated T-cell proliferation may relate to tyrosine phosphorylation of cellular proteins and activation of MAPK p38 [36]. However, Ciesla et al. [37] found that HS inhibited platelet-activating factor-mediated MAPK p38 activation in isolated PMNs from healthy volunteers. Ciesla et al. [38] have also shown that HS could reversibly inhibit cytotoxic responses in isolated human PMNs, an effect that occurred again with repeated HS treatment. Of note, many of these responses can be demonstrated in vitro suggesting that HS has a direct effect on immune cells. It appears that the administration of HS and resultant hypertonicity elicits a cellular signal, which modulates and inhibits the immune cascade normally associated with reperfusion injury. Administration of HS resulting in suppression of this cascade may impact long-term morbidity and survival. However, recent findings suggest that once this cascade is initiated the beneficial effects of hypertonic solutions are diminished.

Supporting the in vitro observations, a number of studies in trauma and hemorrhage rodent models have observed an inhibition of inflammatory responses and reduced tissue injury after HS infusion [16, 17, 25, 39–42]. Some in vivo studies observed that infusion of HS reduced susceptibility to sepsis after hemorrhage, possibly due to inhibition of sepsis-induced P-selectin expression or to bacterial challenge [43–45]. Other studies suggest that the reduced lung or hepatic injury associated with HS after hemorrhage or ischemia/reperfusion in animal models can be attributed to reduced neutrophil priming, activation and respiratory burst [17, 39, 41, 46, 47]. In a mouse hemorrhage/LPS injection model, Pascual et al. [48, 49] found HS infusion reduced PMN adherence to pulmonary endothelium and reduced lung myeloperoxidase activity compared to LR infusion; findings consistent with others [16, 17]. In addition, it has been proposed that HS infusion induces stat3 activation of endogenous IL-10 release as a protective mechanism [40, 50]. Other investigators have proposed that the improved immune function after hemorrhage related to HS infusion is due to its producing a more balanced profile of T-lymphocytes or to its effects on adhesion molecules on the neutrophils [25, 42, 51].

Taken together, these data suggest that initial or early hypertonic saline resuscitation would be of greater benefit than infusion after administration of conventional fluids. The modulation of immune function by HS would possibly reduce secondary complications. Furthermore, the addition of dextran, as in HSD, does not inhibit the immunomodulatory effects of HS in response to hemorrhage.

Bleeding

As noted above, the administration of hypertonic fluids causes an acute increase in blood pressure which, in the presences of uncontrolled bleeding could contribute in increased bleeding, as suggested by Bickell et al. [3, 52–55]. Rapid administration of HSD may rapidly elevate blood pressure, which could disrupt established clots and therefore increase blood loss. However, several studies addressing this issue found that if the standard intravenous set and infusion procedures are used, blood pressure is prevented from reaching unsafe levels [56].

Clinical trials

Over the past decade there have been several reviews of the clinical use of hypertonic fluids [8, 32, 57–63]. The number of reviews greatly exceeds the number of clinical trials. This disparity is partially because of the difficulties associated with studies involving critically ill trauma patients and the requirement for community consent. In many of these reviews, clinical populations have been mixed with data from elective surgery patients combined with data from patients with traumatic injuries. In addition, analyses included intermingled solutions with various NaCl concentrations and different colloids. Therefore, it is incumbent upon the reader to sort through the literature to fully understand the available data. For the present review of the use of hypertonic fluids in clinical studies, we will focus on patients with traumatic injuries treated with HS (7.5% NaCl) or HSD (7.2–7.5% NaCl and 4–6% dextran).

Primary end points

The end points in the evaluation of any resuscitation product must include safety and efficacy. The criteria for the evaluation of efficacy are based on a definitive influence on clinical outcome. While there are numerous physiological measures suggestive of improvement, efficacy must be tied to the ultimate outcome of the patient. If, for example, a fluid improves cardiac output but the patient still dies, efficacy is not improved. Accepted clinical outcomes for evaluation of a resuscitation fluid by regulatory agencies are an improvement in survival, a reduction in morbidity or a decrease in the number of patients requiring allogeneic transfusions [64, 65]. While the importance of the first two end points is obvious, the avoidance of transfusion is based upon the risk associated with receiving allogeneic blood products.

Survival

Survival is the definitive end point of clinical intervention. There have been a number of studies evaluating the use of HS and HSD in patients with traumatic injuries. The focus here will be on 13 randomized studies in which a hypertonic fluid was used as part of the initial care and outcomes were compared to those for SOC. In 11 of the studies of HS or HSD, enrollment was based on injuries due to trauma [66–74]. In the other two studies, criteria included hypovolemic shock [75, 76]. Because 96% and 85% of patients enrolled in these two studies also had traumatic injuries, they are included in the present review. In all 13 studies, there were both blunt injuries (primarily from vehicle accidents), and penetrating injuries (gunshot or stab wounds). Injuries were distributed equally between these two mechanisms of injury in most of the studies.

Table 15.1 Percent survival of patients after treatment with hypertonic saline (HS) or standard of care (SOC) from published clinical studies of trauma patients.

Reference	SOC	HS
Younes [75]	77% (35)	80% (35)
Vassar [73]	63% (27)	47% (32)
Vassar [72]	83% (84)	86% (85)
Fabian (cited in Wade [79])	63% (75)	64% (67)
Fabian (cited in Wade [79])	72% (113)	65% (71)
Vassar [74]	49% (45)	60% (50)
Cooper [91]*	50% (115)	55% (114)

Values in parenthesis are the number of subjects per group.
* Refers to studies where enrollment was limited to patients with traumatic brain injury (TBI).

For HS, seven prospective studies have been extensively reviewed by the Cochrane Collaboration and our group (Table 15.1) [33, 57–59, 62, 77–80]. Findings in all cases were similar, with no evidence of improvement in survival for HS compared with isotonic crystalloids. However, the limitations of the published studies do not rule out important clinical differences.

Whether or not HSD improves survival in patients with traumatic injuries is controversial. For this review, we appraised 11 prospective studies of 748 patients treated with HSD and 797 receiving SOC fluids (Table 15.2). The mean difference in survival was an increase of 3.6% in favor of HSD. However, the evidence was not conclusive, with only one of the studies reporting a significant improvement in survival. In one study with a trend for a decrease in survival, the groups appear to be mismatched as to the severity of injury [74]. Extensive retrospective review of these studies concluded that HSD had favorable effect on survival compared to SOC. But presently, there are no randomized clinical trials demonstrating conclusive evidence of increased survival to support the use of hypertonic colloids in the initial treatment of patients with traumatic injuries.

Of note, there may be specific patients within the traumatic injury population that may benefit

Table 15.2 Percent survival of patients after treatment with hypertonic saline dextran (HSD) or standard of care (SOC) from published clinical studies of trauma patients.

Reference	SOC	HSD
Younes [75]	77% (35)	80% (35)
Maningas [68]	80% (25)	87% (23)
Vassar [73]	46% (24)	48% (23)
Vassar [72]	59% (83)	64% (83)
Mattox [69]	80% (211)	83% (211)
Younes [94]	64% (111)	73% (101)
Vassar [74]	83% (84)	78% (89)
Vassar [71]	49% (45)	56% (50)
Alpar [66]	87% (90)	92% (90)
Rizoli [70]	86% (14)	100% (10)
Bulger [67]	88% (26)	92% (36)

from hypertonic fluids. Recent discussions have suggested that hypertonic fluids for maintaining plasma volume in patients with burns or traumatic brain injuries (TBIs). In the treatment of burn injuries, hypertonic fluids have reduced fluid requirements and prevented edema formation [81–86]. Also, Oda and coworkers [87] recently found that HS decreased fluid requirements and reduced the risk of abdominal compartment syndrome in patients with severe burns (mean = 65% TBSA). The authors noted no difference in multisystem organ failure or survival between the HS and SOC groups. However, another comparative trial reported an increase in mortality, raising questions about the advisability of HS for burn patients [88, 89]. For treatment of TBI, the benefit of HS has drawn greater attention based on the observation of HS administration and decreased intracranial pressure and improved cerebral perfusion pressure [90]. The randomized trial of 7.5% HS for field treatment of patients with TBI failed to demonstrate an improvement in survival or neurological function, though post hoc reviews suggest possible efficacy [71, 79, 91]. Benefits of HS fluid administration retrospectively described in patients who require surgery, blood transfusion, or treatment for TBI suggest that there may be subpopulations in which HS solutions could improve survival.

Morbidity

As mentioned, studies of immunological function in human cells show improvements with the administration of hypertonic solutions [92, 93]. These improvements, coupled with an improvement in organ blood flow during adequate resuscitation, should lead to a reduction in medical complications secondary to hypoperfusion and reperfusion injury. The trend has been for a reduction in the incidence of complications when HS is administered, and in the number of patients in which they are reported. In a study of 422 patients by Mattox et al. [69], 22 had medical complications; seven patients (3%) treated with HSD had complications versus 13 (6%) with complications who received SOC. Of the patients with complications, only one of the seven (14%) who received HSD died, while six (46%) of the SOC-treated patients died. In a study by Vassar et al. [74], deaths from sepsis and organ failure were one for SOC, three for HS, and three for HSD. In addition, Younes et al. [94] reported that the incidence of complications was similar among treatment groups. Recent studies, though of limited numbers of patients, suggest no difference between treatments in rates of infection or multiple organ failure [67, 70]. Though a definitive evaluation of the effect of hypertonic fluids on the incidence of medical complications is still necessary, the trend is toward a reduction or no change in the rate of medical complications in patients administered HS.

Allogenic transfusion

Patients who require the transfusion of whole blood or packed red cells are presumed to be in a life-threatening state of hypovolemia. The necessity for blood replacement is correlated with severity of injury and is more common in patients with penetrating injuries [74]. The amount of blood infused is on the order of 1–2 L [71, 74]. In a meta-analysis of individual patient data from six of the previous studies of HSD, Wade et al. found that the odds ratio (1.60; 95% CV 0.95, 2.81) favored HSD improved survival until discharge in patients requiring blood transfusion [79]. This finding, however, was not statistically significant. Vassar et al. [74] reported the estimated blood loss and replacement requirements of patients undergoing emergent surgical procedures. There was no significant difference in the amount of blood required, 1.5 ± 2.7 L for SOC and 1.2 ± 1.8 L with HSD, but in the HSD group, survival was improved compared to predicted outcome. Younes et al. [75] noted that significantly greater amounts of blood were administered to patients with SOC compared with either HS or HSD. Rizoli and coworkers [70] also noted a trend toward a reduction in blood use with HSD infusion. Bulger et al. [67] reported no difference between treatments in the number of red blood cell units transfused, and the incidence of massive transfusions (>10 units) was similar.

In general patients requiring blood transfusion are believed to be at risk of dying, and the administration of HSD tends to increase the probability of survival in this population [79]. However, while these studies report the mean number of red cell units transfused and suggest a reduction in requirements with HS administration, none have addressed the avoidance of allogeneic transfusions. As the number of transfused units of blood products is decreased, the probability of developing infection is reduced, however, the ideal primary end point is the elimination of the risk by eliminating all transfusions.

Secondary end points

Fluid requirements

Hypertonic fluids may decrease fluid requirements and attenuate edema formation. In the earliest reports by Younes et al. [75, 76], there was a significant reduction in the required volume of both crystalloids and blood in those patients with hypotension who were initially administered HS or HSD. The reduction in fluid requirements was over 40% compared to SOC. This study was conducted in an emergency room where investigators controlled fluid administration to a systolic blood pressure (SBP) of 100 mmHg. In the recent study by Alper and Killampalli [66], fluid requirements were decreased by 30%. The group receiving SOC was administered 6.5 L in comparison with 4.5 L in those treated with HSD. In trials by others the administration of fluids was not as well controlled. However, there was still the trend toward a reduction in early fluid requirements in those who received hypertonic fluids. In patients administered HSD, the trend was a reduction of about 1000 mL during 24-hour fluid administration [68, 69, 71, 72, 76, 94]. No difference in urine output between treatments has been noted [66, 69]. Thus, administration of HS solutions reduces overall resuscitation fluid requirements and net positive fluid balance compared to SOC.

Blood pressure

The majority of the clinical trials with hypertonic fluids enrolled patients who were hypotensive, defined as a SBP of less than 90 mmHg [33]. It is assumed that patients with a blood pressure that is sustained at a low level for an extended period of time will have a poor outcome [95, 96]. This is supported by the work of Vassar et al. [71, 74], in which blood pressure was not increased in response to fluid administration in nonsurvivors to the extent that it was in survivors. If this holds true, the benefits of hypertonic fluids outweigh SOC, as researchers have consistently found a greater increase in blood pressure with HS [68,69,71,75,76,94]. For most patients, the increase in SBP with HS or HSD is on the order of 10 mmHg above that observed with SOC [69, 71, 75, 76, 94]. If it is assumed that an increase in blood pressure is beneficial, resulting in increased survival, the administration of HS or HSD would be favored.

Immune responses

Modulation of immune function has been related to fewer incidents of multiple organ failure, and lower infection rates and subsequent length of ICU and hospital stays. To date, few clinical studies have investigated the immunomodulatory effects of HS or HSD in trauma patients. In normovolemic women, HS infusion increased the number of B-cells and decreased the number of circulating neutrophils compared to LR in a 2-hour study period, suggesting a modest immunologic effect in these women [92]. This agrees with the modest 12% inhibition of CD11b expression in activated neutrophils observed in normal healthy volunteers

[97]. However, these authors speculated that this modest effect could be more pronounced in trauma patients in whom neutrophil-mediated tissue injury is common. In a single blinded study of women undergoing abdominal hysterectomy, infusion of HS did not affect natural killer cell activity, lymphocyte proliferation, or other assays of immune function compared with normal saline, leading the authors to conclude that the recommended therapeutic dose of HS did not affect cellular immune response [98]. More recently, two studies have evaluated the effects of HSD on immune function in patients with traumatic hemorrhagic shock. Infusion of 250 mL of HSD resulted in a transient hypernatremia, but shock-induced neutrophil activation was reduced and L-selectin shedding was induced for 24 hours [70]. HSD also significantly reduced TNF-α production, leading the authors to conclude that HSD promotes a more balanced inflammatory response to hemorrhagic shock. In a randomized, double-blind study of traumatic hypovolemic shock, Bulger et al. [67] also observed reduced neutrophil activation and a more normal monocyte profile 12 hours after HSD infusion compared with those that received LR. Perhaps these data further support the observation that elective surgery patients are not always a good surrogate models for trauma patients.

Safety

Hypertonic fluids raise a number of safety issues [8, 32, 60, 73, 99]. While there has been supposition as to possible complications, on the whole, data are limited. Notably, the focus has been on the HS component rather than the colloids in the combination fluids. This is partly due to the extensive experience associated with use of the various colloids, especially in Europe. The safety concerns of colloid solutions are addressed by others in this book. For this reason, we will direct our discussion to the safety of the hypertonic component of the solutions.

Uncontrolled bleeding

An increase in blood pressure has been purported to induce an increase in bleeding in the presence of uncontrolled hemorrhage [3]. In animal models, administration of fluid to increase blood pressure leads to greater blood loss, and, ultimately death [53, 54, 100]. This occurs in animals with the administration of either HS or HSD. It is of interest that when the amount of blood loss is estimated, and the requirements of resuscitation fluids are examined, there is little difference between HS and SOC fluids [66, 71, 75]. Concerns about uncontrolled bleeding focus particularly on patients with penetrating injuries to major vessels that require surgical intervention to stop the hemorrhage. Oddly, in a number of studies it was actually the patients with penetrating injuries requiring surgery that had the greatest improvement in discharge survival [69, 71]. For example, in a study by Mattox et al. [69], in patients with penetrating injuries requiring surgery the use of HSD was favored ($p = 0.01$) to improve survival over the first 24 hours. In this study at the hospital with the highest enrollment of patients with penetrating injuries requiring surgery, (Ben Taub General in Houston TX), the survival rates were 88% with HSD and 77% with SOC treatment ($p = 0.06$). This is also the institution where studies about the benefits of withholding fluids in the field were conducted and survival in the HSD group was still higher than patients receiving limited fluid [3]. Vassar et al. [71, 74] also noted an improved discharge survival in patients requiring urgent operative treatment if they had received HSD. Thus, if fluids are used for the emergent resuscitation of patients with hypotension and traumatic injuries, hypertonic fluids do not appear to increase bleeding compared to SOC fluids, as hemoglobin concentrations, hematocrit, and estimated blood loss are not different between treatments [69, 71, 72, 74]. Take together these data suggest that this subgroup had a significant improvement in survival with HS infusions irrespective of any additional bleeding.

Another factor contributing to an increase in bleeding would be the hemodilution that occurs with the infusion of hypertonic fluids. Hemodilution would cause a decrease in the concentration of clotting factors and lead to an increase in clotting time contributing to an increase in bleeding. The reported incidence of coagulopathies has been similar among the test solutions [69, 71]. The incidence of massive transfusion was also the same [67]. In studies that have measured prothrombin (PT) and activated partial thromboplastin times (aPTT), no significant differences have been noted between treatments. The dextran component of HSD has also been reported to reduce clotting when administered in large volumes. However, administration of 250 mL of HSD in studies in which the dextran concentration was increased up to 12% showed no difference in clotting factors [71]. In vitro studies of the effects of HS on clot formation and strength suggest that dilutions of over 15% of blood volume have anticoagulant effects [101,102]. However, these levels of dilution far exceed the recommended dose for hypertonic fluids. Therefore, evidence from clinical studies support the in vitro studies that at the recommended dose it appears that the use of HS or HSD does not alter clotting.

Hypernatremia

A consistent observation following the use of HS is hypernatremia. An increase of 10–12 mmol/L in plasma sodium is observed if 250 mL of HS or HSD is administered to a patient with traumatic injuries [66–74]. There have been no adverse neurological reactions or neuropathological abnormalities found at autopsy associated with this increase in plasma sodium concentration [73, 74]. Further, in patients who died in which autopsies were conducted, there were no incidences of central pontine myelinolysis [71, 73, 74]. At present, there are no reports of any adverse effects associated with increases in sodium concentrations of the magnitude reported with the administration of 250 mL of 7.5% NaCl or HSD. However, we have little information about the use of HS solutions in children, who may be more susceptible to the adverse effects of hypernatremia [103, 104].

Acidosis

HS has been postulated to result in acidosis due to hyperchloremia. Following admission to hospital, there appears to be no difference in pH (or base excess) between patients administered HS or SOC [69]. However, Vassar et al. [73] reported that 8 of 106 patients administered hypertonic solutions had significant hyperchloremic acidemia but all eight were moribund before administration of the fluid. As acidosis is present in severely injured trauma patients and in those patients with a period of cardiac arrest, it has been difficult to determine if there is a cause and effect relationship between acidosis and administration of HS. This has led to the recommendation that HS administration be avoided in patients with preexisting acidosis, especially following cardiac arrest [32]. Recently, Bender et al. [105] reported the use of hypertonic saline hetastarch in patients requiring cardiopulmonary resuscitation. The patients were in severe acidosis upon enrollment (mean pH 7.04 ± 0.11), with no change noted after HS infusion. The benefit of HS was more pronounced if the duration of cardiac arrest was greater than 6 minutes, or if the initial cardiac rhythm was asystole or pulseless. These findings suggest that HS for the patient with acidosis may still be of benefit.

Timing of administration

In most of the available studies, hypertonic fluids were administered within 2 hours following injury. In addition, there appears to be a greater benefit if HS is administered as the first fluid in resuscitation [32]. Animal studies support this observation, although the beneficial effects were attenuated with the administration of repeated doses during continued bleeding, possibly due to a reduction in the resultant osmotic gradient with each dose [106]. The rate of administration may also make a difference [56]. Therefore, it is recommended that HS fluids be the initial fluid administered to resuscitate a patient with hypotension and traumatic injuries, at a rate limited by use of a standard intravenous infusion set.

Dose

The dose and rate of administration of hypertonic fluids that is recommended, 250 mL, followed by conventional fluids as needed, is based on survival studies in animals [6, 107]. Issues as to the safety of this dose and administration rate have been raised in intraoperative studies. Rapid administration of hypertonic saline hetastarch to patients with a limited cardiac reserve undergoing cardiac surgery resulted in hypotension, with transient hypovolemic left ventricular failure [108, 109]. In trauma patients, the rate of administration has been limited by the size of the infusion needle and the use of gravity to initiate flow [56, 110, 111]. A more rapid administration of hypertonic fluids has not been evaluated in patients. There is little data to support an increase in volume or rate of administration of the present dose (250 mL), which has been suggested to be effective in the treatment of trauma patients.

The recommended dose does raise a question as to body size. In all studies a uniform dose has been used over a wide range of body weights. Unfortunately, in the clinical trials published to date, body weight has not been reported. As the majority of patients have been young male adults, body weight could vary from 50 to 150 kg, thus the dose by body weight covers a wide range, 5–1.6 mL/kg. Recent studies in children undergoing cardiac surgery demonstrated the dose of 4 mL/kg of HS colloid fluids to be safe and effective [103, 104]. The use of HS improved cardiac output, reduced extravascular lung water, and decreased fluid requirements. This work suggests that adjustment of the dose to 4 mL/kg may be appropriate for patients with body weights less than 60 kg. The present dose of 250 mL favors safety and has not been associated with adverse events in patients with traumatic injuries.

Summary

Presently, there are major ongoing multicenter double blind randomized trials with hypertonic fluids. The Resuscitation Outcomes Consortium (ROC) is conducting two multicenter trials of HS resuscitation in trauma patients. The first study seeks to determine the impact of hypertonic resuscitation on survival for blunt or penetrating trauma in patients in hypovolemic shock. The second will determine the impact of hypertonic resuscitation on long term (6 months) neurologic outcome for blunt trauma patients with severe TBI. Both studies will be three arm, randomized, blinded intervention trials comparing HS/dextran (7.5% saline/6% Dextran 70, HSD), HS alone (7.5% saline, HS), and normal saline as the initial resuscitation fluid administered to these patients in the prehospital setting. These studies will hopefully provide definitive evidence as to the efficacy of hypertonic fluids in the treatment of patients with traumatic injuries and hypovolemia.

Currently, there is no evidence from randomized double-blinded control studies of the primary outcomes of survival, morbidity, or avoidance of allogeneic blood transfusions to support the use of HS fluids in the initial resuscitation of the patient with traumatic injuries. It must be remembered that none of the SOC fluids has been required to demonstrate an improvement in these primary outcomes. However, with the administration of hypertonic fluids there are improvements in secondary clinical end points in comparison to SOC fluids. There is a consistent improvement in blood pressure, a decrease in fluid requirements over the first 24 hours, and improved immune function. Furthermore, retrospective analyses suggest improvements in specific patient populations. These include improved survival in those patients who required emergent surgical care or blood transfusion and who presumably suffered greater injury acuity. Unfortunately, at this time these patient populations cannot be identified in the field at the onset of care for randomization into clinical trials. Clinical studies thus far have raised no major safety issues. At this time, despite extensive and compelling preclinical data and strong preliminary clinical studies, caution should be used in the administration of hypertonic solutions to patients who are hypotensive and have traumatic injuries.

References

1. Kauvar DS, Lefering R, Wade CE. Impact of hemorrhage on trauma outcome: an overview of epidemiology, clinical presentations, and therapeutic considerations. J Trauma 2006;60(6 Suppl.):S3–11.
2. Kauvar DS, Wade CE. The epidemiology and modern management of traumatic hemorrhage: US and international perspectives. Crit Care 2005;9(5 Suppl.):S1–9.
3. Bickell WH, Wall MJ, Jr, Pepe PE, et al. Immediate versus delayed fluid resuscitation for hypotensive

patients with penetrating torso injuries. N Engl J Med 1994;331(17):1105–9.
4. Holcomb JB, Jenkins D, Rhee P, et al. Damage control resuscitation: directly addressing the early coagulopathy of trauma. J Trauma 2007;62(2):307–10.
5. Cotton BA, Guy JS, Morris JA, Jr, Abumrad NN. The cellular, metabolic, and systemic consequences of aggressive fluid resuscitation strategies. Shock 2006;26(2):115–21.
6. Velasco IT, Pontieri V, Rocha e Silva M, Jr, Lopes OU. Hyperosmotic NaCl and severe hemorrhagic shock. Am J Physiol 1980;239(5):H664–73.
7. Maningas PA, Bellamy RF. Hypertonic sodium chloride solutions for the prehospital management of traumatic hemorrhagic shock: a possible improvement in the standard of care? Ann Emerg Med 1986;15(12):1411–14.
8. Kramer GC. Hypertonic resuscitation: physiologic mechanisms and recommendations for trauma care. J Trauma 2003;54(5 Suppl.):S89–99.
9. Drobin D, Hahn RG. Kinetics of isotonic and hypertonic plasma volume expanders. Anesthesiology 2002;96(6):1371–80.
10. Svensen C, Hahn RG. Volume kinetics of Ringer solution, dextran 70, and hypertonic saline in male volunteers. Anesthesiology 1997;87(2):204–12.
11. Svensen C, Sjostrand F, Hahn RG. Volume kinetics of intravenous fluid therapy in the prehospital setting. Prehosp Disaster Med 2001;16(1):9–13.
12. Hannon JP, Wade CE, Bossone CA, et al. Blood gas and acid-base status of conscious pigs subjected to fixed-volume hemorrhage and resuscitated with hypertonic saline dextran. Circ Shock 1990;32(1):19–29.
13. Hannon JP, Wade CE, Bossone CA, et al. Oxygen delivery and demand in conscious pigs subjected to fixed-volume hemorrhage and resuscitated with 7.5% NaCl in 6% Dextran. Circ Shock 1989;29(3):205–17.
14. Wade CE, Hannon JP, Bossone CA, et al. Resuscitation of conscious pigs following hemorrhage: comparative efficacy of small-volume resuscitation. Circ Shock 1989;29(3):193–204.
15. Wade CE, Tillman FJ, Loveday JA, et al. Effect of dehydration on cardiovascular responses and electrolytes after hypertonic saline/dextran treatment for moderate hemorrhage. Ann Emerg Med 1992;21(2):113–9.
16. Angle N, Hoyt DB, Cabello-Passini R, et al. Hypertonic saline resuscitation reduces neutrophil margination by suppressing neutrophil L selectin expression. J Trauma 1998;45(1):7–12; discussion-3.
17. Angle N, Hoyt DB, Coimbra R, et al. Hypertonic saline resuscitation diminishes lung injury by suppressing neutrophil activation after hemorrhagic shock. Shock 1998;9(3):164–70.
18. Junger W, Liu F, Loomis W, Hoyt D. Hypertonic saline enhances cellular immune function. Circ Shock 1994;42(4):190–96.
19. Junger WG, Coimbra R, Liu FC, et al. Hypertonic saline resuscitation: a tool to modulate immune function in trauma patients? Shock 1997;8(4):235–41.
20. Junger WG, Hoyt DB, Davis RE, et al. Hypertonicity regulates the function of human neutrophils by modulating chemoattractant receptor signaling and activating mitogen-activated protein kinase p38. J Clin Invest 1998;101(12):2768–79.
21. Junger WG, Hoyt DB, Hamreus M, et al. Hypertonic saline activates protein tyrosine kinases and mitogen-activated protein kinase p38 in T-cells. J Trauma 1997;42(3):437–43; discussion 43–5.
22. Mazzoni MC, Borgstrom P, Arfors KE, Intaglietta M. Dynamic fluid redistribution in hyperosmotic resuscitation of hypovolemic hemorrhage. Am J Physiol 1988;255(3 Pt 2):H629–37.
23. Mazzoni MC, Borgstrom P, Arfors KE, Intaglietta M. The efficacy of iso- and hyperosmotic fluids as volume expanders in fixed-volume and uncontrolled hemorrhage. Ann Emerg Med 1990;19(4):350–58.
24. Mazzoni MC, Borgstrom P, Intaglietta M, Arfors KE. Capillary narrowing in hemorrhagic shock is rectified by hyperosmotic saline-dextran reinfusion. Circ Shock 1990;31(4):407–18.
25. Rizoli S, Kapus A, Fan J, et al. Immunomodulatory effects of hypertonic resuscitation on the development of lung inflammation following hemorrhagic shock. J Immunol 1998;161(11):6288–96.
26. Steinbauer M, Harris AG, Messmer K. Effects of dextran on microvascular ischemia-reperfusion injury in striated muscle. Am J Physiol 1997;272(4 Pt 2):H1710–6.
27. Thiel M, Buessecker F, Eberhardt K, et al. Effects of hypertonic saline on expression of human polymorphonuclear leukocyte adhesion molecules. J Leukoc Biol 2001;70(2):261–73.
28. Ciesla DJ, Moore EE, Gonzalez RJ, et al. Hypertonic saline inhibits neutrophil (PMN) priming via attenuation of p38 MAPK signaling. Shock 2000;14(3):265–9; discussion 9–70.
29. Ciesla DJ, Moore EE, Zallen G, et al. Hypertonic saline attenuation of polymorphonuclear

neutrophil cytotoxicity: timing is everything. J Trauma 2000;48(3):388–95.
30. Choi SH, Lee SW, Hong YS, et al. Selective inhibition of polymorphonuclear neutrophils by resuscitative concentration of hypertonic saline. Emerg Med J 2006;23(2):119–22.
31. Fahrner SL, Shackford SR, Bourguignon P, et al. Effect of medium tonicity and dextran on neutrophil function in vitro. J Trauma 2002;52(2):285–92.
32. Rocha-e-Silva M, Poli de Figueiredo LF. Small volume hypertonic resuscitation of circulatory shock. Clinics 2005;60(2):159–72.
33. Wade CE, Kramer GC, Grady JJ, et al. Efficacy of hypertonic 7.5% saline and 6% dextran-70 in treating trauma: a meta-analysis of controlled clinical studies. Surgery 1997;122(3):609–16.
34. Coimbra R, Junger WG, Liu FC, et al. Hypertonic/hyperoncotic fluids reverse prostaglandin E2 (PGE2)-induced T-cell suppression. Shock 1995;4(1):45–9.
35. Oreopoulos GD, Bradwell S, Lu Z, et al. Synergistic induction of IL-10 by hypertonic saline solution and lipopolysaccharides in murine peritoneal macrophages. Surgery 2001;130(2):157–65.
36. Junger H, Edelman DB, Junger WG. Hypertonicity promotes survival of corticospinal motoneurons via mitogen-activated protein kinase p38 signaling. J Mol Neurosci 2003;21(2):111–20.
37. Ciesla DJ, Moore EE, Biffl WL, et al. Hypertonic saline attenuation of the neutrophil cytotoxic response is reversed upon restoration of normotonicity and reestablished by repeated hypertonic challenge. Surgery 2001;129(5):567–75.
38. Ciesla DJ, Moore EE, Musters RJ, et al. Hypertonic saline alteration of the PMN cytoskeleton: implications for signal transduction and the cytotoxic response. J Trauma 2001;50(2):206–12.
39. Homma H, Deitch EA, Feketeova E, et al. Small volume resuscitation with hypertonic saline is more effective in ameliorating trauma-hemorrhagic shock-induced lung injury, neutrophil activation and red blood cell dysfunction than pancreatitic protease inhibition. J Trauma 2005;59(2):266–72.
40. Ke QH, Zheng SS, Liang TB, et al. Pretreatment of hypertonic saline can increase endogenous interleukin 10 release to attenuate hepatic ischemia reperfusion injury. Dig Dis Sci 2006;51(12): 2257–63.
41. Powers KA, Zurawska J, Szaszi K, et al. Hypertonic resuscitation of hemorrhagic shock prevents alveolar macrophage activation by preventing systemic oxidative stress due to gut ischemia/reperfusion. Surgery 2005;137(1):66–74.
42. Rizoli SB, Kapus A, Fan J, Li YH, Marshall JC. Rotstein OD. Immunomodulatory effects of hypertonic resuscitation on the development of lung inflammation following hemorrhagic shock. J Immunol 1998; 161(11):6288–96.
43. Coimbra R, Hoyt DB, Junger WG, et al. Hypertonic saline resuscitation decreases susceptibility to sepsis after hemorrhagic shock. J Trauma 1997;42(4):602–6; discussion 6–7.
44. Shields CJ, O'Sullivan AW, Wang JH, et al. Hypertonic saline enhances host response to bacterial challenge by augmenting receptor-independent neutrophil intracellular superoxide formation. Ann Surg 2003;238(2):249–57.
45. Vachharajani V, Vital S, Russell J, Granger DN. Hypertonic saline and the cerebral microcirculation in obese septic mice. Microcirculation 2007;14(3):223–31.
46. Shields CJ, Winter DC, Sookhai S, et al. Hypertonic saline attenuates end-organ damage in an experimental model of acute pancreatitis. Br J Surg 2000;87(10):1336–40.
47. Zallen G, Moore EE, Tamura DY, et al. Hypertonic saline resuscitation abrogates neutrophil priming by mesenteric lymph. J Trauma 2000;48(1):45–8.
48. Pascual JL, Ferri LE, Seely AJ, et al. Hypertonic saline resuscitation of hemorrhagic shock diminishes neutrophil rolling and adherence to endothelium and reduces in vivo vascular leakage. Ann Surg 2002;236(5):634–42.
49. Pascual JL, Khwaja KA, Ferri LE, et al. Hypertonic saline resuscitation attenuates neutrophil lung sequestration and transmigration by diminishing leukocyte-endothelial interactions in a two-hit model of hemorrhagic shock and infection. J Trauma 2003;54(1):121–30; discussion 30–32.
50. Powers KA, Woo J, Khadaroo RG, et al. Hypertonic resuscitation of hemorrhagic shock upregulates the anti-inflammatory response by alveolar macrophages. Surgery 2003;134(2):312–18.
51. Lu YQ, Cai XJ, Gu LH, et al. Hypertonic saline resuscitation maintains a more balanced profile of T-lymphocyte subpopulations in a rat model of hemorrhagic shock. J Zhejiang Univ Sci B 2007;8(1):70–75.
52. Bickell WH, Bruttig SP, Millnamow GA, et al. The detrimental effects of intravenous crystalloid after aortotomy in swine. Surgery 1991;110(3):529–36.
53. Bickell WH, Bruttig SP, Millnamow GA, et al. Use of hypertonic saline/dextran versus lactated

Ringer's solution as a resuscitation fluid after uncontrolled aortic hemorrhage in anesthetized swine. Ann Emerg Med 1992;21(9):1077–85.
54. Bickell WH, Bruttig SP, Wade CE. Hemodynamic response to abdominal aortotomy in the anesthetized swine. Circ Shock 1989;28(4):321–32.
55. Bickell WH, Shaftan GW, Mattox KL. Intravenous fluid administration and uncontrolled hemorrhage. J Trauma 1989;29(3):409.
56. Bruttig SP, O'Benar JD, Wade CE, Dubick MA. Benefit of slow infusion of hypertonic saline/dextran in swine with uncontrolled aortotomy hemorrhage. Shock 2005;24(1):92–6.
57. Bunn F, Roberts I, Tasker R, Akpa E. Hypertonic versus isotonic crystalloid for fluid resuscitation in critically ill patients. Cochrane Database Syst Rev 2000 (4):CD002045.
58. Bunn F, Roberts I, Tasker R, Akpa E. Hypertonic versus isotonic crystalloid for fluid resuscitation in critically ill patients. Cochrane Database Syst Rev 2002 (1):CD002045.
59. Bunn F, Roberts I, Tasker R, Akpa E. Hypertonic versus near isotonic crystalloid for fluid resuscitation in critically ill patients. Cochrane Database Syst Rev 2004 (3):CD002045.
60. Dubick MA, Bruttig SP, Wade CE. Issues of concern regarding the use of hypertonic/hyperoncotic fluid resuscitation of hemorrhagic hypotension. Shock 2006;25(4):321–8.
61. Poli-de-Figueiredo LF, Cruz RJ, Jr, Sannomiya P, Rocha ESM. Mechanisms of action of hypertonic saline resuscitation in severe sepsis and septic shock. Endocr Metab Immune Disord Drug Targets 2006;6(2):201–6.
62. Roberts I, Alderson P, Bunn F, et al. Colloids versus crystalloids for fluid resuscitation in critically ill patients. Cochrane Database Syst Rev 2004 (4):CD000567.
63. Thompson R, Greaves I. Hypertonic saline–hydroxyethyl starch in trauma resuscitation. J R Army Med Corps 2006;152(1):6–12.
64. Silverman T, Aebersold P, Landow L, Lindsey K. Regulatory perspectives on clinic al trials for trauma, transfusion, and hemostasis. Transfusion 2005;45(1 Suppl.):14S–21S.
65. Wade CE, Holcomb JB. Endpoints in clinical trials of fluid resuscitation of patients with traumatic injuries. Transfusion 2005;45(1 Suppl.):4S–8S.
66. Alpar EK, Killampalli VV. Effects of hypertonic dextran in hypovolaemic shock: a prospective clinical trial. Injury 2004;35(5):500–506.
67. Bulger EM, Cuschieri J, Warner K, Maier RV. Hypertonic resuscitation modulates the inflammatory response in patients with traumatic hemorrhagic shock. Ann Surg 2007;245(4):635–41.
68. Maningas PA, Mattox KL, Pepe PE, et al. Hypertonic saline-dextran solutions for the prehospital management of traumatic hypotension. Am J Surg 1989;157(5):528–33; discussion 33–4.
69. Mattox KL, Maningas PA, Moore EE, et al. Prehospital hypertonic saline/dextran infusion for post-traumatic hypotension. The U.S.A. multicenter trial. Ann Surg 1991;213(5):482–91.
70. Rizoli SB, Rhind SG, Shek PN, et al. The immunomodulatory effects of hypertonic saline resuscitation in patients sustaining traumatic hemorrhagic shock: a randomized, controlled, double-blinded trial. Ann Surg 2006;243(1):47–57.
71. Vassar MJ, Fischer RP, O'Brien PE, et al. A multicenter trial for resuscitation of injured patients with 7.5% sodium chloride. The effect of added dextran 70. The multicenter group for the study of hypertonic saline in trauma patients. Arch Surg 1993;128(9):1003–11; discussion 11–3.
72. Vassar MJ, Perry CA, Gannaway WL, Holcroft JW. 7.5% sodium chloride/dextran for resuscitation of trauma patients undergoing helicopter transport. Arch Surg 1991;126(9):1065–72.
73. Vassar MJ, Perry CA, Holcroft JW. Analysis of potential risks associated with 7.5% sodium chloride resuscitation of traumatic shock. Arch Surg 1990;125(10):1309–15.
74. Vassar MJ, Perry CA, Holcroft JW. Prehospital resuscitation of hypotensive trauma patients with 7.5% NaCl versus 7.5% NaCl with added dextran: a controlled trial. J Trauma 1993;34(5):622–32; discussion 32–3.
75. Younes RN, Aun F, Accioly CQ, et al. Hypertonic solutions in the treatment of hypovolemic shock: a prospective, randomized study in patients admitted to the emergency room. Surgery 1992;111(4):380–85.
76. Younes RN, Birolini D. Hypertonic/hyperoncotic solution in hypovolemic patients: experience in the emergency room. Rev Hosp Clin Fac Med Sao Paulo 2002;57(3):124–8.
77. Alderson P, Schierhout G, Roberts I, Bunn F. Colloids versus crystalloids for fluid resuscitation in critically ill patients. Cochrane Database Syst Rev 2000 (2):CD000567.
78. Schierhout G, Roberts I. Fluid resuscitation with colloid or crystalloid solutions in critically ill

patients: a systematic review of randomised trials. BMJ 1998;316(7136):961–4.
79. Wade C, Grady J, Kramer G. Efficacy of hypertonic saline dextran (HSD) in patients with traumatic hypotension: meta-analysis of individual patient data. Acta Anaesthesiol Scand Suppl 1997;110: 77–9.
80. Wade CE, Grady JJ, Kramer GC, et al. Individual patient cohort analysis of the efficacy of hypertonic saline/dextran in patients with traumatic brain injury and hypotension. J Trauma 1997;42(5 Suppl.):S61–5.
81. Caldwell FT, Jr. Hypertonic vs. hypotonic resuscitation. J Trauma 1979;19(11 Suppl.):874.
82. Elgjo GI, Mathew BP, Poli de Figueriedo LF, et al. Resuscitation with hypertonic saline dextran improves cardiac function in vivo and ex vivo after burn injury in sheep. Shock 1998;9(5):375–83.
83. Elgjo GI, Poli de Figueiredo LF, Schenarts PJ, et al. Hypertonic saline dextran produces early (8–12 hrs) fluid sparing in burn resuscitation: a 24-hr prospective, double-blind study in sheep. Crit Care Med 2000;28(1):163–71.
84. Elgjo GI, Traber DL, Hawkins HK, Kramer GC. Burn resuscitation with two doses of 4 mL/kg hypertonic saline dextran provides sustained fluid sparing: a 48-hour prospective study in conscious sheep. J Trauma 2000;49(2):251–63; discussion 63–5.
85. Guha SC, Kinsky MP, Button B, et al. Burn resuscitation: crystalloid versus colloid versus hypertonic saline hyperoncotic colloid in sheep. Crit Care Med 1996;24(11):1849–57.
86. Monafo WW, Chuntrasakul C, Ayvazian VH. Hypertonic sodium solutions in the treatment of burn shock. Am J Surg 1973;126(6):778–83.
87. Oda J, Ueyama M, Yamashita K, et al. Hypertonic lactated saline resuscitation reduces the risk of abdominal compartment syndrome in severely burned patients. J Trauma 2006;60(1):64–71.
88. Huang PP, Stucky FS, Dimick AR, et al. Hypertonic sodium resuscitation is associated with renal failure and death. Ann Surg 1995;221(5):543–54; discussion 54–7.
89. Pruitt BA, Jr. Does hypertonic burn resuscitation make a difference? Crit Care Med 2000;28(1):277–8.
90. Tyagi R, Donaldson K, Loftus CM, Jallo J. Hypertonic saline: a clinical review. Neurosurg Rev 2007.
91. Cooper DJ, Myles PS, McDermott FT, et al. Prehospital hypertonic saline resuscitation of patients with hypotension and severe traumatic brain injury: a randomized controlled trial. JAMA 2004;291(11):1350–7.
92. Kolsen-Petersen JA. Immune effect of hypertonic saline: fact or fiction? Acta Anaesthesiol Scand 2004;48(6):667–78.
93. Rotstein OD. Novel strategies for immunomodulation after trauma: revisiting hypertonic saline as a resuscitation strategy for hemorrhagic shock. J Trauma 2000;49(4):580–83.
94. Younes RN, Aun F, Ching CT, et al. Prognostic factors to predict outcome following the administration of hypertonic/hyperoncotic solution in hypovolemic patients. Shock 1997;7(2):79–83.
95. Eastridge BJ, Owsley J, Sebesta J, et al. Admission physiology criteria after injury on the battlefield predict medical resource utilization and patient mortality. J Trauma 2006;61(4):820–23.
96. Eastridge BJ, Salinas J, McManus JG, et al. Hypotension begins at 110 mm Hg: redefining "hypotension" with data. J Trauma 2007;63(2):291–7; discussion 7–9.
97. Angle N, Cabello-Passini R, Hoyt DB, et al. Hypertonic saline infusion: can it regulate human neutrophil function? Shock 2000;14(5):503–8.
98. Kolsen-Petersen JA, Nielsen JO, Bendtzen K, Tonnesen E. Infusion of hypertonic saline (7.5% NaCl) causes minor immunological changes in normovolaemic women. Acta Anaesthesiol Scand 2004;48(2):224–33.
99. Dubick MA, Wade CE. A review of the efficacy and safety of 7.5% NaCl/6% dextran 70 in experimental animals and in humans. J Trauma 1994;36(3):323–30.
100. Sondeen JL, Coppes VG, Holcomb JB. Blood pressure at which rebleeding occurs after resuscitation in swine with aortic injury. J Trauma 2003;54(5 Suppl.):S110–7.
101. Coats TJ, Heron M. The effect of hypertonic saline dextran on whole blood coagulation. Resuscitation 2004;60(1):101–4.
102. Tan TS, Tan KH, Ng HP, Loh MW. The effects of hypertonic saline solution (7.5%) on coagulation and fibrinolysis: an in vitro assessment using thromboelastography. Anaesthesia 2002;57(7):644–8.
103. Rocha ESR, Caneo LF, Lourenco Filho DD, et al. First use of hypertonic saline dextran in children: a study in safety and effectiveness for atrial septal defect surgery. Shock 2003;20(5):427–30.
104. Schroth M, Plank C, Meissner U, et al. Hypertonic-hyperoncotic solutions improve cardiac function in children after open-heart surgery. Pediatrics 2006;118(1):e76–84.

105. Bender R, Breil M, Heister U, et al. Hypertonic saline during CPR: feasibility and safety of a new protocol of fluid management during resuscitation. Resuscitation 2007;72(1):74–81.
106. O'Benar JD, Bruttig SP, Wade CE, Dubick MA. Hemodynamic and metabolic responses to repeated hemorrhage and resuscitation with hypertonic saline dextran in conscious swine. Shock 1998;10(3):223–8.
107. Wade CE, Dubick MA, Grady JJ. Optimal dose of hypertonic saline/dextran in hemorrhaged swine. J Trauma 2003;55(3):413–16.
108. Prien T. Response to the comments on the contributions "Hypertonic solutions in heart surgery" and "Hypertonic hyperoncotic volume replacement (7.5% NaCl/10% hydroxyethyl starch 200,000/0.5) in patients with coronary artery stenoses" by H. Bohrer and E. Martin. Zentralbl Chir 1993;118(6):374.
109. Prien T, Thulig B, Wusten R, et al. Hypertonic-hyperoncotic volume replacement (7.5% NaCl/10% hydroxyethyl starch 200.000/0.5) in patients with coronary artery stenoses. Zentralbl Chir 1993;118(5):257–63; discussion 64–6.
110. Aprahamian C, Thompson BM, Towne JB, Darin JC. The effect of a paramedic system on mortality of major open intra-abdominal vascular trauma. J Trauma 1983;23(8):687–90.
111. Smith JP, Bodai BI, Hill AS, Frey CF. Prehospital stabilization of critically injured patients: a failed concept. J Trauma 1985;25(1):65–70.

CHAPTER 16
Hyperchloremic Acidosis

Edward Burdett[1] *& Andre Vercueil*[2]
[1] National Hospital of Neurology and Neurosurgery, London, UK
[2] King's College Hospital, London, UK

Introduction

It was in 1934 that Alexis Hartmann first demonstrated that electrolyte imbalances caused by intravenous fluid administration could affect human health and alter clinical outcome; explanations for the resultant acidosis were based on the "dilution" of bicarbonate ions by the infused solution, and the phenomenon of hyperchloremic acidosis was not described until 1953. There has since been increasing interest in a physicochemical approach to acid–base homeostasis in the critical care, anesthesiology and physiology literature, as it provides a model that allows a new insight into diagnosis of acid–base disturbances, and different treatment options based on manipulation of plasma electrolyte levels.

This chapter will demonstrate how high plasma levels of chloride can cause acidosis on the basis of Stewart's physicochemical theory of acid–base balance. We will go on to describe the effects that hyperchloremic acidosis may have on homeostasis and detail the most relevant in vitro data and experiments in both animal and humans demonstrating its etiology, incidence in the clinical population, and effects on different organ systems.

How does hyperchloremia cause acidosis?

Hydrogen ion concentration in aqueous solutions within the human body is tightly controlled in health, and disturbances of acid–base balance are a common phenomenon in the critically ill. The high charge density of hydrogen ions (H^+) has effects on enzyme structure and configuration, and thus their regulation at low concentration is essential. Knowledge of how and why derangements of H^+ concentration occur may help both in the diagnosis and treatment of these acid–base disturbances.

The 1990s saw the development of the Henderson–Hasselbalch equation on the basis of equilibrium theory of carbamate species in human blood. A descriptive approach, it centers on the pH effects of the partial pressure of carbon dioxide ($PaCO_2$) and the concentration of bicarbonate ions in plasma, which are then used to describe different kinds of acid–base disturbances. Siggaard-Andersen later developed the semiquantitative base-excess model after examining titrations of human blood and described a nomogram to determine base excess in the clinical setting [1]. This approach remains the most widely used in clinical practice, as it is relatively easy to understand and apply in common clinical scenarios, although it breaks down at physiological extremes. The theory has been criticized for the primacy of the role of bicarbonate as an independently adjusted variable, and it has been said that base excess quantifies rather than explains acid–base disturbances. The fact that it is an in vitro measurement may mean that it has little relevance in a physiological system.

In 1981 Stewart proposed a quantitative approach to acid–base physiology based on fundamental principles of physical chemistry, with elements of the approaches of Van Slyke [2] and Singer and Hastings [3]. He recognized that *"the*

Alternatives to Blood Transfusion in Transfusion Medicine,
2nd edition. Edited by A. Maniatis, P. Van der Linden,
J.-F. Hardy.

quantitative results of several interacting but independent mechanisms cannot be explained or understood solely in terms of the action of any single one of these mechanisms" [4]. On the basis of the laws of mass action, the conservation of mass, and conservation of charge, he derived three independent variables that are the final determinants of pH and explained how all other variables, including bicarbonate, were dependant on these three independent variables. Two of these were new, namely the strong ion difference (SID), and the total weak acids (A_{tot}).

Knowledge of the quantitative physicochemical approach appears to offer advantages over bicarbonate-centered approaches in understanding the complex acid–base disturbances associated with critical illness and intravenous fluid therapy. In particular it allows the clinician to determine the causative ion and provides a rationale for hyperchloremic acidosis, as well as explaining the alkalosis associated with decreased plasma albumin concentrations.

Stewart's physicochemical approach

It is difficult to briefly describe the approach, and there is value in understanding the equations used to arrive at the final, relatively simple concepts.

Central concepts

- $[H^+]$ in any solution is only determined by the current values of SID, $PaCO_2$ and $[A_{tot}]$ in that solution. These are the three independent variables.
- Changes in dependant variables can only occur as a result of changes in independent variables—dependant variables cannot cause changes in each other.
- Transport of strong ions across cell membranes may influence $[H^+]$
- Reactions are taking place in aqueous solution—water is by far the most concentrated substance in the body (10^9 times that of H^+) and can dissociate, which is of great importance.
- Electrical neutrality must be maintained in aqueous solution—this is important in quantitative analysis as it provides a link between concentrations of nonreacting strong ions and equilibrating weak ones.
- The dissociation equilibria of all incompletely dissociated substances, as derived from the law of mass action, must be satisfied at all times
- Conservation of mass—the amount of each component substance in an aqueous solution remains constant unless it is added or removed from the outside, or it is created or destroyed by reactions within the solutions. This last applies when dissociation and recombination occur and is fundamental when discussing hydrogen ions.

Definitions

- Strong electrolytes—always completely dissociated in solution, so that none of the undissociated parent molecules remain. Na^+, K^+, Ca^{2+}, Mg^{2+}, and Cl^- exist in body fluids as completely ionized entities, and hence are referred to as strong ions. At physiological pH, lactate, sulphate, and β-hydroxybutarate will also act as strong ions, because of their large dissociation constants.

  Strong ion difference (SID)—excess of strong cations in body fluids, SID = [strong cations] − [strong anions].
  - Strong ions are not involved in any chemical reactions in the solution. All that matters is the net positive charge due to the presence of strong ions.
- Arterial PCO_2 ($PaCO_2$)—the body is an open system for CO_2, eliminating the 360 L (14 moles) of CO_2 produced via the lungs per day. Henry's law states that the concentration of dissolved CO_2 is directly proportional to the partial pressure—in venous and interstitial fluid the concentration of dissolved CO_2, expressed as [CO_2 dissolved], is one of the three independent variables.
- Weak electrolytes—substances that only partially dissociate when dissolved in water, and both molecules of parent substance as well as products of dissociation all exist together in solution.
  - $HA \rightarrow H^+ + A^-$, and $[H^+] \times [A^-] = K_a \times [HA]$, where K_a is the dissociation constant
  - Equilibrium requires that rate of dissociation = rate of recombination
- Total concentration of weak acid $[A_{tot}]$—the total concentration of nonvolatile weak acid in any compartment

- $[A_{tot}] = [HA] + [A^-]$, and does not vary with changes in pH. It is an independent variable.
- Nonvolatile weak acids (A^-) in plasma consist mainly of albumin, with a smaller contribution from inorganic phosphate. Interstitial fluid has much lower concentrations of both in health, but capillary leak can alter this. Red blood cells contain hemoglobin as the dominant weak acid.

Stewart analyzed the various components which constitute human fluids in each compartment applying the definitions and central concepts listed. He developed the theme by initially examining water, then strong ion solutions in water, weak acid solutions in water, and finally solutions containing carbon dioxide. This allowed him to develop a set of six simultaneous equations primarily describing the behavior of weak ions, which could be applied to isolated blood plasma and isolated intracellular fluid.

Equations and derivations

Pure water

This is the simplest acid–base system, which can be thought of as the behavior of hydrogen ions in aqueous solution. Water has important properties for Stewart's hypothesis:

- It has a large dielectric constant, and so will dissociate to yield ion-containing solutions.
- $[H^+] \times [OH^-] = K_w[H_2O]$

where K_w is the dissociation constant for water and is dependant on temperature. Because of extremely high $[H_2O]$, relative to the ionized component, it can be thought of as constant and thus

- Water dissociation equilibrium:

$$[H^+] \times [OH^-] = K'_w \qquad (16.1)$$

Strong ions in water

Remember that

SID = [strong cations] − [strong anions]

Consider solutions of ions fully dissociated in water, and thus not participating in any reactions. A simplified solution would contain Na^+, Cl^-, and ions in water. Now some of the central concepts must apply:

- Electroneutrality

$$[Na^+] - [Cl^-] + [H^+] - [OH^-] = 0 \qquad (16.2)$$

Substituting $K'_w/[H^+]$ for $[OH^-]$ from Equation (16.1) yields

$$[Na^+] - [Cl^-] + [H^+] - (K'_w/[H^+]) = 0$$

One can then clear this to yield the quadratic equation

$$[H^+]^2 = ([Na^+] - [Cl^-]) \times [H^+] - K'_w = 0$$

This can then be solved for $[H^+]$

$$[H^+] = \sqrt{K'_w + \frac{([Na^+] - [Cl^-])^2}{4}} - \frac{([Na^+] - [Cl^-])}{2}$$

$$\text{or } [H^+] = \sqrt{K'_w + \frac{[SID]^2}{4}} - \frac{[SID]}{2}$$

From the definitions it can be seen that $[H^+]$ is a function of the SID and that the SID is therefore an independent variable imposed on the system externally.

In body fluids SID is approximately equal to 40 mEq/L.

In extracellular fluid SID $\approx$ ($[Na^+]$ − $[Cl^-]$), while intracellular fluid SID $\approx$ ($[K^+] + [Mg^{2+}]$)

The important conceptual point is that a measured difference in $[H^+]$ only tells us that strong ions have been added or removed from the solution.

Note here that we can begin to see the physiological cause for hyperchloremic acidosis: as the level of chloride is raised relative to the level of sodium, the SID will reduce, affecting the $[H^+]$ equilibrium.

Weak electrolytes in aqueous solution

Weak electrolytes introduce additional equilibria involving OH^- or H^+. In human physiology these are weak acids (HA), and must satisfy the two requirements of dissociation equilibrium and conservation of mass for "A"

- Weak acid dissociation equilibrium:

$$[H^+] \times [A^-] = K_a \times [HA] \qquad (16.3)$$

where K_a is the dissociation constant for HA

- Conservation of mass for "A"

$$[A_{tot}] = [HA] + [A^-] \qquad (16.4)$$

The system must still satisfy the previously described principles

- Water dissociation: $[H^+] \times [OH^-] = K'_w$
- Electroneutrality: $[SID] + [H^+] - [OH^-] - [A^-] = 0$

There are thus four equations with four unknowns which must be simultaneously solved. By a process of systematic substitution, $[H^+]$ can be calculated from the cubic polynomial equation obtained. The important observations are that

- $[H^+]$ is determined by $[A_{tot}]$, K_a, K'_w, and [SID] because they must all be solved simultaneously
- [SID] and $[A_{tot}]$ are therefore independent variables
- [SID] changes occur frequently in body fluids, while weak electrolyte concentrations change little
- [SID] of interstitial fluid is altered locally by ion pumps and the production of lactate
- weak electrolytes are mainly plasma proteins, in particular albumin

Strong ions and CO_2

$[CO_2 \text{ (dissolved)}] = S_c \times pCO_2$ from Henry's law, where S_c is the gas solubility coefficient.

Dissolved CO_2 can be removed from solution by two further reactions

- combination with water to form carbonic acid H_2CO_3, which then dissociates to form H^+ and bicarbonate ions $HCO_3{}^-$
- combination with OH^- ions to form $HCO_3{}^-$

Carbonic acid is in equilibrium with CO_2 (dissolved), therefore

$$[CO_2\text{(dissolved)}] \times [H_2O] = k \times [H_2CO_3]$$

Substituting $S_c \times pCO_2$ for CO_2 (dissolved) and combining all constants,

$[H_2CO_3] = K_h \times pCO_2$ because $[H_2O]$ is so large as to be virtually constant

Substituting H^+ and bicarbonate ions $HCO_3{}^-$ for $[H_2CO_3]$ yields the bicarbonate ion formation equilibrium

$$[H^+] \times [HCO_3^-] = K_c \times pCO_2 \qquad (16.5)$$

which is catalyzed by carbonic anhydrase.

The final equilibrium is the carbonate ion formation equilibrium

$$[H^+] \times [CO_3^{2-}] = K_3 \times [HCO_3^-] \qquad (16.6)$$

Application of the formulae to human plasma and intracellular fluid

Human plasma is effectively an aqueous solution containing strong ions, weak acids and CO_2 (dissolved), and by combining the six formulae derived above it is possible to calculate $[H^+]$ by solving then simultaneously.

1 Water dissociation equilibrium:
$$[H^+] \times [OH^-] = K'_w$$
2 Electroneutrality equation:
$$[SID] + [H^+] - [HCO_3^-] - [A^-] - [CO_3^{2-}] - [OH^-] = 0$$
3 Weak acid dissociation equilibrium:
$$[H^+] \times [A^-] = K_a \times [HA]$$
4 Conservation of mass for "A":
$$[A_{tot}] = [HA] + [A^-]$$
5 Bicarbonate ion formation equilibrium:
$$[H^+] \times [HCO_3^-] = K_c \times pCO_2$$
6 Carbonate ion formation:
$$[H^+] \times [CO_3^{2-}] = K_3 \times [HCO_3^-]$$

This yields a fourth-order polynomial equation:
$$a[H^+]^4 + b[H^+]^3 + c[H^+]^2 + d[H^+] + e = 0$$
where
$a = 1$,
$b = [SID] + K_a$,
$c = \{K_a \times ([SID] - [A_{tot}]) - K'_w - K_c \times pCO_2\}$,
$d = -\{K_a \times (K'_w + K_c \times pCO_2) - K_3 \times K_c \times pCO_2\}$,
$e = -K_a \times K_3 \times K_c \times pCO_2$

It can therefore be seen that the only *independent* variables which determine $[H^+]$ and thus pH are SID, $[A_{tot}]$, and pCO_2, and any change in pH must be due to a change of one of them. This has obvious relevance to the practice of transfusion medicine, given that all available intravenous fluids are solutions of strong ions either as the sole constituent or as the carrier solution.

We can conclude three things from the above. Firstly, the interpretation of acid–base changes using Stewart's physicochemical approach is not intuitive, and requires a detailed knowledge of physiology, chemistry, and mathematics. Secondly that acid–base derangements should not be thought of as due to either metabolic or respiratory causes but can be thought of in a unified way. Thirdly, that the ratio of anions to cations in plasma is fundamental to describing the etiology of hyperchloremic acidosis. We will now go on to describe the evidence available which supports this model and which describe its consequences.

There is a wealth of experimental data describing the most common etiology of hyperchloremic acidosis, namely large sodium chloride loads. This

Table 16.1 Comparison of electrolyte composition of different IV fluids and normal human plasma.

Contents (mmol/L)	Plasma (normal values may vary)	Normal saline	Hartmanns	Plasmalyte 148	Hextend	Gelofusine
Sodium	135–145	154	131	154	140	143
Potassium	4.5–5.0	0	5	<1 5	3	
Chloride	99–105	154	108	125	98	124
Calcium	2.0–2.5	0	2.5	<1	0	2.5
Magnesium	0.7–1.4	0	1	<1	1.5	0.5
Osmolality	290–300	286	254	274	288	307
Osmolarity	291	308	276	310	298.5	305
Lactate	1–2	0	24	0	0	28
Bicarbonate	23–278	0	0	0	50 (acetate/ gluconate)	0
Na:Cl ratio	1.38	1.0	1.21	1.27	1.42	1.15

Manufacturers: normal saline, nonproprietary; Hartmann's solution, nonproprietary; Gelofusine, B. Braun Medical Inc, Germany; Plasmalyte B, Baxter International, Deerfield, IL, USA; Hextend, BioTime Inc, Berkeley, CA, USA.

will be discussed first, before we examine the data identifying the consequences of this syndrome. We will examine the most compelling evidence from in vitro studies, and then go on to discuss the evidence in animal, volunteer, and patient populations.

Etiology of hyperchloremic acidosis

As described above, a reduction in plasma pH may be caused by a reduction in the SID, which in turn is most likely to be due to an upset in the balance of cations and anions. An alteration in the ratio of sodium to chloride in plasma by infusing a solution with a nonphysiological concentration of chloride ions will affect the SID. Should the plasma chloride level rise disproportionately to the plasma sodium level, the SID will be reduced, resulting in acidosis.

There are several factors which may cause hyperchloremic acidosis. It was initially described as a consequence of ammonium chloride poisoning, and some uncommon renal tubular acidosis disorders can now be thought of as chloride ion channelopathies [5], but the most common cause and the one that concerns us in transfusion medicine is iatrogenic sodium chloride overdose, usually due to intravenous infusion of a large volume of normal saline.

Several clinical trials conclude that normal saline infusion is causally related to hyperchloremic acidosis. In a randomized controlled trial in 1994, Macfarlane and Lee [6] described a reduced serum pH in a group of surgical patients given normal saline when compared to a balanced fluid solution containing less chloride. This is a recurring theme; investigating perioperative gynecological patients in 1999, Scheingraber [7] showed that normal saline infusion was independently associated with metabolic acidosis compared to the infusion of a balanced crystalloid solution. There have since been several other studies describing the same phenomenon (Table 16.1).

Of the commercially available IV fluids, very few have a composition close to that of human plasma, with most having an excess of chloride ions. Those that match plasma more closely, e.g., Hartmann's solution, Hextend, and Tetraspan are described as "balanced" salt solutions.

By contrast, 0.9% saline solutions, when viewed from a physicochemical perspective, have a SID of zero, as they have equal numbers of sodium and chloride ions. When they are infused into a physiological milieu in large volumes, they reduce the SID by equilibration with plasma, increasing the plasma Cl^- concentration relative to the plasma Na^+ concentration. As we have seen, this reduction in SID causes an increase in H^+ concentration. This type of hyperchloremic acidosis can be thought of as an infusion-related acidosis.

Consequences of hyperchloremic acidosis

In vitro studies

The ex vivo data supports the hypothesis that a high chloride load affects renal function and coagulation homeostasis. We will describe these in turn.

With regards to the kidney, data supporting an adverse effect of a high chloride load on renal physiology arose in the early 1980s when, without reference to Stewart's physicochemical theory, Wilcox [8] demonstrated that hyperchloremia caused renal vasoconstriction in a specific and dose-dependant manner, and that renal blood flow and glomerular filtration rate were inversely related to the chloride concentration in the Loop of Henle.

Wilcox went on to show that chloride could affect prostaglandin release in the kidney, which he hypothesized could mediate these vascular changes.

In vitro work on coagulation homeostasis has demonstrated a greater derangement on coagulation as measured by thromboelastography (TEG), and reduced platelet function measured by whole blood aggregometry in blood diluted with a colloid product suspended in a normal saline solution compared with blood diluted with the same colloid in a balanced salt solution [9]. This work has been replicated in similar studies [10].

Animal studies

An experimental rat model of salt-sensitive hypertension demonstrated that the blood-pressure increase caused by sodium chloride was not replicated by infusion with sodium bicarbonate, leading investigators to suggest that it was the chloride rather than the sodium which was responsible [11].

Animal models have also shown an association between iatrogenic hyperchloremia and gastrointestinal morbidity, namely, intestinal injury in rats [12] and impaired gastropyloric motility in pigs [13].

Any form of acid–base derangement will affect the function of inflammatory mediators, and there is considerable animal evidence showing pro-inflammatory cytokines being released in response to hyperchloremia, including the interleukins IL-6, IL-10, and tumor necrosis factor. Interestingly this effect was not reproduced with other forms of acidemia; indeed, lactic acidosis seemed to be anti-inflammatory.

Kellum and colleagues, who have published extensively in this area, recently showed in an experimental model of sepsis that dogs treated with lactated Ringer's solution and 5% hydroxyethyl starch diluted in a balanced electrolyte solution had less acidosis and improved survival compared with those treated with normal saline. In a further study, the same authors demonstrated a reduced mean arterial pressure and increased nitrate/nitrite level in septic rats when exposed to hyperchloremia. The effect was more closely correlated to chloride levels than to pH. Kellum has since written that although there is no evidence that correcting acidosis in the critically ill improves outcome, there is evidence that iatrogenic acidosis is harmful [14].

In a rat model of massive hemorrhage, resuscitation with red cells suspended in normal saline caused more acidosis than resuscitation with red cells suspended in lactated Ringer's solution, and resulted in worse survival [15]. These results were replicated in a similar pig model [16] comparing normal saline resuscitation with Ringer's lactate, although the survival difference in this pig model did not achieve statistical significance.

Volunteer studies

In a landmark study, Williams et al. [17] demonstrated an adverse outcome by administration of normal saline to healthy volunteers in her randomized crossover study. The volunteers were given 50 mL/kg of Hartmanns solution or Normal saline over 1 hour. The volunteers given Normal saline displayed a lower blood pH at the end of the hour, and a number of symptoms and signs not present in the group given Hartmanns solution; their time to first urination was longer, and they demonstrated a higher incidence of abdominal pain, nausea, and lassitude and decreased perceived ability at abstract thinking.

The administration of 50 mL/kg is a great deal of fluid to give healthy volunteers—more than 3.5 L over 1 hour for a 75-kg subject. These volumes of fluid are, however, comparable to the volumes given to an under-resuscitated patient undergoing major surgery, or to a critically ill patient in the intensive care unit (ICU).

A more recent trial of similar design [18] replicated these results, and showed a paradoxically greater natriuresis in the group of volunteers given a balanced salt solution when compared to normal saline, even though the saline contained more sodium, suggesting a direct inhibitory chloride effect on the renal tubule, consistent with the earlier in vitro work by Wilcox.

Clinical studies

Most of the clinical data that exists with regards to hyperchloremia is focused on the intraoperative surgical population, a group that often receives a large intravenous fluid load over a relatively short time. Again, the clinical data is most compelling when examining renal function and coagulation.

With regards to renal function, in a randomized controlled trial on 180 cardiac surgical patients, Bennett-Guerrero et al. [19] demonstrated an inferior outcome in several renal variables in the group given a normal saline based regime, namely reduced urine output, increased creatinine rise, need for renal replacement and decreased creatinine clearance when compared to the group given a balanced fluid regime.

A more recent randomized controlled trial in patients undergoing renal transplantation demonstrated an association between normal saline infusion and hyperkalemia and acidemia postoperatively, which was an unexpected finding: traditionally saline has been favored over balanced fluids for patients with renal failure due to the presence of potassium in the latter. The authors suggest that the hyperkalemia associated with normal saline infusion, which caused the trial to be prematurely terminated, may be caused by an extra cellular shift of potassium in response to increasing academia [20]. The acidemia, in turn, is likely to be caused by the reduction in the SID due to the hyperchloremia.

Further data on renal dysfunction is available from a nonsurgical patient group. Merten and Burgess [21] recently observed that renal dysfunction in patients caused by intravenous administration of iodinated contrast agents may be alleviated by intravenous prehydration, but that the type of hydration matters. In their randomized controlled trial of 119 patients undergoing a radiographic procedure involving the use of iodinated contrast, they noted a significantly reduced incidence of renal dysfunction in the patient group given intravenous sodium bicarbonate compared to the group given an equivalent volume of sodium chloride. It is instructive to note that equimolar concentrations of sodium were given to both groups, with the only difference being the presence of either bicarbonate ions or chloride ions as the anion.

In a randomized double-blind controlled trial on elderly surgical patients undergoing elective major noncardiac surgery, Wilkes et al. demonstrated reduced splanchnic perfusion using gastric tonometry in a saline-based fluid group when compared to a balanced fluid group [22]. The study was terminated prematurely due to an increased acidosis in the saline group, but despite this a trend was noted toward more postoperative nausea and vomiting (PONV) in the saline-based group. The authors concluded that the hyperchloremic acidosis from normal saline infusion impairs gastric perfusion. In another recent clinical trial, Moretti et al. demonstrated a significantly increased rate of PONV associated with hyperchloremia following infusion of normal saline-based fluids [23].

In a randomized controlled trial comparing normal saline infusion to lactated Ringer's solution in patients undergoing elective open abdominal aortic aneurysm (AAA) repair, Waters et al. reported an increased requirement for blood products and a trend toward increased blood loss in the normal saline group [24]. Similarly, in a clinical trial involving patients undergoing elective surgery with expected moderate to severe blood loss (>500 mL), Gan et al. demonstrated a nonsignificant increase in hemorrhage and a significantly greater amount of red cells transfused in their normal saline based group when compared to the group given balanced fluids. There were more coagulation related adverse events in the saline-based group in this study [25].

Coagulopathy was again demonstrated, this time as manifested by abnormal TEG, in another clinical trial comparing in perioperative patients the infusion of a hydroxyethyl starch suspended in a normal saline vehicle with a similar starch suspended in a balanced electrolyte vehicle [26].

Although the trial data we have discussed reveals a difference in some aspects of patient morbidity, no clinical trial to date has effectively demonstrated a significant difference in patient mortality or other markers of serious morbidity. For example, in their randomized controlled trial of perioperative elective AAA patients, Waters et al. did not demonstrate a difference in mortality, length of ICU stay, or time on the ventilator between their balanced and normal saline groups, despite an increased acidosis in the normal saline group. Similar findings have been reported in other clinical trials demonstrating differences in surrogate end points: the question remains, however, whether the trials were underpowered for mortality and significant morbidity, or whether no such difference exists.

Hyperchloremia worsens base deficit, which may cause the clinician to give further fluid, wrongly considering the worsening acidosis to be a result of poor perfusion. The extra fluid paradoxically worsens the base deficit; this cycle of iatrogenic injury will lead to inappropriate fluid therapy and fluid overload. This has been demonstrated in several groups of patients receiving large quantities of normal saline with subsequent hyperchloremia, including children with diabetic ketoacidosis and adults undergoing major surgery. An understanding of the quantitative physicochemical approach may aid in diagnosing the cause of these complex acid–base problems, and thus prevent iatrogenic injury.

Conclusion

Hyperchloremia is a potent cause of acidosis. A variety of homeostatic imbalances are caused by hyperchloremia: some of these seem to be due to metabolic acidosis, and some may be due to the excess of chloride ion itself. Animal and human volunteer studies have demonstrated that normal saline infusion can have adverse effects including reduced survival when compared to balanced fluid infusion.

Patient outcome studies have shown significant differences in some morbidity outcomes, in particular renal, gastrointestinal, and coagulation, but have not demonstrated a difference in mortality. This may be due to absence of effect, poor study design, or lack of power from the existing clinical studies.

References

1. Siggaard-Anderson O. *The Acid-Base Status of the Blood*, 4th edn. Munksgaard, Copenhagen, 1974.
2. Peters J, Van Slyke D. *Quantitative Clinical Chemistry*. Williams and Wilkins, Baltimore, MD, 1931.
3. Singer RB, Hastings AB. An improved clinical method for the estimation of the disturbances of the acid-base balance of human blood. Medicine 1948;27:223–42.
4. Stewart PA. Modern quantitative acid-base chemistry. Can J Physiol Pharmacol 1983;61:1444–61.
5. Shayakul C, Alper SL. Defects in processing and trafficking of the AE 1 Cl^-/HCO_3^- exchanger associated with inherited distal renal tubular acidosis. Clin Exp Nephrol 2004;8:1–11.
6. McFarlane C, Lee A. A comparison of Plasmalyte 148 and 0.9% saline for intra-operative fluid replacement. Anaesthesia 1994;49:779–81.
7. Scheingraber S, Rehm M, Sehmisch C, Finsterer U. Rapid saline infusion produces hyperchloraemic acidosis in patients undergoing gynecologic surgery. Anesthesiology 1999;90:1265–70.
8. Wilcox CS. Regulation of renal blood flow by plasma chloride. J Clin Invest 1983;71:726–35.
9. Roche AM, James MFM, Grocott MPW, Mythen MG. Coagulation effects of in vitro serial haemodilution with a balanced electrolyte hetastarch solution compared with a saline-based hetastarch solution and lactated Ringer's solution. Anaesthesia 2002;57(10): 950–55.
10. Roche AM, James MFM, Bennett-Guerrero E, Mythen MG. A head-to-head comparison of the in vitro coagulation effects of saline-based and balanced

electrolyte crystalloid and colloid intravenous fluids. Anesth Analg 2006;102(4):1274–9.
11. Kotchen TA, Luke RG, Ott CE, Galla JH, Whitescarver S. Effect of chloride on renin and blood pressure responses to sodium chloride. Ann Intern Med 1983;98: 817–22.
12. Pedoto A, Nandi J, Oler A, et al. Role of nitric oxide in acidosis-induced intestinal injury in anesthetized rats. J Lab Clin Med 2001;138:270–76.
13. Tournadre JP, Allaouchiche B, Malbert CH, Chassard D. Metabolic acidosis and respiratory acidosis impair gastro-pyloric motility in anesthetized pigs. Anesth Analg 2000;90:74–9.
14. Kellum JA, Song M, Almasri E. Hyperchloremic acidosis increases circulating inflammatory molecules in experimental sepsis. Chest 2004;130(4):962–7.
15. Healey MA, Davis R, Liu FC, Loomis WH, Hoyt DB. Lactated ringer's is superior to normal saline in a model of massive haemorrhage and resuscitation. J Trauma 1998;45(5):894–9.
16. Traverso LW, Lee WP, Langford MJ. Fluid resuscitation after an otherwise fatal hemorrhage: I. Crystalloid solutions. J Trauma 1986;26(2):168–75.
17. Williams EL, Hildebrand KL, McCormick SA, Bedel MJ. The effect of intravenous lactated Ringer's solution versus 0.9% sodium chloride solution on serum osmolality in human volunteers. Anesth Analg 1999; 88:999–1003.
18. Reid F, Lobo DN, Williams RN, et al. (Ab)normal saline and physiological Hartmann's solution: a randomized double-blind crossover study. Clin Sci 2003; 104:17–24.
19. Bennett-Guerrero E, Frumento RJ, Mets B, Manspeizer HE, Hirsh AL. Impact of normal saline based versus balanced-salt intravenous fluid replacement on clinical outcomes: a randomized blinded clinical trial. Anesthesiology 2001;95:A147.
20. O'Malley CM, Frumento RJ, Hardy MA, et al. A randomized, double-blind comparison of lactated Ringer's solution and 0.9% NaCl during renal transplantation. Anesth Analg 2005;100(5):1518–24.
21. Merten GJ, Burgess WP. Prevention of contrast-induced nephropathy with sodium bicarbonate: a randomized controlled trial. JAMA 2004;291:2328–34.
22. Wilkes NJ, Woolf R, Mutch M, et al. The effects of balanced versus saline-based hetastarch and crystalloid solutions on acid-base and electrolyte status and gastric mucosal perfusion in elderly surgical patients. Anesth Analg 2001;93:811–16.
23. Moretti EW, Robertson KM, El-Moalem H, Gan TJ. Intraoperative colloid administration reduces postoperative nausea and vomiting and improves postoperative outcomes compared with crystalloid administration. Anesth Analg 2003;96(2):611–17.
24. Waters JH, Gottlieb A, Schoenwald P, Popovich MJ, Sprung J, Nelson DR. Normal saline versus lactated Ringer's solution for intraoperative fluid management in patients undergoing abdominal aortic aneurysm repair: an outcome study. Anesth Analg 2001; 93:817–22.
25. Gan TJ, Bennett-Guerrero E, Phillips Bute B, et al. Hextend, a physiologically balanced plasma expander for large volume use in major surgery: a randomized phase III clinical trial. Hextend Study Group. Anesth Analg 1999;88(5):992–8.
26. Boldt J, Wolf M, Mengistu A. A new plasma-adapted hydroxyethylstarch preparation: in vitro coagulation studies using thrombelastography and whole blood aggregometry. Anesth Analg 2007;104(2):425–30.

PART 4
Tolerance of Anemia

CHAPTER 17

Basic Principles of Oxygen Transport and Calculations

Jean-Louis Vincent, Pongdhep Theerawit & Davide Simion
Department of Intensive Care, Erasme Hospital, Université Libre de Bruxelles, Brussels, Belgium

Introduction

Oxygen is an essential requirement for normal cell activity involved in the provision of energy by oxidative reactions. If oxygen availability is limited, or there is an imbalance between oxygen delivery and demand such that cellular oxygen requirements are not met, cellular functions will be impaired leading to cellular and organ dysfunction. Maintaining adequate oxygen transport is therefore crucial to prevent cellular dysoxia. To achieve this, a clear understanding of the principles underlying oxygen transport in health and how this may be altered in disease is essential.

Back to basics

Oxygen delivery (DO_2) is the amount of oxygen provided to the tissues per minute. DO_2 is dependent on the cardiac output and the arterial oxygen content (CaO_2) so can be calculated as follows:

$$\begin{aligned} DO_2 &= CO \times CaO_2 \\ &= CO \times (\text{oxygen bound to hemoglobin}) \\ &\quad + (\text{oxygen dissolved in plasma}) \\ &= CO \times (Hb \times SaO_2 \times 1.39) + (PaO_2 \times 0.031) \end{aligned}$$

where Hb is the hemoglobin concentration (g/L), SaO_2 (%) the hemoglobin oxygen saturation, 1.39 the amount of oxygen bound to 1 g of fully saturated hemoglobin and PaO_2 the arterial oxygen tension. In normal conditions, dissolved oxygen contributes minimally to CaO_2 and can effectively be neglected. However, in severe anemia (especially when blood is unavailable), the contribution of the dissolved oxygen to tissue oxygen transport becomes relatively more important if the patient is receiving 100% oxygen. The normal DO_2 is 700–1000 mL/minute.

Oxygen consumption (VO_2) is the amount of oxygen taken up by the tissues per minute and is dependent on the cardiac output and the arterial-venous oxygen difference ($CaO_2 - CvO_2$), so can be calculated as follows:

$$\begin{aligned} VO_2 &= CO \times (CaO_2 - CvO_2) \\ &= CO \times Hb \times (SaO_2 - SvO_2) \times k. \end{aligned}$$

The normal VO_2 is about 200–300 mL/min.

The oxygen extraction ratio (O_2ER) is the amount of oxygen taken up by the tissues in relation to the amount of oxygen provided by them, and can be calculated as follows:

$$\begin{aligned} O_2ER &= \frac{VO_2}{DO_2} \\ &= \frac{CO \times (CaO_2 - CvO_2)}{CO \times CaO_2} \\ &= \frac{CaO_2 - CvO_2}{CaO_2} \end{aligned}$$

The normal O_2ER is 25–30%.

Alternatives to Blood Transfusion in Transfusion Medicine, 2nd edition. Edited by A. Maniatis, P. Van der Linden, J.-F. Hardy.

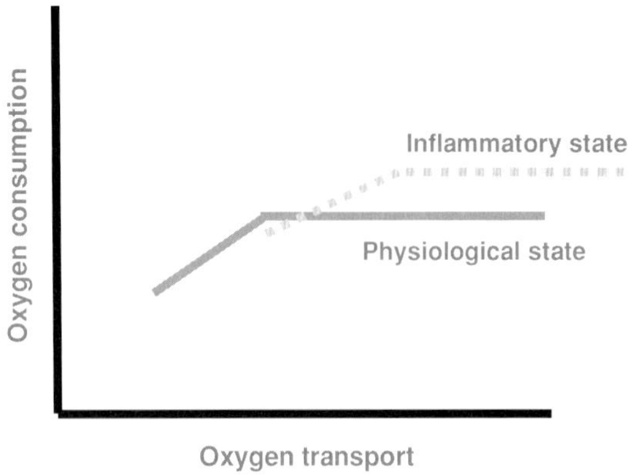

Figure 17.1 The VO_2/DO_2 relationship in physiological (solid line) conditions and in pathophysiological conditions (dotted line).

In physiological conditions, VO_2 is independent of DO_2 because oxygen extraction can adapt to counter changes in DO_2 such that when DO_2 decreases as a result, for example, of a decrease in cardiac output or hemoglobin concentration, O_2ER will increase and VO_2 will remain relatively stable (Figure 17.1). However, if DO_2 decreases below a so-called "critical" point at which O_2ER is unable to increase further, VO_2 will also start to be affected and VO_2 becomes DO_2 dependent. Due to the increased relative importance of the dissolved oxygen in plasma during extreme anemia, hyperoxic ventilation (100% O_2) can significantly decrease the Hbcrit at both systemic and regional levels [1]. In certain conditions, e.g., sepsis, when oxygen extraction capabilities are altered, the DO_2/VO_2 curve is shifted to the right and the critical level of DO_2, at which VO_2 becomes DO_2 dependent, is higher (Figure 17.1, dotted line) [2, 3].

Effects of transfusion on cellular oxygenation

Blood transfusions usually do not increase cellular VO_2. Indeed, VO_2 is generally independent of DO_2 in the absence of profound hemodynamic alterations. VO_2 increases following transfusions only in the presence of hemorrhagic shock [4, 5] and possibly severe respiratory failure [6, 7]. Even DO_2 does not always increase following a blood transfusion.

To understand the effects of blood transfusions on oxygenation, one must clearly separate anemia and hemorrhage (Figure 17.2). Hemorrhage is badly tolerated because of the associated hypovolemia, which decreases venous return and therefore cardiac output. Therefore, treatment of hemorrhage should focus primarily on the correction of hypovolemia. In these conditions, DO_2 increases substantially by the increase in cardiac output. One should also remember that in the initial phase of hemorrhage, the hemoglobin concentration is still normal or only slightly decreased, but will decrease following the plasma reexpansion induced by intravenous solutions or fluid shifts from extravascular compartments, by the phenomenon called "transcapillary refill." It is only when hypovolemia is corrected that cardiac output can increase sufficiently to compensate for the fall in hemoglobin. However, normovolemic anemia can be remarkably well tolerated. Several elements can account for this. First, cardiac output is increased by several mechanisms, including a decrease in blood viscosity and a sympathetic response that increases myocardial contractility and heart rate. Second, there is redistribution of cardiac output towards the vital organs (heart and brain). Third, there is an increase in oxygen extraction by the tissues, manifested by a decrease in mixed venous oxygen saturation (SvO_2).

Transfusions will obviously have opposite effects to anemia, increasing blood viscosity and reducing the adrenergic response. It is intriguing to consider that transfusions may result in a decrease in myocardial contractility. Hence, cardiac output often decreases following transfusions in the normovolemic patient, and the increase in DO_2 can be minor or even absent. For example, Shah et al. [4] observed in resuscitated trauma patients that blood transfusion of one unit of RBC increased hemoglobin from 9.2 ± 0.3 to 10.2 ± 0.3 g/dL, but decreased cardiac output, so that DO_2 did not change.

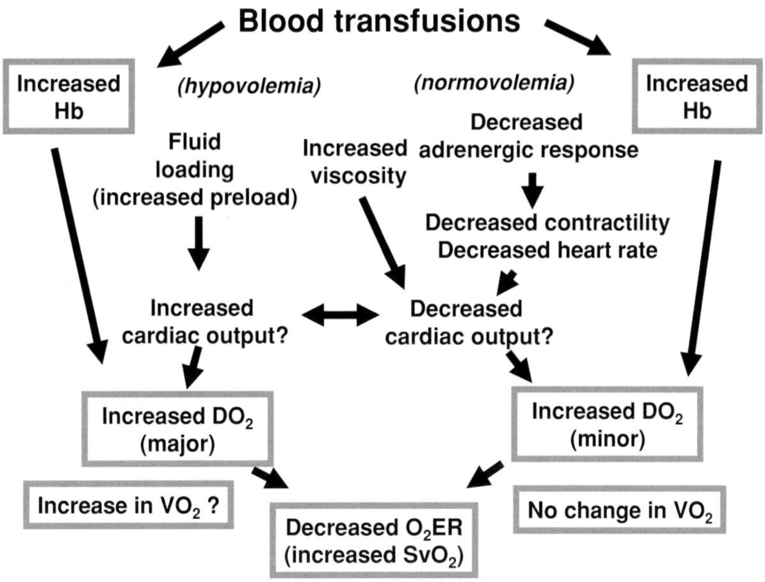

Figure 17.2 Effects of transfusions on DO_2, in relation to the initial volume status.

The effects of transfusions on oxygen extraction

If anemia is associated with a decrease in SvO_2, blood transfusions are also expected to increase SvO_2, i.e., to decrease oxygen extraction. From above, the O_2ER can be calculated from the CaO_2 and CvO_2, and hence also as:

$$O_2ER = \frac{(CaO_2 - CvO_2)}{CaO_2} = \frac{(Hb \times SaO_2 \times C) - (Hb \times SvO_2 \times C)}{Hb \times SvO_2 \times C} = \frac{(SaO_2 - SvO_2)}{SaO_2}$$

Hence, SvO_2 is virtually the reverse of O_2ER in the absence of hypoxemia, i.e., when SaO_2 is close to 1.

It is interesting to note that O_2ER itself is influenced, but not determined, by the hemoglobin concentration. The relationship between cardiac index and O_2ER can be useful to assess the effects of transfusions on DO_2 and VO_2 (Figure 17.3) [8].

The microcirculatory effects of blood transfusions

Even though hemoglobin levels increase in large vessels, capillary hematocrit (or "microhematocrit") may not increase comparably. The

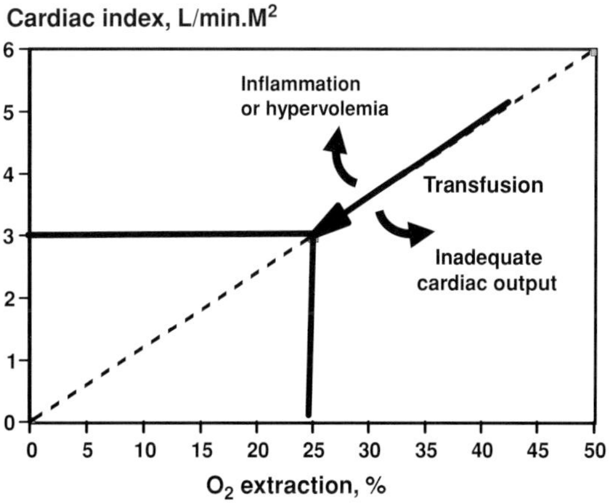

Figure 17.3 Effects of transfusions on the relationship between cardiac index and O_2ER.

microhematocrit is less than the systemic hematocrit because of the Fahraeus effect. Red blood cells, circulating in a vessel with a diameter less than 300 μm, have a mean hematocrit less than the hematocrit present in the supplying vessels. This phenomenon is explained by the concentration of red blood cells in the center of the blood vessel allowing them to move more rapidly. As a result, increasing the systemic hematocrit has very little effect on the capillary hematocrit for levels greater than 20–25%. Moreover, within the microcirculation, the hematocrit is very heterogeneous.

Transfused red blood cells, which have been altered by storage lesions, may not penetrate the microcirculation as well as native red blood cells. The importance of the age of the red blood cell remains controversial as current evidence does not support a clinically relevant relationship between the age of transfused red blood cells and morbidity or mortality [9].

The effects of red blood cells on the microcirculation have not been well defined. Using the orthogonal polarization spectral (OPS) imaging technique, we studied the sublingual microcirculation before and after transfusion in patients with sepsis who were moderately anemic [10]. Microvascular perfusion was not significantly altered by transfusion of 1–2 units of red blood cells, but there was considerable interindividual variation. Further analysis revealed that changes in perfusion were correlated with the initial perfusion, such that transfusion improved perfusion in those patients in whom perfusion was already altered at baseline but not in those with normal perfusion at baseline [10]. Nevertheless, global hemodynamic effects were similar in all patients. Hence, a simple interpretation is that the effect of red blood cell transfusion (altered by storage lesions) in septic patients (in whom red blood cells are altered by the inflammatory response) is dependent on the initial degree of microcirculatory alterations. Other techniques allowing the microcirculation to be visualized or assessed at the bedside, such as near-infrared spectroscopy, could be useful to determine the effects of transfusions.

Conclusion

Maintaining adequate tissue oxygen is a fundamental aspect of the management of all critically ill patients. The effects of blood transfusions on cellular oxygenation are quite complex. Global DO_2 is influenced by cardiac output, hemoglobin, and SaO_2. In this short review, we did not consider the influence of hypoxemia that would make our analysis even more complex. Anemia and blood transfusions both influence not only hemoglobin concentrations but also cardiac output in a quite complex fashion. Blood transfusions do not always increase DO_2 and are even less likely to increase VO_2. They usually decrease the ratio of VO_2 over DO_2, i.e., O_2ER. These global effects may not result in parallel effects on the microcirculation, which are also relevant for the cells and are influenced by many factors related to the host and to the characteristics of the transfused red blood cells. The effects of blood transfusions on oxygen transport are, therefore, difficult to predict.

References

1. Kemming GI, Meisner FG, Kleen M, Meier JM, Tillmanns J, Hutter JW, et al. Hyperoxic ventilation at the critical haematocrit. Resuscitation 2003;56:289–97.
2. Vincent JL, De Backer D. Oxygen transport—the oxygen delivery controversy. Intensive Care Med 2004; 30:1990–96.
3. Squara P. Matching total body oxygen consumption and delivery: a crucial objective? Intensive Care Med 2004;30:2170–79.
4. Shah DM, Gottlieb ME, Rahm RL, Stratton HH, Barie PS, Paloski WH, et al. Failure of red blood cell transfusion to increase oxygen transport or mixed venous PO2 in injured patients. J Trauma 1982;22:741–6.
5. Steffes CP, Bender JS, Levison MA. Blood transfusion and oxygen consumption in surgical sepsis. Crit Care Med 1991;19:512–17.
6. Ronco JJ, Phang PT, Walley KR, Wiggs B, Fenwick JC, Russell JA. Oxygen consumption is independent of changes in oxygen delivery in severe adult respiratory

distress syndrome. Am Rev Respir Dis 1991;143: 1267–73.

7. Piagnerelli M, Vincent JL. Evaluation du seuil transfusionnel érythrocytaire chez les patients de réanimation. Réanimation 2008;17:318–25.
8. Yalavatti GS, DeBacker D, Vincent JL. Assessment of cardiac index in anemic patients. Chest 2000;118: 782–7.
9. Lelubre C, Piagnerelli M, Vincent JL. Association between duration of storage of red blood cells and morbidity and mortality in adult patients: myth or reality? Transfusion 2009;49:1384–94.
10. Sakr Y, Chierego M, Piagnerelli M, Verdant C, Dubois MJ, Koch M, et al. Microvascular response to red blood cell transfusion in patients with severe sepsis. Crit Care Med 2007;35:1639–44.

CHAPTER 18
Assessment of Tissue Oxygenation

Michael Piagnerelli[1], Ann Dierick[2] & Philippe Van der Linden[2]
[1]Department of Intensive Care, Erasme Hospital, Université Libre, de Bruxelles, Brussels, Belgium
[2]Department of Anesthesiology, CHU Brugmann-HUDERF, Université Libre de Bruxelles, Brussels, Belgium

Introduction

Since the first major trial comparing restrictive (7 g/dL of hemoglobin concentration) versus liberal (10 g/dL of hemoglobin concentration) red blood cell (RBC) transfusion practice in euvolemic critically ill patients (the Transfusion Requirement In Critical Care or TRICC study) [1], physicians appear to have adopted lower RBC transfusion triggers [2]. However, transfusion of RBCs is a potentially life-saving therapy in case of major bleeding and remains an essential and frequently performed medical intervention. Recently, different studies reported, in contrast to the TRICC trial, that a higher transfusion trigger may have beneficial effects on outcome. These studies included especially patients with cardiac dysfunction [3, 4], brain injuries [5–7] or sepsis and alterations of the microcirculation [8]. The apparent controversy between these different studies highlights the fact that hemoglobin concentration alone is an insufficient indicator of an individual's need for RBC transfusion, as the adequacy of the hemoglobin concentration in any given situation depends on the tissue's oxygen requirements. This chapter will focus on the tools currently available to the clinician to assess tissue oxygenation during acute normovolemic anemia.

Alternatives to Blood Transfusion in Transfusion Medicine, 2nd edition. Edited by A. Maniatis, P. Van der Linden, J.-F. Hardy.

Physiology of oxygen transport

RBCs are the key element for oxygen (O_2) transport from the air to the mitochondria in the cells [9]. Interestingly, on top of being an O_2 transporter, RBCs are now also considered as an O_2 sensor capable to induce vasodilatation in hypoxic conditions [9–13]. Oxygen transport to the tissues includes two main biophysical principles: convection (bulk flow of blood) and diffusion (random movement of O_2 molecules) [14]. As blood flow passes through the lungs, O_2 diffuses down its partial pressure gradient from the alveoli into the bloodstream where it combines with hemoglobin in the RBCs and is carried by convective transport through the heart and further down to the large and small arteries into the microcirculatory vessels. At this level, the partial pressure gradient favors diffusion from the RBC to the tissue [14, 15]. The microcirculation, including arterioles, capillaries, venules, and lymphatic vessels with a diameter <100 μm is the essential site of O_2 exchange [16]. Within individual organs, the distribution of blood flow and thus RBC supply is, by nature, heterogeneous. Blood flow heterogeneity develops down the arteriolar tree into the microcirculation, where the distribution of flow is actively regulated by changes in vascular resistance and perfusion pressures which originate primarily from arterioles. Even changes in the resistance of the smallest terminal arterioles may be followed by a significant redistribution of RBC flow within the capillary network. Blood flow within the microcirculation is also influenced by different factors such as blood viscosity and its effects on endothelial wall shear stress [17] that may influence the vascular tone through generation of vasoactive substance like nitric oxide.

Oxygen-derived variables

O_2 delivery, O_2 consumption, and O_2 extraction

O_2 delivery (DO_2) represents the amount of O_2 delivered to the tissues per minute, and O_2 uptake (VO_2) represents the total of O_2 consumed in the body per minute. Global DO_2 is the product of the cardiac output and arterial O_2 content (CaO_2). CaO_2 is the product of the arterial O_2 saturation (SaO_2), hemoglobin concentration, and an invariable, reflecting the hemoglobin–O_2 binding capacity.

VO_2 can be directly measured from expired gas analysis taking into account the inspiratory and expiratory concentration of O_2, the CO_2 production, and the minute ventilation using the formula: $VO_2 = VCO_2/RQ$, where RQ is the respiratory quotient. Disadvantages of this technique are complexity of measurement of expiratory gases, need of a patient in stable conditions, and possible errors of measurement when high FiO_2 are required [18].

VO_2 can also be calculated by the Fick method using the formula:

$$VO_2 = CI \times ([Hb] \times 1.39 \times [SaO_2 - SvO_2] + 0.0031 \times [PaO_2 - PvO_2],$$

where CI represents the cardiac index, [Hb] the hemoglobin concentration, 1.39 the O_2 fixation capacity of 1 g of hemoglobin, SaO_2 the arterial O_2 saturation, SvO_2 the mixed venous O_2 saturation, PaO_2 the arterial partial pressure of O_2, and PvO_2 the mixed venous partial pressure of O_2.

In a healthy adult, VO_2 is approximately 250 mL/minute at rest. When DO_2 decreases, VO_2 is maintained by an increased in O_2 extraction (EO_2), since $EO_2 = VO_2/DO_2$ or ($SaO_2 - SvO_2/SaO_2$). EO_2 and SvO_2 are thus linked by a simple equation:

$EO_2 = 1 - SvO_2$. Assuming $SaO_2 = 1$, when SvO_2 is 70%, EO_2 is 30%.

When DO_2 decreases beyond a certain threshold, the increase in EO_2 becomes insufficient to maintain VO_2, which in turn begins to decrease (the "oxygen supply dependency"). This phenomenon indicates that tissue O_2 demand is no longer encountered. Below this point (critical DO_2), the decrease in VO_2 is associated with an increase in lactic acid production [18] and an inadequate supply of ATP relative to cellular requirements. In humans, the critical SvO_2 is approximately 40–50% corresponding to a critical EO_2 of approximately 50–60% [18, 19].

The relationship between VO_2 and DO_2 can be used to assess the adequacy of tissue oxygenation. However, the measurements of all of these parameters involves invasive catheterizations, complex calculations and can be criticized because of the possible mathematical coupling of the data (measurements of CI, hemoglobin concentration, and arterial O_2 concentration used in the calculation of both parameters may alter the physiological relation between them) [20], or cumbersome equipment if metabolic carts are used to measure VO_2.

The relationship between CI and EO_2 ($CI/EO_2 < 10$) may provide a useful means of monitoring tissue oxygenation, especially in anemic cardiac critically ill patients [21]. Indeed, CI/EO_2, which is around 12 (3/0.25) in healthy humans, is relatively stable in the event of isovolemic hemodilution [22, 23]. In patients with hypovolemia or with an altered cardiac function, CI/EO_2 decreases, whereas patients with sepsis may show an increased CI/EO_2 ratio [24].

Venous O_2 saturation

SvO_2 is easily measured at the bedside either intermittently, or continuously with fiber optic modified catheters, although it requires invasive monitoring. Measurement of central venous O_2 saturation ($ScvO_2$) via central venous catheter reflects principally the rate of O_2 extraction at the level of the brain and the upper part of the body [25]. Several factors may limit the interpretation of a SvO_2 or $ScvO_2$ value. Indeed, these parameters only provide information on global EO_2 of a given territory and the ability to extract O_2 varies considerably from one tissue to another [25]. For example, the O_2 saturation of the coronary venous blood is physiologically lower (37%) than that of renal venous blood (92%) [25]. In pathologic conditions such as septic shock, peripheral EO_2 is altered and SvO_2 remains high, being therefore of little help. Moreover, the value of SvO_2 depends on the position of the oxyhemoglobin dissociation curve. For the same PvO_2 value, the SvO_2 will be lower in case of acidosis, which explains the right shift of the hemoglobin–O_2 affinity curve (Bacroft curve) [9]. Nevertheless, this is not clinically relevant if SVO_2 or $SvcO_2$ are continuously or frequently measured with a cooximeter.

Blood lactate concentrations

Lactate is the end product of the glycolysis. A total of 15–20 mEq/kg/day is released by many tissues including RBCs, skeletal muscle, and skin. Lactate is produced from pyruvate degradation through the lactate dehydrogenase enzyme and concentration >2 mEq/L provides generally evidence of inadequate tissue oxygenation [26]. Several studies have shown that blood lactate levels rise when the critical EO_2 level is reached during hemodilution [27–29]. However, elevated blood lactate concentrations do not necessarily reflect anaerobic metabolism secondary to cellular hypoxia. Indeed, tissue hypoxia and anaerobic metabolism cannot be sustained for a long period of time without inducing cell death, as the energy produced by anaerobic metabolism is quite low compared to aerobic metabolism [26]. Mild hyperlactatemia (2–4 mEq/L) in hemodynamically stable septic patients is probably not related to tissue hypoxia [26]. Other mechanisms, including activation of aerobic glycolysis with increased pyruvate availability [30], altered lactate clearance because of liver failure (function and/or perfusion), or increased lactate regional production (lungs in acute lung injury, white blood cells stimulated by endotoxins) may also cause an increase in blood lactate concentration [31, 32]. Lactate levels are easily and rapidly measured at the bedside and the assessment of repeated values with calculation of the early lactate clearance is of more interest than an isolated lactate value [33]. It must also be remembered that blood lactate concentrations represent, as does SvO_2, a global marker of oxygenation and offer no information about local perfusion.

Assessment of the microcirculation

Microcirculation, which includes vessels with a diameter <100 μm, plays a central role in tissue oxygenation, because it is across the walls of the microvessels that O_2 diffuses from the blood to the cells within each tissue. Alterations at this circulatory compartment level are frequently observed in critically ill patients [34, 35]. Reduction of the microcirculation shunting is a new therapy in providing adequate tissue O_2.

Different techniques allowing the assessment of the microcirculation have been recently developed. Nevertheless, all of these techniques need confirmation for their usefulness in measuring tissue oxygenation in the clinical setting.

The orthogonal polarization spectroscopy imaging

The orthogonal polarization spectroscopy (OPS) imaging is a newly developed noninvasive technique that allows direct visualization of the microcirculation [36]. The technique has been described in detail elsewhere [36]. Briefly, polarized light illuminates the area of interest, is then reflected by the background, and is absorbed by hemoglobin.

Specific optical filtration allows the elimination of the light reflected at the surface of the tissue to produce high-contrast reflected light images of the microcirculation. Hence, RBCs appear dark, while white blood cells and platelets may sometimes be visible as refringent bodies. Vessels are only visible if they content RBCs. For this reason, the technique is especially convenient to study tissues characterized by a thin epithelial layer, such as mucosal surfaces (rectum, vaginal, sublingual area) although other microcirculation beds, like at the level of the brain have also been studied [37, 38].

Compared to healthy volunteers, patients with cardiogenic and septic shock exhibited a decreased capillary density and a reduction in the proportion of perfused capillaries [34, 35, 39, 40]. Interestingly, persistence of such microcirculatory alterations has been associated with a poor outcome and this independently of the systemic hemodynamic status [34, 40]. These alterations of the microcirculation, studied by the OPS imaging technique, could be modulated by various therapeutic interventions, including nitric oxide donors and dobutamine administration [41, 42]. Sakr et al. [8] reported recently on the effect of RBCs transfusion in stable septic patients. These authors observed that in patients with altered baseline microcirculation, transfusion was associated with an increased number of perfused capillaries. In contrast, in patients with well-preserved baseline microcirculation, transfusion was associated with a decreased capillary density. This study highlights the possible beneficial role of the assessment of the microcirculation before deciding to transfuse an anemic septic patient. However, this technique presents several limitations: it is time consuming and observer-dependent, and requires a very cooperative or adequately sedated patient. Moreover, as described above, only vessels that contain RBCs can be observed due to the light absorbance of hemoglobin. All of these factors therefore restrict the routine use of this technique. In addition, comparison of the results reported in different studies is sometimes difficult, as different scoring indices of flow have been developed to quantify the alterations of the microcirculation. A recent round table conference proposed to uniform the scoring indices in characterizing the flow and images quality assessment [43]. Nevertheless, heterogeneity in microvascular blood flow and oxygenation exists between organs and may change dramatically during critical periods [44]. In the scope of all this, more investigation into OPS imaging is required before it can be recommended for routine use at the bedside.

Gastric tonometry and the sublingual partial pressure of carbon dioxide ($PslCO_2$)

Gastric tonometry was developed more than 15 years ago, as a tool to evaluate splanchnic perfusion in critically ill patients. According to the Fick equation, the determinants of tissue PCO_2 are tissue CO_2 production and blood flow. In low-flow states tissue hypercapnia is due to stagnation of CO_2 [45]. Therefore, the PCO_2 gap (difference between arterial and gastric intramucosal PCO_2) could provide useful information about splanchnic oxygenation. As the gut appears to be the first organ to suffer during circulatory shock, monitoring of tissue oxygenation at this level may be of great value in critically ill patients. Gastric tonometry has shown that prolonged mucosal acidosis was a sensitive predictor of poor outcome in critically ill patients and resuscitation therapy guided by gastric tonometry could be associated with a decreased mortality in this high-risk population [46]. Bacher et al. [47] studied the effect of moderate isovolemic hemodilution from a hematocrit of 40–34% on gastric mucosal pH during cardiac surgery. These authors observed a better preservation of the gastric mucosal pH in the hemodiluted patients than in those of the control group. However, routine clinical use of this technique is hampered by several methodological problems. The most important one relies on the fact that the increased gradient between mucosal and arterial PCO_2 is not always due to an imbalance between perfusion and metabolism. Indeed, the relationship between carbon dioxide partial pressure and content is not linear when O_2 saturation, hemoglobin, and/or the arterial-venous pH difference change [48, 49]. Some years ago, Weil et al. [50] reported that in hemorrhagic shock, sublingual partial pressure of carbon dioxide ($PslCO_2$) and gastric tonometry revealed parallel alterations, suggesting that both areas can be similarly affected during acute circulatory failure. More recently, several studies reported that $PslCO_2$ measurements may correlate with the severity of shock and outcome in emergency room [51] or in intensive care unit [52, 53]. Also, Creteur et al. [53] observed in 12 patients with septic shock that $PslCO_2$ was correlated with the proportion of well-perfused capillaries as assessed by the OPS imaging technique. Moreover, infusion of dobutamine at 5 μg/kg minute induced an increased capillary perfusion and a decreased $PslCO_2$ gap (Figure 18.1), suggesting that the regional microcirculatory blood flow should be the main determinant of $PslCO_2$

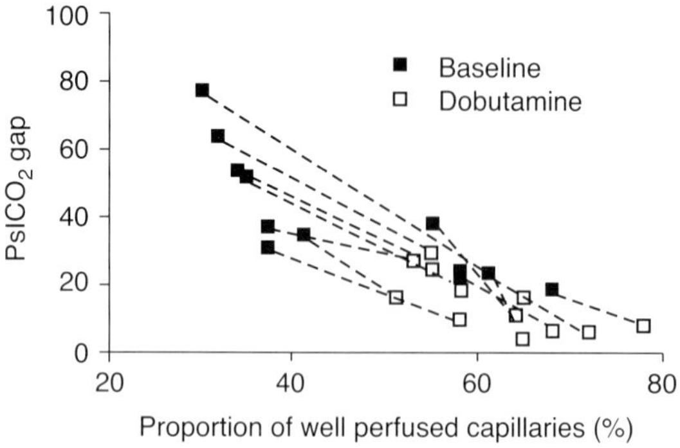

Figure 18.1 Individual effects of a dobutamine infusion (5 μg/kg minute during 90 minutes) on sublingual to arterial PCO_2 gradient ($PslCO_2$ gap; mmHg) and the proportion of well-perfused capillaries investigated by the OPS technique in 12 patients in the early phase of septic shock. Adapted from Creteur et al. [53].

[53]. Although $PslCO_2$ appears a promising technique, its usefulness as a clinical tool in transfusion decision making remains to be demonstrated.

The near-infrared spectroscopy

The near-infrared spectroscopy (NIRS) has been recently proposed as a rapid and noninvasive technique for the measurement of blood flow and tissue oxygenation, both in the muscles and the brain [54–56]. This technique determines tissue O_2 saturation using the principles of light transmission and absorption. Indeed, NIRS measures oxygenated and deoxygenated hemoglobin as well as the redox state of the cytochrome aa3. It determines a parameter, which is an average of O_2 saturation values of arterial, venous, and capillary vascular beds, according to the law of Lambert–Beer [57]. Cytochrome aa3 is the terminal cytochrome of the respiratory chain, responsible for 90% of cellular O_2 consumption through oxidative phosphorylation [58]. Using this technique, muscular blood flow and VO_2 were recently studied in critically ill septic patients after an occlusion test of the brachial artery [55, 59]. In these patients, the relative inability of muscular tissue oxygenation to recover after such an ischemic challenge was associated with a poor outcome. Interpretation of NIRS measurements at the bedside can be hampered by the presence of artifacts, related to light contamination through scatter and absorption. Some clinical studies have assessed the usefulness of the NIRS technique in the context of blood transfusion and hemodilution. Torella and coworkers studied the effects of RBC transfusions in 29 patients undergoing aortic or spinal surgery [60]. They observed an increase in the peripheral O_2 saturation after transfusion, correlating with the volume of blood transfused. In another work, the same authors observed a decrease in gastrocnemius muscle O_2 saturation in 30 patients undergoing acute normovolemic hemodilution to target hemoglobin of 11 g/dL [61]. Further studies are needed to determine if the parameters provided by the NIRS technology can be of clinical interest in evaluating the individual need for blood transfusion in critically ill patients.

Conclusions

Assessment of tissue oxygenation during anemia represents a key factor in evaluating the need for blood transfusion in critically ill patients. Most of the clinical tools provide information on global tissue oxygenation and many of them imply invasive monitoring.

Studying the microcirculation represents probably the best approach to assess the O_2 transport–consumption relationship. New techniques have been developed to directly evaluate the microcirculation (OPS, $PslCO_2$, NIRS). Nevertheless, these techniques are still under investigation and present pitfalls that limit their clinical use. Currently, the decision to transfuse must be individually evaluated with careful consideration of all available oxygenation parameters in conjunction with the patient's clinical and hemodynamic status and comorbidities.

References

1. Hebert PC, Wells G, Blajchman MA, et al. A multicenter, randomized, controlled clinical trial of transfusion requirements in critical care. N Engl J Med 1999;340:409–17.

2. Hébert PC, Fergusson DA, Stather D, et al. Revisiting transfusion practices in critically ill patients. Crit Care Med 2005;33:7–12.
3. Wu WC, Rathore SS, Wang Y, Radford MJ, Krumholz HM. Blood transfusion in elderly patients with acute myocardial infarction. N Engl J Med 2001;345:1230–36.
4. Rao SV, Jollis JG, Harrington RA, et al. Relationship of blood transfusion and clinical outcomes in patients with acute coronary syndromes. JAMA 2004;292:1555–62.
5. Leal-Noval SR, Rincon-Ferrari MD, Marin- Niebla A, et al. Transfusion of erythrocyte concentrates produces a variable increment on cerebral oxygenation in patients with severe traumatic brain injury. Intensive Care Med 2006;32:1733–40.
6. Smith MJ, Stiefel MF, Magge S, et al. Packed red blood cell transfusion increases local cerebral oxygenation. Crit Care Med 2005;33:1104–8.
7. Naidech AM, Jovanovic B, Wartenberg KE, et al. Higher hemoglobin is associated with improved outcome after subarachnoid hemorrhage. Crit Care Med 2007;35:2383–9.
8. Sakr Y, Chierego M, Piagnerelli M, et al. Microvascular response to red blood cell transfusion in patients with severe sepsis. Crit Care Med 2007;35:1639–44.
9. Piagnerelli M, Zouaoui Boudjeltia K, Vanhaeverbeek M, Vincent JL. Red blood cell rheology in sepsis. Intensive Care Med 2003;29:1052–61.
10. Crawford JH, Isbell TS, Huang Z, et al. Hypoxia, red blood cells, and nitrite regulate NO-dependent hypoxic vasodilation. Blood 2006;107:566–74.
11. Rozier MD, Zata VJ, Ellsworth ML. Lactate interferes with ATP release from red blood cells. Am J Physiol Heart Circ Physiol 2007;292:H3038–42.
12. Dietrich HH, Ellsworth ML, Sprague RS, Dacey RG. Red blood cell regulation of microvascular tone through adenosine triphosphate. Am J Physiol Heart Circ Physiol 2000;278:H1294–8.
13. Sprague RS, Stephenson AH, Ellsworth ML. Red not dead: signaling in and from erythrocytes. Trends Endocrinol Metab 2007;18:350–55.
14. Pittman RN. The microcirculation and tissue oxygenation. In: Sibbald WJ, Messmer KFW, Fink MP, Vincent JL (eds) *Tissue Oxygenation in Acute Medicine. Update in Intensive Care Medicine*. Springer, Berlin, Heidelberg, New York, 1998, pp. 36–54.
15. Graf J, Eichelbrönner O, Sibbald WJ. The red blood cell and nitrite oxide. In: Vincent JL (ed.) *Yearbook of Intensive Care and Emergency Medicine*. Springer-Verlag, Berlin, Heidelberg, New York, Tokyo, 1999, pp. 465–75.
16. Tsai AG, Johnson PC, Intaglietta M. Oxygen gradients in the microcirculation. Physiol Rev 2003;83:933–63.
17. Baskurt OK, Yalcin O, Meiselman HJ. Hemorheology and vascular control mechanisms. Clin Hemorheol Microcirc 2004;30:169–78.
18. Vincent JL, De Backer D. Oxygen transport-the oxygen delivery controversy. Intensive Care Med 2004;30:1990–96.
19. Van Woerkens EC, Trouwborst A, van Lanschot JJ. Profound hemodilution: what is the critical level of hemodilution at which oxygen delivery-dependent oxygen consumption stars in an anesthetized human? Anesth Analg 1992;75:818–21.
20. Hanique G, Dugernier T, Laterre PF, Dougnac A, Roeseler J, Reynaert MS. Significance of pathologic oxygen supply dependency in critically ill patients: comparison between measured and calculated methods. Intensive Care Med 1994;20:12–18.
21. Yalavatti GS, De Backer D, Vincent JL. The assessment of cardiac index in anemic patients. Chest 2000;118:782–7.
22. Greattinger JS, Parsons RL, Campbell JA. A correlation of clinical and hemodynamic studies in patients with mild and severe anemia with and without congestive failure. Ann Intern Med 1963;58:617–26.
23. Fontana JL, Welborn L, Mongan PD, Sturm P, Martin G, Bunger R. Oxygen consumption and cardiovascular function in children during profound intraoperative normovolemic hemodilution. Anesth Analg 1995;80:219–25.
24. Silance PG, Simon C, Vincent JL. The relation between cardiac index and oxygen extraction in acutely ill patients. Chest 1994;105:1190–97.
25. Reinhart K, Kuhn HJ, Hartog C, Bredle DL. Continuous central venous and pulmonary artery oxygen saturation monitoring in the critically ill. Intensive Care Med 2004;30:1552–6.
26. De Backer D. Lactic acidosis. Intens Care Med 2003;29:699–702.
27. Shinde SB, Golam KK, Kumar P, Patil ND. Blood lactate levels during cardiopulmonary bypass for valvular heart surgery. Ann Card Anaesth 2005;8:39–44.
28. Ranucci M, De Toffol B, Isgro G, Romitti F, Conti D, Vicentini M. Hyperlactatemia during cardiopulmonary bypass: determinants and impact on postoperative outcome. Crit Care 2006;10:R167.
29. Van Der Linden P, De Hert S, Mathieu N, et al. Tolerance to acute isovolemic hemodilution. Effect of anesthetic depth. Anesthesiology 2003;99:97–104.

30. Levy B, Mansart A, Montemont C, et al. Myocardial lactate deprivation is associated with decreased cardiovascular performance, decreased myocardial energetics, and early death in endotoxic shock. Intensive Care Med 2007;33:495–502.
31. De Backer D, Creteur J, Zhang H, Norrenberg M, Vincent JL. Lactate production by the lungs in acute lung injury. Am J Respir Crit Care Med 1997;156:1099–1104.
32. Haji-Michael PG, Ladrière L, Sener A., Vincent JL, Malaisse WJ. Leukocyte glycolysis and lactate output in animal sepsis and ex vivo human blood. Metabolism 1999;48:779–85.
33. Nguyen HB, Rivers EP, Knoblich BP, et al. Early lactate clearance is associated with improved outcome in severe sepsis and septic shock. Crit Care Med 2004;32:1637–42.
34. De Backer D, Creteur J, Preiser JC, Dubois MJ, Vincent JL. Microvascular blood flow is altered in patients with sepsis. Am J Respir Crit Care Med 2002;166:98–104.
35. Trzeciak S, Dellinger RP, Parillo JE, et al. Microcirculatory alterations in resuscitation and shock investigators. Early microcirculatory perfusion derangements in patients with severe sepsis and septic shock: relationship to hemodynamics, oxygen transport, and survival. Ann Emerg Med 2007;49:88–98.
36. Groner W, Winkelman JW, Harris AG, et al. Orthogonal polarization spectral imaging: a new method for study of the microcirculation. Nat Med 1999;5:1209–12.
37. Mathura KR, Bouma GJ, Ince C. Abnormal microcirculation in brain tumours during surgery. Lancet 2001;358:1698–9.
38. Pennings FA, Ince C, Bouma GJ. Continuous realtime visualization of the human cerebral microcirculation during arteriovenous malformation surgery using orthogonal polarization spectral imaging. Neurosurgery 2006;59:167–71.
39. De Backer D, Creteur J, Dubois MJ, Sakr Y, Vincent JL. Microvascular alterations in patients with acute severe heart failure and cardiogenic shock. Am Heart J 2004;47:91–9.
40. Sakr Y, Dubois MJ, De Backer D, et al. Persistent microcirculatory alterations are associated with organ failure and death in patients with septic shock. Crit Care Med 2004;32:1825–31.
41. De Backer D, Creteur J, Dubois MJ, et al. The effects of dobutamine on microcirculatory alterations in patients with septic shock are independent of its systemic effects. Crit Care Med 2006;34:403–8.
42. Spronk PE, Ince C, Gardien MJ, Mathura KR, Oudemans-van Straaten HM, Zandstra DF. Nitroglycerin in septic shock after intravascular volume resuscitation. Lancet 2002;360:1395–6.
43. De Backer D, Hollenberg S, Boerma C, et al. How to evaluate the microcirculation: report of a round table conference. Crit Care 2007;11:R101.
44. Boerma EC, Van Der Voort PH, Spronk PE, Ince C. Relationship between sublingual and intestinal microcirculatory perfusion in patients with abdominal sepsis. Crit Care Med 2007;35:1055–60.
45. Knuesel R, Jakob S, Brander L, Bracht H, Siegenthaler A, Takala J. Changes in regional flow and pCO(2) gradients during isolated abdominal aortic blood flow reduction. Intensive Care Med 2003;29:2255–65.
46. Gutierrez G, Clark C, Brown SD, Price K, Ortiz L, Nelson C. Effect of dobutamine on oxygen consumption and gastric mucosal pH in septic patients. Am J Respir Crit Care Med 1994;150:324–9.
47. Bacher A, Mayer N, Rajek AM, Haider W. Acute normovolaemic haemodilution does not aggrave gastric mucosal acidosis during cardiac surgery. Intensive Care Med 1998;24:313–21.
48. Jakob SM, Kosonen P, Ruokonen E, Parviainen I, Takala J. The Haldane effect-an alternative explanation for increasing gastric mucosal PCO_2 gradients ? Br J Anaesth 1999;83:740–46.
49. Cerny V, Cvachovec K. Gastric tonometry and intramucosal pH-theorical principles and clinical application. Physiol Res 2000;49:289–97.
50. Jin X, Weil MH, Sun S, Tang W, Bisera J, Mason EJ. Decrease in organ blood flows associated with increases in sublingual PCO_2 during hemorrhagic shock. J Appl Physiol 1998;85:2360–64.
51. Weil MH, Nakagawa Y, Tang W, et al. Sublingual capnometry: a new noninvasive measurement for diagnosis and quantification of severity of circulatory shock. Crit Care Med 1999;27:1225–9.
52. Marik PE, Bankov A. Sublingual capnometry versus traditional markers of tissue oxygenation in critically ill patients. Crit Care Med 2003;31:818–22.
53. Creteur J, De Backer D, Sakr Y, Koch M, Vincent JL. Sublingual capnometry tracks microcirculatory changes in septic patients. Intensive Care Med 2006;32:516–23.
54. Van Beekvelt MC, Colier WN, Wevers RA, Van Engelen BG. Performance of near-infrared spectroscopy in measuring local O_2 consumption and blood flow in skeletal muscle. J Appl Physiol 2001;90:511–19.
55. Creteur J, Carollo T, Soldati G, Buchele G, De Backer D, Vincent JL. The prognostic value of muscle StO2

in septic patients. Intensive Care Med 2007;33:1549–56.

56. Wahr JA, Tremper KK, Samra S, Delpy DT. Near-infrared spectroscopy: theory and applications. J Cardiothorac Vasc Anesth 1996;10:406–18.
57. Delpy DT, Cope M, Van Der Zee P, Arridge S, Wray S, Wyatt J. Estimation of optical pathlength through tissue from direct time of flight measurement. Phys Med Biol 1988;33:1433–42.
58. Jobsis FF. Noninvasive, infrared monitoring of cerebral and myocardial oxygen sufficiency and circulatory parameters. Science 1977;198:1264–7.
59. Girardis M, Rinaldi L, Busani S, Flore I, Mauro S, Pasetto A. Muscle perfusion and oxygen consumption by near-infrared spectroscopy in septic shock and non-septic shock. Intensive Care Med 2003;29:1173–6.
60. Torella F, Haynes SL, McCollum CN. Cerebral and peripheral oxygen saturation during red cell transfusion. J Surg Res 2003;110:217–21.
61. Torella F, Haynes SL, McCollum CN. Cerebral and peripheral near-infrared spectroscopy: an alternative transfusion trigger? Vox Sang 2002;83:254–7.

CHAPTER 19
Tissue Oxygenation and Blood Transfusion

Stefan Suttner & Joachim Boldt
Department of Anesthesiology and Intensive Care Medicine, Klinikum der Stadt Ludwigshafen, Ludwigshafen, Germany

Introduction

Indications for transfusion—transfusion trigger

Transfusion of packed red blood cells (PRBCs) is a potentially life-saving therapy in case of major bleeding and remains an essential and frequently performed medical intervention. The American Association of Blood Banks reports that in 2004 nearly 29 million units of blood components were transfused, including 14 million units of PRBCs [1]. Up to 80% of these transfusions are administered to surgical and critically ill patients. In 1995, Corwin et al. reported that 85% of critically ill patients who remained in the intensive care unit (ICU) longer than 1 week received blood transfusions [2]. The mean volume of PRBCs transfused was 9.5 units per patient. More recently, the prospective, multicenter, observational cohort CRIT study (Anemia and Blood Transfusion in the Critically Ill—Current Clinical Practice in the United States), which included 4892 medical and surgical ICU patients, reported an overall transfusion rate of 44% among patients in the ICU [3]. With an aging population and further advances in medical treatments and procedures requiring blood transfusions, the demand for blood continues to increase. Despite the widespread use of PRBC transfusions, for a variety of reasons, the number of indications in which such transfusions are appropriate is quite limited. In an analysis of nine studies assessing the appropriateness of red cell transfusions, inappropriate rates of 18–55% have been reported [4]. However, substantial variation was found in the criteria for an appropriate or an inappropriate transfusion. In an effort to reduce the perceived overtransfusion of blood and blood components, guidelines for blood transfusion have been issued by several organizations, including a consensus conference of the American National Institutes of Health, the American College of Physicians, the American Society of Anesthesiology, and the Society of Thoracic Surgeons [5–8] (Table 19.1).

These guidelines recommend that PRBCs should be administered only when the hemoglobin (Hb) concentration is low (e.g., less than 6 g/dL in a young, healthy patient), especially when the anemia is acute. Red blood cells (RBCs) are usually unnecessary when the Hb concentration is more than 10 g/dL. The determination of whether intermediate Hb concentrations (i.e., 6–10 g/dL) justify or require PRBC transfusion should be based on any ongoing indication of organ ischemia, potential or actual ongoing bleeding (rate and magnitude), the patient's intravascular volume status, and the patient's risk factors for complications of inadequate oxygenation [8]. The use of a single arbitrary Hb based transfusion trigger for all patients (i.e., Hb of 10 g/dL) is not recommended [8]. Specifically discouraged was the use of transfusion to enhance a sense of well-being of the patient, to promote wound healing, as a prophylactic measure in the absence of signs and symptoms, or to expand intravascular volume in the absence of evidence of

Alternatives to Blood Transfusion in Transfusion Medicine, 2nd edition. Edited by A. Maniatis, P. Van der Linden, J.-F. Hardy.

Table 19.1 American Society of Anesthesiology Guidelines for transfusion of red blood cells (RBCs) in adults [8].

• Transfusion for patients with Hb level of less than 6 g/dL is indicated, especially when anemia is acute
• Transfusion is rarely indicated when the Hb concentration is greater than 10 g/dL
• For stable patients with Hb level between 6 and 10 g/dL, the benefit of transfusion is unclear
• The use of a single Hb "trigger" for all patients is not recommended
• Indications for transfusion of autologous RBCs may be more liberal than for allogeneic RBCs

inadequacy in oxygen-carrying capacity or oxygen delivery.

Useful transfusion triggers should rather consider signs of inadequate tissue oxygenation that may occur at various Hb concentrations depending on the patient's underlying diseases. These "physiological" transfusion triggers can be based on signs and symptoms of impaired global or regional tissue oxygenation. However, before transfusion decisions based on physiological transfusion triggers are made, maintenance of strict normovolemia by the use of crystalloid and colloids has to be ensured [9].

Physiology of oxygen transport

Knowledge of the basic principles of oxygen transport and the physiology of anemia is a prerequisite for meaningful RBC transfusion decisions [10]. Thus, we emphasize some basic principles. The main function of RBCs is O_2 transport from the atmosphere to the mitochondria. The transport of O_2 from the atmosphere to the cell involves two biophysical principles: convection (i.e., bulk flow of blood) and diffusion (i.e., random movement of O_2 molecules). As blood passes through the lung, oxygen diffuses down its partial pressure gradient from the alveoli into the bloodstream where it combines with Hb in the RBCs and is carried by convective transport through the heart and large and small arteries to the microcirculatory vessels where the partial pressure gradient favors diffusion from the RBC to the tissue [11].

The microcirculation usually is defined as that part of the vascular tree comprising blood vessels smaller than 100 μm, including arterioles, capillaries, and venules. Its many branches, which expand the oxygen exchange area and its close proximity to the cells, make the microcirculation ideal for oxygen exchange with surrounding tissue. Within individual organs, a heterogeneous distribution of blood flow, and thus RBC supply, is physiological [11, 12]. Blood flow heterogeneity continues down the arteriolar tree into the microcirculation, where the distribution of flow is actively regulated by changes in vascular resistance and perfusion pressures which originate primarily from arterioles. Even changes in the resistance of the smallest, terminal arterioles may be followed by substantial redistribution of RBC flow within the capillary networks [11, 12]. Blood flow within the microcirculation is also subject to passive control, for example, when altered by rheologic influences and network geometry (Figure 19.1).

The concept of critical oxygen delivery/critical Hb level

The amount of oxygen available to the cell is determined by the adequacy of cardiorespiratory function, Hb concentration, the redistribution of cardiac

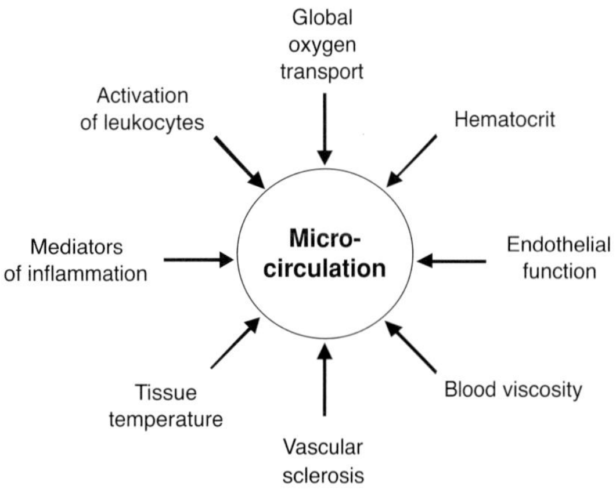

Figure 19.1 Factors influencing microcirculation.

output to the various organs, and to regulation of the microcirculation.

The amount of O_2 delivered, either to the whole body or to specific organs, is the product of blood flow and arterial O_2 content. For the whole body, O_2 delivery (DO_2) is the product of total blood flow or cardiac output (CO) and arterial O_2 content (C_aO_2).

The arterial oxygen content is expressed by the following formula:

$$C_aO_2 = (Hb \cdot 1.39 \cdot S_aO_2) + (0.0031 \cdot p_aO_2)$$

where Hb is the hemoglobin concentration (in g/dL), 1.39 is the oxygen carrying capacity of Hb (in mL O_2/g Hb), S_aO_2 denotes arterial oxygen saturation, and p_aO_2 denotes arterial partial pressure of oxygen; 0.0031 is the solubility coefficient of oxygen in plasma at 37°C (mL O_2/mmHg pO_2). In terms of CaO_2, more than 99% of O_2 is transported by Hb and only a negligible amount is dissolved in the plasma fraction at ambient p_aO_2 in room air. Thus, under most circumstances, DO_2 can be calculated by

$$DO_2 = C_aO_2 \cdot CO$$

It is important to note that blood flow, which is one of the key determinants of DO_2, is regulated not only at the level of the central circulation (as represented by CO in the formula above) but also at the regional level and the microcirculatory level. The latter is primarily determined by the autonomic control of vascular tone and local microvascular responses and to the degree of affinity of the Hb molecule for oxygen.

Under physiological conditions DO_2 exceeds O_2 consumption (VO_2) by a factor of up to 4, resulting in an oxygen extraction ratio (O_2ER) of 20–30%. Consequently, even a marked isolated decrease in Hb concentration with all other determinants remaining constant will still result in sufficient DO_2 to meet tissue oxygen requirements. However, below a critical threshold of Hb concentration there will be a decrease not only in DO_2 but also in VO_2. This relationship between VO_2 and DO_2 is referred to as the concept of critical DO_2 or critical Hb level. Above the critical DO_2/critical Hb level tissue oxygenation is sufficient as represented by a constant VO_2, which is thus "DO_2 independent." By contrast, below the critical DO_2/critical Hb level oxygen demands are no longer met, resulting in a decrease in VO_2. This state is characterized by a "VO_2–DO_2 dependency" and the development of tissue hypoxia (Figure 19.2) [13, 14]. This whole body shift to anaerobic metabolism might be the absolute indicator for RBC transfusion. From a physiological point of view, the expected benefit of a RBC transfusion at this threshold would be an increase in VO_2 and DO_2 and prevention of irreversible cellular injury.

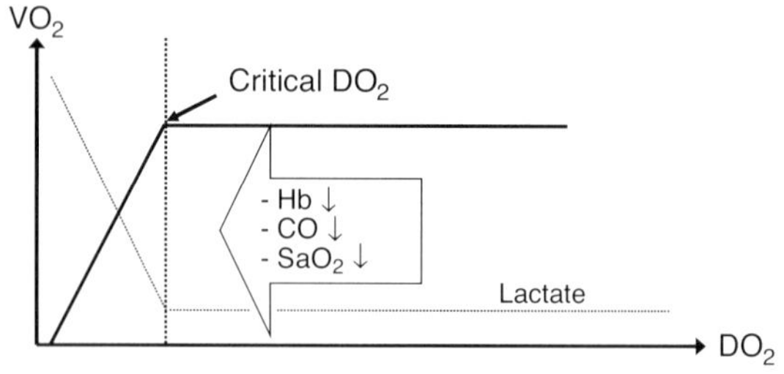

Figure 19.2 Relationship between systemic oxygen delivery and oxygen consumption. The VO_2 decreases only when the DO_2 falls below a critical threshold (critical DO_2); this is associated with an increase in lactate.

The point of systemic critical O_2 delivery/critical Hb level, however, may vary according to the individual patient's ability to tolerate and compensate for anemia [9, 10, 13]. Factors affecting a patient's response to decreased Hb concentration, and thus the factors that should influence the physician's decision to transfuse, include the patient's cardiopulmonary reserve (determined by the presence or absence of cardiac and/or pulmonary disease), the rate and magnitude of blood loss (actual and anticipated), oxygen consumption (affected by body temperature, drugs/anesthetics, sepsis, muscular activity), and atherosclerotic disease (cerebrovascular, cardiovascular, peripheral, renal) [8].

The critical Hb level cannot be defined in a generally applicable way, but it is intriguing to learn that even extreme acute normovolemic hemodilution (ANH) to a Hb concentration of 5 g/dL was well tolerated in otherwise healthy humans [16]. No signs of compromised DO_2, such as a decrease in VO_2 or an increase in lactate, were observed, not even after further compromising DO_2 by acute β-blockade suggesting that a Hb concentration of 5 g/dL was not yet critical [16]. The critical Hb level can only be defined for certain organs, specific situations and disease states, and particular age groups [15]. Anemia is believed to be less well tolerated in older patients, in the critically ill, and in patients with clinical conditions such as coronary, cerebrovascular, or respiratory disease.

Patients with coexisting cardiac diseases may be at particular risk of developing inadequate oxygenation and cardiac complications at low Hb levels even when normovolemic. Anesthetized patients with severe coronary artery disease (CAD) tolerated ANH to a Hb concentration of 9.9 ± 0.2 g/dL without evidence of myocardial ischemia [17]. Increases in cardiac output and oxygen extraction compensated the decrease in arterial oxygen content due to ANH completely. However, the exact Hb level associated with myocardial ischemia is variable and depends on the degree of coronary stenosis and whether it is a one- or a multivessel CAD [16, 17].

Elderly patients (65–88 years of age) without known cardiac disease tolerate moderate ANH to a mean Hb concentration of 8.8 g/dL well and were capable of fully compensating the decrease in arterial oxygen content by increases in cardiac output and oxygen extraction [19]. None of these patients was hemodynamically unstable or showed evidence of myocardial ischemia before retransfusion. Thus, hemodynamic tolerance of low Hb levels was well preserved in elderly patients without clinical evidence of cardiac disease.

However, the above results do not exclude that tissue ischemia could develop earlier in some areas due to a higher regional critical O_2 delivery, especially in acute blood loss and when hypovolemia complicates anemia.

Measuring tissue oxygenation and microcirculatory flow

As mentioned earlier, assessment of the adequacy of oxygen supply to organs and tissues is essential to guide transfusion decisions. Whether RBC transfusion actually restores tissue oxygenation is difficult to determine due to the lack of appropriate clinical monitoring techniques [20, 21]. Monitoring of tissue oxygenation and organ function in the clinical setting is largely based on measuring traditional variables of resuscitation, such as global hemodynamics, pulse oximetry, capillary refill, urine output, or indirect biochemical markers. However, these parameters remain as insensitive indicators of dysoxia and are considered to be poor surrogates for the oxygen availability at tissue levels, since tissue oxygenation is determined by the net balance between cellular oxygen supply and oxygen demand [20, 21]. Furthermore, the fact that continuing regional tissue dysoxia can persist despite the presence of an apparently normal adequate systemic blood flow, pressure, and arterial oxygen content, highlights the need for specific indices of oxygenation at tissue level [22, 23]. Methodologies to detect tissue dysoxia and oxygen debt can grossly be subdivided into two groups, namely techniques directed at the assessment of oxygenation at the systemic level, and monitoring techniques for measurements at the organ level (Table 19.2).

Oxygen delivery, oxygen uptake, and oxygen extraction ratio

The relationship between DO_2 and VO_2 can be used to assess the adequacy of tissue oxygenation. However, measurement of DO_2 and VO_2 requires right heart catheterization to measure cardiac output or is technically demanding and expensive if metabolic carts are used to measure VO_2. However, the interpretation of DO_2/VO_2 relationships has been criticized because of mathematical coupling [23]. However, this is only the case if DO_2 and VO_2 are determined from right heart catheterization.

Mixed venous oxygen saturation

Mixed venous oxygen saturation (SvO_2) can be readily measured from blood gas analysis derived at the bedside either intermittently or continuously with fiberoptic pulmonary artery catheters. Since the pulmonary artery carries blood from all vascular beds of the organism, mixed venous blood may represent the amount of oxygen in systemic circulation that is left after passage through the

Table 19.2 Clinical techniques to monitor tissue oxygenation and microcirculatory flow.

Monitor	Method	Variables	Global/regional	Invasive/noninvasive
Systemic oxygenation	Pulmonary artery catheter	$VO_2/DO_2/ERO_2$	Global	Invasive
Mixed venous O_2 saturation	Pulmonary artery catheter—blood gas analyses	SVO_2	Global	Invasive
Lactate	Laboratory—enzymatic testing	Lactate	Global	Invasive
Gastrointestinal tonometry	Measurement of pCO_2 in an air- or saline-filled balloon	$PrCO_2/pCO_2$ gap pHi	Regional	Minimally invasive
Near-infrared spectroscopy	Absorbance analysis of near-infrared light	Hb/O_2Hb cytochrome aa_3	Regional	Noninvasive
Oxygen electrodes	Polarographic probes	PO_2	Regional	Minimally invasive
Orthogonal polarization spectral imaging	Scattered polarized light	Diameter of vessels, velocity of RBCs, functional capillary density	Regional	Noninvasive
Sidestream darkfield imaging	LEDs emit green light which directly illuminates the tissue microcirculation	Diameter of vessels, velocity of RBCs, functional capillary density	Regional blood flow	Noninvasive

VO_2, oxygen consumption; DO_2, oxygen delivery; ERO_2, oxygen extraction ratio; SvO_2, mixed venous oxygen saturation; $prCO_2$, regional gastric CO_2 tension; pCO_2gap, arterial-to-intramucosal pCO_2 difference; pHi, gastric intramucosal pH; Hb/O_2Hb, deoxygenated/oxygenated Hb; pO_2, partial pressure of oxygen.

tissues. Thus, SvO_2 might serve as a parameter of global oxygenation. Determinants of SvO_2 are SaO_2, systemic VO_2, CO, and Hb concentration, with

$$SvO_2 = \frac{SaO_2 - VO_2}{1.39 \cdot Hb \cdot CO}$$

Accordingly, an increase in VO_2 and a decrease in Hb, CO, and arterial oxygenation will result in a decrease of SvO_2. Interpretation of SvO_2 values might be difficult in conditions where DO_2/VO_2 relationships are altered. For example in sepsis, arterial-venous microcirculatory shunting may increase SvO_2, thus preventing adequate tissue oxygenation, while regional tissue dysoxia is present [22].

Arterial lactate

Lactate is formed from pyruvate by the cytosolic enzyme lactate dehydrogenase and lactate concentrations >2 mmol/L are generally considered as a biochemical indicator of inadequate oxygenation [24]. Circulatory failure and impaired tissue perfusion is the most common cause of lactic acidosis in intensive care patients. However, a number of mechanisms other than impaired tissue oxygenation may cause an increase in blood lactate, including activation in glycolysis, reduced pyruvate dehydrogenase activity, or liver failure [25, 26]. Therefore, understanding the complex process of tissue lactate production and utilization is important to understand the usefulness and potential limitations of monitoring blood lactate levels.

Measurement of global DO_2, VO_2, O_2ER, SvO_2, and blood lactate may all provide means of assessing global oxygenation. They are not sufficient parameters, however, to indicate abnormalities in regional perfusion and oxygen balance.

Gastric mucosal tonometry

The introduction of gastric or sigmoid mucosal tonometry for the measurement of intraluminal carbon dioxide has enabled the clinician to change focus from global oxygen transport to regional tissue oxygenation. Measuring the regional gastric CO_2 tension ($prCO_2$) photometrically with infrared spectrometry via a special gastric tube and calculating the arterial-to-intramucosal pCO_2 difference (pCO_2gap) and gastric intramucosal pH (pHi) provide valuable information about splanchnic perfusion [27–30]. Thus, tonometer measurements might provide an insight in a region of the body that is among the first to develop an inadequacy of tissue oxygenation in circulatory shock and the last to be restored by resuscitation [27]. Gastrointestinal tonometry has been evaluated in various situations during surgery and intensive care [27, 28]. As a result, it has been shown that prolonged acidosis in the gastric mucosa might be a sensitive but not specific predictor of outcome in critically ill patients [27, 28].

Near-infrared spectroscopy

Near-infrared spectroscopy (NIRS) is a continuous noninvasive method applying the principles of light transmission and absorption to determine tissue oxygen saturation. NIRS measures oxygenated and deoxygenated Hb as well as the redox state of cytochrome aa3 (cyt aa3) as an average value of arterial, venous, and capillary blood according to the law of Lambert–Beer. cyt aa3, the terminal cytochrome of the respiratory chain, is responsible for approximately 90% of cellular oxygen consumption through oxidative phosphorylation [31]. Since the redox state of cyt aa3 is primarily determined by available oxygen, a decrease in cellular oxygen delivery results in a reduction of oxidative phosphorylation and a decreased oxidation level of cyt aa3. Monitoring the redox state of cyt aa3 might therefore be a key indicator of an impaired cellular oxidative metabolism and tissue dysoxia. Although NIRS may be applied to almost any organ, it has mainly been used in studies investigating cerebral or muscle oxygenation after different types of hypoxic injuries [31, 32]. The main limitation of NIRS in the clinical setting is the inability to make quantitative measurements because of the contamination of light by scatter and absorption [31, 32]. Moreover, normal values for regional tissue oxygen saturation in organs like the brain or skeletal have not yet been established.

Tissue oxygen tensions

Monitoring tissue oxygen tensions has become feasible for clinical use by the development of miniaturized implantable Clark electrodes. These polarographic oxygen sensors enable us to measure oxygen partial pressure in tissues ($ptiO_2$), organs, and body fluids directly and continuously. $PtiO_2$ values correspond to oxygen availability on a cellular level and provide information about oxygen supply and utilization in specific tissue beds [22]. Tissue oxygen tension has been measured successfully in intensive care as well as during several other surgical procedures [33–37]. Studies on the critical threshold of $ptiO_2$ after traumatic brain injury showed that the absolute level of oxygenation in the cerebral white matter was a reliable predictor of neurological outcome [34, 35]. However, organs like the brain are not readily accessible and thus not suitable for clinical routine monitoring. Monitoring muscle pO_2 might provide an early and reliable indicator of stagnant blood flow and tissue dysoxia. Moreover, it is easily accessible and reacts to hemorrhage, resuscitation, and shock on a similar time scale to that of the gastrointestinal tract. This has been shown clinically and in experimental studies [37–39]. Limiting factors in the use of polarographic oxygen probes are the dependence of electrode currents on tissue temperature, errors in $ptiO_2$ readings due to tissue trauma and edema by electrode insertion, or intravascular misplacement of the oxygen sensors.

Orthogonal polarization spectral imaging

Orthogonal polarization spectral (OPS) imaging is a newly developed noninvasive technique that allows direct visualization of microcirculation [40]. Polarized light is used to illuminate the area of interest. The light is scattered by the tissue and collected by the objective lens. A polarization filter or analyzer, oriented orthogonal to the initial plane of the illumination light, is placed in front of the imaging camera, eliminating the reflected light scattered at or near the surface of the tissue that retains its original polarization or glare. Depolarized light scattered deeper within the tissues passes through the analyzer. High-contrast images of microcirculation are formed by absorbing structures of blood vessels, for example, that are close to the surface and that are illuminated by the depolarized light coming from deeper structures. Because of its specific characteristics, this device is particularly convenient for studying the tissues protected by a thin epithelial layer, such as mucosal surfaces. In critically ill patients, the sublingual area is the most easily investigated mucosal surface.

Using OPS imaging in the sublingual area of patients in shock states, several investigators recently observed that microcirculatory alterations are frequent in critically ill patients [41,42]. Compared with healthy volunteers, patients with cardiogenic and septic shock presented a decrease in capillary density and a decrease in the proportion of the perfused capillaries. Current studies are ongoing to determine the effects of various interventions on microcirculation in humans.

The limitations of the OPS imaging technique include movement artifacts and the presence of various secretions such as saliva and blood. Because OPS imaging techniques use light absorbance by Hb, vessels can be visualized only when these are filled by RBCs. In addition, patients need to be cooperative or adequately sedated to prevent them from biting the device.

A major problem with using monitors of regional tissue oxygenation in clinical practice is that normal and critically abnormal values have not been established. Moreover, heterogeneity in microvascular blood flow and oxygenation that exists between organs as well as at the level of each organ may further increase during shock, sepsis, or other states of critical illness. Consequently, a common dysoxic threshold in vitally important organs such as the brain, the myocardium, the gastrointestinal tract, or any given tissue remains unclear.

Effect of RBC transfusion on tissue oxygenation in experimental and clinical studies

Clinical and animal studies have reported contradictory findings about the oxygenation capacity of stored RBCs [33,43–49] (Table 19.3).

Table 19.3 Clinical studies evaluating the effect of blood transfusion on tissue oxygenation.

Author	Patient group	No. of patients	Tissue O_2 monitor	Effect of blood transfusion
Leal-Noval [35]	Hemodynamically stable, nonbleeding patients with severe traumatic brain injury	60	Brain pO_2	Transfusion of 1–2 units of RBCs improved cerebral pO_2
Zygun DA [36]	Anemic patients with severe traumatic brain injury	30	Brain pO_2 and cerebral metabolism	Transfusion of 2 units of RBCs improved cerebral pO_2 and metabolism
Marik PE [46]	Critically ill patients with sepsis	23	Gastric mucosal tonometry	Transfusion of 3 units of RBCs led to a decrease of pHi
Sakr Y [50]	Critically ill patients with severe sepsis	35	OPS	Transfusion 1–2 units of RBCs had no effect on microcirculatory flow
Smith MJ [49]	Volume-resuscitated patients with subarachnoid hemorrhage	35	Brain pO_2	Transfusion of RBCs improved cerebral pO_2
Silverman H [45]	Critically ill patients with sepsis	21	Gastric mucosal tonometry	Transfusion of 2 units of RBCs had no effect on pHi
Suttner S [33]	Volume-resuscitated patients after elective coronary artery bypass grafting	51	Skeletal muscle pO_2	Transfusion of 2 units of RBCs had no effect on skeletal muscle pO_2
Walsh TS [48]	Critically ill patients with significant organ failure, but no evidence of hemorrhage	22	Gastric mucosal tonometry	Transfusion of 2 units of RBCs had no effect on global and regional oxygenation

OPS, orthogonal polarization spectral imaging; pHi, intramucosal pH.

In a recent clinical study, Suttner et al. used systemic O_2 transport variables and skeletal muscle O_2 tension to assess global and regional oxygenation status of 51 volume-resuscitated, mechanically ventilated patients after elective coronary artery bypass grafting following transfusion of one or two units of allogeneic RBCs [33]. The authors further tested the hypothesis that increasing O_2-carrying capacity by 100% O_2 ventilation would be equally effective or even superior to red cell transfusion in improving tissue oxygenation in the immediate postoperative period. Tissue oxygen tension was measured continuously using implantable polarographic microprobes. Transfusion of stored allogeneic blood was only efficacious in improving systemic O_2 delivery, whereas VO_2 and skeletal muscle O_2 tension remained unchanged. Augmentation of blood O_2 content by 100% O_2 ventilation also failed to increase VO_2, but was followed by an immediate increase in systemic DO_2 and skeletal muscle pO_2. This improved oxygenation status was due to an increase in convective oxygen transport with an increased driving gradient for diffusion of plasma-dissolved oxygen into the tissues. However, the study was restricted to hemodynamically stable, low-risk patients without excessive bleeding. Therefore, the results of this study may not be extended to patients who exhibit a pathological O_2 supply dependency or have perfusion failure (i.e., circulatory or septic shock).

Other clinical investigations used gastric tonometry to study the effects of transfusions on gastric intramucosal pH [29, 30]. In these studies, a large interindividual variability in the response to RBC transfusions was observed.

Silverman and Tuma compared the effectiveness of dobutamine administration with the effectiveness of transfusion in increasing gastric intramucosal pH [45]. Although dobutamine administration significantly increased a low baseline intramucosal pH, transfusion with PRBCs failed to have any effect on intramucosal pH in the patients evaluated. Marik and Sibbald's study also failed to show a beneficial effect of red cell transfusion on measured systemic oxygen uptake and gastric intramucosal pH in septic patients with elevated lactate levels [46]. On retrospective analysis they found a decrease in gastric intramucosal pH after transfusion of three RBC units that were stored for more than 15 days, reflecting an inadequacy of splanchnic oxygenation. They concluded that poorly deformable cells cause microcirculatory occlusions, and further postulated that these occlusions lead to tissue ischemia. Thus, the age of RBC units may be an important factor influencing the efficacy of RBC transfusion to improve tissue oxygenation.

Long-term blood storage decreases RBC concentrations of adenosine triphosphate and 2,3-diphosphoglycerate, resulting in decreased erythrocyte membrane deformability and increased affinity of Hb for O_2 [44]. These "storage" effects may interfere with the ability of RBCs to transport and unload O_2 at the capillary level [47]. Therefore, it has been proposed to transfuse fresh rather than stored erythrocytes.

Contradictory results were reported by Walsh et al., who evaluated changes in tonometric indices of gastric mucosal oxygenation and global oxygenation parameters in 22 ventilated critically ill patients with significant organ failure, but no evidence of hemorrhage [48]. The patients received two units of leukodepleted red cells in a double-blind, randomized fashion that were either fresh (stored <5 days) or had prolonged storage time (>20 days). In this study, the authors were not able to detect any adverse consequences on gastric intramucosal pH and changes in the arterial-gastric mucosal carbon dioxide gap with a storage time >20 days as compared to patients receiving RBCs <5 days. Possible explanations for the differences in results are that the patients in the Marik study were at an earlier stage of sepsis and more oxygen supply dependent or that the Walsh et al. used leukodepleted RBC and transfused only two RBC units, whereas Marik and Sibbald used three. Recently, Weiskopf et al. showed that transfusion of erythrocytes stored for less than 5 hours ("fresh") or more than 3 weeks ("old") to increase Hb from 5 to 7 g/dL equally reversed neuropsychological deficits in unmedicated healthy volunteers [51]. The equal efficacy of fresh blood and blood stored for 23 days was found despite significant decreases of 2,3-diphosphoglycerate and P50, the partial pressure of oxygen at pH 7.4 and partial pressure of carbon dioxide 40 mmHg, at which the oxyhemoglobin saturation is 50%. This study strongly indicates that "old" and "fresh" RBCs are equally efficacious in restoring inadequate oxygenation.

Only two clinical studies found beneficial effects of RBC transfusion on tissue oxygenation [45, 49]. In a prospective observational study, Smith et al. continuously monitored local brain tissue oxygen partial pressure during transfusion of allogeneic RBC units to volume-resuscitated patients with subarachnoid hemorrhage or traumatic brain injury, without cardiac disease [49]. An increase in brain tissue oxygen partial pressure was observed in 26 of the 35 patients (74%). The mean increase in brain tissue oxygen partial pressure for all patients was 3.2 ± 8.8 mmHg, a 15% change from baseline. This mean increase appears to be independent of cerebral perfusion pressure, Hb oxygen saturation, and inspiratory fraction of oxygen. In nine patients, brain tissue oxygen partial pressure decreased after RBC transfusion.

Another prospective observational study investigated the long-term influence of erythrocyte transfusion on cerebral oxygenation in hemodynamically stable, nonbleeding patients with severe traumatic brain injury and monitored through intracranial pressure and brain tissue partial pressure of oxygen catheters [35] Transfusion of 1–2 units of RBCs was associated with a variable increase in brain tissue partial pressure of oxygen during a 6-hour period, with a peak at 3 hours in 78% of the patients. Low baseline brain tissue partial pressures of oxygen (<15 mmHg) defined those patients who benefited the most from erythrocyte transfusion.

Conclusion

The use of a single arbitrary Hb based transfusion trigger for RBC transfusions for all patients (i.e., Hb concentration of 10 g/dL) is not recommended. Useful transfusion triggers should rather consider signs of inadequate tissue oxygenation that may occur at various Hb concentrations depending on the patient's underlying diseases. These "physiological" transfusion triggers can be based on signs and symptoms of impaired global or regional tissue oxygenation. However, clinical monitoring techniques that indicate failing tissue oxygenation have often not proved easy, reproducible, and sensitive to regional tissue hypoxia. Current evidence from studies of the influence of allogeneic blood transfusion on tissue oxygenation is seriously hampered by the absence of a significant number of adequately powered randomized controlled trials. Small clinical and animal studies report contradictory findings about the oxygenation capacity of stored RBCs. However, including measures of tissue oxygenation into transfusion decisions may enable a more individual use of allogeneic PRBCs in specific situations.

Key points

1 Transfusion of allogeneic PRBCs is a frequently performed and potentially life-saving therapy.
2 RBC transfusions are indicated only to avoid or to treat tissue hypoxia.
3 Whether RBC transfusion actually restores tissue oxygenation is difficult to determine owing to the lack of appropriate clinical monitoring techniques.
4 Clinical and animal studies report contradictory findings about the oxygenation capacity of stored RBCs.
5 Including measures of tissue oxygenation into transfusion decisions may enable a more individual use of allogeneic PRBCs in specific situations.

References

1. About blood and cellular therapies, www.aabb.org/Content/About_Blood/FAQ/bloodfaq.htm (accessed June 01, 2007).
2. Corwin HL, Parsonnet KC, Gettinger A. RBC transfusion in the ICU: is there a reason? Chest 1995;108:767–71.
3. Corwin HL, Gettinger A, Pearl R. The CRIT study: anemia and blood transfusion in the critically ill—current clinical practice in the United States. Crit Care Med 2004;32:39–52.
4. Hasley PB, Lave JR, Kapoor WN. The necessary and the unnecessary transfusion: a critical review of reported appropriateness rates and criteria for red cell transfusions. Transfusion 1994;34:110–15.

5. Office of Medical Applications of Research, National Institutes of Health. Perioperative red blood cell transfusion. JAMA 1988;260:2700–703.
6. American College of Physicians. Practice strategies for elective red blood cell transfusion. Ann Intern Med 1992;116:403–6.
7. Society of Thoracic Surgeons Blood Conservation Guideline Task Force, Ferraris VA, Ferraris SP, et al. Perioperative blood transfusion and blood conservation in cardiac surgery: The Society of Thoracic Surgeons and The Society of Cardiovascular Anesthesiologists clinical practice guideline. Ann Thorac Surg 2007;83:S27–86.
8. American Society of Anesthesiologists Task Force on Perioperative Blood Transfusion and Adjuvant Therapies. Practice guidelines for perioperative blood transfusion and adjuvant therapies: an updated report by the American Society of Anesthesiologists Task Force on perioperative blood transfusion and adjuvant therapies. Anesthesiology 2006;105:198–208.
9. Madjdpour C, Spahn DR, Weiskopf RB. Anemia and perioperative red blood cell transfusion: a matter of tolerance. Crit Care Med 2006;34:S102–8.
10. Van Der Linden P. Transfusion strategy. Eur J Anaesthesiol 2001;18:495–8.
11. Pittmann RN. The microcirculation and tissue oxygenation. In: Sibbald WJ, Messmer K, Fink MP (eds) *Tissue Oxygenation in Acute Medicine*. Springer, Berlin, Heidelberg, New York, 1998, pp. 36–54.
12. Ellis CG, Wrigley SM, Groom AC. Heterogeneity of red blood cell perfusion in capillary networks supplied by a singe arteriole in resting skeletal muscle. Circ Res 1994;75:357–68.
13. van Woerkens EC, Trouwborst A, van Lanschot JJ. Profound hemodilution: what is the critical level of hemodilution at which oxygen delivery-dependent oxygen consumption starts in an anesthetized human? Anesth Analg 1992;75:818–21.
14. Weiskopf RB, Viele MK, Feiner J, et al. Human cardiovascular and metabolic response to acute, severe isovolemic anemia. JAMA 1998;28:217–21.
15. Ronco JJ, Fenwick JC, Tweedale MG, et al. Identification of the critical oxygen delivery for anaerobic metabolism in critically ill septic and nonseptic humans. JAMA 1993;270:1724–30.
16. Lieberman JA, Weiskopf RB, Kelley SD, et al. Critical oxygen delivery in conscious humans is less than 7.3 mL $O_2 \times kg^{-1} \times min^{-1}$. Anesthesiology 2000;92: 407–13.
17. Spahn DR, Leone BJ, Reves JG, Pasch T. Cardiovascular and coronary physiology of acute isovolemic hemodilution: a review of nonoxygen-carrying and oxygen-carrying solutions. Anesth Analg 1994;78:1000–1021.
18. Spahn DR, Schmid ER, Seifert B, Pasch T. Hemodilution tolerance in patients with coronary artery disease who are receiving chronic beta-adrenergic blocker therapy. Anesth Analg 1996;82:687–94.
19. Spahn DR, Zollinger A, Schlumpf RB, et al. Hemodilution tolerance in elderly patients without known cardiac disease. Anesth Analg 1996;82:681–6.
20. Ince C. Microcirculation in distress: a new resuscitation end point? Crit Care Med 2004;32:1963–4.
21. Raat NJ, Ince C. Oxygenating the microcirculation: the perspective from blood transfusion and blood storage. Vox Sang 2007;93:12–8.
22. Vallet B, Tavernier B, Lund N. Assessment of tissue oxygenation in the critically ill. Eur J Anaesth 2000; 17:221–9.
23. Siegemund M, van Bommel J, Ince C. Assessment of regional tissue oxygenation. Intensive Care Med 1999;25:1044–66.
24. Hanique G, Dugernier T, Laterre PF, Dougnac A, Roeseler J, Reynaert MS. Significance of pathologic oxygen supply dependency in critically ill patients: comparison between measured and calculated methods. Intensive Care Med 1994;20:12–18.
25. Ince C, Sinaasappel M. Microcirculatory oxygenation and shunting in sepsis and shock. Crit Care Med 1999; 27:1369–77.
26. Bakker J, Coffernils M, Leon M, Gris O, Vincent JL. Blood lactate levels are superior to oxygen-derived variables in predicting outcome in human septic shock. Chest 1994;99:956–62.
27. De Backer D, Creteur J, Silva E, Vincent JL. The hepatosplanchnic area is not a common source of lactate in patients with severe sepsis. Crit Care Med 2001; 29:256–61.
28. Russell JA. Gastric tonometry: does it work? Intensive Care Med 1997;23:3–6.
29. Mythen MG, Webb AR. The role of gut mucosal hypoperfusion in the pathogenesis of postoperative organ dysfunction. Intensive Care Med 1994;20: 203–9.
30. Kolkman JJ, Otte JA, Groeneveld ABJ. Gastrointestinal luminal pCO_2 tonometry: an update on physiology, methodology and clinical applications. Br J Anaesth 2000;84:74–86.
31. Jobsis FF. Non-invasive infrared monitoring of cerebral and myocardial sufficiency and circulatory parameters. Science 1977;198:1264–7.

32. Guery BPH, Mangalaboyi J, Menager P, Mordon S, Vallet B, Chopin C. Redox status of cytochrome a,a3: a non-invasive indicator of dysoxia in regional hypoxic or ischemic hypoxia. Crit Care Med 1999;27: 576–82.
33. Suttner S, Piper SN, Kumle B, et al. The influence of allogeneic red-cell transfusion compared with 100% oxygen ventilation on systemic oxygen transport and skeletal muscle oxygen tension after cardiac surgery. Anesth Analg 2004;99:2–11.
34. Valadka AB, Gopinath SP, Contant CF, Uzura M, Robertson CS. Relationship of brain tissue pO_2 to outcome after severe head injury. Crit Care Med 1998; 26:1576–81.
35. Leal-Noval SR, Rincon-Ferrari MD, Marin-Niebla A, et al. Transfusion of erythrocyte concentrates produces a variable increment on cerebral oxygenation in patients with severe traumatic brain injury: a preliminary study. Intensive Care Med 2006;32:1733–40.
36. Zygun DA, Nortje J, Hutchinson PJ, Timofeev I, Menon DK, Gupta AK. The effect of red blood cell transfusion on cerebral oxygenation and metabolism after severe traumatic brain injury. Crit Care Med 2009;37:1074–8.
37. Boekstegers P, Weidenhöfer S, Kapsner T, Werdan K. Skeletal muscle partial pressure of oxygen in patients with sepsis. Crit Care Med 1994;22:640–50.
38. McKinley BA, Ware DN, Marvin RG, Moore FA. Skeletal muscle pH, pCO_2, and pO_2 during resuscitation of severe hemorrhagic shock. J Trauma 1998; 45:633–6.
39. McKinley BA, Butler BD. Comparison of skeletal muscle pO_2, pCO_2, and pH with gastric tonometric pCO_2 and pH in hemorrhagic shock. Crit Care Med 1999;27:1869.
40. Groner W, Winkelman JW, Harris AG, et al. Orthogonal polarization spectral imaging: a new method for study of the microcirculation. Nat Med 2000; 5:1209–13.
41. De Backer D, Creteur J, Preiser JC, Dubois MJ, Vincent JL. Microvascular blood flow is altered in patients with sepsis. Am J Respir Crit Care Med 2002; 166:98–104.
42. Sakr Y, Dubois MJ, De Backer D, Creteur J, Vincent JL. Persistent microcirculatory alterations are associated with organ failure and death in patients with septic shock. Crit Care Med 2004;32:1825–31.
43. Van Der Linden P, De Hert S, Belisle S, et al. Comparative effects of red blood cell transfusion and increasing blood flow on tissue oxygenation in supply-dependent conditions. Am J Respir Crit Care Med 2001;163:1605–8.
44. Fitzgerald RD, Martin CM, Dietz GE, et al. Transfusing red blood cells stored in citrate phosphate dextrose adenine-1 for 28 days fails to improve tissue oxygenation in rats. Crit Care Med 1997;25:726–32.
45. Silverman H, Tuma P. Gastric tonometry in patients with sepsis: effects of dobutamine infusions and packed red blood cell transfusions. Chest 1992; 102:184–8.
46. Marik PE, Sibbald WJ. Effect of stored-blood transfusion on oxygen delivery in patients with sepsis. JAMA 1993;269:3024–9.
47. Chin-Yee I, Arya N, D'Almeida M. The red cell storage lesion and its implications for transfusion. Transfus Sci 1997;18:447–58.
48. Walsh TS, McArdle F, McLellan SA, et al. Does the storage time of transfused red blood cells influence regional or global indexes of tissue oxygenation in anemic critically ill patients? Crit Care Med 2004; 32:364–71.
49. Smith MJ, Stiefel MF, Magge S, et al. Packed red blood cell transfusion increases local cerebral oxygenation. Crit Care Med 2005;33:1104–8.
50. Sakr Y, Chierego M, Piagnerelli M, et al. Microvascular response to red blood cell transfusion in patients with severe sepsis. Crit Care Med 2007;35:1639–44.
51. Weiskopf RB, Feiner J, Hopf H, et al. Fresh blood and age stored blood are equally efficacious in immediately reversing anemia-induced brain oxygenation deficits in humans. Anesthesiology 2006;104: 911–20.

CHAPTER 20
Anemia and Cardiovascular Disease

Antonis S. Manolis[1], *Spyridon Koulouris*[1], *Kostas Triantafyllou*[1,2], *Dimitris Sakellariou*[1], *Sokratis Pastromas*[1] *& Helen Melita*[3]

[1]First Department of Cardiology, Evangelismos General Hospital of Athens, Athens, Greece
[2]Hôpital Bichat Paris, France
[3]Central Laboratories, Onassis Cardiac Surgery Center, Athens, Greece

Introduction

Anemia is a well-recognized risk factor in a variety of medical conditions, including cardiovascular disease (CVD), where a close link between anemia and the development of CVD is being increasingly appreciated over the recent years.

Classically, chronic anemia has been associated with high-output heart failure (HF) especially when hemoglobin (Hgb) levels are ≤8 mg/dL [1]. This type of HF is characterized by (i) reduced afterload due to decreased systemic vascular resistance and reduced blood viscosity (due to a decrease in erythrocyte number and hematocrit); (ii) increased preload due to an increase in venous return; and (iii) increased left ventricular (LV) systolic performance due to increase both in preload and in sympathetic activity [2, 3]. Mechanisms inducing arterial dilatation include (i) hypoxic vasodilation due to hypoxia-generated metabolites; and (ii) flow-mediated vasodilation due to increased blood flow, an effect mediated by endothelial cells and endothelium-derived nitric oxide (NO) [4]. Beyond vasodilation, increase of the vascular bed due to recruitment of new vessels and formation of collaterals and arteriovenous shunts seems to play an additional minor role [5]. Ensuing pathophysiologic changes including tissue hypoxia, volume overload with its attendant LV hypertrophy, and LV dilation, may ultimately lead to circulatory decompensation especially in the presence of associated pathological conditions, such as hypertension, diabetes mellitus (DM), and uremia (Figure 20.1) [6–12].

In patients with end-stage renal disease (ESRD), a significant correlation between LV volume and mass with the severity and duration of anemia independently from age, DM, and hypertension has been repeatedly demonstrated [13, 14]. But even in patients with milder forms of renal impairment, a decrease in Hgb level is a better predictor of LV hypertrophy (LVH) than systolic blood pressure [15–19]. This holds true for the general population as well, as was shown in the Framingham Heart study [16], and in the Atherosclerosis Risk in Communities (ARIC) study [20]. In the ARIC study, which investigated 14,410 individuals without CVD at baseline, anemia defined by Hgb <13 g/dL in men and <12 g/dL in women was independently associated with 1.4 times higher risk of myocardial infarction (MI), coronary angioplasty (PCI), coronary artery bypass surgery (CABG) or definite coronary death in the entire cohort during a mean follow up of approximately 6 years [20].

Beyond its potentially causative role in the development of CVD both in subjects with or without cardiovascular risk factors and in patients with renal insufficiency, anemia also seems to aggravate the prognosis of those who already suffer from cardiovascular complications. Patients with *congestive HF* are the most characteristic example. Anemia is common among patients with HF, and the prevalence of anemia increases with the severity of HF, decline in renal function, and with increased age of

Alternatives to Blood Transfusion in Transfusion Medicine, 2nd edition. Edited by A. Maniatis, P. Van der Linden, J.-F. Hardy.

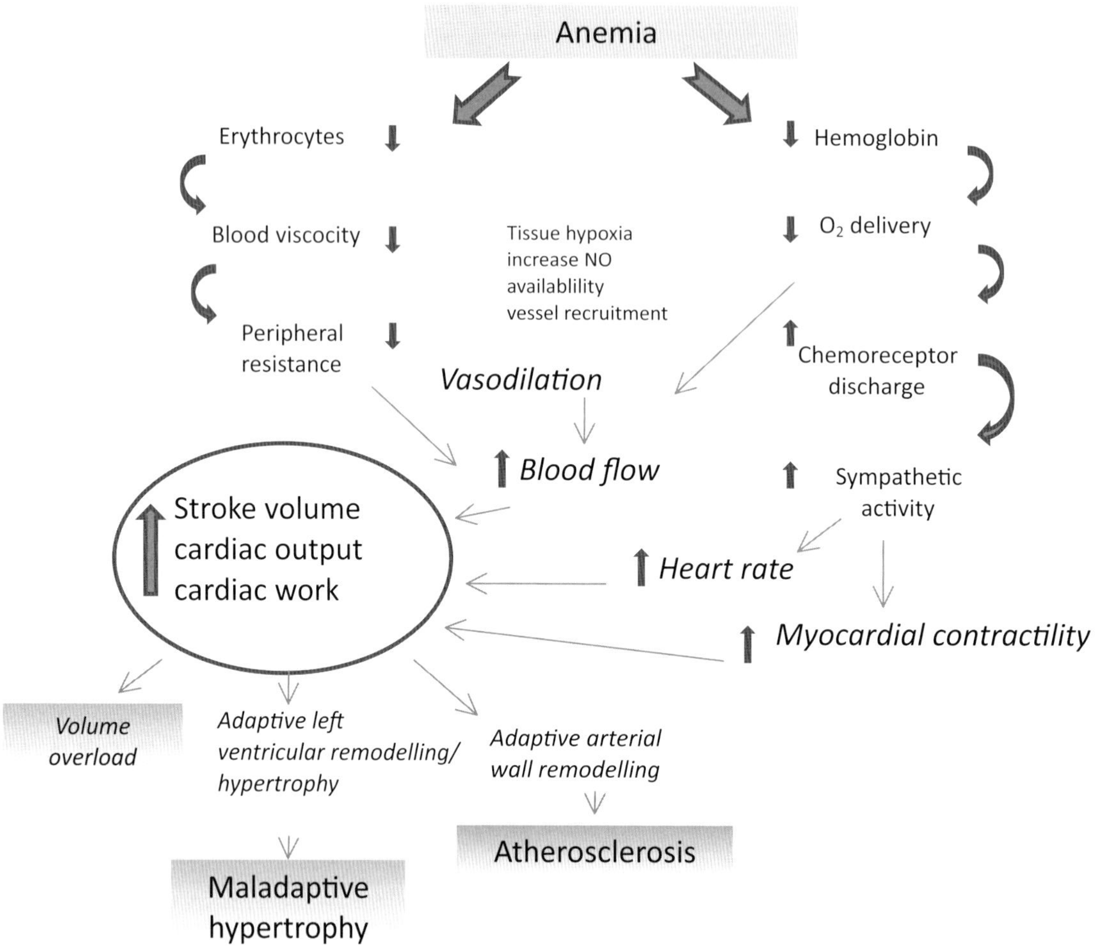

Figure 20.1 Proposed pathophysiologic mechanisms linking anemia to the development of cardiovascular disease.

the population and possibly with associated comorbidities such as diabetes, renal dysfunction, poor diet, and gastrointestinal blood loss [21, 22].

Anemia may precipitate *myocardial ischemia* as well. The myocardium has a high oxygen-extraction ratio and can augment oxygen delivery only by increasing coronary blood flow. Such an increase may not be possible in patients with fixed coronary stenoses. In the normal healthy heart, oxygen consumption and oxygen extraction are relatively constant at hematocrit levels between 20 and 60% [23]. Indeed, considerable experimental data suggest that a Hgb level of 7 g/dL is tolerated without myocardial ischemia if there is no obstructive coronary artery disease (CAD). With coronary artery obstruction, however, ischemia can occur with even mild anemia [24].

The impact of anemia therapy on outcomes in CVD has been intensively investigated over the recent years. Definitive evidence is still lacking and anemia correction has not been incorporated into the routine clinical practice yet. The simplest way of correcting anemia through blood transfusions, although guided by common sense, has been shown to be potentially harmful especially when used liberally and aggressively as a treatment strategy [25]. On the contrary, the administration of erythropoietin (EPO) seems promising, especially for the anemic patients with chronic kidney dysfunction (CKD), HF, or both [26]. However, concerns have also been raised about the safety of this type of treatment, since EPO has been associated with an increased risk of hypertension and thrombosis [27, 28].

In this setting, further investigation regarding the most appropriate "transfusion trigger" and "target" levels of hematocrit as well as the role of nonblood-based alternatives (i.e., EPO and its recombinants) for improving oxygen delivery in anemia is warranted. Ongoing large clinical trials (Trial to Reduce Cardiovascular Events with Aranesp—TREAT, Reduction of Events with Darbepoetin alfa in Heart Failure trial—RED-HF) are expected to provide us with some answers [29, 30].

Anemia in heart failure

Prevalence and prognostic implications

Heart failure (HF) is a significant burden for health care systems and is expected to increase considering the aging of the population. Despite recent diagnostic and therapeutic advances it still portends a poor prognosis [31]. Such disappointing findings may be partly explainable by the underutilization of mortality reducing therapies, such as ACE inhibitors, β-blockers, and aldosterone antagonists [32]. Among other reasons for the poor prognosis of HF, outstands the high prevalence of untreated anemia, which only recently attracted attention [31, 33]. Epidemiologic studies demonstrated that lower Hgb levels in HF are related to female gender, older age, poor kidney function, lower body weight, inflammation, and advanced disease status [34].

Different estimates of anemia prevalence among HF patients give percentages ranging from 9 to 79.1%, depending on the definition used for anemia, as well as HF severity and etiology in the studied population [35, 36]. In general, a physician should expect at least mild anemia to coexist in 30–50% of HF patients [37–39].

Beyond being common, anemia portends increased disease severity, more adverse events, inferior quality of life and ominous prognosis. It coexists more often with NYHA functional class III or IV, lower peak oxygen consumption (VO_2 max), and impaired renal function [36, 40]. Most importantly, multiple reports show that it is an independent predictor of morbidity and mortality in HF patients [19, 37–39, 41–43]. However, it is not yet clear whether anemia is a pathophysiologic factor that worsens HF or merely a marker of more severe disease.

Mechanisms of anemia in heart failure

The cardiorenal anemia syndrome

The pathogenesis of anemia coexisting with HF is variable and difficult to elucidate. Pathophysiological correlates and other comorbidities can be both a cause as well as a consequence of anemia. Renal damage due to prolonged renal ischemia among HF patients with low cardiac output is a common mechanism related to anemia. The term *cardiorenal anemia syndrome* suggests this interplay among HF, renal dysfunction, and anemia (Figure 20.2) [44]. Each of these three conditions deteriorates and is deteriorated by the other two and the three together form a vicious cycle. The syndrome is more common among older patients with a remarkably low LV ejection fraction (LVEF). Of note, HF and renal failure have also common etiologies such as DM, hypertension and vascular disease. Chronic renal insufficiency is a risk factor in itself for CVD, especially when anemia is present [45]. In patients with CKD, anemia promotes LVH, which is in turn an established risk factor for HF and sudden death [46].

The *cardiorenal anemia syndrome* can be better understood when EPO is considered. EPO is an hypoxia-induced hormone synthesized by peritubular cells in the cortex-medullary border of the adult kidney. Its levels can be elevated above normal values in many anemic patients with HF in proportion to the severity of symptoms, but this elevation is unlikely to compensate for the degree of prevailing renal hypoxia [47]. In such cases the inverse correlation between EPO and Hgb levels is modest, indicating a blunted response or even resistance to

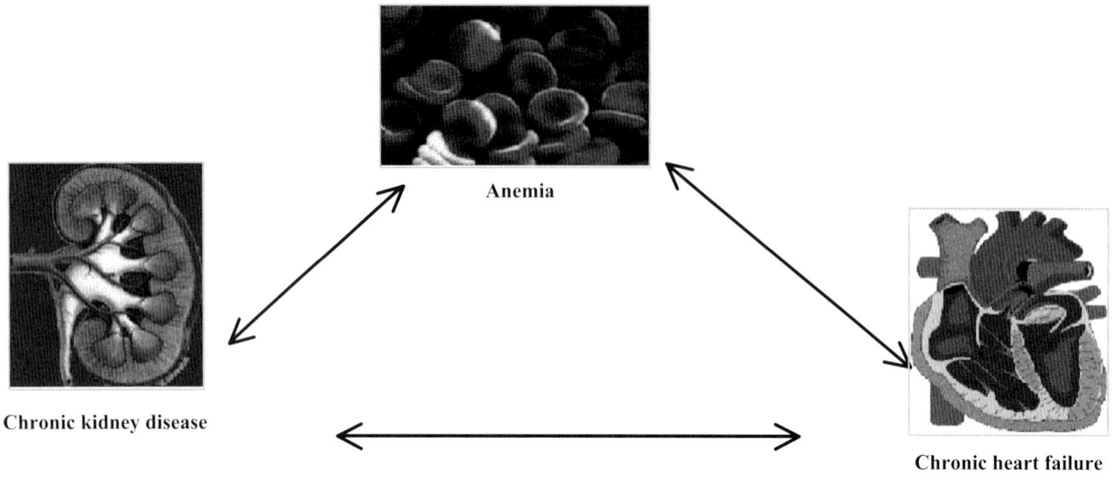

Figure 20.2 The vicious circle of "cardiorenal anemia syndrome."

EPO, which explains anemia. Elevated EPO levels in HF patients are associated with an adverse prognosis independent of Hgb levels [48]. Of course, if severe enough, coexisting renal failure will lead to EPO underproduction.

The combination of HF, renal insufficiency, and anemia seems to have an additive effect on morbidity and mortality. It has been estimated that each of these three factors increases the risk of death or ESRD by 50–100% and the three together raise the chances by up to 300% [49]. In the recently published ANCHOR study, Hgb levels and CKD have been shown to independently predict substantially increased risks of death and hospitalization among HF patients. Of note, mortality and hospitalizations increased in a graded fashion for Hgb values <13 g/dL and creatinine clearance values <45 mL/minute/1.73 m^2 [32] and Hgb was an independent predictor of outcomes at all levels of kidney function [39].

Other mechanisms

Hemodilution

Activation of the sympathetic, the renin–angiotensin–aldosterone and vasopressin systems that characterize HF lead to sodium and water retention. Hemodilution seems to be present in about 40% of HF patients but in the majority of cases the RBC volume may also be reduced [50, 51].

ACE inhibitors

ACE inhibitors are widely used in HF but may cause the hematocrit to fall by 2–5%. Suppression of angiotensin II production by ACE inhibitors in high doses may inhibit EPO synthesis [52]. Angiotensin II can stimulate erythroid progenitor cell growth in vitro while captopril inhibits it [53]. ACE inhibitors have also been shown to reduce production of interleukin-12, a cytokine known to stimulate erythropoiesis [54]. ACE inhibitors may also cause some degree of EPO resistance particularly at high doses [55]. Whether angiotensin receptor blockers (ARBs) have a similar effect is uncertain due to a paucity of data.

Hematinic deficiency

Treatment of the disease underlying HF, principally CAD with agents such as aspirin and warfarin, can contribute to iron loss and anemia due to gastrointestinal blood loss. Iron deficiency can be found in 21% of anemic HF patients [38]. Poor nutrition, cardiac cachexia, uremic gastritis, and malabsorption also predispose to iron as well as folate and B_{12} deficiencies.

Proinflammatory cytokines

Heart failure is characterized by an inflammatory milieu and proinflammatory cytokines seem to contribute to anemia [56, 57]. Substantial evidence implicates tumor necrosis factor-α (TNF-α) and interleukins (IL) 1 and 6 in the disruption of erythropoiesis, which is also frequently seen in other inflammatory conditions [57]. In HF patients, an inverse relationship has been demonstrated between cytokines and plasma Hgb levels [58]. TNF-α secreted by the failing heart can cause anemia by reducing EPO production in the kidneys, by EPO resistance at the bone marrow level and by disrupting the supply of iron necessary for erythropoiesis through inhibition of its release from the reticuloendothelial system [59, 60]. Inflammatory cytokines might also antagonize the action of EPO at a cellular level [61, 62].

Anemia correction treatment among patients with heart failure

The encouraging results of anemia correction by the use of recombinant EPO in other settings of chronic disease, such as CKD, inspired its use to treat anemia in HF [63]. Several groups have already tested the efficacy of EPO to correct anemia and improve outcomes in anemic HF patients. Initial studies were characterized by small patient numbers, differences in population characteristics and duration of follow-up. The first by Silverberg et al. was uncontrolled and examined the effects of anemia correction among 26 patients suffering from severe NYHA class IV HF with mean serum creatinine of 2 mg/dL [36]. The therapeutic targets were Hgb >12 g/dL and serum ferritin >400 μg/L. They were pursued by using a regimen of 2000 IU/week of EPO along with 200 mg of intravenous iron per week adjusted according to the response. Patients were treated for 7.2 ± 5.5 months and the clinical outcome was characterized by improved functional capacity, a modest increase of LVEF, and a dramatic decrease of hospitalizations.

The same and other groups continued this work with randomized controlled and uncontrolled studies in patients with HF and showed that anemia correction was similarly useful in HF patients with and without DM [64–68]. All the results were in the same direction with improvement of functional capacity indices (VO_2 max, 6-minute walk test, total exercise time) and better quality of life, and a decrease in hospitalizations. One study also showed a significant fall in plasma B-type natriuretic peptide (BNP) levels. Two recent randomized, double-blind, placebo-controlled studies comprising 475 patients with HF and anemia tested the effects of darbepoetin alfa [69]. Although Hgb levels increased with darbepoetin compared to placebo, improvement in symptoms was not significant. Of note, there was a nonsignificant trend toward decreased mortality in the darbepoetin arm. The effect of darbepoetin treatment on morbidity and mortality of this type of patients is expected to be determined by the ongoing randomized controlled RED-HF study, which will enroll 3400 patients [30].

When correcting anemia with EPO in HF patients, consideration should be given to the optimal target. Concerns are raised by three published studies comparing aggressive versus moderate anemia correction in patients with CKD [70–73]. There were trends toward higher risk of death and MI for patients assigned to the higher target hematocrit. Although the safety of aggressive anemia correction is still an ongoing debate, the raised concerns are important for HF patients. Theoretically, by raising Hgb concentration, tissue oxygen delivery increases, but at the cost of increased blood viscosity and potentially thrombotic events. However, there is evidence that at least anemia correction to a target hematocrit of 36% is safe [73].

Beyond studies using EPO in order to improve outcomes in anemic HF patients, others have evaluated the effect of iron supplementation alone among HF patients with iron deficiency anemia. A small uncontrolled, open-label study tested the effects of an intravenous iron sucrose regimen in 16 such patients, which succeeded in correcting anemia and was related to symptomatic improvement and increased exercise capacity during three months of follow-up [74]. In the FERRIC-HF, a randomized single-blinded study, intravenous iron sucrose treatment was tested in 35 HF patients with iron deficiency with or without anemia. The active treatment was linked to improved NYHA class and VO_2 max increase especially in anemic patients [69]. The IRON-HF study, a large multicenter, randomized, double-blind, placebo-controlled trial is ongoing and will seek better answers concerning the expected clinical benefits of iron supplementation alone in HF patients with iron deficiency anemia [75].

To conclude, there is substantial evidence that correction of anemia can improve outcomes of patients with HF. Studies reported so far show that by increasing Hgb levels one should expect improved functional capacity, fewer hospitalizations, stabilized renal function, and less diuretic use. These results were mainly derived from studies testing treatment by EPO in patients with advanced HF and modestly impaired renal function (cardiorenal anemia syndrome). Some evidence also recently appeared that even iron supplementation alone, for the subgroup of HF patients with iron deficiency anemia, can improve functional status. However, many questions remain unanswered and further research is needed in order to optimize treatment regimens and determine if anemia correction in HF patients can not only lead to increased exercise capacity but also to survival benefits.

Anemia and acute coronary syndromes

Abnormal hemoglobin levels are quite frequently encountered among patients with an acute coronary syndrome (ACS). In one retrospective analysis of acute MI admissions to nonFederal hospitals in New Jersey in 1986 (prethrombolytic era, $n = 15\,584$) and 1996 (thrombolytic era, $n = 14\,757$), anemia was detected in 6.4 and 10.2% ($p < 0.0001$) of patients respectively [76]. In more recent studies the incidence of anemia has been reported even higher (18–24.6%) [77–79]. The increased incidence of either occult or clinically apparent blood loss due to the use of both more aggressive antiplatelet regimens (clopidogrel, IIb/IIIa inhibitors) and more invasive revascularization procedures may account for this increase. Anemia in ACS seems also to be associated with advancing age, DM, and renal dysfunction [77].

ACS which include ST-segment-elevation MI, nonST-segment-elevation MI, and unstable angina, develop as a consequence of an intrinsic mismatch between myocardial oxygen supply and demand. Anemia exacerbates this imbalance by causing a decrease in oxygen-carrying capacity. Indeed, anemic dogs have shown ischemic ST-segment changes and locally depressed cardiac function at higher hemoglobin levels with experimentally created coronary stenosis varying from 50 to 80% [80]. However, despite this clear-cut pathophysiologic substrate, clinical data have been rather inconsistent in supporting the adverse effect of anemia on the outcome of patients presenting with ACS. Older studies both from the prethrombolytic and thrombolytic era failed to establish an independent long-term prognostic role of anemia in patients with acute MI. Most of them were small, had short duration follow-up, or focused on a specific group of patients [70, 81–83]. The higher unadjusted mortality observed among patients with acute MI and anemia was attributed to older age, higher comorbidity, and more LV dysfunction [76].

However, more recent data have shown that hemoglobin levels are independently associated with short and long-term prognosis of patients presenting with ACS. In a retrospective study, 1841 consecutive patients admitted with the diagnosis of acute MI were categorized according to the hemoglobin level on admission (10 g/dL or less, or greater than 10 g/dL). The 30-day mortality was 21.6% in patients with Hgb levels on admission <10 g/dL and 9.3% in patients with Hgb levels >10 g/dL. More importantly, this relationship between low Hgb levels and 30-day mortality remained significant after adjustment for other risk factors (HR 1.76, CI 1.08–2.85; $p = 0.02$) [84].

More powerful data offered an analysis of the 30-day cardiovascular outcome in patients comprising the 16 Thrombolysis in Myocardial Infarction (TIMI) trials database. In patients with ST-elevation MI, when those with Hgb values between 14 and 15 g/dL were used as the reference, cardiovascular mortality increased as Hgb levels fell below 14 g/dL, with an adjusted odds ratio of 1.21 for each 1 g/dL decrement in Hgb. In patients with nonST-elevation ACS, with those with Hgb 15–16 g/dL used as the reference, the likelihood of cardiovascular death, MI, or recurrent ischemia increased as Hgb fell below 11 g/dL, with an adjusted OR of 1.45 for each 1 g/dL decrement in Hgb [85].

Moreover, in a more recent prospective study of 1410 consecutive patients with ACS the presence of anemia was an independent predictive factor of mortality and had an incremental predictive value to the calculation of 30-day survival probability [86].

Regarding the impact of anemia on the long-term prognosis of patients presenting with ACS, recent data, albeit limited, suggest a significant prognostic role as well. In a 20-year follow-up study of 193 men presented with ACS, a Hgb level <13 g/dL was associated with an almost twofold increase in the risk of death or MI [87]. Studying a much larger database of 1038 patients with ACS, Vaglio et al. [88] were also able to show a similar importance of anemia in the 2-year outcome. More importantly, they were able to demonstrate a graded response. Thus, mild anemia (hematocrit levels 33.1–39%) was associated with a 1.5 increase in death rate, while more severe anemia was associated with a 2.5 increase of the risk. A similar graded relationship was found in a cohort of older patients (mean age 73 years) hospitalized for acute MI. The mortality at 1 year was 18.6% for individuals with a hematocrit ≥40%; 23.5% (relative risk: 1.35) for hematocrit 36–39%; 30.7% (relative risk 1.94) for hematocrit between 30 and 35%, and 35.8% (relative risk: 3.16) for those with a hematocrit <30%. An interaction between anemia and CKD was also noted in this particular study suggesting a possible joint role of these two risk factors for mortality after a MI [89]. In the subpopulation of patients who undergo revascularization procedures, anemia seems to retain its prognostic significance. As shown by Nikolsky et al. [90], baseline anemia in patients undergoing primary PCI for acute MI was found to be an independent predictor of both in-hospital and 1-year mortality.

The pathophysiology underlying the frequent development of anemia in patients with ACS has not been clearly defined. Nevertheless, the contribution of blood loss offers a reasonable explanation. The use of clopidogrel, for example, has been associated with increased incidence of bleeding in patients with ACS who undergo invasive procedures [91]. In general, severe bleeding can be estimated as being between <1 and 10% in patients with nonST elevation MI or unstable angina [92]. On the contrary, bleeding is more frequent in patients with ST-elevation acute MI probably due to the additional use of thromolytic regimens [93].

Of note, as serum ferritin is an acute-phase reactant, a reduction in ferritin due to iron deficiency can be masked by the acute systemic inflammatory response characterizing the ACS [77]. Other factors may be the frequent coexistence of DM and CKD in patients with myocardial ischemia both associated with reduced EPO production and impaired hemopoetic response in this hormone [94]; also bone marrow suppression by the acute inflammatory response [95] or drugs [96] and more rarely nutritional deficiencies [77]. However, blood loss seems to be the most important factor and is probably the major contributor to the adverse prognosis associated with anemia in patients with ACS [97,98]. Not only may blood loss predispose to anemia but also anemia seems to predispose patients with acute MI to the development of bleeding [99].

Since anemia has been linked to a worse prognosis in patients with ACS, correction through blood transfusion has been studied as a strategy aiming to abrogate the adverse outcomes. Indeed, Wu et al. [81] showed that blood transfusion reduced short-term mortality in eldlerly patients with ACS who had a hematocrit up to 33% on admission. However, blood transfusions in this setting have been associated with higher mortality in most of the studies [100,101]. Wu et al. showed to the contrary that blood transfusion to increase Hb concentration within "normal range" may improve survival In a recent study, transfusions increased the risk of an adverse outcome by 2.5 times even after correcting for the presence of anemia and other significant risk factors [102]. In a prospective database of patients with acute MI, Aronson et al. [103] calculated an adjusted hazard ratio for mortality of 1.9 in transfused patients. Nevertheless, transfusion had a protective effect in patients with hemoglobin ≤8 mg/dL. Similarly, in the CRUSADE trial blood transfusion had an adverse effect in patients with nonST elevation ACS and Hct > 27% [104]. However, this effect was neutralized in patients with lower Hct levels. Thus, current evidence seems not to support routine use of blood transfusion in anemic patients with ACS, with the possible exception of those with very low Hb levels. Proposed mechanisms of the adverse effects of blood transfusion include an immunomodulatory effect leading to a graft-versus-host reaction, an increase in mediators of inflammation, alterations in handling of NO by stored red blood cells [105] as well as decreased RBC deformability in stored blood [106, 107] which can promote vasoconstriction thereby triggering or worsening ischemia and finally volume expansion and increasing blood viscosity [108]. Given the fact that blood transfusion seems to be of limited value in patients with an ACS, other alternative therapies like the use of EPO are currently being tested in clinical trials [109].

Chronic renal disease and anemia in CVD

Over the past decades the incidence of CVD and CKD are rising steadily. About 20 million of the US population (11%) has CKD [110, 111] whereas about 400,000 of the adult US population (0.1%) have end-stage renal disease (ESRD). Congestive HF is also quite prevalent among the general population. Although the annual incidence of HF in those >65 years of age is about 10 per 1000 persons [112], a report from the Hemodialysis (HEMO) study [113] indicated that the prevalence in ESRD is about 40%.

Cardiovascular disease, especially atherosclerosis, stroke, and MI, has long been recognized as the most common cause of mortality in adult patients with CKD [114] accounting for approximately 50% of deaths in patients with ESRD in the US between 1997 and 2001 [115]. Indeed, CVD mortality rates in ESRD patients are 30 times higher than in the general population [116]. Also, only 15% have normal LV structure and function at dialysis initiation [117].

It is well established that HF and CKD are inexorably linked (one can cause or worsen the other). The connector between this relationship seems to be a third factor often seen in both conditions. This factor is anemia. Anemia can be caused by both the HF and the CKD and this anemia can act back and further damage both. These three diseases make a vicious circle called the cardiorenal anemia syndrome [118, 119] (Figure 20.2). Correction of anemia may be crucial in the prevention of the progression of both HF and CKD.

The cardiorenal anemia syndrome

The high prevalence of CVD in patients with CKD is widely reported over the past several years [19, 120–124]. Almost 25% of the whole cardiac output is used for kidney perfusion. Kidney function is believed to be impaired when glomelural filtration rate (GFR) falls below 60 mL/minute/1.73 m^2. In a large epidemiologic study by Go et al. [125] which included 100,000 individuals, there was noted an increase in age-adjusted risk of mortality and incidence of CVD as the renal function worsened. Specifically, this risk in patients with GFR between 45 and 59 mL/minute/1.73 m^2 was 17% and in patients with GFR <15 mL/minute/1.73 m^2 it was 343%. Decreasing renal function results in serious changes in several homeostatic mechanisms including coagulation, fibrinolysis, endothelial function, anemia, arrhythmias, calcium–phosphorous balance, renin–angiotensin–aldosterone system, and lipid metabolism [126].

Heart abnormalities in CKD

The pathogenesis of CVD in patients with CKD comprises causes that are the same as in the general population (e.g., smoking, hyperlipidemia), factors that cause renal failure and also have adverse effects on the heart (e.g., DM) and factors that are independent of the underlying cause of renal insufficiency (e.g., hypertension, uremia per se). The clinical manifestations of CVD in CKD can be stable or unstable angina, MI, arrhythmias, or congestive HF. In ESRD, at the onset of hemodialysis, 50% of patients have symptoms or clinical signs of CVD [115] and almost 80% have ECG abnormalities [127].

The main pathophysiologic mechanisms of heart disorders in CKD patients include enhanced atherosclerosis, metabolic abnormalities of the heart, overactivity of sympathetic nervous system, microvascular disease, LVH, and cardiomyocyte abnormalities.

Enhanced atherosclerosis

The high prevalence of atherosclerotic lesions in uremic patients has been amply documented by autopsy studies [128, 129]. The prevalence of calcified plaques is 4 times higher in uremic patients. In a recent study, very rapid appearance of advanced coronary lesions was demonstrated in young adults with childhood-onset chronic renal failure [130]. Oxidative stress seems to play a major role in the production of atherosclerotic plaques in CKD. Highly reactive oxygen radicals as O_2- superoxide, hydroxy radicals, hydroxy peroxide, or peroxinitrite were found in high concentrations in patients with renal failure [131]. Even in early stages of the disease, elevated plasma concentrations of C-reactive protein (CRP), interleukin-6 and advanced oxidation protein products, interleukin-1 (IL-1) receptor antagonists and soluble TNF receptors were found [130]. Thus, uremia per se is a proinflammatory condition, independent of dialysis [133]. Inflammation markers, such as CRP, seem to be independent risk factors for cardiovascular mortality in the general population [134] as well as in the dialysis patients [135]. Hyperphosphatemia is another factor that probably plays a role in the atherosclerotic plaque progression. In dialysis patients a pre-dialysis serum phosphate concentration of >6.5 mg/dL increases all-cause [136] and cardiac mortality [137]. High concentration of phosphorus is deleterious even in patients without renal failure as it is a predictor of the narrowing of coronary arteries [138].

Metabolic abnormalities of the heart

The heart in uremic patients seems to have several metabolic abnormalities. As shown in animals [139] when they are in low flow circumstances, a decay of ATP and generation of adenosine are observed, leading to a reduction of energy stores. Under hypoxic conditions, the heart is forced to generate ATP through glycolysis which needs a high glucose concentration, and in the uremic cardiomyocyte it is this insulin-dependent glucose entry that is compromised [140, 141]. The beneficial effect of intensive insulin therapy which was observed in diabetic patients after acute myocardial infarction (MI) in the DIGAMI study [142], as well as in critically ill patients in general and especially in those with acute renal failure [143] may be explained by this mechanism. Moreover, in the cardiomyocyte of patients with CKD, an abnormal calcium cycling and contractile function occurs [144], as well as an increased rate of apoptosis [145].

Overactivity of the sympathetic nervous system

Chemoreceptors and baroreceptors are activated in the damaged kidney, even when GFR is still normal [146, 147]. Activating signals from these receptors then convene to the hypothalamus where they cause an increase in sympathetic tone. Sympathetic overactivity will increase inotropy and, consequently, oxygen demand and is therefore unwanted in patients with ischemic heart disease. This sympathetic overexpression may be one of the major reasons of poor outcome of patients with ESRD after a MI [148]. Thus, the role of β-blockers is very important in uremic patients and their use is continuously increasing. In a prospective study, carvedilol was shown to improve survival in dialysis patients with impaired cardiac function due to dilated cardiomyopathy [149, 150]. Furthermore, in the CIBIS II trial in the subgroup of chronic HF patients with renal failure, the protective effect of bisoprolol was the same as in the other patients [151]. In the DOPPS study although only a minority of dialyzed patients with CAD received β-blockers, their survival was higher by 13% [152]. Over the past several years β-blockers are being increasingly employed in patients with CKD, whether diabetic or not [153].

Microvessel disease

The heart capillaries in uremic patients have reduced length and thus their growth is not in accordance with the cardiomyocyte hypertrophy [154]. Therefore, there is an increased distance through which oxygen must diffuse from the capillary lumen to the interior of the cardiomyocyte. This will expose the cardiomyocyte to hypoxia whenever the oxygen supply of the heart is critically low, for instance when coronary blood flow decreases. Moreover, abnormalities in vascular remodeling may occur in patients with CKD [155].

Left ventricular hypertrophy

LVH is present from the early stages of CKD [156]. The cause of LVH in renal disease relates to a chronic increase in stroke work and the work of the LV per minute, which are the results of pressure and volume overload [157].

Cardiac disorders caused by anemia

It is known from several years that severe anemia can cause HF even in individuals without cardiac abnormalities [6]. In Figure 20.1 there is shown the pathogenetic mechanism of HF due to anemia [158–169]. In a recent study [170] in a large population of over 1,000,000 elderly patients, anemia conferred a twofold relative risk to develop HF during the next year compared to those with a normal hematocrit.

Almost all the HF parameters are worse in anemic HF patients [40, 171]. Specifically, they have more hospitalizations, worse NYHA functional class, lower LVEF, and exercise tolerance as expressed by reduced VO_2 peak, higher level of BNP, higher heart rate, more severe peripheral edema, higher pulmonary capillary wedge pressures, and a greater resistance to therapy as judged by the need for higher doses of diuretics. They also have increased levels of proinflammatory cytokines such as TNF-α and interleukin 6 (IL 6), a higher prevalence of cardiac cachexia, and a more rapid progression of renal failure.

Approximately one third of HF patients have Hgb <12 g/dL [172]. The presence of anemia is associated with more severe HF as expressed by NYHA functional class. In multiple studies, anemia has emerged as an independent risk factor of morbidity and mortality, but also a therapeutic target in HF patients [172–179]. The degree of anemia in HF may also play a role in hospital mortality and hospital costs [180].

Anemia causes in HF & CKD

Over the past several years a lot of pathophysiologic mechanisms of anemia in patients with HF and CKD have been proposed, among which prevail HF itself and its drug therapy (ACE inhibitors or ARBs), the associated renal dysfunction, coexisting DM, production of proinflammatory cytokines such as TNF-α or of other substances from the heart myocytes of patients with HF that inhibit erythropoiesis [96, 181–189]. Aspirin, taken by the majority of HF patients, may also cause microscopic blood loss from the gastrointestinal system and thus produce anemia. Proteinuria which is also common in HF patients can cause anemia by the loss of EPO, iron, and transferrin in great amounts from the urine [187]. Finally, hemodilution is another possible explanation of anemia in HF.

Benefits of anemia treatment

The close relationship of anemia with poor prognosis made the correction of anemia a therapeutic target in HF and CKD patients. Administration of recombinant EPO and IV or peros iron was first used in HF patients in 2000 [36]. The correction of anemia to a Hgb level >12.5 g/dL by IV iron at a dose of 200 mg/week (ferric sucrose) and EPO 2000 IU/week in patients with severe HF improved symptoms and quality of life of these patients, evidenced by improvement of the NYHA functional class, increased LVEF, reduced number and days of hospitalization, reduced doses of oral and IV diuretics required, and improved self-assessed shortness of breath and fatigue. It was also noted that after correction of anemia, creatinine clearance was stabilized when before correction it had been falling at about 1 mL/minute every month [190]. The first randomized blind placebo-controlled study of EPO therapy in 22 patients with anemia and severe HF was performed in 2003 and had favorable results [51]. Other more recent studies had similar results [67, 74].

Nevertheless, the use of recombinant human EPO has some adverse effects. These adverse effects include the development or worsening of systemic hypertension, access site thrombosis in dialysis patients with arteriovenous shunts and generally increased thrombosis risk. Thus, the optimal hemoglobin level in patients with CKD is not yet known and the benefits must be judged and weighed against the risks of EPO use.

The CREATE study [72, 191] tried to investigate the effect of early anemia correction in patients with CKD on the cardiovascular risk which was assessed as the time to first cardiovascular event, including angina, acute congestive HF, MI, arrhythmias, sudden death, stroke, transient cerebrovascular ischemia, and manifestation of peripheral vascular disease. It included 603 patients with CKD not yet requiring renal replacement therapy (creatinine clearance 15–35 mL/minute) and moderate anemia (Hgb, 11.0–12.5 g/dL). Patients were randomized to early treatment or late treatment with epoetin beta administered subcutaneously. The early treatment group started epoetin therapy immediately, aiming for a target Hgb level of 13–15 g/dL. The late treatment group only started epoetin therapy once the Hgb level had declined to below 10.5 g/dL (target Hgb level 10.5–11.5 g/dL). After 3 years of follow-up, no difference was observed between the two groups in the cardiovascular events.

Another study, the CHOIR study, in patients with CKD was planned in order to find the "optimal" level of hemoglobin [71]. This study included 1432 patients with CKD who received epoetin alfa for the correction of their anemia. Patients were divided in two groups. The first group received a dose of epoetin alfa targeted to achieve a Hgb level of 13.5 g/dL and the other group received a dose targeted to achieve a level of 11.3 g/dL. The primary end point was a composite of death, MI, hospitalization for congestive HF, and stroke. After a follow-up period of 16 months, the group with high target Hgb had more cardiovascular events and no difference in the quality of life was observed between the two groups.

The PRESAM study included 4333 predialysis patients with CKD. It was observed that the use of EPO in the pre-dialysis period was associated with a lower incidence of HF, angina pectoris, and MI during this period [192]. Moreover, the mortality rate, and the hospitalization rate after dialysis was started, was also shown to be lower in those who received EPO in the predialysis period.

In a recent meta-analysis [193] of nine randomized trials which included 5143 patients with CKD, it was observed that there was a significantly higher risk of all-cause mortality and arteriovenous access thrombosis in the higher Hgb target group than in the lower Hgb target. The authors concluded that there is risk of major adverse events—including death—when Hgb is raised to 12–16 g/dL in CKD patients which is in the normal range for healthy individuals and suggests that there should be considered an upper limit for target Hgb concentrations in the next guidelines for anemia management in CKD which until now recommend the maintenance of Hgb concentration at 11g/dL. Similar results were found in a previous meta-analysis. This was a meta-analysis of controlled studies of anemia treatment in pre-dialysis and dialysis patients. It was concluded that the benefit of maintaining Hgb of up to 12 g/dL was associated with a lower all-cause mortality but there is no evidence of benefit by increasing Hgb above this level [194].

All these data clearly suggest that anemia indeed does play a role in the worsening of HF, but large randomized placebo-controlled studies are needed to confirm this. Furthermore, more studies are required on total correction of anemia in HF, CKD, and ESRD. These studies should ideally include patients with a wide range in Hgb levels and last for several years to recognize dysfunctions, which are slow in occurring.

Diabetes and anemia

Anemia is quite common in patients with DM and often goes unrecognized. Although data from prospective surveys are lacking, cross-sectional studies have shown a prevalence at least two times higher than that of the general population [181, 195]. A further and sharp increase of anemia prevalence has been observed in diabetics with micro- or macrovascular complications, especially those with various degrees of renal impairment. The prevalence of anemia seems to increase progressively with worsening renal failure[196]. In patients with diabetic nephropathy, frequencies of up to 70% have been reported [197]. Moreover, anemia is more common in diabetic nephropathy than in other renal diseases. For example, the Third National Health and Nutrition Examination Survey found that people in the general population with DM were nearly twice as likely to have anemia as people without DM but with a similar degree of renal impairment [198]. Finally, anemia develops earlier and is more severe in patients with DM than in patients with renal impairment from other causes [182]. The etiology of anemia in DM is complex, but a major factor seems to be the inability of the kidney to increase the circulating concentrations of EPO as a response to falling hemoglobin (functional EPO deficiency) [199]. This seems to happen even in the absence of overt diabetic nephropathy [200]. Additional, nonrenal factors include reduced erythrocyte survival [201], chronic systemic inflammation [202], occult blood loss, and hematinic deficiencies [203]. It has been reported that up to one-third of patients with DM have reduced iron availability [204]. Finally, drugs used for the treatment of DM and its complications may also precipitate anemia through various mechanisms. Thiazolidinendiones, for example, can cause a dilutional benign anemia through fluid retention and increase in plasma volume [205]. Metformin intake on the contrary has been associated with a decrease in both folic acid and vitamin B12 absorption [206]. The precise mechanism by which DM impairs renal EPO response remains unidentified. Although functional EPO deficiency is linked to renal dysfunction, the defect appears to be beyond that seen in other renal diseases. The predominance of damage to specific cells and vascular architecture of the renal tubulointerstitium, and the resulting systemic inflammation, autonomic neuropathy, and induction of inhibitors of EPO release, have all been suggested as contributors to impaired renal EPO production and release [207].

Anemia has been clearly associated with the presence and the progression of both microvascular and macrovascular complications in DM. Diabetic patients with anemia had an increased risk of nephropathy [208, 208], retinopathy [209], neuropathy [210], impaired wound healing [211], and macrovascular disease. Some of the risk of macrovascular disease may be attributed to nephropathy, a common cause of both anemia and CVD. However, anemia per se may also be independently associated with accelerated vascular disease [212]. Moreover, in diabetic patients with macrovascular disease anemia further worsens prognosis [19, 213]. Tissue hypoxia may be the common denominator linking anemia to organ-specific dysfunction and may account for the interaction between anemia and hyperglycemia on the progression of diabetic microvascular and macrovascular complications. Given that, anemia should be considered a nontraditional risk factor and its treatment might prevent or slow progression of DM complications. Small studies have shown that symptoms such as fatigue and exercise tolerance, and poor quality of life are improved when anemia is corrected with the administration of iron and EPO [214]. Signs and symptoms of HF have also been shown to improve in patients with DM and HF [65]. However, definitive data of the effect of anemia correction on morbidity and mortality are lacking. A recently completed clinical trial failed to show any regression in left ventricular hypetrophy after administration of epoetin beta for correction of anemia to an Hb target level of 13–15 g/dL in diabetic patients with chronic kidney disease [215]. Nevertheless, normalization of Hb level prevented an additional increase in left ventricular hypertrophy, was safe, and improved quality of life in these patients. More large-outcome studies are now in progress and are expected to provide us with valuable information on the benefits of anemia correction in patients with either DM alone or DM with renal dysfunction [201].

Risk of anemia in CABG and valve surgery

Both preoperative and perioperative anemias are major components of the high-risk profile of patients who are candidates for cardiac surgery [216]. Clearly, bleeding and the addition of nonhematic fluids during cardiopulmonary bypass (CPB) leading to hemodilution are the main causes of anemia in the surgical patient. Beyond blood loss during the procedure, activation of the contact coagulation factors during extracorporeal circulation causes activation of the complex fibrinolytic system with subsequent hemorrhagic diathesis [217, 218]. Moreover, CPB shortens RBC life by increasing fragility [219, 220]. On the contrary, the current practice of CPB, which entails the addition of 1.5–2 L or more of crystalloid and colloid fluids (used to prime the CPB circuit), frequently results in marked hemodilution, often to hematocrit concentrations <20% [221]. Finally, drugs most commonly the antithrombotic and antiplatelet agents contribute to the development of bleeding and consequent anemia [216].

Anemia has an adverse impact on the prognosis of patients who undergo cardiac surgery. Data from a large US registry of CABG patients have shown that the lowest hematocrit during CPB is significantly associated with increased risk of in-hospital mortality, intra- or postoperative placement of an intra-aortic balloon pump and return to CPB after attempted weaning [222]. Others have shown an independent, nonlinear relationship between nadir hematocrit concentration during CPB and acute renal failure necessitating dialysis support [221]. The risk of stroke is also increased in these patients [223].

Several strategies have been developed to prevent and treat perioperative anemia in cardiac surgery. However, transfusion of RBCs remains the mainstay of treatment. The lower cutoff point of Hgb levels for deciding to transfuse remained a controversial issue for many years. It was initially believed that a Hgb concentration of 10 g/dL (hematocrit 30%) was essential in surgical patients and that transfusion should be undertaken whenever necessary to achieve it [224]. This concept was essentially challenged in the 1980s not by the appearance of new evidence but by the realization that human immunodeficiency virus (HIV) was transmissible by blood transfusion. Physiology studies showed that oxygen delivery in acute normovolaemic anemia was similar at a Hgb concentration of 7 g/dL to that at 13 g/dL. On the strength of this observation, and the knowledge that many severely anemic patients (for example those with renal failure) can safely be brought through anesthesia and surgery, a consensus conference encouraged the belief that a Hgb level of 7 g/dL was generally acceptable [225].

In the past decade, more evidence about the lowest tolerable Hgb level has become available. Experimental animals can survive hemodilution to a hematocrit value of 4% [226]. Human studies are rare in this field, but it has been shown recently that 32 resting healthy subjects tolerated acute normovolemic anemia to a Hgb level of 5 g/dL without a rise in plasma lactate levels, although two subjects developed significant ST segment changes on Holter ECG monitors [227]. However, patients who have surgery for cardiac disease may not tolerate these low levels of hemoglobin. In a series of 4470 patients admitted to Canadian intensive care units, a tendency to increased mortality was observed in patients with cardiac disease when Hgb values fell below 9.5 g/dL, a trend which could be reversed by blood transfusion [228].

Given the fact that CABG and other cardiac procedures are among the most frequently performed operations and account for ~10% of all RBC units transfused [229] as well the important hazards associated with blood transfusion, recently published guidelines for cardiac surgery have indicated that: "...With hemoglobin levels below 6 g/dL, RBC transfusion is reasonable, as this can be lifesaving. Transfusion is reasonable in most postoperative patients whose hemoglobin is <7 g/dL, but no high-level evidence supports this recommendation. (Level of evidence C) ..." [216].

Alternative to blood transfusion strategies are currently been investigated as well. These strategies include drugs like antifibrinolytic agents: aprotinin is not more available), Desmopressin is no more recommended for cardiac surgery patients, recombinant factor VIIA[230–232] not demonstrated and EPO[233–235] remains a matter of debate, new devices that aid blood concentration and finally, new perfusion techniques like intraoperative autotransfusion, intraoperative autologous donation, preoperative autologous blood donation, postoperative shed blood reinfusion, etc. [216].

Conclusion

A close association between anemia and the development of CVD is being increasingly recognized over the recent years. In the general population, anemia is associated with increased cardiovascular morbidity. There seems to be a potentially causative role in the development of CVD both in subjects with or without cardiovascular risk factors and in patients with renal dysfunction. Anemia also seems to aggravate the prognosis of patients who already suffer from cardiovascular complications, such as those with congestive HF. Anemia is quite common among patients with HF, encountered in frequencies hovering around 30%. Anemia may also precipitate myocardial ischemia, particularly in patients with CAD, whereby ischemia can occur with even mild degree of anemia.

The impact of anemia therapy on outcomes in CVD has been intensively investigated over the recent years. Definitive evidence is still lacking and anemia correction has not been incorporated into the routine clinical practice yet. Correcting anemia through blood transfusions, although guided by common sense, has been shown to be potentially harmful especially when used liberally and aggressively as a treatment strategy. On the contrary, the administration of EPO seems promising, especially for the anemic patients with CKD, HF, or both. However, concerns have been raised about the safety of this type of treatment, since EPO has been associated with an increased risk of hypertension and thrombosis.

References

1. Givertz MM, Colucci WS, Braunwald E. Clinical aspects of heart failure, pulmonary edema, high-output failure. In: Zipes DP, Libby P, Bonow RO, Braunwald E (eds) *Braunwald's Heart Disease*, 7th edn. Elsevier Saunders, Philadelphia, 2005, pp. 539–68.
2. Beard JL, Tobin BW, Smith SM. Effects of iron repletion and correction of anemia on norepinephrine turnover and thyroid metabolism in iron deficiency. Proc Soc Exp Biol Med 1990;193:306–12.
3. Muller R, Steffen HM, Brunner R, et al. Changes in alpha adrenergic system and increase in blood pressure with recombinant human erythropoietin (rHuEpo) therapy for renal anemia. Clin Invest Med 1991;14:614–22.
4. Anand IS, Chandrashekhar Y, Wander GS, et al. Endothelium-derived relaxing factor is important in mediating high output state in chronic anemia. J Am Coll Cardiol 1995;25:1402–7.
5. Martin C, Yu AY, Jiang BH, et al. Cardiac hypertrophy in chronically anemic sheep: increased vascularization is associated with increased myocardial expression of vascular endothelial growth factor and hypoxia-inducible factor 1. Am J Obstet Gynecol 1998;178:527–34.
6. Anand IS, Chandrashekhar Y, Ferrari R, et al. Pathogenesis of oedema in chronic severe anemia: studies of body water and sodium, renal function, haemodynamic variables, and plasma hormones. Br Heart J 1993;70:357–62.
7. Grossman W. Cardiac hypertrophy: useful adaptation or pathological process? Am J Med 1980;69:576–84.
8. Varat MA, Adolph RJ, Fowler NO. Cardiovascular effects of anemia. Am Heart J 1972;83:415–26.
9. Kamiya A, Togawa T. Adaptive regulation of wall shear stress to flow change in the canine carotid artery. Am J Physiol 1980;239:H14–21.
10. Metivier F, Marchais SJ, Guerin AP, et al. Pathophysiology of anaemia: focus on the heart and blood vessels. Nephrol Dial Transplant 2000;15(Suppl. 3):14–18.
11. Gibbons GH, Dzau VJ. The emerging concept of vascular remodeling. N Engl J Med 1994;330:1431–8.
12. Katz AM. Cardiomyopathy of overload. A major determinant of prognosis in congestive heart failure. N Engl J Med 1990;322:100–111.
13. London GM, Fabiani F, Marchais SJ, et al. Uremic cardiomyopathy: an inadequate left ventricular hypertrophy. Kidney Int 1987;3(1):973–80.
14. Foley RN, Parfrey PS, Hamett JD, et al. The impact of anaemia on cardiomyopathy, morbidity and mortality in end- stage renal disease. Am J Kidney Dis 1996;28:53–61.
15. Levin A, Thompson CR, Ethier J, et al. Left ventricular mass index increase in early renal disease: impact of decline in hemoglobin. Am J Kidney Dis 1999;34:125–34.
16. Amin GM, Tighiouart H, Weiner DE, et al. Hematocrit and left ventricular mass: The Framingham Heart Study. J Am Coll Cardiol 2004;43:1276–82.
17. Abramson JL, Jurkovitz CT, Vaccarino V, et al. Chronic kidney disease, anemia, and incident stroke in a middle-aged, communitybased population: the ARIC study. Kidney Int 2003;64:610–15.

18. Al-Ahmad A, Rand WM, Manjunath G, et al. Reduced kidney function and anemia as risk factors for mortality in patients with left ventricular dysfunction. J Am Coll Cardiol 2001;38:955–62.
19. McClellan WM, Flanders WD, Langston RD, et al. Anemia and renal insufficiency are independent risk factors for death among patients with congestive heart failure admitted to community hospitals: a population-based study. J Am Soc Nephrol 2002;13:1928–36.
20. Sarnak MS, Tighiouart H, Manjunath G, et al. Anemia as a risk factor for cardiovascular disease in the Atherosclerosis Risk in Communities (ARIC) Study. J Am Coll Cardiol 2002;40:27–33.
21. Lindenfeld J. Prevalence of anemia and effects on mortality in patients with heart failure. Am Heart J 2005;149:408–13.
22. Mehta PA, Cowie MR. Epidemiology and pathophysiology of heart failure. Medicine 2006;34(6):210–214.
23. Fortune JB, Feustel PJ, Saifi J, et al. Influence of hematocrit on cardiopulmonary function after acute hemorrhage. J Trauma 1987;27:243–7.
24. Hebert PC, Yetisir E, Martin C, et al. Transfusion requirements in Critical Care Investigators for the Canadian Critical Care Trials Group. Is a low transfusion threshold safe in critically ill patients with cardiovascular diseases? Crit Care Med 2001;29:227–34.
25. Hebert PC, Wells G, Blajchman MA, et al. A multicenter, randomized controlled clinical trial of transfusion requirements in critical care. N Engl J Med 1999;340:409–41.
26. Komajda M. Anemia in chronic heart failure: should we treat it and how? J Am Coll Cardiol 2007;49(7):763–4.
27. Muirhead N, Bargman J, Burgess E, et al. Evidence-based recommendations for the clinical use of recombinant human erythropoietin. Am J Kidney Dis 1995;26(Suppl. 1):S1–24.
28. Churchill DN, Muirhead N, Goldstein M, et al. Probability of thrombosis of vascular access among hemodialysis patients treated with recombinant human erythropoietin. J Am Soc Nephrol 1994;4:1809–13.
29. Mix TC, Brenner RM, Cooper ME, et al. Rationale—trial to reduce cardiovascular events with aranesp therapy (TREAT): evolving the management of cardiovascular risk in patients with chronic kidney disease. Am Heart J 2005;149:408–13.
30. Young JB, Anand IS, Diaz R, et al. Reduction of events with darbepoetin alfa in heart failure (RED-HF)TM trial. J Card Fail 2006;12(Suppl. 1): S77.
31. Levy D, Kenchaiah S, Larson MG, et al. Long term trends in the incidence of and survival with heart failure. N Engl J Med 2002;347:1397–402.
32. Cleland FGF, Cohen-Solal A, Aguillar JC, et al. Management of heart failure in primary care (The IMPROVEMENT of heart failure programme): an international survey. Lancet 2002;360:1631–9.
33. Tang WHW, Miller H, Partin M, et al. Anemia in ambulatory patients with chronic heart failure: a single center clinical experience derived from electronic medical records. J Am Coll Cardiol 2003;41(Suppl.):157A.
34. Okonko DO, Anker SD. Anemia in chronic heart failure: pathogenetic mechanisms. J Card Fail 2004;10(Suppl. 1):S5–9.
35. Maggioni AP, Anand I, Gottlieb SO, et al. Effects of valsartan on morbidity and mortality in patients with heart failure not receiving angiotensin-converting enzyme inhibitors. J Am Coll Cardiol 2002;40:1414–21.
36. Silverberg DS, Wexler D, Blum M, et al. The use of subcutaneous erythropoietin and intravenous iron for the treatment of the anemia of severe, resistant congestive heart failure improves cardiac and renal function and functional cardiac class, and markedly reduces hospitalizations. J Am Coll Cardiol 2000;35:1737–44.
37. Komajda M, Anker SD, Charleswort A, et al. The impact of new onset anemia on morbidity and mortality in chronic heart failure: results from COMET. Eur Heart J 2006;27:1440–46.
38. Ezekowitz JA, McAlister FA, Armstrong PW. Anemia is common in heart failure and is associated with poor outcomes. Circulation 2003;107; 223–5.
39. Go AS, Yang J, Ackerson LM, et al. Hemoglobin level, chronic kidney disease, and the risks of death and hospitalization in adults with chronic heart failure: the Anemia in Chronic Heart Failure: Outcomes and Resource Utilization (ANCHOR) study. Circulation 2006;113:2713–23.
40. Horwich TB, Fonarow GC, Hamilton MA, et al. Anemia is associated with worse symptoms, greater impairment in functional capacity and a significant increase in mortality in patients with advanced heart failure. J Am Coll Cardiol 2002;39:1780–86.
41. Salem DN, Levey AS, Sarnak MJ. Reduced kidney function and anemia as risk factors for mortality in

patients with left ventricular dysfunction. J Am Coll Cardiol 2001;38:955–62.
42. Anand I, McMurray JJ, Whitmore J, et al. Anemia and its relationship to clinical outcome in heart failure. Circulation 2004;110:149–54.
43. Kosiborod M, Smith GL, Radford MJ, et al. The prognostic importance of anemia in patients with heart failure. Am J Med 2003;114:112–9.
44. Silverberg DS, Wexler D, Blum M, et al. Erythropoietin should be part of congestive heart failure management. Kidney Int 2003;64(Suppl. 87):S40–47.
45. Jurkovitz CT, Abramson JL, Vaccarino LV, et al. Association of high serum creatinine and anemia increases the risk of coronary events: results from the prospective community-based atherosclerosis risk in communities (ARIC) study. J Am Soc Nephrol 2003;14:2919–25.
46. McMahon, LP, Roger SD, Levin A. Development, prevention, and potential reversal of left ventricular hypertrophy in chronic kidney disease. J Am Soc Nephrol 2004;15:1640–47.
47. Volpe M, Tritto C, Testa U, et al. Blood levels of erythropoietin in congestive heart failure and correlation with clinical, hemodynamic, and hormonal profiles. Am J Cardiol 1994;74:468–73.
48. Van Der Meer P, Voors AA, Lipsic E, et al. Prognostic value of plasma erythropoietin on mortality in patients with chronic heart failure. J Am Coll Cardiol 2004;44:63–7.
49. Gilbertson D, Li S, Murray AM. Competing risks of death *vs* ESRD in Medicare beneficiaries age 65+ with chronic kidney disease, CHF, and anemia. J Am Soc Nephrol 2002;13(Suppl.):A848.
50. Androne AS, Katz SD, Lund L, et al. Hemodilution is common in patients with advanced heart failure. Circulation 2003;107; 226–9.
51. Mancini DM, Katz SD, Lang CC, et al. Effect of erythropoietin on exercise capacity in patients with moderate to severe chronic heart failure. Circulation 2003;107:294–9.
52. Chatterjee B, Nydegger UE, Mohacsi P. Serum erythropoietin in heart failure patients treated with ACE-inhibitors or AT(1) antagonists. Eur J Heart Fail 2000;2:393–8.
53. Mrug M, Stopka T, Julian BA, et al. Angiotensin II stimulates proliferation of normal early erythroid progenitors. J Clin Invest 1997;100:2310–14.
54. Macdougall IC. The role of ACE inhibitors and angiotensin II receptor blockers in the response to epoetin. Nephrol Dial Transplant 1999;14:1836–41.
55. Erturk S, Ates K, Duman N, et al. Unresponsiveness to recombinant human erythropoietin in haemodialysis patients: possible implications of angiotensin converting enzyme inhibitors. Nephrol Dial Transplant 1996;11:396–7.
56. Iversen PO, Woldbaek PR, Tonnessen T, et al. Decreased hematopoiesis in bone marrow of mice with congestive heart failure. Am J Physiol Regul Integr Comp Physiol 2002;282:R166–72.
57. Weiss G. Pathogenesis and treatment of anaemia of chronic disease. Blood Rev 2002;16:87–96.
58. Bolger AP, Doehner W, Sharma R, et al. Anemia in chronic heart failure: the relationship to inflammatory cytokine expression and prognostic importance. Circulation 2002;106(Suppl.):570–71.
59. Torre-Amione G, Bozkurt B, Deswal A, et al. An overview of tumor necrosis factor alpha and the failing human heart. Curr Opin Cardiol 1999;14: 206–10.
60. Sharma R, Anker SD. Cytokines, apoptosis and cachexia: the potential for TNF antagonism. Int J Cardiol 2002;85:161–71.
61. Cromie N, Lee C, Struthers AD. Anaemia in chronic heart failure: what is its frequency in the UK and its underlying causes? Heart 2002;87:377–8.
62. Casadevall N. Cellular mechanism of resistance to erythropoietin. Nephrol Dial Transplant 1995;10: 27–30.
63. Locatelli F, Alijama P, Barany P, et al. European Best Practice Guidelines Group. Revised European best practice guidelines for the management of anaemia in patients with chronic renal failure. Nephrol Dial Transplant 2004;19(Suppl. 2):ii1–47.
64. Silverberg DS, Wexler D, Sheps D, et al. The effect of correction of mild anemia in severe, resistant congestive heart failure using subcutaneous erythropoietin and intravenous iron: a randomized controlled study. J Am Coll Cardiol 2001;37:1775–80.
65. Silverberg DS, Wexler D, Blum M, et al. The effect of correction of anemia in diabetics and non-diabetics with severe resistant heart failure by subcutaneous erythropoietin and intravenous iron. Nephrol Dial Transplant 2003;18:141–6.
66. Silverberg DS, Wexler D, Blum M, et al. Effects of treatment with epoetin beta on outcomes in patients with anaemia and chronic heart failure. Kidney Blood Press Res 2005;28:41–7.
67. Palazzuoli A, Silverberg D, Iovine F, et al. Erythropoietin improves anemia, exercise tolerance and renal function and reduces B-type natriuretic

peptide and hospitalization in patients with heart failure and anemia. Am Heart J 2006;152:1096. e9–15.

68. Ponikowski P, Anker SD, Szachniewicz J, et al. Effect of darbepoetin alfa on exercise tolerance in anemic patients with symptomatic chronic heart failure: a randomized, double-blind, placebo-controlled trial. J Am Coll Cardiol 2007;49:753–62.
69. Coletta AP, Tin L, Loh PH, et al. Clinical trials update from the European Society of Cardiology heart failure meeting: TNT subgroup analysis, darbepoetin alfa, FERRIC-HF and KW-3902. Eur J Heart Fail 2006;8:547–9.
70. Besarab A, Bolton WK, Browne JK, et al. The effects of normal as compared with low hematocrit values in patients with cardiac disease who are receiving hemodialysis and epoetin. N Engl J Med 1998;39:584–90.
71. Singh AK, Szczech L, Tang KL, et al. Correction of anemia with epoetin alfa in chronic kidney disease. N Engl J Med 2006;355:2085–98.
72. Drüeke TB, Locatelli F, Clyne N, et al. Normalization of hemoglobin level in patients with chronic kidney disease and anemia. N Engl J Med 2006;355:2071–84.
73. Ma JZ, Ebben J, Xia H, et al. Hematocrit level and associated mortality in hemodialysis patients. J Am Soc Nephrol 1999;10:610–19.
74. Bolger AP, Bartlett FR, Penston HS, et al. Intravenous iron alone for the treatment of anemia in patients with chronic heart failure. J Am Coll Cardiol 2006;48:1225–7.
75. Beck-da-Silva L, Rohde LE, Pereira-Barretto AC, et al. Rationale and design of the IRON-HF study: a randomized trial to assess the effects of iron supplementation in heart failure patients with anemia. J Card Fail 2007;13:14–17.
76. Al Falluji N, Lawrence-Nelson J, Kostis JB, et al. Effect of anemia on 1-year mortality in patients with acute myocardial infarction. Am Heart J 2002;144:636–41.
77. Bindra K, Berry C, Rogers J, et al. Abnormal hemoglobin levels in acute coronary syndromes. Q J Med 2006;99:851–62.
78. Arant CB, Wessel TR, Olson MB, et al. Hemoglobin level is an independent predictor for adverse cardiovascular outcomes in women undergoing evaluation for chest pain—results from the national heart, lung, and blood institute women's ischemia syndrome evaluation study. J Am Coll Cardiol 2004;43:2009–14.
79. Nikolsky E, Mehran R, Aymong ED, et al. Impact of anemia on outcomes of patients undergoing percutaneous coronary interventions. Am J Cardiol 2004;94:1023–7.
80. Yoshikawa H, Powell WJ Jr, Bland JH, et al. The effect of acute anemia on experimental myocardial ischemia. Am J Cardiol 1973;32:670–78.
81. Wu WC, Rathore SS, Radford MJ, et al. Blood transfusion in elderly patients with acute myocardial infarction. New Engl J Med 2001;345:1230–36.
82. Carson JL, Duff A, Poses RM, et al. Effect of anemia and cardiovascular disease on surgical mortality and morbidity. Lancet 1996;348:1055–60.
83. Carson JL, Duff A, Berlin JA, et al. Perioperative blood transfusion and postoperative mortality. JAMA 1998;279:199–205.
84. Lipsic E, Van Der Horstc ICC, Voorsa AA, et al. Hemoglobin levels and 30-day mortality in patients after myocardial infarction. Int J Cardiol 2005;100:289–92.
85. Sabatine MS, Morrow DA, Giugliano R, et al. Association of hemoglobin levels with clinical outcomes in acute coronary syndromes. Circulation 2005;111:2042–9.
86. Meneveau N, Schiele F, Seronde MF, et al. Anemia for risk assessment of patients with acute coronary syndromes. Am J Cardiol 2009;103:442–7.
87. Cavusoglu E, Chopra V, Gupta A, et al. Usefulness of anemia in men an independent predictor of two-year cardiovascular outcome in patients presenting with acute coronary syndrome. Am J Cardiol 2006;98:580–84.
88. Vaglio J, Safley DM, Rahman M, et al. Relation of anemia at discharge to survival after acute coronary syndromes. Am J Cardiol 2005;96:496–9.
89. Langston R, Presley R, Flanders WD, et al. Renal insufficiency and anemia are independent risk factors for death among patients with acute myocardial infarction. Kidney Int 2003;64:1398–405.
90. Nikolsky E, Aymong ED, Halkin A, et al. Impact of anemia in patients with acute myocardial infarction undergoing primary percutaneous coronary intervention: analysis from the Controlled Abciximab and Device Investigation to Lower Late Angioplasty Complications (CADILLAC) Trial. J Am Coll Cardiol 2004;44:547–53.
91. Berry C, Kelly J, Cobbe SM, et al. Comparison of femoral bleeding complications after coronary angiography versus percutaneous coronary intervention. Am J Cardiol 2004;94:361–3.

92. Rao SV, Eikelboom JA, GrangerCB, et al. Bleeding and blood transfusion issues in non-ST-segment elevation acute coronary syndromes. Eur Heart J 2007;28:1193–204.
93. LeMay MR, Wells GA, Labinaz M, et al. Combined angioplasty and pharmacological intervention versus thrombolysis alone in acute myocardial infarction (CAPITAL AMI Study). J Am Coll Cardiol 2005;46(3):417–24.
94. Thomas MC, Cooper ME, Tsalamandris C, et al. Anemia with impaired erythropoietin response in diabetic patients. Arch Int Med 2005;165:466–9.
95. Means RT. Advances in the anemia of chronic disease. Int J Hematol 1999;70:7–12.
96. Ishani A, Weinhandl E, Zhao ZH, et al. Angiotensin-converting enzyme inhibitor as a risk factor for the development of anemia, and the impact of incident anemia on mortality in patients with left ventricular dysfunction. J Am Coll Cardiol 2005;45:391–9.
97. Eikelboom JW, Mehta SR, Anand SS, et al. Adverse impact of bleeding on prognosis in patients with acute coronary syndromes. Circulation 2006;114:774–82.
98. Manoukian SV, Feit F, Mehran R, et al. Impact of major bleeding on 30-day mortality and clinical outcomes in patients with acute coronary syndromes. An analysis from the ACUITY trial. J Am Coll Cardiol 2007;49:1362–8.
99. Dauerman HL, Lessard D, Yarzebski J, et al. Bleeding complications in patients with anemia and acute myocardial infarction. Am J Cardiol 2005;96(10):1379–83.
100. Yang X, Alexander KP, Chen AY, et al. CRUSADE Investigators. The implications of blood transfusions for patients with non-ST-segment elevation acute coronary syndromes: results from the CRUSADE national quality improvement initiative. J Am Coll Cardiol 2005;46:1490–95.
101. Rao SV, Jollis JG, Harrington RA, et al. The relationship of blood transfusion and clinical outcomes in patients with acute coronary syndromes. JAMA 2004;292:1555–62.
102. Singla I, Zahid M, Good CB, et al. Impact of blood transfusions in patients presenting with anemia and suspected acute coronary syndrome. Am J Cardiol 2007;99:1119–21.
103. Aronson D, Dann EJ, Bonstein L, et al. Impact of red blood cell transfusion on clinical outcomes in patients with acute myocardial infraction. Am J Cardiol 2008;102(8):1116–17.
104. Alexander KP, Chen AY, Wang TY, et al. Transfusion practice and outcomes in non-STsegment elevation acute coronary syndromes. Am Heart J 2008;155(6):1047–53.
105. Stamler JS, Jia L, Eu JP, et al. Blood flow regulation by S-nitrosohemoglobin in the physiological oxygen gradient. Science 1997;276:2034–7.
106. Weed RI, LaCelle PL, Merrill EW. Erythrocyte metabolism and cellular deformability. Vox Sang 1969;17:32–3.
107. Longster GH, Buckley T, Sikorski J, et al. Scanning electron microscope studies of red cell morphology. Changes occurring in red cell shape during storage and post transfusion. Vox Sang 1972;22:161–70.
108. Perrotta PL, Snyder EL. Non-infectious complications of transfusion therapy. Blood Rev 2001;15:69–83.
109. Belonje AM, Voors AA, van Gilst WH, et al. HEBE III investigators. Effects of erythropoietin after an acute myocardial infarction: rationale and study design of a prospective, randomized, clinical trial (HEBE III). Am Heart J 2008;155:817–22.
110. United States Renal Data System. *USRDS 2005, Annual Data Report*. National Institute of Health, National Institute of Diabetes and Digestive and Kidney Diseases, Bethesda, MD, 2005.
111. National Kidney Foundation. K/DOQI clinical practice guidelines for chronic kidney disease evaluation, classification and stratification. Am J Kidney Dis 2002;39(Suppl. 1):S1–266.
112. Redfield MM, Jacobsen SJ, Burnett JC, et al. Burden of systolic and diastolic ventricular dysfunction in the community: appreciating the scope of the heart failure epidemic. JAMA 2003;289:194–202.
113. Cheung AK, Sarnak MJ, Yan G, et al. Cardiac diseases in maintenance hemodialysis patients: results of the HEMO Study. Kidney Int 2004;65:2380–89.
114. Chavers BM, Li S, Collins AJ, Herzog CA. Cardiovascular disease in paediatric chronic dialysis patients. Kidney Int 2002;62:648–53.
115. Groothoff J, Gruppen M, de Groot E, Offringa M. Cardiovascular disease as a late complication of end-stage renal disease in children. Perit Dial Int 2005;25(Suppl. 3):S123–6.
116. Collins AJ, Li S, Ma JZ, Herzog C. Cardiovascular disease in end-stage renal disease patients. Am J Kidney Dis 2001;38(Suppl. 1):S26–9.
117. Foley RN, Parfrey PS, Harnett JD, et al. Clinical and echocardiographic disease in patients starting end-stage renal disease therapy. Kidney Int 1995;47:186–92.

118. Silverberg DS, Wexler D, Blum M, Iaina A. The cardio renal anaemia syndrome: correcting anaemia in patients with resistant congestive heart failure can improve both cardiac and renal function and reduces hospitalization. Clin Nephrol 2003;60(Suppl. 1):S93–102.
119. Silverberg DS, Wexler D, Blum M, et al. The interaction between heart failure, renal failure and anaemia- the cardiorenal anaemia syndrome. Blood Purif 2004;22:277–28.
120. McAlister FA, Ezekowitz J, Tonelli M, Armstrong PW. Renal insufficiency and heart failure: prognostic and therapeutic implications from a prospective cohort study. Circulation 2004;109:1004–9.
121. Dries DL, Exner DV, Domanski MJ, Greenberg B, Stevenson IW. The prognostic implications of renal insufficiency in asymptomatic and symptomatic patients with left ventricular systolic dysfunction. J Am Coll Cardiol 2000;35:681–9.
122. Stack AG, Bloembergen WE. A cross-section study of the prevalence and clinical correlates of congestive failure among incident US dialysis patients. Am J Kidney Dis 2001;38:991–1000.
123. Brenner BM, Cooper ME, de Zeeuw D, et al., for the RENAAL Study Investigators. Effects of losartan on renal and cardiovascular outcomes in patients with type 2 diabetes and nephropathy. N Engl J Med 2001;345:861–9.
124. Adams KF, Fonarow GC, Emerman CL, et al. Characteristics and outcomes of patients hospitalized for heart failure in the United States: rationale, design, and preliminary observations from the first 100,000 cases in the Acute Decompensated Heart Failure National Registry (ADHERE). Am Heart J 2005;149:209–16.
125. Go AS, Chertow GM, Fan D, et al. Chronic kidney disease and the risks of death, cardiovascular events, and hospitalization. N Engl J Med 2004;351:1296–305.
126. McCullough PA. Cardio renal risk: an important clinical intersection. Rev Cardiovasc Med 2002;3:71–76.
127. Greaves SC, Gamble GD, Collins JF, et al. Determinants of left ventricular hypertrophy and systolic dysfunction in chronic renal failure. Am J Kidney Dis 1994;24:768–76.
128. Clyne N, Lins LE, Pehrsson SK. Occurrence and significance of heart disease in uraemia. Scand J Urol Nephrol 1986;20:307–11.
129. Ansari A, Kaupke CJ, Vaziri ND, Miller R, Barbari A. Cardiac pathology in patients with end-stage renal disease maintained on hemodialysis. Int J Artif Organs 1993;16:31–6.
130. Oh J, Wunsch R, Turzer M, et al. Advanced coronary and carotid arteriopathy in young adults with childhood-onset chronic renal failure. Circulation 2002;106:100–105.
131. Boaz M, Smetana S, Weinstein T, et al. Secondary prevention with antioxidants of cardiovascular disease in endstage renal disease (SPACE): randomised placebo-controlled trial. Lancet 2000;356:1213–8.
132. Witko-Sarsat V, Friedlander M, Nguyen Khoa T, et al. Advanced oxidation protein products as novel mediators of inflammation and monocyte activation in chronic renal failure. J Immunol 1998;161:2524–32.
133. Stenvinkel P, Heimburger O, Paultre F, et al. Strong association between malnutrition, inflammation, and atherosclerosis in chronic renal failure. Kidney Int 1999;55:1899–911.
134. Ridker PM, Hennekens CH, Buring JE, Rifai N. C-reactive protein and other markers of inflammation in the prediction of cardiovascular disease in women. N Engl J Med 2000;342:836–43.
135. Zimmermann J, Herrlinger S, Pruy A, et al. Inflammation enhances cardiovascular risk and mortality in hemodialysis patients. Kidney Int 1999;55:648–58.
136. Block GA, Hulbert-Shearon TE, Levin NW, Port FK. Association of serum phosphorus and calciumx-phosphate product with mortality risk in chronic hemodialysis patients: a national study. Am J Kidney Dis 1998;31:607–17.
137. Ganesh SK, Stack AG, Levin NW, et al. Association of elevated serum PO(4), CaxPO(4) product, and parathyroid hormone with cardiac mortality risk in chronic hemodialysis patients. J Am Soc Nephrol 2001;12:2131–8.
138. Narang R, Ridout D, Nonis C, Kooner JS. Serum calcium, phosphorus and albumin levels in relation to the angiographic severity of coronary artery disease. Int J Cardiol 1997;60:73–9.
139. Raine AE, Seymour AM, Robert AFC, et al. Impairment of cardiac function and energetics in experimental renal failure. J Clin Invest 1993;92:2934–40.
140. Ritz E, Koch M. Morbidity and mortality due to hypertension in patients with renal failure. Am J Kidney Dis 1993;21:113–8.
141. Amann K, Ritz C, Adamczak M, Ritz E. Why is coronary heart disease of uraemic patients so frequent and so devastating? Nephrol Dial Transplant 2003;18:631–40.

142. Malmberg K. Prospective randomised study of intensive insulin treatment on long term survival after acute myocardial infarction in patients with diabetes mellitus. DIGAMI (Diabetes Mellitus, Insulin Glucose Infusion in Acute Myocardial Infarction) Study Group. BMJ 1997;314:1512–5.
143. Van Den Berghe G, Wouters P, Weekers F, et al. Intensive insulin therapy in the critically ill patients. N Engl J Med 2001;345:1359–67.
144. Periyasamy SM, Chen J, Cooney D, et al. Effects of uremic serum on isolated cardiac myocyte calcium cycling and contractile function. Kidney Int 2001;60:2367–76.
145. Anversa P, Nadal-Ginard B. Myocyte renewal and ventricular remodelling. Nature 2002;415:240–43.
146. Rump LC, Amann K, Orth S, Ritz E. Sympathetic overactivity in renal disease: a window to understand progression and cardiovascular complications of uraemia? Nephrol Dial Transplant 2000;15:1735–8.
147. Klein IH, Ligtenberg G, Oey PL, Koomans HA, Blankestijn PJ. Sympathetic activity is increased in polycystic kidney disease and is associated with hypertension. J Am Soc Nephrol 2001;12:2427–33.
148. Herzog CA, Ma JZ, Collins AJ. Poor long-term survival after acute myocardial infarction among patients on long-term dialysis. N Engl J Med 1998;339:799–805.
149. Cice G, Ferrara L, Di Benedetto A. Dilated cardiomyopathy in dialysis patients—beneficial effects of carvedilol: a double-blind, placebo-controlled trial. J Am Coll Cardiol 2001;37:407–11.
150. Cice G, Ferrara L, D'Andrea A. Carvedilol increases two year survival in dialysis patients with dilated cardiomyopathy. J Am Coll Cardiol 2003;41:1438–44.
151. Erdmann E, Lechat P, Verkenne P, et al. Results from post-hoc analyses of the CIBIS II trial: effect of bisoprolol on high-risk patient groups with chronic heart failure. Eur J Heart Fail 2001;3:469–79.
152. Bragg JL, Mason NA, Maroni BJ, Held PJ, Young EW. Beta-adrenergic antagonist utilization among hemodialysis (HD) patients. J Am Soc Nephrol 2001;12:321A.
153. Zuanetti G, Maggioni AP, Keane W, Ritz E. Nephrologists neglect administration of betablockers to dialysed diabetic patients. Nephrol Dial Transplant 1997;12:2497–500.
154. Amann K, Breitbach M, Ritz E, Mall G. Myocyte/capillary mismatch in the heart of uremic patients. J Am Soc Nephrol 1998;9:1018–22.
155. Amann K, Miltenberger-Miltenyi G, Simonaviciene A, et al. Remodeling of resistance arteries in renal failure: effect of endothelin receptor blockade. J Am Soc Nephrol 2001;12:2040–50.
156. Levin A, Singer J, Thompson CR, Ross H, Lewis M. Prevalent left ventricular hypertrophy in the predialysis population: identifying opportunities for intervention. Am J Kidney Dis 1996;27:347–54.
157. London GM. Cardiovascular disease in chronic renal failure: Pathophysiologic aspects. Semin Dial 2003;16(2):85–94.
158. Bongartz LG, Cramer MJ, Doevendans PA, et al. The severe cardiorenal syndrome:"Guyton revisited". Eur Heart J 2005;26:11–7.
159. Johnson DB, Dell'Italia LJ. Cardiac hypertrophy and failure in hypertension. Curr Opin Nephrol Hypertens 1996;5:186–91.
160. Katz AM. The cardiomyopathy of overload: an unnatural growth response in the hypertrophied heart. Ann Intern Med 1994;121:363–71.
161. Aessopos A, Deftereos S, Farmakis D, et al. Cardiovascular echocardiographic study. Clin Invest Med 2004;27:265–73.
162. Astor BC, Arnett DK, Brown A, Coresh J. Association of kidney function with left ventricular morphology among African Americans: the Atherosclerotic Risk in Communities (ARIC) study. Am J Kidney Dis 2004;43:836–45.
163. Olivetti G, Lagrasta C, Quaini F, et al. Capillary growth in anaemia induced ventricular remodelling in the rat heart. Circ Res 1989;65:1182–92.
164. Olivetti G, Quaini F, Lagrasta C, et al. Myocyte cellular hypertophy and hyperplasia contribute to ventricular wall modelling in anaemia induced cardiac hypertrophy in rats. Am J Pathol 1992;141:227–39.
165. Rossi MA, Carillo SV. Electron microscopic study on the cardiac hypertrophy induced by iron deficiency in the rat. Br J Exp Pathol 1983;64:373–87.
166. Rakusan K, Cicutti N, Kolar F. Effect of anaemia on cardiac function, microvascular structure and capillary hematocrit in rat hearts. Am J Physiol Heart Circ Physiol 2001;280:H1407–14.
167. Schunkert H, Hense HW. A heart price to pay for anaemia. Nephrol Dial Transplant 2001;16:445–8.
168. Davis LE, Hohimer AR. Hemodynamics and organ flow in fetal sheep subjected to chronic anaemia. Am J Physiol 1991;261:R152–8.
169. Davis LE, Hohimer R, Brace RA. Changes in left thoracic lymph flow during progressive anaemia in the ovine fetus. Am J Obstet Gynecol 1996;174:1469–76.

170. Sandgren E, Murray AM, Herzog CA, et al. Anemia and new-onset congestive heart failure in the general Medicare population. J Card Fail 2005;11:99–105.
171. Low I, Grutzmacher P, Bergmann M, Schoeppe W. Echocardiographic findings in patients on maintenance hemodialysis substituted with recombinant human erythropoietin. Clin Nephrol 1989;31:26–30.
172. Silverberg DS, Wexler D, Iaina A. The role of anemia in the progression of congestive heart failure. Is there a place for erythropoietin and intravenous iron? J Nephrol 2004;17:749–61.
173. Felker GM, et al. Anemia as a risk factor and therapeutic target in heart failure. J Am Coll Cardiol 2004;44:959–66.
174. Obialo CI. Cardiorenal consideration as a risk factor for heart failure. Am J Cardiol 2007;99(Suppl.):21D–24.
175. Wexler D, Silverberg DS, Sheps D, et al. Prevalence of anaemia in patients admitted to hospital with a primary diagnosis of congestive heart failure. Int J Cardiol 2004;96:79–7.
176. Tanner H, Moschovitis G, Kuster GM, et al. The prevalence of anemia in chronic heart failure. Int J Cardiol 2002;86:115–21.
177. Herzog CA, Muster HA, Li S, Collins AJ. Impact of congestive heart failure, chronic kidney disease and anemia on survival in the medicare population. J Card Fail 10:467–72.
178. Gregory DD, Sarnak MJ, Konstam MA, et al. Impact of chronic kidney disease and anaemia on hospitalization expense in patients with left ventricular dysfunction. Am J Cardiol 2003;92: 1300–305.
179. Felker GM, Gattis WA, Leimberger JD, et al. Usefulness of anaemia as a predictor of death and rehospitalization in patients with decompensated heart failure. Am J Cardiol 2003;92:625–8.
180. Nordyke RJ, Kim JJ, Goldberg GA, et al. Impact of anaemia on hospitalization time, charges and mortality in patients with heart failure. Value Health 2004;7:464–71.
181. Thomas MC, MacIsaac RJ, Tsalamandris C. Anemia in patients with type 1 diabetes. J Clin Endocrinol Metab 2004;89:4359–63.
182. El-Achkar TM, Ohmit SE, McCullough PA, et al. Higher prevalence of anaemia with diabetes mellitus in moderate kidney insufficiency: the Kidney Early Evaluation Program. Kidney Int 2005;67:1483–8.
183. Herrera-Garza EH, Stetson SJ, Cubillos-Garzon A, et al. Tumor necrosis factor: a mediator of disease progression in the failing human heart. Chest 1999;115:1170–74.
184. Deicher R, Horl WH. Hepcidin: a molecular link between inflammation and anaemia. Nephrol Dial-Transplant 2004;19:521–4.
185. Rivera S, Liu L, Nemeth E, et al. Hepcidin excess induces the sequestration of iron and exacerbates tumor-associated anaemia. Blood 2005;105:1797–802.
186. Detivaud L, Nemeth E, Boudjema K, et al. Hepcidin levels in humans are correlated with hepatic iron stores, hemoglobin levels and hepatic function. Blood 2005;10:746–8.
187. Vaziri ND. Erythropoietin and transferrin metabolism in nephrotic syndrome. Am J Kidney Dis 2001;38:1–8.
188. Macdougall IC. The role of ACE inhibitors and angiotensin II receptor blockers in the response to erythropoietin. Nephrol Dial Transplant 1999;14:1836–41.
189. Odabas AR, Cetinkaya R, Selcuk Y, et al. The effect of high dose losartan on erythropoietin resistance in patients undergoing hemodialysis. Panminerva Med 2003;45:59–62.
190. Silverberg DS, Wexler D, Blum M, et al. Aggressive therapy of Congestive Heart Failure and associated chronic renal failure with medications and correction of anaemia stops or slows the progression of both diseases. Perit Dial Int 2001;21(Suppl. 3):S236–40.
191. Macdougal IC. CREATE: new strategies for early anaemia management in renal insufficiency. Nephrol Dial Transplant 2003;18(Suppl. 2):ii13–6.
192. Valderabano F, Horl W, Macdougall IC, et al. Predialysis survey on anaemia management. Nephrol Dial Transplant 2003;18:89–100.
193. Phrommintikul A, Haas SJ, Elsik M, Krum H. Mortality and target haemoglobin concentrations in anaemic patients with chronic kidney disease treated with erythropoietin: a meta-analysis. Lancet 2007;369:381–8.
194. Strippoli GFM, Craig JC, Manno C, Schena FP. Hemoglobin targets for the anaemia of chronic kidney disease: a meta-analysis of randomized, controlled studies. J Am Soc Nephrol 2004;15:3154–65.
195. Thomas MC, MacIsaac RJ, Tsalamandris C, et al. Unrecognized anemia in patients with diabetes: A cross-sectional survey. Diabetes Care 2003;26:1164–9.

196. New JP, Aung T, Baker PG, et al. The high prevalence of unrecognized anaemia in patients with diabetes and chronic kidney disease: a population-based study. Diabet Med 2008; 25:564–9.
197. KEEP 2004 Data Report. Am J Kidney Dis 2005;45(Suppl. 2):S8–13 and S76–7.
198. Astor BC, Muntner P, Levin A, et al. Association of kidney function with anemia: the Third National Health and Nutrition Examination Survey (1988–1994). Arch Intern Med 2002;162:1401–8.
199. Thomas MC, Tsalamandris C, MacIsaac R, et al. Functional erythropoietin deficiency in patients with type 2 diabetes and anaemia. Diabet Med 2006;23:502–9.
200. Thomas S, Rampersa M. Anemia in diabetes. Acta Diabetol 2004;41:S13–17.
201. Jones RL, Peterson CM. Hematologic alterations in diabetes mellitus. Am J Med 1981;70:339–52.
202. Coccia MA, Cooke K, Stoney G, et al. Novel erythropoiesis stimulating protein (darbepoetin alfa) alleviates anaemia associated with chronic inflammatory disease in a rodent model. Exp Hematol 2001;29:1201–9.
203. Thomas MC, Tsalamandris C, MacIssaac R, et al. Anemia in diabetes; an emerging complication of microvascular disease. Curr Diab Rev 2005;1:107–26.
204. Thomas MC, Cooper ME, Rossing K, et al. Anaemia in diabetes: is there a rationale to TREAT? Diabetologia 2006;49:1151–7.
205. Bell DSH. A comparison of agents used to manage type 2 diabetes. Need for reappraisal of traditional approaches. Treat Endocrinol 2004;3(2):67–76.
206. Wulffele MG, Koy A, Lehert P, et al. Effects of short term treatment with metformin on serum concentrations of homocysteine, folate and vitamin B12 in type 2 diabetes mellitus:a randomized placebo-controlled trial. J Intern Med 2004;25(2):302–3.
207. Ueda H, Ishimura E, Shoji T, et al. Factors affecting progression of renal failure in patients with type 2 diabetes. Diabetes Care 2003;26:1530–34.
208. Yokoyama H, Tomonaga O, Hirayama M, et al. Predictors of the progression of diabetic nephropathy and the beneficial effect of angiotensin-converting enzyme inhibitors in NIDDM patients. Diabetologia 1997;40:405–41.
209. Qiao Q, Keinanen-Kiukaanniemi S, Laara E. The relationship between hemoglobin levels and diabetic retinopathy. J Clin Epidemiol 1997;50:153–8.
210. Bosman DR, Winkler AS, Marsden JT, et al. Anemia with erythropoietin deficiency occurs early in diabetic nephropathy. Diabetes Care 2001;24:495–9.
211. Roman RM, Lobo PI, Taylor RP, et al. Prospective study of the immune effects of normalizing the hemoglobin concentration in hemodialysis patients who receive recombinant human erythropoietin. J Am Soc Nephrol 2004;15:1339–46.
212. Srivastava PM, Thomas MC, Calafiore P, et al. Diastolic dysfunction is associated with anaemia in patients with Type II diabetes. Clin Sci (Lond) 2006;110:109–11.
213. Lavery LA, Van Houtum WH, Armstrong DG. Institutionalization following diabetes-related lower extremity amputation. Am J Med 1997;103(5):383–8.
214. Ross SD, Fahrbach K, Frame D, et al. The effect of anemia treatment on selected health-related quality-of-life domains: a systematic review. Clin Ther 2003;25:1786–805.
215. Ritz E, Laville M, Bilous RW, et al. Target level for hemoglobin correction in patients with diabetes and CKD: primary results of the Anemia Correction in Diabetes (ACORD) study. Am J Kidney Dis 2007;49:194–207.
216. The Society of Thoracic Surgeons Blood Conservation Guideline Task Force and The Society of Cardiovascular Anesthesiologists Special Task Force on Blood Transfusion. Perioperative blood transfusion and blood conservation in cardiac surgery: The Society of Thoracic Surgeons and The Society of Cardiovascular Anesthesiologists Clinical Practice Guideline. Ann Thorac Surg 2007;83:S27–86.
217. Journois D, Mauriat P, Pouard P, et al. Assessment of coagulation factor activation during cardiopulmonary bypass with a new monoclonal antibody. J Cardiothorac Vasc Anesth 1994;8:157–61.
218. Brody JI, Pickering NJ, Fink GB. Concentrations of Factor VIII-related antigen and Factor XIII during open heart surgery. Transfusion 1986;26:478–84.
219. Yamaguchi H, Allers M, Roberts D. The effect on the red cell deformability during cardiopulmonary bypass. Scand J Thorac Cardiovasc Surg 1984;18:119–21.
220. Cohen E, Neustein SM, Silvay G. Profound anemia following cardiac surgery. J Cardiothorac Vasc Anesth 1993;7:721–3.
221. Karkouti K, Beattie WS, Wijeysundera DN. Hemodilution during cardiopulmonary bypass is an independent risk factor for acute renal failure in adult cardiac surgery. J Thorac Cardiovasc Surg 2005;129:391–400.

222. DeFoe GR, Ross CS, Olmstead EM, et al. Lowest hematocrit on bypass and adverse outcomes associated with coronary artery bypass grafting. Ann Thorac Surg 2001;71:769–76.
223. Floyd TF, McGarvey M, Ochroch A, et al. Perioperative changes in cerebral blood flow after cardiac surgery: Influence of anemia and aging. Ann Thorac Surg 2003;76:2037–42.
224. Sunder-Plassmann L, Kloevekorn WP, Holpe K, et al. The physiological significance of acutely induced hemodilution. In: Ditzel J, Lewis DH (eds) *6th European Conference for Microcirculation*. Karger, Basel, 1971, pp. 23–28.
225. Consensus Conference. Perioperative red blood cell transfusion. JAMA 1988;260:2700–703.
226. Wilkerson DK, Rosen AL, Sehgal LR, et al. Limits of cardiac compensation in anemic baboons. Surgery 1988;103:665–70.
227. Weiskopf RB, Viele MK, Feiner J, et al. Human cardiovascular and metabolic response to acute, severe, isovolemic anemia. JAMA 1998;279:217–21.
228. Hebert PC, Wells G, Tweeddale M, et al. Does transfusion practice affect mortality in critically ill patients? Am J Resp Crit Care Med 1998;279:199–205.
229. Graves EJ. National hospital discharge survey: annual summary 1991. Vital Health Stat 1993;114:1–62.
230. Karkouti K, Beattie WS, Wijeysundera DN, et al. Recombinant factor VIIa for intractable blood loss after cardiac surgery: a propensity score-matched case-control analysis. Transfusion 2005;45:26–34.
231. Von Heymann C, Redlich U, Jain U, et al. Recombinant activated factor VII for refractory bleeding after cardiac surgery: a retrospective analysis of safety and efficacy. Crit Care Med 2005;33:2241–6.
232. Romagnoli S, Bevilacqua S, Gelsomino S, et al. Small-dose recombinant activated factor VII (NovoSeven) in cardiac surgery. Anesth Analg 2006;102:1320–26.
233. Monk TG. Preoperative recombinant human erythropoietin in anemic surgical patients. Crit Care 2004;8(Suppl. 2):45–8.
234. Sowade O, Warnke H, Scigalla P, et al. Avoidance of allogeneic blood transfusions by treatment with epoetin beta (recombinant human erythropoietin) in patients undergoing open heart surgery. Blood 1997;89:411–18.
235. D'Ambra MN, Gray RJ, Hillman R, et al. Effect of recombinant human erythropoietin on transfusion risk in coronary bypass patients. Ann Thorac Surg 1997;64:1686–93.

PART 5
Perioperative Hemostasis

CHAPTER 21
Monitoring of Hemostasis in the Perioperative Setting

Sibylle A. Kozek-Langenecker & Eva Schaden
Department of Anesthesiology and Pain Management, Medical University of Vienna, Vienna, Austria

Introduction

The aim of perioperative monitoring of hemostasis is to increase the safety of patients undergoing surgical procedures. Massive bleeding can either be anticipated (during major surgery with a high risk of bleeding) or unexpected. Management requires (1) preoperative risk evaluation and preoperative optimization (e.g., discontinuation or modification of anticoagulant drugs, prophylactic coagulation therapy); and (2) intraoperative causal diagnosis of the complex pathophysiology of massive bleeding as well as early goal-directed therapy. Risk evaluation and risk reduction for postoperative hypercoagulability and thrombosis also needs to be considered in the perioperative management of patients. The present review focuses on bleeding history, routine coagulation testing, and viscoelastic point-of-care hemostasis monitoring as the diagnostic basis for perioperative prothrombotic interventions.

Preoperative evaluation and preparation

The preoperative assessment of the bleeding history of the patient and of his/her relatives remains the most important tool for making a correct diagnosis of both mild and severe inherited or acquired bleeding disorders which may increase the risk of operative bleeding [1]. Standardized questionnaires have been designed in order to assess the type of bleeding (mucosal vs nonmucosal) and the timing of bleeding (immediate vs delayed, since early childhood vs late in life) among other items such as use of anticoagulant or antiplatelet drugs [2, 3]. Preoperative clinical examination may also reveal hematoma, petechiae, or wound healing defects indicating bleeding disorders. Preoperative patient evaluation should be done well enough in advance to elective surgery to correct bleeding risk factors.

The most common cause of clinical nonsurgical bleeding relates to abnormalities in platelet function, with von Willebrand syndrome being considered the most frequent inherited bleeding disorder [4, 5]. Recommended baseline screening tests involve routine coagulation tests investigating the plasmatic coagulation profile, as well as tests of platelet function [3]. If bleeding history is positive (abnormal), further laboratory investigation of hemostasis is indicated and requires a stepwise approach [6]. If bleeding history is normal, further laboratory investigations of hemostasis are only indicated if the patient is scheduled for surgery with a high risk of bleeding or if there is a relevant comorbidity (Figure 21.1).

If preoperative evaluation anticipates an increased operative bleeding risk, preoperative patient preparation includes discontinuation or modification of anticoagulant drugs if clinically possible [7, 8], prophylactic therapy to promote coagulation (e.g., antifibrinolytic drugs, desmopressin, vitamin K), and to prevent/decrease allogeneic transfusion

Alternatives to Blood Transfusion in Transfusion Medicine, 2nd edition. Edited by A. Maniatis, P. Van der Linden, J.-F. Hardy.

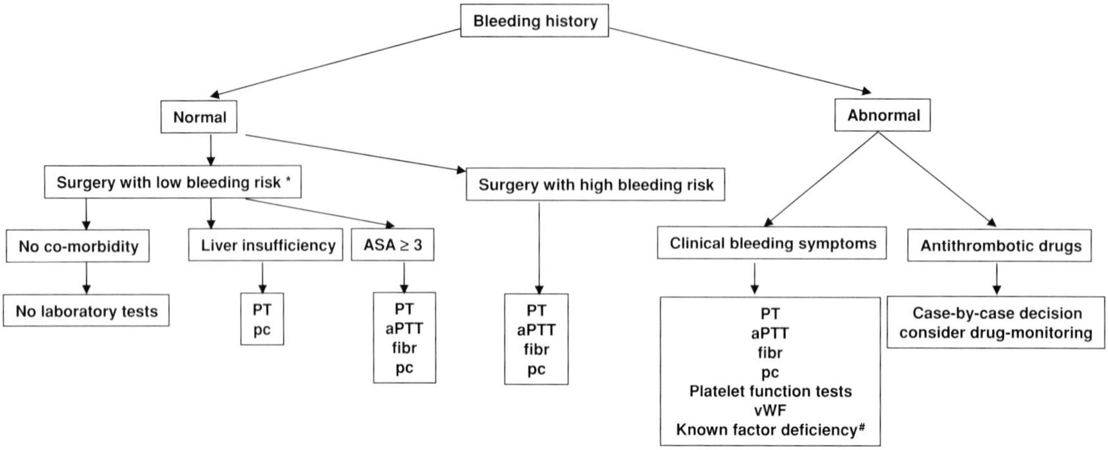

Figure 21.1 Preoperative monitoring of hemostasis. PT, prothrombin time; pc, platelet count; aPTT, activated partial thromboplastin time; fibr, fibrinogen level; vWF, von Willebrand factor. * or no evidence for usefulness of laboratory tests; #, e.g., factor VIII in hemophilia A.

requirements (e.g., erythropoietin, autologous blood predonation) [1]. The risks and benefits of instituting preoperative optimization in patients on anticoagulant or dual antiplatelet drugs should be assessed on a case-by-case basis and may involve specific drug monitoring [7, 9, 10].

Intraoperative monitoring

Periodic visual assessment of the surgical field and communication with the surgical team is recommended as standard practice to detect impending or established coagulopathy, and entails the assessment of the amount of blood lost and the presence of microvascular bleeding from mucosal lesions, serosal surfaces, catheter insertion sites, and wounds. The diagnosis of intra- and postoperative coagulopathy in massive transfusion needs to be verified by appropriate coagulation tests [1]. Meanwhile, surgical attempts to control a visible source of hemorrhage are required (e.g., ligation, embolization, packing). Monitoring for "basic coagulation support" further includes *temperature monitoring* for maintaining normothermia and *blood gas analysis* for correction of acidosis, anemia, and hypocalcemia. Monitoring for "advanced coagulation support" involves routine coagulation testing, rotational thromboelastometry (ROTEM), thromboelastography (TEG), and platelet function testing.

Routine coagulation testing

Even though these tests were not developed to predict bleeding or guide coagulation management in the surgical setting, most centers in clinical practice draw blood perioperatively for the following routine coagulation tests ("routine coagulation panel"):

• *Activated partial thromboplastin time (aPTT)*: The aPTT was developed to monitor heparinization in the treatment of thromboembolic disorders, to characterize clotting factors, and for research purposes on hemophilia. Activation of coagulation factors, formerly known as the "intrinsic coagulation cascade," is performed by incubating plasma with partial thromboplastins, calcium, and kaolin powder. The endpoint of measurement is the formation of fibrin strands. Empiric cutoff value for therapeutic intervention (fresh frozen plasma (FFP) 15–30 mL/kg or prothrombin concentrate (PCC)) in major surgery is an aPTT > 50 seconds.

• *Prothrombin time (PT)*: This test was developed to monitor and adjust the doses of coumarins.

Activation of coagulation factors, formerly known as the "extrinsic coagulation cascade," is performed by incubating plasma with tissue thromboplastin and calcium. The time until fibrin strand formation is determined. Standardization of the PT for laboratory control of oral anticoagulant treatment is based on the responsiveness of one type of thromboplastin, measured by its international sensitivity index, and conversion into the international normalized ratio (INR). Empiric cutoff value for therapeutic intervention (FFP or PCC) is a PT <65%.

• *Platelet count*: Platelet counting is routinely performed by automated machines. The number of platelets, however, does not reflect the quality of platelet function. Empiric cutoff value for platelet transfusion is a platelet count <50–100 G/L.

• *Fibrinogen concentration*: Fibrinogen plays a major role in routine coagulation tests such as PT and aPTT. In the conventional Clauss method where thrombin is added to plasma, the fibrinogen concentration is proportional to the coagulation time measured. This test is affected by heparin and fibrinogen degradation products. Excessive bleeding has been reported at fibrinogen levels below 50–100 mg/dL [1, 11].

• *Second-level coagulation tests*: Because of long turnaround times and limited availability in many laboratories, coagulation factor levels and molecular markers of the coagulation and fibrinolytic system are rarely assayed in the acute perioperative setting. Patients with inherited coagulation defects may exsanguinate with trauma or major surgery unless specific factor replacement is provided (such as factor VIII, IX, von Willebrand factor concentrate) necessitating second-level coagulation tests.

Routine coagulation monitoring: predictor of bleeding and mortality

Severe aPTT prolongations >1.8 times normal are associated with bleeding [11, 12]. Similarly, INR elevations in trauma patients are only indicative of a risk of generalized bleeding if they are >1.5–1.8 times normal and are associated with an elevated aPTT [11, 13]. A severely prolonged activated clotting time (ACT) may indicate exhaustion of the coagulation system's reserve [14]. In trauma victims, an initially abnormal PT increases the adjusted odds of dying by 35%, a prolonged aPTT by 326% [15].

Although severely abnormal PTs and aPTTs are predictors of mortality, the poor predictive power of moderately impaired routine coagulation tests has repeatedly been argued as a major limitation of these tests [12]. In a multiple regression model, platelet count was not an independent predictor of mortality in emergency medicine [15]. The decline of platelet count is a highly individual phenomenon, some patients being able to recruit platelets from storage pools. Most patients approach the critical platelet count after losing two blood volumes [16].

Limitations of routine coagulation tests

In the perioperative setting where events may proceed at a fast and dramatic pace, real-time monitoring of the patient's coagulation profile and repeated laboratory tests are vital in view of administrating proper replacement therapy. However, results of routine coagulation tests performed at the hospital's central laboratory are generally only available with a delay of at least 30 minutes (sample preparation including centrifugation and buffering, transportation of blood samples, and test results) [17]. Hardy et al. [18] concluded that bedside monitors of hemostasis are needed urgently for the management of operative and trauma-associated bleeding. The bedside determination of PT and aPTT in whole blood using the CoaguCheck (Roche Diagnostics, Switzerland) aimed at overcoming this limitation; however, correlation with central laboratory test results is inadequate.

Routine coagulation tests are performed in plasma at a standardized temperature of 37°C, without the presence of platelets and other blood cells. Accordingly, routine laboratory tests cannot assess the effect of hypothermia on hemostasis in hypothermic patients, neither can they diagnose fibrinolysis and platelet dysfunction. Since the hemostatic response to injury or surgery is a complex interaction of plasma proteins, platelets, and the vessel wall (cell-based model of hemostasis), it cannot be evaluated by tests performed in plasma. Although aPTT, PT, fibrinogen concentration, and platelet count determination are well-validated tests, methodological problems include variable sensitivity of test reagents, high variability between laboratories and investigators, as well as insufficient standardization.

Routine tests pick up abnormalities of hemostasis due to single or multiple deficiencies of coagulation factors, but do not identify them. The PT is a more reliable marker of critically low coagulation factor levels than the aPTT, possibly due to the high rate of false negative aPTT results when acute phase reactant factor VIII is elevated [13]. Several studies demonstrate a poor correlation between the amount of blood products given and the severity of coagulation defects [11, 12]. Obviously, simplistic formulas or flow charts for predicting factor deficiencies from blood loss are not applicable [19]. PT and aPTT assess only the speed of fibrin strand formation, but not the mechanical and functional properties of the clot over time. Functional fibrin polymerization may be impaired despite normal fibrinogen concentration. Colloidal solutions may impair determination of fibrinogen concentration [20].

The most important limitation of routine coagulation tests is the fact that the predominant pathophysiological mechanism of bleeding in the complex scenario of trauma-associated coagulopathy or massive intraoperative blood loss cannot be differentiated: a prolonged aPTT may be because of "intrinsic coagulation factor" deficiency requiring specific substitution, fibrinogen deficiency requiring fibrinogen substitution, hypothermia requiring rewarming, heparinization requiring protamine reversal, or hyperfibrinolysis requiring antifibrinolytic drugs. Thus, an incorrect differential diagnosis may lead to therapeutic mismanagement. Due to the complex nature of hemorrhage in this setting, physicians require coagulation monitoring strategies sensitive to all major possible pathophysiological mechanisms [18, 21, 22]. Near-patient (point-of-care) coagulation monitoring devices have become available and are likely to overcome several limitations of routine (laboratory) coagulation testing.

Near-patient coagulation monitoring

Thromboelastography and rotational thromboelastometry

The viscoelastic whole blood test was invented by Hartert in 1948 and has recently been included in the panel of laboratory monitoring for coagulopathy by the American Society of Anesthesiologists [1]. Thromboelastography (TEG)/rotational thromboelastometry (ROTEM) measures the viscoelastic properties of nonanticoagulated or (citrate) anticoagulated blood after induction of clotting under low shear conditions, resembling the rheologic properties in venous vessels in vivo. The pattern of changes in viscoelasticity reflect the kinetics of all stages of thrombus formation (*r* and *k* time, CT and CFT), the stability and firmness of the clot, which is a function of platelet–fibrin interaction, and fibrin polymerization (MA, MCF), as well as dissolution (fibrinolysis) [23] (Figure 21.2). TEG/ROTEM is a fibrinolysis-sensitive assay and allows for diagnosis of hyperfibrinolysis in bleeding patients [24]. Standardized operating procedures required for quality control testing are available. A multicenter investigation yielded consistent values between centers and provided general reference ranges for the ROTEM [25]. Interpretation of TEG/ROTEM results is simplified by both graphical and numerical presentation of results, highlighting of abnormal results, and computerized analysis of the trace. While conventional TEG has been described as an insufficient monitor in trauma patients because of unclear interpretation and limited run-to-run variation [26], the ROTEM (Pentapharm GmbH, Germany) improved the original TEG (Haemoscope Inc., USA) procedure by reducing the interference with vibrations and limited transportability. Addition of different coagulation-activating agents and/or platelet inhibiting agents allows the detection and quantification of specific coagulation defects such as (1) *defect in clot firmness* due to fibrinogen deficiency (being an early

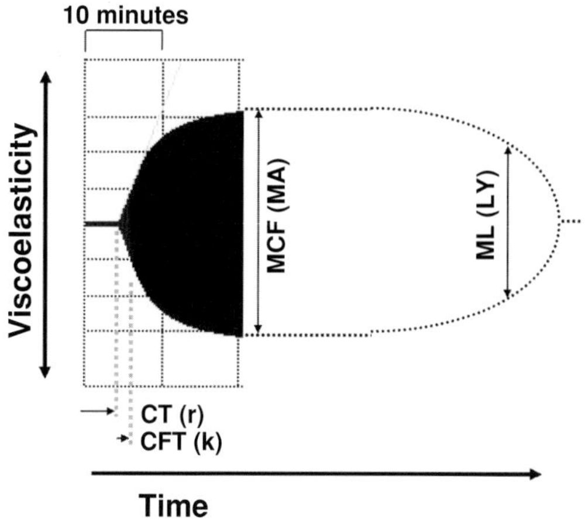

Figure 21.2 Parameters of thromboelastometry and thromboelastography. The pattern of changes in viscoelasticity reflect the kinetics of all stages of thrombus formation (CT and CFT, *r* and *k* times), firmness of the clot, which is a function of platelet–fibrin interaction and fibrin polymerization (MCF, MA), as well as dissolution (fibrinolysis; ML, LY). Thromboelastometric parameters: CFT, clot formation time (seconds); CT, clotting time (seconds); MCF, maximum clot firmness (mm); ML, maximum lysis (%). Thromboelastographic parameters: k = coagulation time (seconds); LY, lysis index (%); MA, maximum amplitude (MA); r = reaction time (seconds).

phenomenon) and thrombocytopenia; (2) *impaired clot stability* due to hyperfibrinolysis and factor XIII deficiency (being a late phenomenon); and (3) *prolonged clot generation* due to various coagulation factor deficiencies or heparin. ROTEM not only provides a global picture of the injured patient's hemostatic status but also permits differential diagnosis of the major underlying *pathophysiological mechanism* of coagulopathy. Normal viscoelastic test results are unlikely to coincide with bleeding (high negative predictive value) [27]. As a consequence, another important implication of TEG/ROTEM monitoring is the immediate initiation of surgical reexploration if no hemostatic cause of bleeding is observed.

Test modifications and differential diagnosis

EXTEM is a baseline test that uses recombinant tissue factor to activate coagulation (comparable to the PT) that causes rapid generation of the clot. The maximum clot firmness (MCF_{EXTEM}) gives information on the maximum clot strength and stability, which is largely dependent on platelet count and fibrinogen level. Prepared disposable wells containing cytochalasin D, a platelet inhibitor, are used in the FIBTEM test. MCF_{FIBTEM} represents the contribution of fibrinogen to the clot strength. Critical MCF cutoff values appear within 15 minutes after test initiation (depending on hemostatic function). A low MCF_{FIBTEM} is indicative of the need to administer fibrinogen concentrates. A normal MCF_{FIBTEM} ($\geq$12 mm) in the presence of a low MCF_{EXTEM} (<50 mm) indicates the need for platelet substitution. Thus, comparing MCF_{FIBTEM} to MCF_{EXTEM} permits differentiation of a low platelet count from dys- or hypofibrinogenemia.

Practical consideration: FIBTEM and EXTEM should be performed simultaneously as first line ROTEM tests in surgical patients. Some experts recommend analysis of A10 (clot strength 10 minutes after start of ROTEM) instead of the MCF because this variable is obtained more rapidly. This approach allows timely therapeutic decisions. $A10_{FIBTEM}$ <6 mm triggers administration of high dose fibrinogen concentrate (60 mg/kg), $A10_{FIBTEM}$ between 6 and 11 mm triggers administration of 30 mg/kg.

The clotting time (CT_{EXTEM}) gives information about the initial activation and dynamics of clot formation, thus allowing analysis of factor deficiencies (and the detection of anticoagulants). The critical cutoff value for CT, indicating the necessity to administer PCC or FFP, appears about 100 seconds after test initiation.

EXTEM allows for the visual diagnosis of hyperfibrinolysis when a typical tapering trace is shown. In addition, wells containing aprotinin (APTEM) permit the quantitive assessment of fibrinolysis and the estimation of the therapeutic benefit from an antifibrinolytic agent such as tranexamic acid. Any improvement in CT, CFT, and MCF in APTEM compared to EXTEM unmasks low-grade hyperfibrinolysis (e.g., $CT_{APTEM}/CT_{EXTEM} < 0.8$). Risks associated with antifibrinolytic drugs have to be considered [10]. If detected in the ROTEM or TEG, first line therapy is aimed at correcting hyperfibrinolysis, followed by replacement of consumed coagulation factors.

INTEM uses ellagic acid contact activator (comparable to the reagent used for aPTT) to analyze the general coagulation status. Wells containing heparinase (HEPTEM) or ecarin can be used to detect specific anticoagulant effects. The comparison of CT_{INTEM} and CT_{HEPTEM} permits the quantification of heparinization and estimation of the therapeutic benefit from protamine reversal [28].

Practical consideration: INTEM and HEPTEM should be performed as first line ROTEM tests in heparinized (cardiac) patients and as second line ROTEM tests in all other surgical patients if (endogenous or exogenous) heparinization is suggested to complicate bleeding. CT_{INTEM} >240 seconds and CT_{HEPTEM}/CT_{INTEM} <0.66 triggers protamine administration.

The described test modifications and their potential intraoperative implications are summarized in Figure 21.3. Each routine test is specific for some portion of the hemostatic mechanism and none can be used alone. Similarly, ROTEM test combinations (EXTEM, FIBTEM, APTEM) are required as a basic diagnostic panel in the presence of massive bleeding.

Another test modification that can be performed for further differential diagnosis is the incubation of blood in the EXTEM assay with coagulation factor XIII (0.2 international units). A reversal of maximum lysis (to the normal range) from ML_{EXTEM} and ML_{APTEM} of 20–25% indicates factor XIII deficiency. A test modification containing factor XIII is not yet commercially available, but coagulation factor XIII concentrates are available to spike ROTEM test cuvettes and to diagnose this bleeding mechanism.

TEG/TEM measurements can be performed at the actual body core temperature of the patient at adjusted test temperatures between 22 and 42°C, thus allowing quantitative analysis of the anticoagulant effect induced by hypothermia [29]. Test temperature adjustments, however, should not be conducted in the OR because physicians may be tempted to treat abnormal test results with coagulation factor substitution while only rewarming is indicated.

Practical considerations

TEG/ROTEM measurements should be performed at baseline (before surgery), when clinically abnormal bleeding occurs, and after therapeutic interventions. Tests should be initiated immediately after blood withdrawal. TEG/ROTEM are easy to use by nonlaboratory personnel in the emergency unit or the OR. Performance of TEG/ROTEM in the central laboratory by trained laboratory personnel reduces the possibility of handling errors; online data transmission to a monitor in the OR permits timely coagulation management.

Point-of-care coagulation monitoring using TEG/ROTEM increases knowledge and vigilance of anesthesiologists for hemostasis and coagulopathy. Clinical users' meetings promote the exchange of experience and speed up transfer of knowledge.

Management algorithm for coagulation therapy

Routine laboratory-based transfusion algorithms are superior to treatment based solely on the clinician's experience [18, 30]. Normal values of routine coagulation tests and in vivo bleeding time as a trigger for antifibrinolytic drugs (indication by exclusion) [31], does not allow the appropriate management of coagulation, based on pathophysiological criteria. TEG-guided administration of clotting factors was superior to routine coagulation testing [32]. The institution of transfusion algorithms based on thromboelastographic parameters reduced transfusion requirements (and in some study designs also blood loss) in both routine and high-risk cardiac surgery in adults and children and in liver transplantation [33–40]. Transfusion requirements after, compared with before, the implementation of the ROTEM were significantly lower and clinically more relevant [41]. TEG was found to be an early predictor of transfusion in blunt injury patients [42].

ROTEM cutoff values recommended by experts (not yet evidence-based) are higher for traumatized patients with ongoing bleeding than for patients undergoing elective surgery such as liver transplantation and cardiac surgery and in the absence of active bleeding [43, 44]. It must be kept in mind that the excessive support of the hemostatic system in

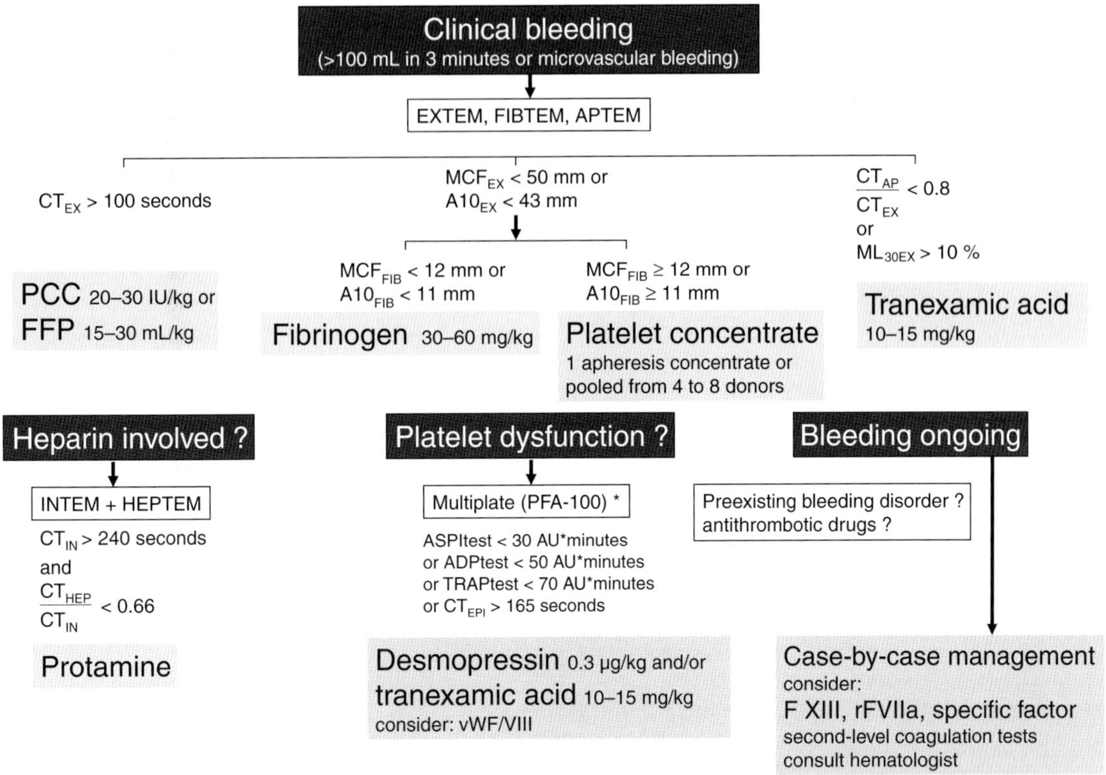

Figure 21.3 Intraoperative monitoring of hemostasis and therapeutic consequences. Basic panel consists of EXTEM (= EX), FIBTEM (= FIB), APTEM (= AP). Depending on the results and medical history, INTEM (= IN), HEPTEM (= HEP), platelet function testing and second line tests (e.g., factor VIII in hemophilia) are recommended. ADP, adenosine diphosphate; ASPI, arachidonic acid; AU, aggregation units; CT, clotting time; EPI, epinephrine; FFP, fresh frozen plasma; MCF, maximum clot firmness; ML, maximum lysis; PCC, prothrombin complex concentrate; PFA-100, Platelet Function Analyzer; TRAP, thrombin receptor activator peptide. * only qualitative assessment of TRAP test if platelet count <50–100 G/L or $MCF_{EX} < 50$ mm.

the pre- and intraoperative period may precipitate patients in a prothrombotic state postoperatively with the risk of myocardial infarction, pulmonary embolism, or deep vein thrombosis. Close coagulation monitoring with the ROTEM and PFA-100 to achieve sufficient but not overwhelming multimodal anticoagulation has been recommended in patients with cardiac assist devices [45].

Limitations of point-of-care algorithms based on TEG/ROTEM

Point-of-care monitoring with the ROTEM is still an evolving field. Concomitant training, education, and quality control are critical. Another limitation of these point-of-care tests is their limited robustness. Future studies in emergency medicine are warranted to validate critical cutoff values for procoagulant therapy and transfusion. Not only the amount of bleeding, but also the site will determine cutoff values. Acceptance of the method not only by anesthesiologists but also by hematologists has to be gained and, most important, the improvements in patient outcomes as well as health cost reductions have to be demonstrated. It needs to be determined if goal-directed coagulation management based on a point-of-care algorithm can help prevent coagulopathy during massive transfusion.

Because of the inability to detect platelet function disorders such as von Willebrand syndrome and antiplatelet drug effects (except for the novel TEG aggregation test Platelet Mapping), more specific tests are recommended in platelet-dependent bleeding.

It may be helpful to assign a hematologist or transfusion specialist to a multidisciplinary team treating acutely bleeding patients if proper blood component therapy cannot be achieved by the OR team, including anesthesiologists trained in coagulation management and point-of-care monitoring.

Platelet function tests

Widespread adoption of antiplatelet agents into everyday clinical practice has revolutionized contemporary care of cardiovascular patients. The bleeding risks these drugs pose perioperatively will become increasingly important [46, 47]. Platelet function tests are first-level tests in the preoperative evaluation of patients with a positive bleeding history [3,5] (Figure 21.1) and second-level tests in actively bleeding patients if antiplatelet therapy, inherited or acquired platelet defects, or extracorporeal circulation are involved, and if ROTEM and "routine coagulation panel" tests cannot reveal a defect in hemostasis responsible for bleeding (Figure 21.3).

There is still no simple reliable method for measuring platelet function. Static tests such as the measure of β-thromboglobulin capture only one single point in time and cannot accurately reflect the dynamic processes encountered intraoperatively. Dynamic tests such as the in vivo bleeding time reflect the time-dependent contribution of platelets to overall clot formation. The in vivo bleeding time is an older test method in which the time until cessation of bleeding after incision of the skin by a specific device is determined. However, the bleeding time is poorly standardized, temperature and drug dependent (catecholamines), influenced by vascular disorders, lacks specificity and sensitivity, and is not predictive of bleeding [48]. The bleeding time increases nonspecifically during surgery and transfusion [49], and does not allow the differentiation between bleeding and nonbleeding patients [12].

Several platelet function analyzers test the platelet's response to an agonist. The Platelet Function Analyzer PFA-100 (Dade) provides a measure of platelet function in citrated whole blood. The device measures platelet function at high shear rates. A blood sample of 800 μL is added to a reservoir well in a disposable cartridge. The instrument aspirates the blood sample under a constant vacuum through a capillary and a microscopic aperture within a membrane coated with platelet agonists, collagen, and either epinephrine or adenosine diphosphate (ADP). This leads to the attachment, activation, and aggregation of platelets and formation of a platelet plug. The time taken to occlude the aperture is known as the closure time and is a function of platelet count and reactivity, von Willebrand factor activity, and hematocrit [50]. This method rapidly identifies aspirin effects and platelet disorders prior to surgery [3, 5, 51]. In patients with preoperatively identified platelet dysfunctions, shortening of the PFA-closure time after desmopressin infusion should be assessed ("desmopressin response test"). In cardiac surgical patients, the preoperative PFA-100 closure time correlated with postoperative blood loss in some studies [52], but not in others [53]. A Medline search on the use of the PFA-100 during massive transfusion failed to retrieve any relevant references. Major limitations of the PFA-100 as an intraoperative point-of-care system in massive transfusion include its strong dependence on platelet count (>100 G/L) and hematocrit (>30%). Trigger values are PFA-closure time >165 seconds in epinephrine cartridges.

Optical and impedance platelet aggregometry assess platelet reactivity by measuring changes in luminescence or impedance upon platelet agonist stimulation. Originally, these techniques have only been performed in specialized laboratories by experienced technicians. The need for preparation of platelet rich plasma limited widespread application of optical aggregometry (Born). Further limitations are the dependence to temperature, stirring rate, and limited standardization. Nevertheless, optical aggregometry remains the accepted "gold standard" for the detection of platelet dysfunction.

The novel impedance aggregometer Multiplate (Dynabyte) is a significant step forward and avoids several methodological problems of the original platelet aggregometer, especially by using whole blood, disposable test cuvettes, various commercially available test reagents at standardized concentrations (collagen, arachidonic acid, ADP, thrombin receptor activator peptide (TRAP), ristocetin), an automated pipetting system, and a direct thrombin inhibitor as anticoagulant with minimal per se effects on platelet function. The Multiplate could potentially provide the differential diagnostic information required for the management of acute bleeding problems. This device has been used successfully in the diagnosis of antiplatelet drug effects, and the prediction of blood loss in cardiac surgery [54, 55]. Although aggregometry has recently been reviewed as evidence-based coagulation monitoring [33], the Multiplate assay has not been validated for low platelet counts and, thus, its use in hemorrhagic thrombocytopenia remains to be determined.

A modified thromboelastographic assay, the Platelet Mapping Assay (Haemoscope) has been introduced to monitor platelet function: heparin-anticoagulated whole blood is clotted by a reptilase-factor XIIIa activator mixture [56]. This MA_0 (maximum amplitude) is proportionate to platelet activation and is compared to the $MA_{ADP/AA}$ in clotted blood with additional ADP or arachidonic acid activation, as well as to the MA_{KH} in citrated blood with kaolin activation and heparinase addition. Platelet reactivity is calculated by the following formula:

$$MA\% = 100 \times MA_{ADP/AA} - MA_0/MA_{KH} - MA_0$$

This assay permits monitoring of NSAID inhibition [57] and of the reversal of clopidogrel and NSAID inhibition of platelet function before surgery [58].

Numerous other platelet monitoring techniques assessing the platelet's response to various agonists are emerging such as the Hemostatus (Medtronic), Rapid Platelet Function Analyser (Ultegra, Accumetrics), Clot Signature Analyzer (CSA; Xylum), PlateletWorks (ICHOR, Helena Bio Sience), Hemodyne Platelet Analysis System (Hemodyne Inc.), and Cone and Plate Analyser (CPA "Impact"; Diamed). These tests as well as flow cytometric assays have not yet been broadly adopted in the treatment of platelet-related bleeding.

Summary and conclusions

In the preoperative setting, laboratory investigation of hemostasis is indicated if the bleeding history is abnormal. A stepwise approach including routine coagulation tests such as aPTT, PT, and platelet function is recommended.

In the operative setting associated with clinical bleeding, bedside and repeated monitoring of the patient's coagulation profile is vital for proper procoagulant therapy. Limitations of routine coagulation tests are multifold in early goal-directed coagulation management, such as delay of data reporting, diagnostic gap for hyperfibrinolysis, hypothermia effects, and platelet dysfunction. Near-patient coagulation monitoring using ROTEM or TEG provides a global picture of the hemostatic status. Specific test kits such as EXTEM and FIBTEM allow the detection of specific coagulation defects: reduced clot firmness because of fibrinogen deficiency (being an early phenomenon in bleeding) and thrombocytopenia, impaired clot stability because of hyperfibrinolysis and factor XIII deficiency, and prolonged clot generation due to various coagulation factor deficiencies or heparin. ROTEM/TEG-guided administration of clotting factors has been found superior to therapy based on the clinician's experience and routine coagulation testing. Platelet function tests are useful as second-level tests in bleeding patients if antiplatelet therapy, inherited or acquired platelet defects, or extracorporeal circulation are involved.

Future studies are warranted to validate critical cutoff values for procoagulant therapy and beneficial effects on clinical outcome, as well as to analyze cost-efficiency of near-patient monitoring of hemostasis in the perioperative setting.

References

1. Practice guidelines for perioperative blood transfusion and adjuvant therapies. An updated report by the American Society of Anesthesiologists Task Force on

perioperative blood transfusion and adjuvant therapies. Anesthesiology 2006;105:198–208.
2. Pfanner G, Koscielny J, Pernerstorfer T, et al. Preoperative evaluation of the bleeding history. Recommendations of the working group on perioperative coagulation of the Austrian Society for Anaesthesia, Resuscitation and Intensive Care. Anaesthesist 2007;56:604–11.
3. Koscielny J, von Tempelhoff GF, Ziemer S, et al. A practical concept for preoperative management of patients with impaired primary hemostasis. Clin Appl Thromb Hemost 2004;10:155–66.
4. Rodeghiero F, Castaman G. Congenital von Willebrand disease type I: definition, phenotypes, clinical and laboratory assessment. Best Pract Res Clin Haematol 2001;14:321–35.
5. Lillicrap D, Nair SC, Srivastava A, et al. Laboratory issues in bleeding disorders. Haemophilia 2006;12(Suppl. 3):68–75.
6. Eberl W, Wendt I, Schroeder H. Preoperative coagulation screening prior to adenoidectomy and tonsillectomy. Klin Padiatr 2005;217:20–24.
7. Metzler H, Huber K, Kozek-Langenecker S, Vicenzi MN, Munch A. Coronary stents, dual antiplatelet therapy and peri-operative problems. Anaesthesist 2007;56:401–10.
8. Kozek-Langenecker S, Fries D, Gütl M, et al. Locoregional anesthesia and coagulation inhibitors. Recommendations of the Task Force on Perioperative Coagulation of the Austrian Society for Anesthesiology and Intensive Care Medicine. Anaesthesist 2005;54:476–84.
9. Kozek-Langenecker SA. Antikoagulanzien und deren Reversierung (German). Anästh Intensive Med 2007;48:S153–8.
10. Mangano DT, Tudor IC, Dietzel C. The risk associated with aprotinin in cardiac surgery. N Engl J Med 2006;354:353–65.
11. Ciavarella D, Reed R, Counts R, et al. Clotting factor levels and the risk of diffuse microvascular bleeding in the massively transfused patient. Br J Haematol 1987;67:365–8.
12. Counts RB, Haisch C, Simon TL, et al. Hemostasis in massively transfused trauma patients. Ann Surg 1979;190:91–9.
13. Yuan S, Ferrell C, Chandler WL. Comparing the prothrombin time INR versus the APTT to evaluate the coagulopathy of acute trauma. Thromb Res 2007:120:29–37.
14. Aucar JA, Norman P, Whitten E, et al. Intraoperative detection of traumatic coagulopathy using the activated coagulation time. Shock 2003;19:404–7.
15. MacLeod JB, Lynn M, McKenney MG, et al. Early coagulopathy predicts mortality in trauma. J Trauma 2003;55:39–44.
16. Hiippala ST, Myllyla GJ, Vahtera EM. Hemostatic factors and replacement of major blood loss with plasma-poor red cell concentrates. Anesth Analg 1995;81:360–65.
17. Ketchum L, Hess JR, Hiippala S. Indications for early fresh frozen plasma, cryoprecipitate, and platelet transfusion in trauma. J Trauma 2006;60:S51–58.
18. Hardy JF, de Moerloose P, Samama CM. Massive transfusion and coagulopathy: pathophysiology and implications for clinical management. Can J Anaesth 2006;53:S40–58.
19. Erber WN. Massive blood transfusion in the elective surgical setting. Transfus Apher Sci 2002;27:83–92.
20. Hiippala S. Dextran and hydroxyethyl starch interfere with fibrinogen assays. Blood Coagul Fibrinolysis 1995;6:743–6.
21. Kozek-Langenecker S. Monitoring of hemostasis in emergency medicine. In: Vincent JL (ed.) *Yearbook of Intensive Care and Emergency Medicine*. Springer Verlag, Berlin-Heidelberg, 2007, pp. 847–60.
22. Kozek-Langenecker S. Management of massive operative blood loss. Minerva Anestesiol 2007;73:401–15.
23. Di Benedetto P, Baciarello M, Cabetti L, et al. Thrombelastography. Present and future perspectives in clinical practice. Minerva Anestesiol 2003;69:501–9.
24. Luddington RJ. Thrombelastography/thromboelastometry. Clin Lab Haematol 2005;27:81–90.
25. Lang T, Bauters A, Braun SL, et al. Multi-centre investigation on reference ranges for ROTEM thromboelastometry. Blood Coagul Fibrinolysis 2005;16:301–10.
26. Hess JR, Lawson JH. The coagulopathy of trauma versus disseminated intravascular coagulation. J Trauma 2006;60:S12–19.
27. Cammerer U, Dietrich W, Rampf T, et al. The predictive value of modified computerized thromboelastography and platelet function analysis for postoperative blood loss in routine cardiac surgery. Anesth Analg 2003;96:51–7, table of contents.
28. Mittermayr M, Margreiter J, Velik-Salchner C, et al. Effects of protamine and heparin can be detected and easily differentiated by modified thrombelastography (Rotem): an in vitro study. Br J Anaesth 2005;95:310–16.
29. Kettner S, Kozek S, Groeztner J, et al. Effects of hypothermia on thrombelastography in patients undergoing cardiopulmonary bypass. Br J Anaesth 1998;80:313–17.

30. DeLoughery TG. Coagulation defects in trauma patients: etiology, recognition, and therapy. Crit Care Clin 2004;20:13–24.
31. Capraro L, Kuitunen A, Salmenpera M, Kekomaki R. On-site coagulation monitoring does not affect hemostatic outcome after cardiac surgery. Acta Anaesthesiol Scand 2001;45:200–206.
32. Chowdhury P, Saayman AG, Paulus U, et al. Efficacy of standard dose and 30 ml/kg fresh frozen plasma in correcting laboratory parameters of haemostasis in critically ill patients. Br J Haematol 2004;125:69–73.
33. Shore-Lesserson L. Evidence based coagulation monitors: heparin monitoring, thromboelastography, and platelet function. Semin Cardiothorac Vasc Anesth 2005;9:41–52.
34. Shore-Lesserson L, Manspeizer HE, DePerio M, et al. Thromboelastography-guided transfusion algorithm reduces transfusions in complex cardiac surgery. Anesth Analg 1999;88:312–19.
35. Avidan MS, Alcock EL, Da Fonseca J, et al. Comparison of structured use of routine laboratory tests or near-patient assessment with clinical judgement in the management of bleeding after cardiac surgery. Br J Anaesth 2004;92:178–86.
36. Royston D, von Kier S. Reduced haemostatic factor transfusion using heparinase-modified thrombelastography during cardiopulmonary bypass. Br J Anaesth 2001;86:575–8.
37. Nuttall GA, Oliver WC, Santrach PJ, et al. Efficacy of a simple intraoperative transfusion algorithm for nonerythrocyte component utilization after cardiopulmonary bypass. Anesthesiology 2001;94:773–81; discussion 775A–776A.
38. Spiess BD, Gillies BS, Chandler W, Verrier E. Changes in transfusion therapy and reexploration rate after institution of a blood management program in cardiac surgical patients. J Cardiothorac Vasc Anesth 1995;9:168–73.
39. Miller BE, Guzzetta NA, Tosone SR, Levy JH. Rapid evaluation of coagulopathies after cardiopulmonary bypass in children using modified thromboelastography. Anesth Analg 2000;90:1324–30.
40. Kang Y. Coagulation and liver transplantation: current concepts. Liver Transpl Surg 1997;3:465–7.
41. Anderson L, Quasim I, Soutar R, et al. An audit of red cell and blood product use after the institution of thromboelastometry in a cardiac intensive care unit. Transfus Med 2006;16:31–9.
42. Kaufmann CR, Dwyer KM, Crews JD, et al. Usefulness of thrombelastography in assessment of trauma patient coagulation. J Trauma 1997;42:716–20; discussion 720–2.
43. Goerlinger K, Dirkmann D, Kiss G, et al. ROTEM-baed management for diagnosis and treatment of acute haemorrhage during liver transplantation. A322. Eur J Anaesthesiol 2006;23:85.
44. Coakley M, Reddy K, Mackie I, Mallett S. Transfusion triggers in orthotopic liver transplantation: a comparison of the thromboelastometry analyzer, the thromboelastogram, and conventional coagulation tests. J Cardiothorac Vasc Anesth 2006;20:548–53.
45. Fries D, Innerhofer P, Streif W, et al. Coagulation monitoring and management of anticoagulation during cardiac assist device support. Ann Thorac Surg 2003;76:1593–7.
46. Merritt JC, Bhatt DL. The efficacy and safety of perioperative antiplatelet therapy. J Thromb Thrombolysis 2004;17:21–7.
47. Tanaka KA, Szlam F, Kelly AB, et al. Clopidogrel (Plavix) and cardiac surgical patients: implications for platelet function monitoring and postoperative bleeding. Platelets 2004;15:325–32.
48. Rodgers R. Bleeding time tables: a tabular summary of pertinent literature. Semin Thromb Hemost 1990;16:21–38.
49. Mannucci PM, Federici AB, Sirchia G. Hemostasis testing during massive blood replacement. A study of 172 cases. Vox Sang 1982;42:113–23.
50. Escolar G, Cases A, Vinas M, et al. Evaluation of acquired platelet dysfunctions in uremic and cirrhotic patients using the platelet function analyzer (PFA-100): influence of hematocrit elevation. Haematologica 1999;84:614–19.
51. Barrowcliffe TW, Cattaneo M, Podda GM, et al. New approaches for measuring coagulation. Haemophilia 2006;12(Suppl. 3):76–81.
52. Wahba A, Sander S, Birnbaum DE. Are in-vitro platelet function tests useful in predicting blood loss following open heart surgery? Thorac Cardiovasc Surg 1998;46:228–31.
53. Forestier F, Coiffic A, Mouton C, et al. Platelet function point-of-care tests in post-bypass cardiac surgery: are they relevant? Br J Anaesth 2002;89:715–21.
54. Bauriedel G, Skowasch D, Schneider M, et al. Antiplatelet effects of angiotensin-converting enzyme inhibitors compared with aspirin and clopidogrel: a pilot study with whole-blood aggregometry. Am Heart J 2003;145:343–8.
55. Wheeler GL, Braden GA, Steinhubl SR, et al. The Ultegra rapid platelet-function assay: comparison to standard platelet function assays in patients

undergoing percutaneous coronary intervention with abciximab therapy. Am Heart J 2002;143:602–11.
56. Craft RM, Chavez JJ, Bresee SJ, et al. A novel modification of the Thrombelastograph assay, isolating platelet function, correlates with optical platelet aggregation. J Lab Clin Med 2004;143:301–9.
57. Scharbert G, Gebhardt K, Sow Z, et al. Point-of-care platelet function tests: detection of platelet inhibition induced by nonopioid analgesic drugs. Blood Coagul Fibrinolysis 2007;18:775–80.
58. Craft RM, Chavez JJ, Snider CC, et al. Comparison of modified Thrombelastograph and Plateletworks whole blood assays to optical platelet aggregation for monitoring reversal of clopidogrel inhibition in elective surgery patients. J Lab Clin Med 2005;145:309–15.

CHAPTER 22

Antifibrinolytics in Open-Heart Surgery

Wulf Dietrich
Institute for Research in Cardiac Anesthesia and Working Group of Perioperative Hemostasis, Departments of Anesthesiology and Transfusion Medicine, University of Munich, Munich, Germany

Cardiopulmonary bypass (CPB) is associated with impaired hemostasis, which may lead to increased perioperative bleeding. Therefore, postoperative hemorrhage is a common complication in open-heart surgery. On the other hand, CPB and all major operations are characterized by a marked prothrombotic state in the postoperative period. Postoperative complications like MI, stroke, or pulmonary embolism are associated with prothrombotic activity. Thrombin plays an important part in this activation of coagulation [1], which is also linked to the activation of inflammation [2].

An increased perioperative bleeding tendency may lead to reexploration, which increases the risk of the surgical procedure. Allogeneic blood requirement varies significantly among institutions [3]. However, the overall transfusion rate in open-heart surgery is 50–60% [4]. Because of the risks associated with the use of allogeneic blood products, the shortage of donor blood and the costs of allogeneic blood products, blood conservation has become a priority during cardiac surgery. Furthermore, attenuation of the perioperative activation of coagulation, especially the exaggerated generation of thrombin, is desirable.

Different strategies have been developed to reduce the bleeding tendency and inflammatory reactions associated with cardiac surgery. One approach is the prophylactic administration of antifibrinolytic therapy. The most thoroughly evaluated antifibrinolytic agent is aprotinin. However, this drug was withdrawn from the market in 2007 and is no longer clinically available. Other antifibrinolytics are the so-called lysine analogs like epsilon-aminocaproic acid or tranexamic acid, which are widely used in cardiac surgery to reduce bleeding.

Antifibrinolytics have also been used in other surgical procedures besides cardiac operations. It was reported that bleeding and allogeneic blood requirements were reduced in orthopedic surgery [5,6] or liver transplantation [7,8]. It is conceivable that antifibrinolytic treatment may be effective in all procedures where hemostatic activation is responsible for increased perioperative bleeding. Cardiac surgery provides a controlled, reproducible, and powerful hemostatic stimulus and may, therefore, serve as a model for the consequences of increased hemostatic activation. One has to bear in mind that all pharmacological interventions into the intricate network of hemostasis may result in unwanted side effects. For example, inhibition of fibrinolysis may shift the hemostatic balance to the prothrombotic side.

The aim of this overview is to describe the activation of hemostasis during CPB, to discuss the mode of action of different antifibrinolytics, and to present some clinical results of the use of these drugs. Although aprotinin is no longer available since it was withdrawn from the market for safety concerns, it is still discussed in this review because it represents an example of the effects of nonspecific protease inhibition during major surgery.

Alternatives to Blood Transfusion in Transfusion Medicine, 2nd edition. Edited by A. Maniatis, P. Van der Linden, J.-F. Hardy.

Activation of hemostasis during CPB

Platelet dysfunction is the main cause of nonsurgical bleeding after open-heart surgery [9]. It was thought that platelets are mainly mechanically activated by the contact with the nonendothelial, artificial surfaces of the heart-lung machine, the roller pumps, the suction lines, and the oxygenator [10]. However, currently it is evident that activation of plasmatic coagulation factors during major surgery and especially thrombin generation causes platelet activation and platelet dysfunction. The hemostatic system is activated via two pathways: the contact of blood with the negatively charged surfaces of the extracorporeal circuit results in the activation of the contact phase of hemostasis. prekallikrein is converted to kallikrein, which, in the presence of high molecular weight kininogen, activates Factor XII (Hageman Factor). This process finally leads to the activation of the clotting cascade and the formation of thrombin [11]. The process of hemostatic activation is controlled by amplification and inhibitory cascades of proteolytic enzymes. The vast majority of those are mediated by serine proteases [12].

The extrinsic system of coagulation, on the other hand, is also activated via the release of tissue factor during open-heart surgery [13]. This is the main cause of hemostatic activation in noncardiac surgery. It is still under debate, which of these pathways is the main activator of coagulation during CPB [14]. However, the end point of both pathways is thrombin generation. Thrombin is the pivotal enzyme in this process of activation [1]. Thrombin not only converts fibrinogen to fibrin, but is also the most powerful platelet activator, which activates the endothelium and fibrinolysis via the release of tPA from the endothelium, stimulates neutrophils and monocytes, and influences the smooth muscle cells [1]. Thus, activation of the plasmatic hemostatic system leads also to massive platelet activation. Fibrinolysis is also activated via the intrinsic pathway of hemostasis because of contact phase activation. Plasmin also activates platelets [15].

Several connecting points exist between hemostasis and inflammatory response [2] and both systems cannot be considered different processes. The endothelium [16] is the first link between inflammation and coagulation, since damaged endothelium during and after CPB represents a surface where proteins involved in both coagulation and the development of inflammation are expressed [17].

Heparin, which is commonly used during CPB, inhibits thrombin formation only incompletely [18]. Therefore, the key point of the activation of the hemostatic system is thrombin generation and the ability to attenuate this generation in a more effective way.

Mode of action of aprotinin

The nonspecific serine protease inhibitor aprotinin was discovered 1936 by Kraut and Kunitz [19]. This inhibitor, extracted from bovine lung tissue, consists of 58 amino acids and the stability of the single-chain is ensured by three disulfide bridges. In a dose-dependent manner, it inhibits virtually all serine proteases. Most of the enzymes of the hemostatic system are serine-proteases. The preeminent characteristic of aprotinin is the potential to inhibit plasmin—the final enzyme of fibrinolysis. Thus, despite being a nonspecific protease inhibitor, aprotinin is often characterized as being an antifibrinolytic. However, aprotinin reduces also thrombin generation during CPB [20] and attenuates the inflammatory response to major operations [21]. The activity of aprotinin is often expressed in kallikrein inhibiting units (KIU). The concentration of aprotinin required to inhibit serine proteases varies from 50 KIU/mL for plasmin to 200 KIU/mL for plasma kallikrein [19]. Aprotinin has a biphasic elimination and its half-life is approximately 1 hour [22]. All studies on aprotinin report attenuation or almost total suppression of fibrinolytic activation during CPB. On the other hand, there is no influence on the extrinsic part of fibrinolysis: no differences in tPA concentration could be detected [11].

Aprotinin obtained its drug approval in Central Europe at the end of the 1950s with the indication to attenuate hyperfibrinolytic conditions. Aprotinin was applied in numerous indications with suspected hyperfibrinolysis, especially for the treatment of pancreatitis; however, a clinical benefit of antifibrinolytic treatment could not be demonstrated at that time [23].

In cardiac surgery, John Kirklin's group in Alabama pursued the mechanism of the so-called postperfusion syndrome and demonstrated that the interaction of blood with the artificial, nonendothelialized surfaces of the heart-lung machine-circuit led to the activation of several markers of inflammation, especially of the complement cascade. In the Hammersmith hospital in London, S. Westaby and D. Royston's team tried to attenuate the inflammatory response after CPB by the proteinase inhibitor aprotinin in around 10-fold higher dosages compared with previously applied dosages for other indications. Unexpectedly, they observed an abnormally dry operating field in their cardiosurgical patients. This was the hour of birth of the high-dose aprotinin dosage or the Hammersmith regimen. Soon after the first publication by Royston [24] of a series of 22 patients undergoing repeat cardiac surgery, which reported an almost unbelievable reduction in blood loss and transfusion requirement, the drug, which was already approved, became very popular in Europe. Randomized and observational studies confirmed its blood sparing effect [23]. Later on, it was even criticized that too many redundant trial addressed efficacy questions already definitively answered by previous studies [25].

Aprotinin was approved in the United States by the FDA for repeat CABG surgery 1993 after controlled, randomized US studies had proven its efficacy. Later on, it was also approved for primary CABG with an increased risk of bleeding, but not for valves, pediatric, or major aortic surgery.

The efficacy of the drug was proven after the initial studies in several meta-analyses [26] and finally in a Cochrane report [27]. However, these studies were not aimed or powered enough to confirm the safety of this treatment.

There is further evidence that aprotinin not only inhibits fibrinolysis but also clotting activation. Thrombin generation, measured by prothrombin fragment $F_{1.2}$ [28] as well as thrombin activity, measured as thrombin–antithrombin III complex [29], is reduced by high-dose aprotinin. Though these results are not as uniform as the results on fibrinolytic activation, there is considerable evidence that aprotinin also acts as an anticoagulant [20, 21]. Thus, a very important aspect of aprotinin's mode of action is the reduced thrombin generation secondary to its use.

In clinically applied dosages, aprotinin has no direct platelet protective function. However, platelet activation is tightly linked to activation of hemostasis [30]. Less thrombin and plasmin generation due to aprotinin treatment finally leads to better preserved platelet function which is described with the use of aprotinin [31, 32]

Because aprotinin—by inhibiting kallikrein activation—attenuates contact phase activation, the intrinsic pathway of fibrinolysis is inhibited [33]. Additionally, other physiologic cascade systems of the body, which depend on contact phase activation, are also influenced by the use of high-dose aprotinin. Some results suggest [21] that the inflammatory response to CPB may be decreased by the use of aprotinin. Bradykinin may be one of the mediators modulating perioperative inflammation and bleeding tendency. Aprotinin inhibits the response to bradykinin. This was demonstrated in a rat model, where tranexamic acid had no significant effect on vascular permeability caused by bradykinin, whereas aprotinin decreased vascular permeability significantly [34].

Lysine analogs

The synthetic antifibrinolytics tranexamic acid and epsilon-aminocaproic acid inhibit fibrinolysis by binding to the high-affinity lysine binding-side of plasminogen and plasmin [35], thus blocking the action of plasmin on fibrin. Compared to epsilon-aminocaproic acid, tranexamic acid has the greater efficacy, a longer half-life and stronger plasminogen binding. Tranexamic acid has a molecular weight of 157 Da and is 5–10 times more potent than epsilon-aminocaproic acid, and its half-life in vivo is 80 minutes. The synthetic antifibrinolytics inhibit fibrinolysis at the level of plasminogen as well as plasmin, but there is some evidence that they act more at the level of plasminogen: Eberle

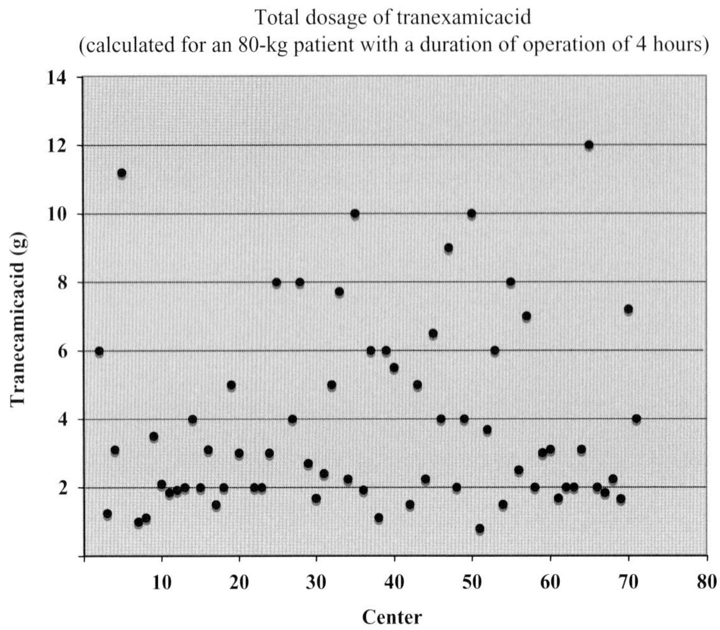

Figure 22.1 This figure shows the result of a survey about the dosage and use of tranexamic acid in 72 German heart centers. The total dosage of tranexamic acid in patients with CAD—for some centers calculated from a per kg dosage for an 80-kg patient—showed a wide variation. Even given the fact that these are survey and not study data, these results demonstrate the urgent need for dosage studies of tranexamic acid.

[36] found increased antiplasmin–plasmin complexes by the use of epsilon-aminocaproic acid compared to aprotinin. Similar results were found by others [37]. This indicates that plasminogen is inhibited by the lysine analogs but the still remaining plasmin generation must be inhibited by physiologic inhibitors.

In contrast to aprotinin, the synthetic antifibrinolytics have no influence on the activation of coagulation; there was no significant alteration in the generation of thrombin–antithrombin complexes [38] or prothrombin fragment $F_{1.2}$ [39] by the use of synthetic antifibrinolytics. Since plasmin acts as a weak platelet agonist, the inhibition of plasmin activity by synthetic antifibrinolytics may also reduce platelet activation and promote hemostasis [40]. The mode of action of lysine analogs in cardiac surgery has been poorly investigated. These drugs solely inhibit fibrinolysis and it is conceivable that this activity shifts the balance of hemostasis toward coagulation [41]. It was hypothesized that a transiently high plasma concentration of epsilon-aminocaproic acid might be conducive to accelerated thrombus formation [42]. The inflammatory response to CPB is also not altered by lysine analogs [43]. The most effective dosage of lysine analogs is not well-defined: while large studies from Canada applied dosages between 6 [44] and 10 g [45], studies from the United States used much lower dosages from 1 to 2 g [35]. In Europe, there is also a wide variation: survey in Germany yielded dosages between 0.5 and 12 g tranexamic acid in cardiac surgery. These results are given in Figure 22.1.

In comparison, lysine analogs and aprotinin both inhibit activation of fibrinolysis during CPB effectively [46]. While the lysine analogs specifically inhibit plasminogen and plasmin activation, aprotinin exhibits a more nonspecific inhibitory capacity. Not only fibrinolysis but also clotting activation is inhibited by aprotinin. While lysine analogs are pure antifibrinolytics, aprotinin is an nonspecific proteinase inhibitor.

Clinical results

The primary end point of most studies investigating antifibrinolytics during cardiac surgery was blood loss and use of allogeneic blood products, which are both clinically and economically significant end points. There is no doubt that the prophylactic use of antifibrinolytics reduces postoperative hemorrhage in patients undergoing open-heart surgery. A Cochrane report [47], which analyzed the relative effectiveness and adverse effect profile lysine analogs and aprotinin, emphasized the effectiveness of both drugs. Adverse events of these drugs were not reported in this report.

Aprotinin was subject to more than 100 randomized clinical trials to study its effectiveness. The updated Cochrane report [27] and a large meta-analysis [48] demonstrated the effectiveness of aprotinin to reduce the need for transfusions and reexploration after cardiac surgery. Epsilon-aminocaproic acid and tranexamic acid were not studied as extensively. Some clinical trials compared the clinical effect of aprotinin and tranexamic acid directly [46, 49]. One trial [46] found a slightly increased efficacy of aprotinin in terms of transfusion requirements, but the clinical significance of this difference was questionable. The recent guidelines of the Society of Thoracic Surgeons and the Society of Cardiovascular Anesthesiologist gave an IA recommendation for both lysine analogs and aprotinin for use in cardiac surgery [50].

All studies done with aprotinin in open-heart surgery revealed that high-dose aprotinin significantly reduces perioperative blood loss and allogeneic blood requirement by 30–80% [51]. Additionally, the percentage of patients not requiring allogeneic blood transfusion was increased by approximately 50% [27]. Comparable results were reported for patients treated with aprotinin in a half-dose, low-dose, or pump prime only regimen [52]. Comparing low-dose and full-dose aprotinin, it could be demonstrated [53] that full-dose aprotinin was superior compared to low-dose in reducing perioperative blood loss and allogeneic blood requirement.

Because the dosage regimens for all drugs vary among the studies, an assessment of comparative efficacy is difficult. High- and low-dose aprotinin significantly reduce postoperative bleeding tendency and transfusion requirement, but the higher dosage regimen seems to be more effective compared to the lower one [54]. Results are less consistent for other antifibrinolytics. Similar reductions of postoperative bleeding tendency were found with a variety of lower dose regimens of aprotinin in comparison to epsilon-aminocaproic acid or tranexamic acid [46].

Aprotinin—early safety concerns

A drug, which shows such a striking efficacy and influence on coagulation like aprotinin, raises concerns about unwanted side effects. Soon after its approval, the first reports on adverse events with the use of aprotinin were published. These first reports of adverse events were related to hypercoagulability [55], renal function [56], and hypersensitivity [57].

Hypercoagulability

The largest study on graft patency found a slight risk of occluded saphenous vein grafts in aprotinin-treated patients [58]. Prothrombotic risks were not the focus of the recent safety discussions. For a discussion of this topic, the reader should refer to the review by Westaby [59].

Renal function

Aprotinin is excreted by the kidney and metabolized in the proximal tubule. Since this is an active process, concerns about the possible nephrotoxicity of aprotinin came up very early after its introduction in cardiac surgery. These concerns could not be substantiated in vitro studies [60], however, clinical studies reported impaired renal function with the use of aprotinin [55, 61]. A slight reversible impairment of renal function after high-dose aprotinin had been demonstrated already in one of the earlier European studies [62] and confirmed by one of the US investigations [63].

Systematic reviews of studies investigating the effect of aprotinin on blood loss and transfusion requirements did not confirm these safety concerns. A Cochrane report described a similar incidence of renal dysfunction in aprotinin treated patients and control subjects [47]. These findings were corroborated in patients undergoing CABG surgery [26]. Admittedly, the end point of almost all studies included in these reviews was blood loss and not renal safety and the number of patients might have been insufficient to detect small differences in renal outcome or uncommon adverse events.

In May 2007, the most comprehensive meta-analysis by Brown et al. [48] analyzed clinical outcomes from 138 trials including approximately 6000 patients treated with either high- or low-dose aprotinin. All dosages were effective in reducing bleeding and transfusion, but only high-dose aprotinin reduced the rate of reexploration (relative risk, 0.49; 95% CI, 0.33–0.73). There were no significant risks or benefits for any agent for mortality, stroke, myocardial infarction, or renal failure. However, high-dose aprotinin significantly increased the risk of renal dysfunction (relative risk, 1.47; 95% CI, 1.12–1.94), 12.9% versus 8.4%. The discussion about severity of renal impairment due to aprotinin is still ongoing [44, 64, 65].

Antigenicity

Aprotinin is a protein derived from bovine lungs. As such it has the potential to stimulate the production of antibodies. Already very early, anaphylactic reactions to aprotinin had been described in patients with a reexposure to the drug. It has been demonstrated that the formation of IgG antibodies is responsible for these sometimes fatal reactions [66]. However, these antibodies disappear over time and after a time interval of 6 months, a reexposure to the drug is possible if its use is indicated [57]. It can be speculated that a considerable number of patients were threatened or died by the inappropriate use of aprotinin during reexposures.

There are no data reported on the risks associated with the use of lysine analogs.

The safety of aprotinin has been heavily questioned in 2006 by studies from Karkouti et al. and Mangano et al. Karkouti analyzed the single-center institutional database and compared out of a pool of 10,870 patients the outcome data of 449 patients treated with aprotinin with 449 matched patients treated with tranexamic acid [67]. The analysis did not demonstrate differences in the incidence of postoperative renal failure requiring dialysis ($p = 0.3$), however, in patients with abnormal preoperative renal function it revealed a significant difference in the incidence of postoperative dysfunction in 23/126 patients with tranexamic acid (18%) and 34/110 (31%) in aprotinin patients ($p = 0.03$). Otherwise, there were no differences in outcome. These results were in accordance with the updated Cochrane report on the use of aprotinin published in 2007 [27].

In an observational, retrospective, multinational database analysis Mangano and colleagues [68] reported the outcome data of 4374 patients undergoing coronary revascularization and found a doubling in the risk of renal events among patients treated with aprotinin (OR 1.89, 95 CI 1.01–3.55; $p = 0.04$). Among patients undergoing complex surgery ($n = 1361$), aprotinin treatment was associated with increased renal dysfunction and renal failure requiring dialysis. Postoperative renal dialysis was observed in 5% of the aprotinin group compared with 1% in the control group and adverse renal outcome was reported in 8% (aprotinin) compared to 3% in patients without aprotinin. In an unadjusted analysis, the authors postulated a dose-dependent effect of aprotinin on renal events (high-dose aprotinin 18% vs 7% in the low-dose group; $p < 0.001$). The authors found an additional risk of aprotinin treatment on cardiovascular events, mainly in primary surgery: OR 1.42 (1.09–1.86; $p = 0.01$) for primary surgery and OR 1.08 (0.75–1.57; $p = 0.67$) for complex surgery, cerebrovascular events OR 2.15 (1.14–4.06; $p = 0.02$) for primary surgery and OR 1.29 (0.71–2.35; $p = 0.41$) for complex surgery, but not on short-term mortality ($p = 0.66$). They also postulated no effect of aprotinin on blood loss and blood transfusion; however, unfortunately, they did not include total allogeneic blood transfusions in their analysis but only intraoperative transfusions. Apparently, patients treated with aprotinin were at higher preoperative risk compared to patients treated with lysine analogs or control patients. Since the indication for aprotinin use was not standardized within the database and the drug was not on the market in all participating countries or not approved for the investigated indication, a selection bias cannot be ruled out. A thorough rebuttal of these results can be found in the publication by Royston et al. [69].

A later analysis of the same dataset claimed an increase in long-term mortality in aprotinin treated patients [70], but left the question open as to why a drug with a short half-life, which did not cause short-term mortality [68], may affect long-term survival. Otherwise, this observation may support the suspicion that aprotinin treated patients were sicker patients and, thus, had a shorter life expectancy.

The Mangano study provoked intensive and controversial discussion [71–75]. Concurrently, the studies by Karkouti and Mangano were subject to two Renal and Cardiovascular Advisory Board meetings of the FDA in September 2006 and 2007. The FDA recommended a change of the packet insert with a new black box warning and asked for new studies. However, the FDA had no sufficient safety concerns to recommend withdrawal of the drug from the market or limit its indications.

The demise of aprotinin

The end of aprotinin was the BART (**B**lood Conservation using **A**ntifibrinolytics: A **R**andomized **T**rial in high-risk cardiac surgery patients) study [44]; this was a multicenter, not industry-sponsored, prospective study from Canada including 2331 high-risk cardiac surgical patients. Patients were randomly assigned to receive aprotinin ($n = 781$) or the lysine analogs tranexamic acid ($n = 770$) or epsilon-amino caproic acid ($n = 780$). The primary endpoint of this study was massive postoperative bleeding. This trial was terminated early because of a consistent trend toward a higher mortality in aprotinin treated patients. The 30-day mortality rate from any cause was 6.0% in the aprotinin group as compared with 3.9% in patients with tranexamic acid (relative risk 1.55; 95% CI 0.99–2.42) and 4% in the epsilon-aminocaproic group (relative risk 1.52; 95% CI 0.98–2.36). If both lysine analog groups were combined, the relative risk of death was 1.53 (95% CI 1.06–2.22). However, the death rate in the ICU was not statistically significantly different. On the other hand, massive bleeding was reduced in the aprotinin group (9.5%) as compared with the other groups (each 12.1%), relative risk 0.79 (95% CI 0.56–1.09). The number of patients transfused with blood products (red blood cells, platelets, cryoprecipitates, and fresh frozen plasma) was significantly lower in the aprotinin group in almost all comparisons. Adverse events like stroke, myocardial infarction, renal failure, or new renal failure were not statistically significant different among the groups.

This detailed listing of the BART results demonstrates the difficulty in interpreting the results: there was a trend toward a higher mortality in the aprotinin group, but the mortality in the ICU was comparable. Likewise, the recorded morbidity, especially renal and cardiac morbidity, was not different (some of the retrospective analyses found increased renal morbidity with aprotinin [76]). Thus, the cause of death remains, presently, speculative. On the other hand, the reduction of massive transfusion and the incidence of allogeneic blood products in the aprotinin group did not result in any benefit for these patients, as it would be expected from other studies investigating the influence of blood transfusion on outcome [77].

The BART Data Safety Monitoring Board recommended after the second interim analysis that randomization of patients to receive aprotinin should be stopped prematurely on October 16, 2007. Immediately upon this notification, the manufacturer withdrew the drug from the market.

Conclusion

The prophylactic perioperative use of antifibrinolytics in open-heart surgery essentially reduces hemorrhage and allogeneic blood requirement. Lysine analogs are effective, but we still need more safety data and more information about the most effective dosage of these drugs. It seems evident that aprotinin has some negative impact on renal function. Whether other detrimental effects are caused by, or associated with, aprotinin remains debatable. One must accept that aprotinin is off the market and is not likely to come back. Ironically, the drug is missed sorely for indications it had never been approved for, like pediatric cardiac surgery [78], aortic surgery [59], or multiple or septic valve replacements. Aprotinin may serve as example for the efficacy of nonspecific protease inhibition. New protease inhibitors are on the horizon [79], however, not only efficacy data but, as the aprotinin story teaches us, safety data for these new drugs are critically important.

References

1. Edmunds LH, Jr, Colman RW. Thrombin during cardiopulmonary bypass. Ann Thorac Surg 2006;82: 2315–22.
2. Esmon CT. The impact of the inflammatory response on coagulation. Thromb Res 2004;114:321–7.
3. Snyder-Ramos SA, Mohnle P, Weng YS, et al. The ongoing variability in blood transfusion practices in cardiac surgery. Transfusion 2008;48:1284–99.
4. Ott E, Mazer CD, Tudor IC, et al. Coronary artery bypass graft surgery–care globalization: the impact of national care on fatal and nonfatal outcome. J Thorac Cardiovasc Surg 2007;133:1242–51.
5. Capdevila X, Calvet Y, Biboulet P, Biron C, Rubenovitch J, dAthis F. Aprotinin decreases blood loss and homologous transfusions in patients undergoing major orthopedic surgery. Anesthesiology 1998;88: 50–57.
6. Murkin JM, Haig GM, Beer KJ, et al. Aprotinin decreases exposure to allogeneic blood during primary unilateral total hip replacement. J Bone Joint Surg Am 2000;82:75–684.
7. Lentschener C, Roche K, Ozier Y. A review of aprotinin in orthotopic liver transplantation: can its harmful effects offset its beneficial effects? Anesth Analg 2005;100:1248–55.
8. Ickx BE, Van Der Linden PJ, Melot C, et al. Comparison of the effects of aprotinin and tranexamic acid on blood loss and red blood cell transfusion requirements during the late stages of liver transplantation. Transfusion 2006;46:595–605.
9. Edmunds LHJ, Ellison N, Colman RW, et al. Platelet function during open heart surgery: comparison of membrane and bubble oxygenators and bubble oxygenators. J Thorac Cardiovasc Surg 1982;83: 805–12.
10. Kirklin JK. Prospects for understanding and eliminating the deleterious effects of cardiopulmonary bypass. Ann Thorac Surg 1991;51:529–31.
11. Dietrich W, Spannagl M, Jochum M, et al. Influence of high-dose aprotinin treatment on blood loss and coagulation pattern in patients undergoing myocardial revascularization. Anesthesiology 1990;73:1119–26.
12. Royston BD, Royston D, Coade SB, Morgan DM, Pearson JD. Aprotinin does not inhibit the release of PGI2 or vWF from cultured human endothelial cells. Thromb Haemost 1992;67:172–5.
13. Boisclair MD, Lane DA, Philippou H, et al. Mechanisms of thrombin generation during surgery and cardiopulmonary bypass. Blood 1993;82:3350–57.
14. Hunt BJ, Parratt RN, Segal HC, Sheikh S, Kallis P, Yacoub M. Activation of coagulation and fibrinolysis during cardiothoracic operations. Ann Thorac Surg 1998;65:712–18.
15. Lu H, Soria C, Li H, et al. Role of active center and lysine binding sites of plasmin in plasmin-induced platelet activation and disaggregation. In: *Thrombosis and Haemostasis*. F.K. Schattauer Verlagsgesellschaft mbH, Stuttgart, 1991, pp. 67–72.
16. Verrier ED, Boyle EM. Endothelial cell injury in cardiovascular surgery. Ann Thorac Surg 1996;62: 915–22.
17. Boyle EM, Pohlman TH, Johnson MC, Verrier ED. Endothelial cell injury in cardiovascular surgery: the systemic inflammatory response. Ann Thorac Surg 1997;63:277–84.
18. Weitz JL, Hudoba M, Massel D, Maraganore J, Hirsh J. Clot-bound thrombin is protected from inhibition by heparin-antithrombin III but is susceptible to inactivation by antithrombin III – independent inhibitors. J Clin Invest 1990;86:385–91.
19. Fritz H, Wunderer G. Biochemistry and applications of aprotinin, the kallikrein inhibitor from bovine organs. Arzneim Forsch/Drug Res 1983;33:479–94.
20. Dietrich W. Reducing thrombin formation during cardiopulmonary bypass: is there a benefit of the additional anticoagulant action of aprotinin? J Cardiovasc Pharmacol 1996;27:S50–57.
21. Landis RC, Haskard DO, Taylor KM. New antiinflammatory and platelet-preserving effects of aprotinin. Ann Thorac Surg 2001;72:S1808–13.
22. Levy JH, Bailey JM, Salmenpera M. Pharmacokinetics of aprotinin in preoperative cardiac surgical patients. Anesthesiology 1994;80:1013–18.
23. Royston D. High-dose aprotinin therapy: a review of the first five years' experience. J Cardiothorac Vasc Anesth 1992;6:76–100.
24. Royston D, Taylor KM, Bidstrup BP, Sapsford RN. Effect of aprotinin on need for blood transfusion after repeat open-heart surgery. Lancet 1987;ii:1289–91.
25. Fergusson D, Glass KC, Hutton B, Shapiro S. Randomized controlled trials of aprotinin in cardiac surgery: could clinical equipoise have stopped the bleeding? Clin Trials 2005;2:218–29.

26. Sedrakyan A, Treasure T, Elefteriades JA. Effect of aprotinin on clinical outcomes in coronary artery bypass graft surgery: a systematic review and meta-analysis of randomized clinical trials. J Thorac Cardiovasc Surg 2004;128:442–8.
27. Henry DA, Carless P, Moxey A, et al. Anti-fibrinolytic use for minimising perioperative allogeneic blood transfusion. Cochrane Database Syst Rev 2007; CD001886.
28. Dietrich W, Dilthey G, Spannagl M, Jochum M, Braun SL, Richter JA. Influence of high-dose aprotinin on anticoagulation, heparin requirement, and celite- and kaolin-activated clotting time in heparin-pretreated patients undergoing open-heart surgery: a double-blind, placebo-controlled study. Anesthesiology 1995;83:679–89.
29. Lu H, Soria C, Commin PL, et al. Hemostasis in patients undergoing extracorporeal circulation: the effect of aprotinin (Trasylol). Thromb Haemost 1991;66:633–7.
30. Butenas S, Branda RF, van't Veer C, Cawthern KM, Mann KG. Platelets and phospholipids in tissue factor-initiated thrombin generation. Thromb Haemost 2001;86:660–67.
31. Kozek-Langenecker SA, Mohammad SF, Masaki T, Green W, Kamerath C, Cheung AK. The effects of aprotonin on platelets in vitro using whole blood flow cytometry. Anesth Analg 2000;90:12–16.
32. Poston RS, Gu J, White C, et al. Perioperative management of aspirin resistance after off-pump coronary artery bypass grafting: possible role for aprotinin. Transfusion 2008;48:39S–46S.
33. Spannagl M, Dooijewaard G, Dietrich W, Kluft C. Protection of single-chain urokinase-type plasminogen activator (scu-PA) in aprotinin treated cardiac surgical patients undergoing cardiopulmonary bypass. Thromb Haemost 1995;73:825–8.
34. OBrien JG, Battistini B, Farmer P, et al. Aprotinin, an antifibrinolytic drug, attenuates bradykinin-induced permeability in conscious rats via platelets and neutrophils. Can J Physiol Pharmacol 1997;75:741–9.
35. Horrow JC, Van Riper DF, Strong MD, et al. The dose-response relationship of tranexamic acid. Anesthesiology 1995;82:383–92.
36. Eberle B, Mayer E, Hafner G, et al. High-dose epsilon-aminocaproic acid versus aprotinin: antifibrinolytic efficacy in first-time coronary operations. Ann Thorac Surg 1998;65:667–73.
37. Blauhut B, Harringer W, Bettelheim P, Doran JE, Spath P, Lundsgaard-Hansen P. Comparison of the effects of aprotinin and tranexamic acid on blood loss and related variables after cardiopulmonary bypass. J Thorac Cardiovasc Surg 1994;108:1083–91.
38. Slaughter TF, Faghih F, Greenberg CS, Leslie JB, Sladen RN. The effects of epsilon-aminocaproic acid on fibrinolysis and thrombin generation during cardiac surgery. Anesth Analg 1997;85:1221–6.
39. Hardy JF, Belisle S, Dupont C, et al. Prophylactic tranexamic acid and epsilon-aminocaproic acid for primary myocardial revascularization. Ann Thorac Surg 1998;65:371–6.
40. Soslau G, Horrow J, Brodsky I. Effect of tranexamic acid on platelet ADP during extracorporeal circulation. Am J Hematol 1991;38:113–19.
41. Bennett Guerrero E, Sorohan JG, Canada AT, et al. Epsilon-aminocaproic acid plasma levels during cardiopulmonary bypass. Anesth Analg 1997;85:248–51.
42. Dentz ME, Slaughter TF, Mark JB. Early thrombus formation on heparin-bonded pulmonary artery catheters in patients receiving epsilon aminocaproic acid. Anesthesiology 1995;82:583–6.
43. Hill GE, Robbins RA. Aprotinin but not tranexamic acid inhibits cytokine-induced inducible nitric oxide synthase expression. Anesth Analg 1997;84:1198–202.
44. Fergusson DA, Hebert PC, Mazer CD, et al. A comparison of aprotinin and lysine analogues in high-risk cardiac surgery. N Engl J Med 2008;358:2319–31.
45. Karski JM, Teasdale SJ, Norman P, et al. Prevention of bleeding after cardiopulmonary bypass with high-dose tranexamic acid. Double-blind, randomized clinical trial. J Thorac Cardiovasc Surg 1995;110: 835–42.
46. Dietrich W, Spannagl M, Boehm J, et al. Tranexamic acid and aprotinin in primary cardiac operations: an analysis of 220 cardiac surgical patients treated with tranexamic acid or aprotinin. Anesth Analg 2008;107:1469–78.
47. Henry DA, Moxey AJ, Carless PA, et al. Anti-fibrinolytic use for minimising perioperative allogeneic blood transfusion (Cochrane Review). The Cochrane Library 2003.
48. Brown JR, Birkmeyer NJ, O'Connor GT. Meta-analysis comparing the effectiveness and adverse outcomes of antifibrinolytic agents in cardiac surgery. Circulation 2007;115:2801–13.
49. Mongan PD, Brown RS, Thwaites BK. Tranexamic acid and aprotinin reduce postoperative bleeding and transfusions during primary coronary revascularization. Anesth Analg 1998;87:258–65.
50. Ferraris VA, Ferraris SP, Saha SP, et al. Perioperative blood transfusion and blood conservation in

cardiac surgery: the Society of Thoracic Surgeons and The Society of Cardiovascular Anesthesiologists clinical practice guideline. Ann Thorac Surg 2007;83: S27–86.

51. Dietrich W. Aprotinin: 1 year on. Curr Opin Anaesthesiol 2009;22:121–7.
52. Levy JH, Pifarre R, Schaff HV, et al. A multicenter, double-blind, placebo-controlled trial of aprotinin for reducing blood loss and the requirement for donor-blood transfusion in patients undergoing repeat coronary artery bypass grafting. Circulation 1995;92:2236–44.
53. Dietrich W, Schopf K, Spannagl M, Jochum M, Braun SL, Meisner H. Influence of high-and low-dose aprotinin on activation of hemostasis in open heart operations. Ann Thorac Surg 1998;65:70–77.
54. Dietrich W, Busley R, Kriner M. High-dose aprotinin in cardiac surgery: is high-dose high enough? An analysis of 8281 cardiac surgical patients treated with aprotinin. Anesth Analg 2006;103:1074–81.
55. Cosgrove DM, Heric B, Lytle BW, et al. Aprotinin therapy for reoperative myocardial revascularization – a placebo-controlled study. Ann Thorac Surg 1992;54:1031–8.
56. Sundt TM, Kouchoukos NT, Saffitz JE, Murphy SF, Wareing TH, Stahl DJ. Renal dysfunction and intravascular coagulation with aprotinin and hypothermic circulatory arrest. Ann Thorac Surg 1993;55: 1418–24.
57. Dietrich W, Ebell A, Busley R, Boulesteix AL. Aprotinin and anaphylaxis: analysis of 12,403 exposures to aprotinin in cardiac surgery. Ann Thorac Surg 2007;84:1144–50.
58. Alderman EL, Levy JH, Rich JB, et al. Analyses of coronary graft patency after aprotinin use: results from the international multicenter aprotinin graft patency experience (IMAGE) trial. J Thorac Cardiovasc Surg 1998;116:716–29.
59. Westaby S. Aprotinin: twenty-five years of claim and counterclaim. J Thorac Cardiovasc Surg 2008;135: 487–91.
60. Horl WH. Aprotinin and renal function in patients undergoing cardiac surgery. Br J Anaesth 2000;84: 3–5.
61. DAmbra MN, Akins CW, Blackstone EH, et al. Aprotinin in primary valve replacement and reconstruction: a multicenter, double-blind, placebo-controlled trial. J Thorac Cardiovasc Surg 1996;112: 1081–9.
62. Blauhut B, Gross C, Necek S, Doran JE, Spath P, Lundsgaard-Hansen P. Effects of high-dose aprotinin on blood loss, platelet function, fibrinolysis, complement, and renal function after cardiopulmonary bypass. J Thorac Cardiovasc Surg 1991;101: 958–67.
63. Lemmer JH, Stanford W, Bonney SL, et al. Aprotinin for coronary artery bypass grafting: effect on postoperative renal function. Ann Thorac Surg 1995;59: 132–6.
64. Manrique A, Jooste EH, Kuch BA, et al. The association of renal dysfunction and the use of aprotinin in patients undergoing congenital cardiac surgery requiring cardiopulmonary bypass. Anesth Analg 2009;109:45–52.
65. Dietrich W, Busley R, Boulesteix AL. Effects of aprotinin dosage on renal function: an analysis of 8548 cardiac surgical patients treated with different dosages of aprotinin. Anesthesiology 2008;108:189–98.
66. Dietrich W, Späth P, Zühlsdorf M, et al. Anaphylactic reactions to aprotinin reexposure in cardiac surgery – relation to antiaprotinin immunoglobulin G and E antibodies. Anesthesiology 2001;95:64–71.
67. Karkouti K, Beattie WS, Dattilo KM, et al. A propensity score case-control comparison of aprotinin and tranexamic acid in high-transfusion-risk cardiac surgery. Transfusion 2006;46:327–38.
68. Mangano DT, Tudor IC, Dietzel C. The risk associated with aprotinin in cardiac surgery. N Engl J Med 2006;354:353–65.
69. Royston D, van Haaften N, De Vooght P. Aprotinin; friend or foe? A review of recent medical literature. Eur J Anaesthesiol 2007;24:6–14.
70. Mangano DT, Miao Y, Vuylsteke A, et al. Mortality associated with aprotinin during 5 years following coronary artery bypass graft surgery. Jama 2007;297: 471–9.
71. Brown JR, Birkmeyer NJ, O'Connor GT. Aprotinin in cardiac surgery. N Engl J Med 2006;354: 1953–7.
72. D'Ambra MN. Aprotinin in cardiac surgery. N Engl J Med 2006;354:1953–7.
73. Ferraris VA, Bridges CR, Anderson RP. Aprotinin in cardiac surgery. N Engl J Med 2006;354: 1953–7.
74. Levy JH, Ramsay JG, Guyton RA. Aprotinin in cardiac surgery. N Engl J Med 2006;354:1953–7.
75. Sedrakyan A, Atkins D, Treasure T. The risk of aprotinin: a conflict of evidence. Lancet 2006;367: 1376–7.
76. Shaw AD, Stafford-Smith M, White WD, et al. The effect of aprotinin on outcome after coronary-artery bypass grafting. N Engl J Med 2008;358:784–93.

77. Koch CG, Li L, Duncan AI, et al. Morbidity and mortality risk associated with red blood cell and blood-component transfusion in isolated coronary artery bypass grafting. Crit Care Med 2006;34: 1608–16.
78. Murugesan C, Banakal SK, Garg R, Keshavamurthy S, Muralidhar K. The efficacy of aprotinin in arterial switch operations in infants. Anesth Analg 2008;107: 783–7.
79. Dietrich W, Nicklisch S, Koster A, Spannagl M, Giersiefen H, van de Locht A. CU-2010 – a novel small molecule protease inhibitor with antifibrinolytic and anticoagulant properties. Anesthesiology 2009;110:123–30.

CHAPTER 23

Efficacy and Safety of Recombinant Activated Factor VII to Control Bleeding in Nonhemophiliac Patients

Jean-François Hardy[1], *Sylvain Bélisle*[1] *& Philippe Van der Linden*[2]
[1]Department of Anesthesiology, University of Montreal, Québec, Canada
[2]Department of Anesthesiology, Université Libre de Bruxelles, Brussels, Belgium

Endogenous activated factor VII plays a crucial role in the coagulation process. The clotting drug NovoSeven® (Novo Nordisk A/S, Bagsvaerd, Denmark) is structurally nearly identical to endogenous factor VIIa and produced by recombination from a baby hamster kidney cell line. Supra-physiologic concentrations of activated factor VII are achieved by the administration of pharmacological doses of recombinant activated factor VII (rFVIIa). rFVIIa plays a central role in coagulation according to the newer, cell-based concepts of coagulation that have emerged recently [1]. To generate thrombin, rFVIIa needs either tissue factor (TF) or activated platelets (TF-independent generation).

During initiation of coagulation, TF exposed on the subendothelium forms a complex with circulating factor VIIa. The TF-FVIIa complex activates factor X and leads to the generation of a small quantity of thrombin. This small quantity of thrombin activates platelets and co-factors, "priming" the system for the subsequent generation of large amounts of thrombin. Factor IX, also activated during the initiation phase, acts as a procoagulant signal and initiates, on the surface of platelets, the cascade leading to the "thrombin burst," i.e., the generation of sufficient thrombin to cleave enough fibrinogen to result in a strong clot. Ultimately, the process is completed when fibrin is cross-linked to enhance durability and when platelets retract, stabilizing the platelet plug.

At least two mechanisms, either TF dependent or independent, may explain the hemostatic effect of rFVIIa administered to (previously normal) patients with uncontrolled hemorrhage [2]. If TF is available to complex rFVIIa, it seems likely that thrombin generation will be mediated by a TF-dependent pathway, given the marked affinity of FVIIa for TF. If TF is separated from the bloodstream by the growing hemostatic plug, rFVIIa may enhance coagulation by directly stimulating factor X on the surface of platelets, resulting in the "thrombin burst" necessary for the formation of a stable clot. It is most likely that both mechanisms are involved. Theoretically, the TF-dependent activation remains localized and the TF-independent activation of FX is not supported by endothelial cells, preventing the systemic initiation of coagulation.

Currently, rFVIIa is approved for the prevention and the treatment of bleeding in patients with hemophilia who present antibodies to factors VIII or IX. Numerous case reports and case series have been published describing its successful use in patients with no prior defect of hemostasis to control bleeding secondary to trauma or major surgery. Over the past 5 years, the estimated number of patients treated with rFVIIa has grown rapidly, mainly for off-license indications.

Alternatives to Blood Transfusion in Transfusion Medicine, 2nd edition. Edited by A. Maniatis, P. Van der Linden, J.-F. Hardy.

Before its introduction in general clinical use, a new treatment has to be proven both effective and safe. The gold standard in establishing the benefits and harms of a novel therapeutic intervention is the randomized controlled trial (RCT). In this chapter, which extends our previous work published elsewhere [3], we reassess all published RCTs that have evaluated the hemostatic efficacy and/or safety of rFVIIa in nonhemophiliac patients. In total, at the time of writing, 18 placebo-controlled double-blind RCTs have been published in 17 articles on the use of rFVIIa to control bleeding in nonhemophiliac patients. rFVIIa was administered either prophylactically to prevent (9 RCTs, 938 randomized patients) [4–12] or therapeutically to treat (9 RCTs, 2012 randomized patients) [13–20] excessive bleeding.

We searched MEDLINE for RCTs published either in English or French on the use of rFVIIa (activated recombinant factor VII/NovoSeven®) outside hemophilia. To be included in this review, studies had to be prospective, randomized, blinded, and placebo-controlled and had to evaluate the efficacy and safety of rFVIIa in nonhemophiliac patients. Retrospective, nonrandomized, open label, nonplacebo-controlled studies were excluded, as were those conducted in patients with hemophilia. Case series, retrospective reviews and registers were considered only for discussion purposes.

Eighteen trials published in 17 articles were identified. Trials dealt either with the prophylactic or the therapeutic use of rFVIIa to prevent or treat excessive bleeding in a variety of clinical contexts. Main data were summarized and are presented in Tables 23.1 and 23.2.

Efficacy of rFVIIa for the prevention of excessive bleeding and the reduction of transfusions

Table 23.1 summarizes the main characteristics and the key findings of the nine trials that have evaluated the prophylactic use of rFVIIa outside hemophilia. In over half of the trials, rFVIIa was not efficacious [5, 6, 8, 9, 11].

The trial by Lodge on the use of rFVIIa to reduce bleeding and transfusions in liver transplantation found a statistically significant but small difference in the proportion of transfused patients [7]. At best, the percentage of patients avoiding transfusions altogether was 10% (6/62 in the 60 μg/kg group; Table 23.1). Use of red blood cells (RBC), fresh frozen plasma (FFP) and platelet concentrates (PC) was similar in all groups and there were no other clinically important differences between groups.

The authors of a pilot study on the use of rFVIIa to reduce allogeneic transfusions in patients undergoing complex noncoronary cardiac surgery with cardiopulmonary bypass stated that "rFVIIa significantly reduces the need for allogeneic transfusion" [10]. However, one patient in the rFVIIa group was excluded from the "per protocol analysis" following unblinding of treatment allocation because of the sudden onset of mediastinal hemorrhage 2 hours after surgery while the patient was in the intensive care unit. The patient consumed 72 units of allogeneic blood products, two further doses of rFVIIa, and returned to the operating room on two occasions before a posterior aortic tear was discovered. When the results were analyzed by intention-to-treat (also presented in the article), the results of the pilot study were negative [10].

The latest trial on the prophylactic use of rFVIIa evaluated the efficacy of the drug to reduce transfusions in burn patients undergoing excision and skin grafting. Interpretation of the results is difficult as they are presented as "Total blood products transfused/full thickness burn wound excised and grafted (% total body surface area)" [12]. We were unable to determine how this applies clinically to a burn patient coming to the operating room for excision and skin grafting and the percent of total body surface area at which the use of rFVIIa becomes beneficial. The effect of treatment on intraoperative bleeding is not reported and all the other outcomes of interest were similar in both groups (Table 23.1).

The study by Friederich et al. showed that rFVIIa reduced perioperative blood loss and eliminated the need for transfusion in patients undergoing retropublic prostatectomy [4]. Nevertheless, most clinicians would consider that blood losses in the

Table 23.1 Main characteristics and key results of trials evaluating the prophylactic use of rFVIIa outside hemophilia.

Author (year)	Clinical setting	No. of patients (placebo/drug)	Dosage scheme	Effects on bleeding (placebo/drug)*	Effects on transfusions (placebo/drug)*	Other outcomes of interest	Adverse events (placebo/drug)
Friederich (2003) [4]	Radical prostatectomy	36 (12/24)	Dose escalation study: 20 μg/kg followed by 40 μg/kg	TBL: 2688 mL vs 1235 mL vs 1089 mL ($p = 0.001$)	NTP: 7/12 vs 3/8 vs 0/16 ($p = 0.001$)	Shorter duration of operation; no effect on LOS	No AEs reported
Lodge (2005) [5]	Major liver resection	204 randomized	Placebo vs 20 μg/kg vs 80 μg/kg; repeated after 5 hours	TBL: 1422 mL vs 1372 mL vs 1073 mL ($p = 0.07$)	NTP: 23/63 vs 26/63 vs 15/59 ($p = 0.09$)	Reduction in Hct smaller in 80 μg/kg ($p = 0.04$)	3 TE events in each group
		185 (63/122) operated as planned					
Shao (2006) [6]	Partial hepatectomy	234 randomized	Placebo vs 50 μg/kg vs 100 μg/kg); repeated every 2 hours (max 4 doses)	TBL: 500 mL vs 800 mL vs 500 mL (medians; $p = 0.77$)	NTP: 29/38 vs 36/51 vs 27/36 ($p = 0.59$)	Not reported	SAEs: 2/76 vs 2/68 vs 5/74 ($p =$ ns)
		221 (76/145) operated as planned			No difference in any ABP transfused		
Lodge (2005) [7]	Liver transplantation	209 randomized	Placebo vs 60 μg/kg vs 120 μg/kg; repeated every 2 hours and on wound closure	No difference in intraoperative blood loss (data not presented)	NTP: 61/61 vs 56/62 vs 52/56 ($p = 0.0331$)	No difference in ICU stay or total LOS	SAEs: 12/62 vs 17/63 vs 16/58 ($p =$ ns); no increased TE events
		182 (61/121) operated as planned			Use of RBC, FFP, and PC similar in all groups		
Planinsic (2005) [8]	Liver transplantation	87 randomized	Placebo vs 20 μg/kg vs 40 μg/kg vs 80 μg/kg; single dose administered	Not reported	Use of RBC (allogeneic and autologous), FFP, and PC similar in all groups	No difference in ICU stay	No difference in SAEs; No difference in TE events: 2/19 vs 2/18 vs 1/24 vs 8/22
		82 (19/63) operated as planned					

Raobaikady (2005) [9]	Reconstruction surgery for traumatic pelvic fracture	48 (24/24) randomized and analyzed	Placebo vs 90 μg/kg; repeated after 2 hours if Hb <8.0 g/dL	TBL: 2070 mL vs 1535 mL ($p = 0.79$)	NTP: 16/24 vs 11/24 ($p = 0.24$)	No difference in duration of operation, ICU stay or total LOS	No adverse events considered related to study drug
				CBL: 2146 mL vs 2787 mL ($p = 0.50$)	Total RBC transfused: 706 mL vs 289 mL ($p = 0.33$)		
Diprose (2005) [10]	Adult complex noncoronary cardiac surgery with CPB	20 (10/10) randomized	Placebo vs 90 μg/kg after neutralization of heparin with protamine	Mediastinal drainage: 630 mL vs 330 mL	NTP: 8/10 vs 3/10 ($p = 0.21$)	No difference in time on ventilator, ICU stay or total LOS	No difference in SAEs (stroke, MI or death)
					Use of RBC, FFP, and PC similar in both groups		
Ekert (2006) [11]	Pediatric congenital heart surgery with CPB	82 enrolled	Placebo vs 40 μg/kg after protamine administration; repeated after 20 minutes and in ICU as needed (3 doses max)	TBL: 12.7 mL/kg vs 15.2 mL/kg ($p = 0.103$)	NTP during surgery 15/36 vs 13/40 ($p = 0.15$)	Time to chest closure longer in treatment group: 99 minutes vs 55 minutes ($p = 0.0263$)	No difference in SAEs; no thrombotic or embolic events in both groups
		76 (36/40) treated as planned			NTP postoperatively 29/35 vs 30/40 ($p = 0.45$)		
Johansson (2007) [12]	Excision and skin grafting in burn patients	18 (9/9) randomized	Placebo vs 40 μg/kg at skin incision and 90 minutes later	Not reported	Total blood products transfused (adjusted for percentage full thickness burn wound excised and grafted): 2.2 vs 0.9 ($p = 0.0013$)	No difference in duration of operation, ICU stay or total LOS	No adverse events considered related to study drug

*Results presented as (1) means or number of patients unless specified otherwise and (2) placebo vs increasing doses of rFVIIa (as presented in the "Dosage scheme" column).

TBL, total blood loss; NTP, number of transfused patients; LOS, length of stay; TE, thromboembolic event; ABP, allogeneic blood products; AE, adverse event; SAE, serious adverse event; ICU, intensive care unit; ns, not significant; RBC, red blood cells; FFP, fresh frozen plasma; PC, platelet concentrates; Hb, hemoglobin concentration; CBL calculated blood loss; CPB, cardiopulmonary bypass; MI, myocardial infarction.

Table 23.2 Main characteristics and key results of trials evaluating the therapeutic use of rFVIIa outside hemophilia.

Author (year)	Clinical setting	No. of patients (placebo/drug)	Dosage scheme	Effects on bleeding (placebo/drug)*	Effects on transfusions (placebo/drug)*	Other outcomes of interest	Adverse events (placebo/drug)
Bosch (2004) [13]	Upper gastrointestinal bleeding	245 randomized	Placebo vs 100 μg/kg (8 doses total)	No effect on composite end point (control of bleeding within 24 hours, prevention of rebleeding and death within 5 days)	Use of RBC similar in both groups: 1.3 vs 1.5 units ($p = 0.73$)	No difference in ICU or total LOS	7 TE events in each group
		242 (121/121) dosed				No difference in emergency and elective procedures	No difference in mortality
Boffard (2005) [14]	Blunt trauma	158 randomized	Placebo vs 200, 100, and 100 μg/kg (3 doses total)	Not reported (difficult to measure accurately in trauma patients)	Use of RBC similar in both groups: 7.2 vs 7.8 (median; $p = 0.07$)	Reduction in the incidence of ARDS in treatment group: 12/74 vs 3/69 ($p = 0.03$)	No difference in SAEs, TE events and mortality
		143 (74/69) analyzed			Use of FFP, PC, and cryoprecipitates similar in both groups		
	Penetrating trauma	143 randomized		Not reported (difficult to measure accurately in trauma patients)	Use of RBC similar in both groups: 4.8 vs 4.0 (median; $p = 0.24$)	Trend toward a reduced incidence of MOF in treatment group: 7/64 vs 2/70 ($p = 0.09$)	No difference in SAEs, TE events and mortality
		134 (64/70) analyzed			Use of FFP, PC, and cryoprecipitates similar in both groups		

Mayer (2005) [15]	Intracerebral hemorrhage	48 randomized	Dose escalation study: placebo vs 10, 20, 40, 80, 120, 160 μg/kg	No difference in% changes in ICH volumes	Not reported (not relevant to the study)	Neurological outcomes similar in all groups	No difference in SAEs, TE events and mortality
		47 (11/36) analyzed		No difference in total hemorrhage volumes (ICH + IVH)			
Mayer (2005) [16]	Intracerebral hemorrhage	400 randomized	Placebo vs 40 μg/kg vs 80 μg/kg vs 160 μg/kg	Significant decreases in ICH, ICH + IVH, and ICH + IVH + edema volumes in treatment groups; significant dose–response relationship	Not reported (not relevant to the study)	Improved neurological outcomes in treatment groups	Arterial TE events: 0/96 vs 16/303 ($p = 0.01$)
		399 (96/303) analyzed					Mortality at 3 months: 28/96 vs 56/303 ($p = 0.02$)
Chuansumrit (2005) [17]	Dengue fever in children	28 randomized	Placebo vs 100 μg/kg; dose repeated after 30 minutes if ineffective	Initial improvement of bleeding in treatment group; bleeding control similar at 6, 12, and 24 hours	Patients transfused RBC (3/9 vs 5/16) and FFP (2/9 vs 4/16) similar in both groups (p = ns)	No difference in LOS	No evidence of TE events
		25 (9/16) analyzed			Nonsignificant decrease in the number of patients transfused PC in the treatment group: 3/9 vs 1/16 ($p = 0.1$)		

(Continued)

Table 23.2 *(Continued)*

Author (year)	Clinical setting	No. of patients (placebo/drug)	Dosage scheme	Effects on bleeding (placebo/drug)*	Effects on transfusions (placebo/drug)*	Other outcomes of interest	Adverse events (placebo/drug)
Pihusch (2005) [18]	Hematopoietic stem cell transplantation	100 (23/77) randomized	Placebo vs 40 μg/kg vs 80 μg/kg vs 160 μg/kg; dose repeated every 6 hours for 36 hours	No significant effect of increasing dose on bleeding score at 38 hours	Use of RBC, FFP, and PC similar in all groups		No difference in SAEs, TE events and mortality
Sachs (2007) [19]	Spinal surgery	49 (13/36) randomized upon reaching bleeding trigger	Placebo vs 30 μg/kg vs 60 μg/kg vs 120 μg/kg; dose repeated every 2 hours (3 doses total)	TBL: 2270 mL vs 1909 mL vs 1262 mL vs 1868 mL (p = ns)	Total transfusion volume (allogeneic and autologous RBC + cell saver + FFP + cryoprecipitates + PC): 1421 mL vs 979 mL vs 711 mL vs 1041 mL (p = ns)		No difference in SAEs, TE events and mortality
Mayer (2008) [19]	Intracerebral hemorrhage	841 (268/573) randomized	Placebo vs 20 μg/kg vs 80 μg/kg	Significant reduction in the increase of ICH volume in treatment groups	Not reported (not relevant to the study)	Proportion of patients with poor clinical outcomes similar in all groups	Arterial TE events: 9% (80 μg/kg) vs 4% (placebo) $p = 0.04$; no difference in mortality

*Results presented as (1) mean or number of patients unless specified otherwise and (2) placebo vs increasing doses of rFVIIa (as presented in the "Dosage scheme" column.

TBL, total blood loss; RBC, red blood cells; FFP, fresh frozen plasma; PC, platelet concentrates; ICU, intensive care unit; LOS, length of stay; SAE, serious adverse event; TE, thromboembolic event; ARDS, acute respiratory distress syndrome; MOF, multiple organ failure; ICH, intracerebral hemorrhage; IVH, intraventricular hemorrhage; ns, not significant.

placebo group were much greater (median 2688 mL) than those encountered in contemporary clinical practice [21], specially in light of the recent advancements in minimally invasive surgical techniques [22, 23]. Accordingly, the usefulness of rFVIIa to reduce bleeding and transfusions in patients undergoing retropubic prostatectomy described in 2003 would probably not apply today.

In summary, the role of rFVIIa to *prevent* excessive bleeding and reduce transfusions in a variety of patients at risk of hemorrhage during surgery has not been demonstrated convincingly.

Efficacy of rFVIIa for the treatment of excessive bleeding and the reduction of transfusions

Table 23.2 summarizes the main characteristics and the key findings of the nine trials (published in eight articles: two studies [14] were published simultaneously) that have evaluated the therapeutic use of rFVIIa outside hemophilia. Three studies evaluated surgical indications while six explored medical indications.

rFVIIa was used as adjunctive therapy for the control of bleeding in severely injured trauma patients in two randomized, placebo-controlled, double-blind clinical trials (one in blunt trauma and one in penetrating trauma). The primary end point of the study "was the number of RBC units (autologous RBCs, allogeneic RBCs, and whole blood) transfused during the 48-hour period after the first dose of trial product." Whether in blunt or penetrating trauma, use of RBC, FFP, and PC was similar in placebo and treatment groups when all patients are considered (intention-to-treat analysis; Table 23.2). There was a significant reduction of transfusions in the blunt trauma patients treated with rFVIIa who were alive at 48 hours (post hoc analysis).

The other surgical trial evaluated the effect of rFVIIa in spinal surgery patients who reached a bleeding trigger (10% blood loss; expected total losses ≥20% total blood volume) during the operation [19]. Mean blood losses and transfusion volume were not different between groups. When adjusted for duration of surgery, number of vertebral segments fused and estimated blood volume, blood loss, and transfusion volume were reduced significantly in treated patients. However, as presented, the results do not allow us to determine in which patients (according to estimated blood volume, planned duration of surgery, and number of vertebral segments fused) the use of rFVIIa may be beneficial.

Positive findings on the therapeutic use of rFVIIa were observed in patients with intracerebral hemorrhage (ICH) [16] In their initial study, Mayer et al. showed that the administration of rFVIIa within four hours after the onset of symptoms of ICH is associated with a reduced growth of the hematoma, and a decrease in 90-day mortality. In addition, an improvement in functional outcomes at 90 days as assessed by four neurologic outcome scales (Modified Rankin Scale, Barthel Index, Extended Glasgow Outcome Scale, and National Institutes of Health Stroke Scale) was observed in the treatment groups, despite an increase in the frequency of thromboembolic events (see below). Unfortunately, these positive results were not confirmed by a subsequent large multicenter, phase III trial involving 841 patients [20].

Three other studies report the use of rFVIIa to treat excessive bleeding in a medical context. The first was in cirrhotic patients presenting with upper gastrointestinal bleeding [13], the second in children with Dengue fever [17] and the third in adults after hematopoietic stem cell transplantation [18]. In all cases, bleeding control and transfusion requirements were similar in both groups.

Finally, a phase II study in cardiac surgery was stopped in November 2007 after enrollment of 172 patients into two dose cohorts of 40 and 80 μg/kg, but without enrolling patients into the final dose cohort (http://clinicaltrials.gov/ct2/show?cond=%22Postoperative+Hemorrhage%22&rank=2). The decision to conclude the study was "based on the wish to accurately reflect current clinical practice with respect to NovoSeven® dosing" (Novo Nordisk announcement, December 2007). As of January 2009 the study remains unpublished.

In summary, the role of rFVIIa to *treat* excessive (or critical, in the case of ICH) bleeding and reduce transfusions in a variety of medical and surgical conditions has not been demonstrated convincingly.

Safety of rFVIIa when used for the prevention or the treatment of excessive bleeding and the reduction of transfusions

The incidence of adverse (including thromboembolic) events was not increased in the nine trials evaluating the prophylactic use of rFVIIa (Table 23.1). With two exceptions, the incidence of adverse events was also not increased in the nine trials evaluating the therapeutic use of rFVIIa (Table 23.2).

An increase in the incidence of arterial thrombotic events was observed in the ICH trial published by Mayer in 2005 [16]. Total (venous and arterial) serious adverse thromboembolic events occurred in 2% of patients receiving placebo and in 7% of all patients treated with rFVIIa ($p = 0.12$). The incidence of venous thromboembolic events was the same (2%) in both groups. However, the incidence of arterial serious adverse thromboembolic events (myocardial ischemic events and cerebral infarctions) was increased in rFVIIa patients (0% vs 5%; $p = 0.01$). The incidence of fatal or disabling thromboembolic events related to treatment was the same (2%) in both groups. Despite the use of smaller doses, a similar increase of arterial TE events was demonstrated in the most recent ICH trial by the same authors [20]. Pooled data from three ICH trials supported the increased risk of arterial thromboembolic events with rFVIIa, particularly at higher doses (120–160 μg/kg) [24].

The majority of studies excluded patients at risk of thrombosis such as those with known hypercoagulopathy, history of pulmonary embolism, or deep vein thrombosis, stable/unstable angina pectoris, myocardial infarction, intermittent claudication, transient ischemic attack/ischemic stroke; signs of cardiac ischemia, etc. In one case, midway through the trial, a change was made "to exclude patients with any history of thrombotic vaso-occlusive disease" [16]. Such strict exclusion criteria may have contributed to the 12% enrollment rate of screened patients mentioned in that trial [16] and raise the possibility that the incidence of adverse thrombotic events might be higher in a broader ICH patient population [25].

In summary, the observations made in 16 of the 18 published RCTs on the use of rFVIIa to prevent or to treat excessive bleeding in nonhemophilia patients do not report an excess of serious (particularly thrombotic) adverse events. The use of rFVIIa in highly selected ICH patients with minimal (but critical) bleeding was associated with an increased risk of arterial thrombosis [16, 20].

Comments

The role of rFVIIa to prevent or to treat excessive (or critical, in the case of ICH) bleeding and reduce transfusions in a variety of patients at risk of hemorrhage during surgery has not been demonstrated convincingly. The most impressive benefits of the therapeutic use of rFVIIa were in patients with ICH but these results were not confirmed in a recent phase III trial. Thus, the generalized administration of rFVIIa to nonhemophiliac patients at risk of excessive (or critical) bleeding cannot be recommended today.

Our findings concur with those of the meta-analysis published by Stanworth et al. [26] that included 13 trials. Six trials examined the prophylactic use of rFVIIa and seven examined the therapeutic use of the drug. The authors conclude that the effectiveness of rFVIIa as a more general hemostatic drug, either prophylactically or therapeutically, remains uncertain compared to its role in the management of patients with hemophilia and that its use should be restricted to clinical trials. The results of three additional studies on prophylaxis [6, 11, 12] and of the two on treatment [19, 20] with rFVIIa are in line with the conclusions of Stanworth's meta-analysis.

Recently, another meta-analysis evaluated the efficacy and safety of rFVIIa in major surgical procedures [27]. The systematic review included seven trials [4–10] while the efficacy analysis was conducted in five [4, 5, 7, 9, 10]. The review concluded that patients receiving rFVIIa had a reduced risk of allogeneic red cell transfusion but the authors were unable to comment on transfusion needs or perioperative bleeding. The selection of studies and the very positive results of the 40 μg/kg group in the Friederich trial [4] may help explain the discrepancy between meta-analyses.

Numerous case reports, case series, and registers have suggested that rFVIIa may be efficacious for the prophylaxis or for the treatment of severe bleeding in different clinical contexts. [28–36] Observational studies report success rates that vary from 69% [33] up to 80% [32, 35]. It is rather interesting to note that these rates are similar to those reported in trials evaluating the therapeutic potential of rFVIIa. When aggregating the data on the control of bleeding in the three RCTs that reported this variable [13, 17, 18], the number of patients with reduced bleeding was 158/210 or 75.2% in the rFVIIa group vs 130/172 or 75.6% in the control group [26]. Thus, whatever the circumstances, approximately 75% of patients appear to respond to treatment, whether it is rFVIIa or placebo.

Notwithstanding the interest of case reports, case series and registers, the gold standard in establishing the benefits and the harms of a technology is the RCT [37]. The RCT is a study in which subjects are randomized to an intervention or control and followed systematically for occurrence of outcome. Randomization and blinding of intervention avoid observator bias, which would, otherwise, be inevitable. Thus, as opposed to observational, single arm interventional studies or those using historical controls, the RCT is the only study design where causality, both for benefits and for harms, can be established. Unfortunately, and contrary to the hopes raised by case reports, case series, and registers, results of published RCTs have failed to demonstrate convincingly the efficacy of rFVIIa outside hemophilia.

Why have such disappointing results been observed? Possible explanations are numerous and include inadequate doses of the drug or inappropriate timing of administration, a suboptimal clotting environment at the time of drug administration, and adherence to a transfusion protocol for red cells and hemostatic blood components. In studies evaluating the prophylactic use of rFVIIa, doses varied between 20 and 120 μg/kg and were either not repeated or repeated at intervals of 2 or 5 hours (Table 23.1). Surprisingly, the study reporting unquestionable efficacy of rFVIIa used the smallest doses administered only once in the early operative phase [4]. Despite the use of more generally accepted dosages (of the order of 90 μg/kg) repeated at a time interval in relation with rFVIIa's half-life of 2–3 hours [38, 39], all the other trials generated results that were either negative [5, 6, 8, 9, 11] or difficult to interpret clinically [7, 10, 12]. In studies evaluating the therapeutic use of rFVIIa, doses were, in general, higher and repeated more frequently. This is congruent with the known pharmacokinetic profile of rFVIIa whereby clearance is increased and half-life is shortened in the presence of bleeding [38, 40, 41]. While doses higher than 50 μg/kg appear to be more efficacious [27], the level of FVII required to achieve hemostasis in different clinical circumstances remains uncertain [39, 42].

An important consideration when treating hemorrhage pertains to the maintenance of an optimal hemostatic environment. Hematocrits as high as 35% may be required to sustain hemostasis in bleeding patients undergoing massive transfusion [43]. Erythrocytes modulate the biochemical and functional responsiveness of activated platelets, suggesting that erythrocytes contribute to thrombosis and hemostasis and supporting the concept that thrombus formation is a multicellular event [44–46]. Another mechanism by which erythrocytes modulate hemostasis is the rheological effect of red cells on the margination of platelets [47], enhancing the near-wall concentration of platelets up to about seven times the average concentration [48]. Maintaining adequate levels of circulating platelets is important given (a) our current knowledge of hemostasis, in which platelets play a pivotal role [42] and (b) the findings from studies [49–52] showing that survival is improved in massively transfused patients who received increased numbers of platelet concentrates.

We used the intent-to-treat principle to evaluate the results of RCTs [37]. Inclusion of only those subjects who followed the protocol as planned (*per protocol* analysis) introduces a number of biases. Subjects who are lost to follow-up or who refuse treatment (despite consenting initially) are likely to be different in important ways from other subjects. The intent-to-treat principle takes into account the inherent difficulties of a treatment. Excluding patients in whom treatment was difficult or impossible will bias the overall results on the efficacy of an intervention. Finally, some important outcomes cannot be predicted at the time of randomization (had they been predicted, the patient would not have been included in the study). For example, it is impossible to determine ahead of time which patient(s) will present with overt surgical bleeding after a cardiac operation [10] or those who will be alive at 48 hours after trauma [14]. Thus, the results of the analysis by intent-to-treat truly reflect the efficacy of an intervention in the conditions of the study.

Prevention of excessive bleeding and transfusions can be achieved by different pharmacological and nonpharmacological interventions. Obviously, to be adopted in clinical practice, an intervention must be efficacious but safety remains a major concern. When administered at pharmacological doses, blood levels of activated factor VII are 1000 times greater than normal. As mentioned previously, rFVIIa augments thrombin generation by TF dependent and independent pathways; enhances the adhesion, deposition, and activation of platelets (thrombin dependent); and inhibits fibrinolysis [42, 53–55]. By definition, any therapy that promotes hemostasis is likely to induce thrombosis. Thus, a favorable balance between hemostasis (the desired effect) and thrombosis (an unwanted, potentially serious adverse event) may be difficult to achieve. In theory, since they are mediated by TF, the effects of rFVIIa should remain localized [56]. Nevertheless, Stanworth et al. observed a trend toward an increase in thromboembolic events associated with the use of rFVIIa either prophylactically (pooled RR 1.25; 95% CI 0.76–2.07) or therapeutically (pooled RR 1.50; 95% CI 0.86–2.62) [26].

Tissue factor may be expressed at sites other than the site of hemorrhage, resulting in undesirable thrombotic events [57]. In animals with no hemostatic defect and a carotid artery lesion, rFVIIa increases the incidence of thrombosis [58, 59]. This may help explain the increased incidence of arterial serious adverse thromboembolic events observed in ICH patients [16]. The "potential increased risk of arterial thromboembolic adverse events with use of NovoSeven, including myocardial ischemia, myocardial infarction, cerebral ischemia and/or infarction" (http://www.fda.gov/medwatch/safety/2005/safety05.htm#NovoSeven) that occurred despite very strict exclusion criteria, as mentioned earlier, raises the possibility that the incidence of adverse thrombotic events might be higher in a broader ICH patient population [25].

A review of the Adverse Event Reporting System (AERS) of the United States Food and Drug Administration (FDA) documented a total of 431 AE reports for rFVIIa between 1999 and 2004 [60]. Of these, 168 reports described 185 thromboembolic events, the majority of which (151) were for unlabeled indications. Reported adverse events included cerebrovascular accident ($n = 39$), acute myocardial infarction ($n = 34$), other arterial thromboses ($n = 26$), pulmonary embolism ($n = 32$), other venous thromboses ($n = 42$), and clotted devices ($n = 10$). In 72% of the 50 reported deaths, the probable cause of death was the thromboembolic event. A major concern was that the use of rFVIIa and spontaneous reporting of AEs increased steadily during the study period while reporting of AEs originating from controlled trials decreased. The authors concluded that RCTs are needed to establish the safety and efficacy of rFVIIa in patients without hemophilia and we believe this conclusion still applies.

Summary and recommendations

In summary, published RCTs do not support the efficacy of rFVIIa to control bleeding and reduce transfusions in various patient populations, either prophylactically or therapeutically. In addition, the safety of rFVIIa remains a major concern [60]. The lack of adequately powered, randomized studies evaluating rFVIIa limits the capacity to draw firm conclusions on its optimal role in our therapeutic armamentarium, whether for the prevention or for the treatment of coagulopathy. Consequently and while awaiting the unambiguous demonstration of its benefits, confirmation of its safety, determination of the optimal dosage, and appropriate timing of administration, the generalized use of rFVIIa to prevent or to control bleeding in nonhemophiliac patients cannot be recommended.

Unfortunately, off-label use of the drug has increased markedly, despite some evidence that the drug may increase the risk of thrombotic events and death, a situation described as "the scientifically unsound creep of prescribing indications" by Hébert and Stanbrook in 2007 [61].

In spite of the lack of formal evidence for efficacy and or safety, the off-label use of a drug like rFVIIa may be, on occasion, appropriate when the anesthesiologist, critical care physician, or surgeon determine that this is the best option for their patient in light of the available evidence [61]. The decision to administer a potent hemostatic such as rFVIIa outside its recognized prescribing indications should, however, always be discussed with the patient (or the patient's family as would be the case for surgical hemorrhage). Patients should be informed about knowledge gaps and pertinent risks [61], which are both important in the case of rFVIIa.

Accordingly, rFVIIa may be considered with caution in patients with refractory life-threatening hemorrhage when all conventional measures (including embolization, surgery, rewarming the patient, etc.) have failed [62]. It should be considered as an adjunct to, rather than in replacement of, such measures. Inasmuch as possible, an optimal hemostatic environment must be ensured. Thus, FVIIa should be considered relatively late in the management of excessive bleeding. Introduction of rFVIIa at a very early stage of hemorrhage will expose an unnecessarily large number of patients to an extraordinarily expensive therapy whose efficacy remains unclear. On the contrary, criteria such as the Sequential Organ Failure Assessment and response to the initial dose of rFVIIa may help determine when treatment is futile [63].

Finally, all patients exposed to rFVIIa should be included in ongoing registers. While registers cannot demonstrate the efficacy or the safety of a drug, they may be helpful to identify specific clinical circumstances in which rFVIIa could be useful and, thus, assist in planning future RCTs on the benefits and risks of rFVIIa used to control bleeding in nonhemophiliac patients.

References

1. Roberts HR, Monroe DM, Oliver JA, Chang JY, Hoffman M. Newer concepts of blood coagulation. Haemophilia 1998;4(4):331–4.
2. Lisman T, de Groot P. Mechanism of action of recombinant activated factor VII. TATM 2003;5(5):S5–10.
3. Hardy JF, Belisle S, Van Der Linden P. Efficacy and safety of recombinant activated factor VII to control bleeding in nonhemophiliac patients: a review of 17 randomized controlled trials. Ann Thorac Surg 2008;86(3):1038–48.
4. Friederich PW, Henny CP, Messelink EJ, et al. Effect of recombinant activated factor VII on perioperative blood loss in patients undergoing retropubic prostatectomy: a double-blind placebo-controlled randomised trial. Lancet 2003;361(9353):201–5.
5. Lodge JP, Jonas S, Oussoultzoglou E, et al. Recombinant coagulation factor VIIa in major liver resection: a randomized, placebo-controlled, double-blind clinical trial. Anesthesiology 2005;102(2):269–75.
6. Shao YF, Yang JM, Chau GY, et al. Safety and hemostatic effect of recombinant activated factor VII in cirrhotic patients undergoing partial hepatectomy: a multicenter, randomized, double-blind, placebo-controlled trial. Am J Surg 2006;191(2):245–9.
7. Lodge JP, Jonas S, Jones RM, et al. Efficacy and safety of repeated perioperative doses of recombinant factor VIIa in liver transplantation. Liver Transpl 2005;11(8):973–9.
8. Planinsic RM, Van Der Meer J, Testa G, et al. Safety and efficacy of a single bolus administration of recombinant factor VIIa in liver transplantation due to chronic liver disease. Liver Transpl 2005;11(8):895–900.
9. Raobaikady R, Redman J, Ball JA, Maloney G, Grounds RM. Use of activated recombinant coagulation factor VII in patients undergoing reconstruction surgery for traumatic fracture of pelvis or pelvis and acetabulum: a double-blind, randomized, placebo-controlled trial. Br J Anaesth 2005;94(5):586–91.
10. Diprose P, Herbertson MJ, O'Shaughnessy D, Gill RS. Activated recombinant factor VII after cardiopulmonary bypass reduces allogeneic transfusion in

complex non-coronary cardiac surgery: randomized double-blind placebo-controlled pilot study. Br J Anaesth 2005;95(5):596–602.
11. Ekert H, Brizard C, Eyers R, Cochrane A, Henning R. Elective administration in infants of low-dose recombinant activated factor VII (rFVIIa) in cardiopulmonary bypass surgery for congenital heart disease does not shorten time to chest closure or reduce blood loss and need for transfusions: a randomized, double-blind, parallel group, placebo-controlled study of rFVIIa and standard haemostatic replacement therapy versus standard haemostatic replacement therapy. Blood Coagul Fibrinolysis 2006;17(5):389–95.
12. Johansson PI, Eriksen K, Nielsen SL, Rojkjaer R, Alsbjorn B. Recombinant FVIIa decreases perioperative blood transfusion requirement in burn patients undergoing excision and skin grafting—results of a single centre pilot study. Burns 2007;33(4):435–40.
13. Bosch J, Thabut D, Bendtsen F, et al. Recombinant factor VIIa for upper gastrointestinal bleeding in patients with cirrhosis: a randomized, double-blind trial. Gastroenterology 2004;127(4):1123–30.
14. Boffard KD, Riou B, Warren B, et al. Recombinant factor VIIa as adjunctive therapy for bleeding control in severely injured trauma patients: two parallel randomized, placebo-controlled, double-blind clinical trials. J Trauma 2005;59(1):8–15; discussion-8.
15. Mayer SA, Brun NC, Broderick J, et al. Safety and feasibility of recombinant factor VIIa for acute intracerebral hemorrhage. Stroke 2005;36(1):74–9.
16. Mayer SA, Brun NC, Begtrup K, et al. Recombinant activated factor VII for acute intracerebral hemorrhage. N Engl J Med 2005;352(8):777–85.
17. Chuansumrit A, Wangruangsatid S, Lektrakul Y, Chua MN, Zeta Capeding MR, Bech OM. Control of bleeding in children with Dengue hemorrhagic fever using recombinant activated factor VII: a randomized, double-blind, placebo-controlled study. Blood Coagul Fibrinolysis 2005;16(8):549–55.
18. Pihusch M, Bacigalupo A, Szer J, et al. Recombinant activated factor VII in treatment of bleeding complications following hematopoietic stem cell transplantation. J Thromb Haemost 2005;3(9):1935–44.
19. Sachs B, Delacy D, Green J, et al. Recombinant activated factor VII in spinal surgery: a multicenter, randomized, double-blind, placebo-controlled, dose-escalation trial. Spine 2007;32(21):2285–93.
20. Mayer SA, Brun NC, Begtrup K, et al. Efficacy and safety of recombinant activated factor VII for acute intracerebral hemorrhage. N Engl J Med 2008;358(20):2127–37.
21. Moul JW, Sun L, Wu H, et al. Factors associated with blood loss during radical prostatectomy for localized prostate cancer in the prostate-specific antigen (PSA)-era: an overview of the Department of Defense (DOD) Center for Prostate Disease Research (CPDR) national database. Urol Oncol 2003;21(6):447–55.
22. Maffezzini M, Campodonico F, Capponi G, Canepa G, Gavazzi L, Calcagno T. Results and complications with the mini-laparotomic incision in 52 consecutive radical retropubic prostatectomies. Arch Ital Urol Androl 2006;78(2):61–3.
23. Farnham SB, Webster TM, Herrell SD, Smith JA, Jr. Intraoperative blood loss and transfusion requirements for robotic-assisted radical prostatectomy versus radical retropubic prostatectomy. Urology 2006;67(2):360–63.
24. Diringer MN, Skolnick BE, Mayer SA, et al. Risk of thromboembolic events in controlled trials of rFVIIa in spontaneous intracerebral hemorrhage. Stroke 2008;39(3):850–56.
25. Sheth KN. Recombinant activated factor VII for acute intracerebral hemorrhage. N Engl J Med 2005;352(20):2133–4; author reply-4.
26. Stanworth SJ, Birchall J, Doree CJ, Hyde C. Recombinant factor VIIa for the prevention and treatment of bleeding in patients without haemophilia. Cochrane Database Syst Rev 2007; (2):CD005011.
27. Ranucci M, Isgro G, Soro G, Conti D, De Toffol B. Efficacy and safety of recombinant activated factor VII in major surgical procedures: systematic review and meta-analysis of randomized clinical trials. Arch Surg 2008;143(3):296–304.
28. Levi M, Peters M, Buller HR. Efficacy and safety of recombinant factor VIIa for treatment of severe bleeding: a systematic review. Crit Care Med 2005;33(4):883–90.
29. Agarwal N, Spahr JE, Rodgers GM. Successful management of intra-abdominal hemorrhage in the presence of severe alcoholic liver disease with activated recombinant factor VII (rFVIIa; NovoSeven): a case report and review of the literature on approved and off-label use of rFVIIa. Blood Coagul Fibrinolysis 2007;18(2):205–7.
30. Grounds M. Recombinant factor VIIa (rFVIIa) and its use in severe bleeding in surgery and trauma: a review. Blood Rev 2003;17(Suppl. 1):S11–21.
31. Warren O, Mandal K, Hadjianastassiou V, et al. Recombinant activated factor VII in cardiac surgery: a systematic review. Ann Thorac Surg 2007;83(2):707–14.

32. Sobieszczyk S, Breborowicz GH, Platicanov V, Tanchev S, Kessler CM. Recombinant factor VIIa in the management of postpartum bleeds: an audit of clinical use. Acta Obstet Gynecol Scand 2006;85(10):1239–47.
33. Isbister J, Phillips L, Dunkley S, Jankelowitz G, McNeil J, Cameron P. Recombinant activated factor VII in critical bleeding: experience from the Australian and New Zealand Haemostasis Register. Intern Med J 2008;38(3):156–65.
34. Grounds RM, Seebach C, Knothe C, et al. Use of recombinant activated factor VII (Novoseven) in trauma and surgery: analysis of outcomes reported to an international registry. J Intensive Care Med 2006;21(1):27–39.
35. Alfirevic Z, Elbourne D, Pavord S, et al. Use of recombinant activated factor VII in primary postpartum hemorrhage: the Northern European registry 2000–2004. Obstet Gynecol 2007;110(6):1270–78.
36. Laffan M, O'Connell NM, Perry DJ, Hodgson AJ, O'Shaughnessy D, Smith OP. Analysis and results of the recombinant factor VIIa extended-use registry. Blood Coagul Fibrinolysis 2003; 14(Suppl. 1):S35–8.
37. Browner WS. Clinical research. A simple recipe for doing it well. Anesthesiology 1994;80(4):923–8.
38. Lindley CM, Sawyer WT, Macik BG, et al. Pharmacokinetics and pharmacodynamics of recombinant factor VIIa. Clin Pharmacol Ther 1994;55(6):638–48.
39. Ludlam CA. The evidence behind inhibitor treatment with recombinant factor VIIa. Pathophysiol Haemost Thromb 2002;32(Suppl. 1):13–18.
40. Klitgaard T, Nielsen TG. Overview of the human pharmacokinetics of recombinant activated factor VII. Br J Clin Pharmacol 2008;65(1):3–11.
41. Klitgaard T, Tabanera y Palacios R, Boffard KD, et al. Pharmacokinetics of recombinant activated factor VII in trauma patients with severe bleeding. Crit Care 2006;10(4):R104.
42. Hedner U, Erhardtsen E. Potential role for rFVIIa in transfusion medicine. Transfusion 2002;42(1):114–24.
43. Hardy JF, De Moerloose P, Samama M. Massive transfusion and coagulopathy: pathophysiology and implications for clinical management. Can J Anaesth 2004;51(4):293–310.
44. Valles J, Santos MT, Aznar J, et al. Erythrocytes metabolically enhance collagen-induced platelet responsiveness via increased thromboxane production, adenosine diphosphate release, and recruitment. Blood 1991;78(1):154–62.
45. Santos MT, Valles J, Marcus AJ, et al. Enhancement of platelet reactivity and modulation of eicosanoid production by intact erythrocytes. A new approach to platelet activation and recruitment. J Clin Invest 1991;87(2):571–80.
46. Valles J, Santos MT, Aznar J, et al. Platelet-erythrocyte interactions enhance alpha(IIb)beta(3) integrin receptor activation and P-selectin expression during platelet recruitment: down-regulation by aspirin ex vivo. Blood 2002;99(11):3978–84.
47. Eberst ME, Berkowitz LR. Hemostasis in renal disease: pathophysiology and management. Am J Med 1994;96(2):168–79.
48. Uijttewaal WS, Nijhof EJ, Bronkhorst PJ, Den Hartog E, Heethaar RM. Near-wall excess of platelets induced by lateral migration of erythrocytes in flowing blood. Am J Physiol 1993;264(4 Pt 2):H1239–44.
49. Cinat ME, Wallace WC, Nastanski F, et al. Improved survival following massive transfusion in patients who have undergone trauma. Arch Surg 1999;134(9):964–8.
50. Cosgriff N, Moore EE, Sauaia A, Kenny-Moynihan M, Burch JM, Galloway B. Predicting life-threatening coagulopathy in the massively transfused trauma patient: hypothermia and acidoses revisited. J Trauma 1997;42(5):857–61.
51. Johansson PI, Hansen MB, Sorensen H. Transfusion practice in massively bleeding patients: time for a change? Vox Sang 2005;89(2):92–6.
52. Johansson PI, Stensballe J, Rosenberg I, Hilslov TL, Jorgensen L, Secher NH. Proactive administration of platelets and plasma for patients with a ruptured abdominal aortic aneurysm: evaluating a change in transfusion practice. Transfusion 2007;47(4):593–8.
53. Hedner U, Ezban M. Tissue factor and factor VIIa as therapeutic targets in disorders of hemostasis. Annu Rev Med 2008;59:29–41.
54. Gerotziafas GT, Chakroun T, Depasse F, Arzoglou P, Samama MM, Elalamy I. The role of platelets and recombinant factor VIIa on thrombin generation, platelet activation and clot formation. Thromb Haemost 2004;91(5):977–85.
55. Lisman T, Adelmeijer J, Cauwenberghs S, Van Pampus EC, Heemskerk JW, De Groot PG. Recombinant factor VIIa enhances platelet adhesion and activation under flow conditions at normal and reduced platelet count. J Thromb Haemost 2005;3(4):742–51.
56. Roberts HR, Monroe DM, 3rd, Hoffman M. Safety profile of recombinant factor VIIa. Semin Hematol 2004;41(1 Suppl. 1):101–8.

57. Warren OJ, Darzi AW, Athanasiou T. Recombinant activated factor VII in cardiac surgery—first, do no harm. J Cardiothorac Surg 2007;2: 50.
58. Charbonneau S, Girard F, Boudreault D, Ruel M, Blais N, Hardy JF. Recombinant human activated factor VII is thrombogenic in a rabbit model of cyclic flow reduction and does not reduce intra-abdominal bleeding. Thromb Haemost 2007;97(2):296–303.
59. Godier A, Mazoyer E, Cymbalista F, Cupa M, Samama CM. Recombinant activated factor VII efficacy and safety in a model of bleeding and thrombosis in hypothermic rabbits: a blind study. J Thromb Haemost 2007;5(2):244–9.
60. O'Connell KA, Wood JJ, Wise RP, Lozier JN, Braun MM. Thromboembolic adverse events after use of recombinant human coagulation factor VIIa. JAMA 2006;295(3):293–8.
61. Hebert PC, Stanbrook M. Indication creep: physician beware. CMAJ 2007;177(7):697, 9.
62. Spahn DR, Tucci MA, Makris M. Is recombinant FVIIa the magic bullet in the treatment of major bleeding? Br J Anaesth 2005;94(5):553–5.
63. Bowles KM, Callaghan CJ, Taylor AL, et al. Predicting response to recombinant factor VIIa in nonhaemophiliac patients with severe haemorrhage. Br J Anaesth 2006;97(4):476–81.

PART 6
Transfusion Triggers

CHAPTER 24
Role of Hemoglobin/Hematocrit

Kristine J. Guleserian[1], Hae W. Kim[2], Bruce Pearce[3], Arkadiy Pitman[3] & A. Gerson Greenburg[4]

[1]Cardiothoracic Surgery, Children's Medical Center, UT Southwestern Medical Center, Dallas, USA
[2]Brown University School of Medicine, Providence, RI, USA
[3]Biopure Corporation, Cambridge, MA, USA
[4]Brown University School of Medicine, Providence, USA; Medical Affairs, Biopure Corporation, Cambridge, USA

Introduction

In 1988 the National Institutes of Health held a consensus conference addressing perioperative human red blood cell product transfusion practice [1]. The objective of the conference was the elucidation of the risks and potential benefits of blood product transfusion and a reassessment of "current" transfusion practices. The conference also served to provide scientific-based recommendations for transfusion practice that would ultimately replace the traditional "10/30 rule" (a hemoglobin concentration of 10 g/dL and hematocrit level of 30%) established by Adams and Lundy in 1942 [2]. Indeed the "transfusion trigger" hemoglobin was lowered by consensus from 10 to 7 g/dL and a more directed assessment of individual clinical needs and symptoms as the basis for transfusion was stressed rather than reliance on a single laboratory value.

Since the NIH consensus recommendations were established there have been multiple attempts to determine whether there exists an "optimal" or "minimally acceptable" hemoglobin level on which to base a universal "transfusion trigger" [3–6]. Investigations have recently focused on deriving a "transfusion trigger" from a variety of measured and derived physiologic parameters related to oxygen delivery physiology [7–10]. Cardiopulmonary disease, age, gender, and underlying acute and chronic diseases as well as current pharmacologic treatment must be considered while establishing transfusion guidelines [11–18]. The question will remain: what is the role of the hemoglobin concentration and hematocrit level in determining the transfusion trigger?

History

A comprehensive view of the history of red cell transfusion is neither possible nor desirable in the context of this work. A few highlights will provide a background for the reader to appreciate the essentially empirical nature of the "transfusion trigger" decision as it has evolved over the last millennium [19–21]. Although there are reports of blood transfusion dating back to the fourteenth century AD, the first documented transfusions were carried out in seventeenth century England and France from animals to humans in an attempt to combat mental illness. Over a century later, autotransfusion for postpartum hemorrhage was introduced by James Blundell in 1818. However until the turn of the century, before allogeneic blood transfusion was possible, physicians were forced to accept low hemoglobin levels because there was no means to alter them. By 1900 ABO blood groups were identified by Karl Landsteiner and a biologic basis for transfusion therapy was initially established.

Alternatives to Blood Transfusion in Transfusion Medicine, 2nd edition. Edited by A. Maniatis, P. Van der Linden, J.-F. Hardy.

With the onset of World War I, whole blood transfusion became available because of significant improvements in blood storage and collection. At the same time, the concept of hemorrhagic shock and the need to correct the underlying hypovolemia was recognized by George Crile. The importance of blood volume was further elucidated by the investigations of Thomas Addison and Ernest Starling. Principles of sepsis and sterility were introduced through the late nineteenth century work of Joseph Lister.

By 1937 the first blood bank was in full operation at Cook County Hospital in Chicago, Illinois. Shortly thereafter, in 1939, the Rh group was discovered and more accurate crossmatching procedures were available. During the height of World War II blood transfusion was a common practice. Complications such as transfusion reactions and transmission of hepatitis were recognized if not fully understood. There followed a 30-year period of exploration into transfusion medicine with emphasis on component therapy—generally considered a useful guiding therapeutic principle—and product safety as the main objectives. Indications for transfusions, especially red cells, and transfusion triggers were mostly ignored because the resource was not considered to pose a significant risk. That all changed in the early 1980s when transfusion related HIV transmission was observed. The medical community at that time suddenly began to reassess the benefits and potential risks of transfusion practice and to emphasize red blood cell conservation techniques and alternative therapies. The latter included not only the development of red cell substitutes but also the decision processes and indications for all aspects of transfusion. It was the events of this time and concerns raised about red cell transfusions that the "10/30 rule" as a transfusion trigger was at long last challenged.

The "10/30 rule"

In 1942 Adams and Lundy recommended preoperative blood transfusion in all patients "when the concentration of hemoglobin is less than 8 to 10 grams per 100 cubic centimeters" [2]. Their recommendation was based the premise that the effects of anemia on the oxygen-carrying capacity of blood resulted in inadequate oxygen transport to the tissues; however, they failed to provide corroborative scientific support for this recommendation. Clark and colleagues subsequently proposed that patients with anemia of "chronic shock" would benefit from preoperative transfusion. Nevertheless by defining an optimal hemoglobin level as 10 g/dL, they established the doctrine of the "transfusion trigger" or the "10/30 rule" for transfusion, which has consequently persisted into current clinical practice [22].

Scientific support of the 10 g/dL hemoglobin as the "optimal hemoglobin" level as 10 g/dL has been provided by Stehling and Zauder. Using in vitro rheologic studies, they demonstrated that oxygen delivery (DO_2) peaks at hematocrit levels of 30% and declines with progressive hemodilution [23]. Of course, hemodilution decreases oxygen carrying capacity as a direct function of hemoglobin concentration and thus in some sense is rheology dependent. Oxygen delivery would be expected to decrease absent any increase in cardiac output necessary to assure adequate tissue perfusion. The "optimal hemoglobin" may then be defined as the hemoglobin concentration at which organ function is at its peak while avoiding the adverse effects of either too low or too high a hemoglobin concentration. In several experimental animal models, oxygen transport, and survival have been shown to be optimal at hematocrit levels of 30–40% [24–26]. Czer and Shoemaker found the optimal hematocrit level to be 32% in the critically ill patient population even after taking into consideration variations in volume status because this particular patient population experienced acute blood loss from trauma or emergency surgery. They also observed that patients could tolerate hematocrit levels of 18% when compensatory mechanisms were normal suggesting that the "optimal hemoglobin" level was not the same as the minimally acceptable hemoglobin level [27].

Is the optimal hemoglobin the minimally acceptable hemoglobin?

For many years the "optimal hemoglobin" was considered to be the same as the "minimally acceptable" or "tolerable" hemoglobin; the terms were used interchangeably. Little was known about the minimally acceptable hemoglobin level until the 1930s when Carrel and Linbergh demonstrated isolated organ survival and growth in a severely anemic (i.e., low hemoglobin concentration) environment. Their work defined the hemoglobin level of 3 g/dL as the "minimally acceptable" or "tolerable" hemoglobin in their models [19]. In an animal model of extreme anemia (hemoglobin concentration of 3–5 g/dL), Takaori and Safar documented long-term survival in 80% of dogs subjected to normovolemic hemodilution [28]. Extrapolation to humans was not readily apparent.

In 1987 Wilkerson illustrated evidence of cardiac compensation in response to decreased hemoglobin in a baboon model with hematocrit levels of 10% and observed survival even at hematocrit levels of 4% [29]. More recently in 1991, Spence and colleagues found that a hemoglobin level of less than 3 g/dL was an independent predictor of poor outcome [30]. In 1978 Geha and Baue studied the effect of graded coronary stenosis and coronary flow during acute normovolemic hemodilution (hematocrit of 20%) and demonstrated cardiac ischemia and compromise in left ventricular performance with significant coronary stenosis (>67% narrowing of left anterior descending artery), while confirming tolerance of acute normovolemic anemia in animals with no or insignificant coronary stenosis [31]. Thus "survival" relative to minimal hemoglobin concentration is dependent upon variable comorbidities but optimal hemoglobin concentration is a broader and more clinically relevant issue.

Many studies initially carried out to establish an optimal hemoglobin level have shown that lower hemoglobin levels are tolerable. In several studies, Spence and Carson evaluated the role of anemia and the risk of postoperative morbidity and mortality in a Jehovah's Witness population. The first study of 125 patients undergoing emergency or elective surgery showed a significantly higher preoperative hemoglobin level in survivors compared to those who died (11.8 vs 7.6 g/dL, $p < 0.002$).

Operative mortality for patients with hemoglobin levels between 0 and 6 g/dL, 6.1 and 8 g/dL, 8.1 and 10 g/dL, and greater than 10 g/dL was 61.5, 33.3, 0, and 7.1% respectively. Additionally, there was no reported mortality in patients with preoperative hemoglobin levels greater than 8 g/dL with operative blood loss of less than 500 mL [32]. The second study demonstrated no operative mortality in 113 elective operations with hemoglobin levels as low as 6 g/dL as long as blood loss remained less than 500 mL [33].

Should the "tolerable" hemoglobin level then be considered the "acceptable" level to establish a transfusion trigger? Although many patients can and do tolerate hemoglobin levels significantly lower than 10 g/dL, this does not imply that that a tolerable hemoglobin level should be the acceptable level used as a transfusion trigger. In some patients, however, it may be. Similarly, although a hemoglobin level of 10 g/dL has been considered optimal, it is unnecessary and potentially harmful to transfuse all patients to this level. The risk of transfusion versus no transfusion must always be considered [34–37].

An alternative to hemoglobin concentration as the "transfusion trigger"

If the hemoglobin concentration is rejected as the indication for transfusion is there another set of variables that reflect tissue perfusion that may be more critical? Moving from the static state measure hemoglobin concentration absent even a blood volume measurement element to the more dynamic state of oxygen delivery physiology may provide just the set of data needed to create a "transfusion trigger" applicable to the modern era [38]. It should be obvious that any such decision process, relying on physiologic and metabolic data obtained with the aid of invasive monitoring, will have a more limited application. The process then becomes site specific in the sense that monitoring equipment and access to blood gas analysis is required. It will not, obviously, apply to many routine transfusion decisions where practice standards prevail and are notorious for being highly variable [39–43]. These decision points may change over time with physician and surgeon education. The accumulation of data showing that a hemoglobin concentration as low as 7 g/dL is equally safe to a higher one-absent a patient with significant cardiovascular disease-strongly supports this approach [11,44,45]. To avoid allogeneic RBC transfusion is considered desirable if the sequelae of not transfusing are no more frequent or of no greater severity than the risk of a complication from the transfusion itself. This is a general principle necessary as criteria to evaluate efficacy and cost of alternatives to conventional red cell transfusion practice. In every decision process the need to consider the alternative to not acting plays a role. In the case of the red cell transfusion decision, the risks of not transfusing a patient with cardiovascular disease may outweigh the risks of a less frequent but potentially more severe transfusion reaction including the transmission of infectious diseases. The transfusion decision must be an active one for there are "risks" associated with either option.

Physiology of oxygen delivery

Oxygen delivery physiology is a rather complex issue, especially when it is applied to patient management. It relates to tissue perfusion in a very real and direct way. Adequate tissue perfusion is the primary goal of resuscitation and maintenance of physiologic function. Without adequate tissue perfusion the machinery of life, basic cell function, and oxidative phosphorylation is disrupted; if the perfusion deficit persists sufficiently long cell death, organ death, and organism death will follow. Tissue perfusion has been studied from the cellular level to the "global" or systemic level. Studies of isolated vascular beds lend understanding to basic physiologic processes and are important in establishing the basis for some of the specific metabolic deviations seen in patients. It is given that there is a relationship between these "microevents" and the more global oxygen delivery parameters we can measure and manipulate but the magnitude and accuracy of the relationship is still not fully appreciated.

In the clinical arena we can appreciate a relationship of global oxygen delivery variables to not only physiologic parameters of tissue perfusion but to overall survival as well. A "transfusion trigger" defined in terms of oxygen delivery physiology is reasonably supported by a growing body of data [7–9].

Absent the ability to evaluate specific organ or tissue oxygen utilization the more "global oxygen delivery" measures can be obtained. Ideally, cardiac output, heart rate, A-VO2 difference, pH, base excess, and lactate can be measured. Additional variables can then be calculated or derived. For now some of these variables require invasive monitoring to place catheters for sampling and are thus associated with some increased risk to the patient. "Global" in this context really refers to systemic hemodynamics and oxygen delivery physiology for that is the most clinically relevant measure available today.

Global oxygen delivery is the product of cardiac output (best expressed as cardiac index) and arterial oxygen content. Arterial oxygen content is measured or derived from an arterial blood gas sample where the key elements are hemoglobin concentration, partial pressure of oxygen (PO_2) and oxygen saturation (SaO_2); the hemoglobin concentration is a major component of this variable. In that context hemoglobin concentration is directly related to oxygen delivery.

Global oxygen consumption is the difference between the product of cardiac output or index and mixed venous oxygen content and global oxygen delivery. The oxygen extraction ratio (OER) is the number resulting from dividing oxygen consumption by the global oxygen delivery. Consumption is expressed as a percentage of delivery and normally runs 25–30%.

There is another interesting relationship noted between oxygen delivery and oxygen consumption that has been defined and validated both clinically and experimentally. Oxygen consumption is "flow dependent"—that is, it increases with oxygen delivery—until a plateau or change in slope of the curve occurs at which point it is said to be "flow independent." The point where this occurs is called the "critical oxygen delivery point" and it reflects adequate tissue perfusion. Values above this imply oxygen supply in excess of need and values below this point imply a need to increase tissue perfusion.

Corresponding to this critical oxygen delivery point the OER begins to increase at around 30–40% and increases exponentially as the relationship is defined in the flow-dependent portion of the curve. Moreover, an increase in the serum lactate can be appreciated near this point as well. Increases in serum lactate that parallel the increases in OER have been documented. This is not unexpected given the relationship between cellular hypoxia, lactate, and the OER.

Thus it would appear that the critical oxygen delivery point, defined in terms of oxygen delivery physiology, reflects in many ways adequate tissue perfusion. Given this logical construct, the transfusion trigger may be this point which is noted to be 9–12 mL O_2/kg body weight. This oxygen delivery approximation may be a more accurate estimate of a true transfusion trigger than any single static measure of hemoglobin concentration.

It must be noted that as the hemoglobin concentration decreases, even in isovolemic hemodilution models, cardiac output will of necessity increase to effect a uniform level of global oxygen delivery. This rather simple model does not consider the autoregulatory aspects of the various vascular beds but rather assumes uniform global oxygen delivery to be good for overall tissue perfusion. Limiting the ability to increase cardiac output will be patient's age, the presence of coronary artery disease, and the presence of beta-blockers or other cardiac drugs [11, 46, 47]. Absent the ability to compensate for a decrease in hemoglobin concentration, the result could be inadequate tissue perfusion and all of the sequelae attendant thereto in terms of detrimental effects. Thus, a transfusion of red blood cells to increase the oxygen carrying capacity of the blood—an increase in oxygen content—and to normalize oxygen delivery will place fewer demands on an already compromised cardiac pump. It must be noted that, in this context, increasing cardiac output is an oxygen-consuming process. A significant portion of any increase in global oxygen delivery is a necessity and will be utilized by the heart itself to increase cardiac output. As a result, the less of an increase in system oxygen delivery will be realized than can be easily calculated or assumed. This concept of evaluating cardiac efficiency and power are just getting underway and may eventually play a role in further refining a physiologically defined "transfusion trigger."

Individual patients and clinical conditions

Most patients with normally functioning cardiovascular compensatory mechanisms will tolerate acute anemia, a moderate decrease in hemoglobin concentration, without event, providing normovolemia is maintained. The signs and symptoms of decreased red blood cell mass are relatively insensitive parameters for use as a transfusion trigger. Signs and symptoms of anemia (hypotension, tachycardia, tachypnea, dizziness, fatigue, etc.) are variable depending on the patient's age, body temperature, medications, rate of volume loss and comorbidities. Muller [48] documented that hemodynamic symptoms are usually not observed until the hemoglobin and hematocrit levels fall to 6 g/dL and 20%, respectively, and that adults were more likely than children to experience these changes. Only 54% had tachycardia, 32% had hypotension, 27% had dyspnea, and 35% had impaired levels of consciousness in the study population of 100 children and 71 adults [48]. Similar results were reported by Carmel and Shulman who found symptoms of chest pain, dyspnea, syncope, or lethargy in 55% of 122 medical students with a mean hemoglobin of 5.5 g/dL [49]. Weiskopf and colleagues also showed that acute isovolemic anemia to a hemoglobin level of 5 g/dL does not result in inadequate tissue oxygenation, assessed by plasma lactate and oxygen consumption, in a population of 33 conscious, healthy resting humans

[50]. However, application of this observation to the complex disease or older patient population should be done cautiously and with deliberation. Elective isovolemic hemodilution in normal healthy volunteers is not the same as the technique applied to an older population with coronary artery disease, hypertension, systemic arteriosclerosis, and a variety of pharmacologic agents.

Is there really a transfusion trigger?

The arbitrary transfusion trigger of a hemoglobin level of 10 gm/dL dating back to 1942 was based on the scientific knowledge and perceptions available at that time. Numerous attempts have been made since then to validate a lower hemoglobin transfusion trigger; however, the hemoglobin level alone has proved to be an unreliable indicator. Multiple sets of guidelines have been proposed with most reaching the conclusion that there is little evidence to support specific recommendation [1, 5, 15, 16, 51]. Indeed, all have essentially established "expert opinion" as the standard because the data is unreliable or nonexistent. In the ICU/OR environment transfusion decisions based on oxygen delivery, measured and derived variables are possible and apparently used although the results and implications may be argued [3, 52]. In all, the data are inadequate to make a standard set of guidelines on the basis of a specific transfusion trigger. Neither the optimal nor the minimally acceptable hemoglobin can be regarded as the transfusion trigger as they either over or underestimate the transfusion need.

Clinical symptoms of cardiac compromise or inadequate oxygen delivery have not correlated well with hemoglobin levels. Use of a symptomatic transfusion strategy has been proposed by Carson and colleagues on the basis of a cohort study of 8787 hip fracture patients in which there was no apparent effect on mortality in patients with hemoglobin levels as low as 8 g/dL, even those with cardiovascular disease [45]. In 1998 Carson and colleagues found transfusion of fewer units of red blood cells (0 vs 2 units, $p < 0.001$) and lower mean hemoglobin levels (9.3 ± 1.2 vs 10.3 ± 0.9 g/dL) but no statistically significant difference in 60-day mortality (11.9% vs 4.8%, relative risk 2.5; 95% CI, 0.5–12.2) with symptomatic transfusion in a randomized pilot study comparing symptomatic versus hemoglobin-level-driven red blood cell transfusions in a population of 84 hip fracture patients undergoing surgical repair [53]. There are few large prospective studies investigating hemoglobin level and concomitant medical problems, such as cardiac disease, pulmonary disease, or sepsis, with regard to mortality, morbidity or functional status [54]. Much larger more definitive trials are certainly needed.

The need for perioperative red blood cell transfusion should be based on individual needs in specific clinical settings according to each patient's clinical condition and ability to tolerate anemia. At hemoglobin levels below 7 (or 6) g/dL cardiac output increases sharply placing extra demands on the myocardium [50, 55]; if the hemoglobin concentration is reduced acutely most anemic patients will require transfusion. In otherwise healthy patients with a hemoglobin level of 10 g/dL or greater, red cell transfusion is rare, if ever indicated. Literature about "healthy individuals" provides a basis for understanding the hemodynamic and cardiopulmonary parameters associated with acute anemia—a decrease in hemoglobin concentration usually associated with a decrease in blood volume [50]. However, these data may not translate into applications in clinical practice in a population of "sick individuals." The decision to transfuse should therefore take into account the rapidity of blood loss and other preexisting conditions such as chronic anemia, impaired cardiopulmonary reserve, and cerebrovascular or peripheral circulatory disease.

The transfusion trigger should not be defined by a simple static variable (i.e., hemoglobin concentration) which is only a part of the oxygen delivery equation but not the sole determinant of this key set of variables. The transfusion trigger is an individualized "transfusion trigger" defined by the patient's needs as assessed by hemodynamics, symptoms, metabolic status, and tissue perfusion status reflected in global oxygen dynamics. It is for these reasons that individualized approach is strongly recommended.

> **Key points**
>
> - Hemoglobin concentration alone should not be a "transfusion trigger."
> - Transfusion should be based on the patient's clinical condition and tolerance of anemia with particular attention to comorbid cardiovascular and pulmonary disease.
> - An individual approach to transfusion practice is strongly recommended.

References

1. Consensus Conference. Perioperative red blood cell trans-fusion. JAMA 1988;260:2700–703.
2. Adams RC, Lundy JS. Anesthesia in cases of poor surgical risks some suggestions for decreasing the risk. Surg Gynecol Obstet 1942;74:1011–19.
3. Hebert PC, Wells G, Blachman MA, et al. A multicenter, randomized, controlled clinical trial of transfusion requirements in critical care. N Engl J Med 1999;340:409–17.
4. Hill SR, Carless PA, Henry DA, et al. Transfusion thresholds and other strategies for guiding allogeneic red blood cell transfusion. Cochrane Database Syst Rev 2002; CD002042.
5. Walsh TS, Garrioch M, Maciver C, et al. Red cell requirements for intensive care units adhering to evidence-based transfusion guidelines. Transfusion 2004;44:1405–11.
6. Hardy JF. Current status of transfusion triggers for red blood cell concentrates. Transfus Aphresis Sci 2004;31:55–66.
7. Greenburg AG. A physiologic basis for red blood cell transfusion decision. Am J Surg 1995;170(Suppl. 6A): 44S–8.
8. Torella F, Haynes SL, McCollum CN. Cerebral and peripheral near-infrared spectroscopy: an alternative transfusion trigger? Vox Sang 2002;83 (3): 254–7.
9. Spahn DR. Physiologic transfusion triggers. Anesthesiology 2006;104:905–6.
10. Sehgal LR, Zebala LP, Takagi I, et al. Evaluation of oxygen extraction ratio as a physiologic transfusion trigger in coronary artery bypass graft surgery patients. Transfusion 2001;41:591–5.
11. Carson JL, Reynolds RC. In search of the transfusion threshold. Hematology 2005;10:86–8.
12. Friedman BA, Burns TL, Schork MA. An analysis of blood transfusion of surgical patients by sex: a question for the transfusion. Transfusion 1980;20: 179–88.
13. Goodnough LT, Verbrugge D, Vizmeg K et al. Identifying elective orthopedic surgical patients transfused with amounts of blood in excess of need. The transfusion trigger revisited. Transfusion 1992;32:648–53.
14. Stainsby D, MacLenna S, Thomas. Guidelines on the management of massive blood loss. Br J Hematol 2006;135:634–41.
15. American Society of Anesthesiologists task force on perioperative blood transfusion and adjuvant therapy. Practice guidelines for perioperative blood transfusion and adjuvant therapies. Anesthesiology 2006;105:198–208.
16. The Society of Thoracic Surgeons blood conservation guideline task force. Perioperative blood transfusion and blood conservation in cardiac surgery: the society of thoracic surgeons and the society of cardiovascular anesthesiologists clinical practice guideline. Ann Thorac Surg 2007;83:27–86.
17. Wu WC, Schifftner TL, Henderson WG, et al. Preoperative hematocrit levels and postoperative outcomes in older patients undergoing noncardiac surgery. JAMA 2007;297:2481–8.
18. Rao SV, Jollis JG, Harrington RA, et al. Relationship of blood transfusion and clinical outcomes in patients with acute coronary syndromes. JAMA 2004;292:1555–62.
19. Diamond LK. A history of blood transfusion. In: Wintrobe MM (ed.) *Blood, Pure and Eloquent*. McGraw-Hill, New York, 1980, pp. 659–83.
20. Keynes G. The history of blood transfusion. In: *Blood Transfusion*. John Wright & Sons, Bristol, 1949, pp. 1–50.
21. Giangrande PL. The history of blood transfusion. Br J Haematol 2000;110:758–67.
22. Clark JH, Nelson W, Lyons C, et al. Chronic shock: the problem of reduced blood volume in the chronically ill patient. Ann Surg 1947;125:618–23.
23. Stehling L, Zauder HL. Acute normovolemic hemodilution. Transfusion 1991;31:857–68.
24. Chapler CK, Cain SM. The physiologic reserve in oxygen carrying capacity. Studies in experimental hemodilution. Can J Physiol Pharmacol 1986;64: 7–12.
25. Schwartz S, Frantz RA, Shoemaker WC. Sequential hemodynamic and oxygen transport responses in

hypovolemia, anemia, and hypoxia. Am J Physiol 1981;241:HH64–72.
26. Robertie PG, Gravlee GP. Safe limits of hemodilution and recommendations for erythrocyte transfusion. Int Anesthesiol Clin 1990;28:197–204.
27. Czer LSC, Shoemaker WC. Optimal hematocrit value in critically ill postoperative patients. Surg Gynecol Obstet 1978;147:363–8.
28. Takaori M, Safar P. Adaptation to sever acute hemodilution with dextran-75 in dogs. Arch Surg 1966;92 (5): 743–8.
29. Wilkerson DK, Rosen AL, Sehgal LR, et al. Limits of cardiac compensation in anemic baboons. Surgery 1988;103:665–70.
30. Spence RK, Costabile JP, Young GS, et al. Is hemoglobin level alone a reliable predictor of outcome in the severely anemic surgical patient? Am Surg 1992;58:92–5.
31. Geha AS, Baue AE. Graded coronary stenosis and coronary flow during acute normovolemic anemia. World J Surg 1978;2:645–52.
32. Spence RK, Carson JA, Poses R, et al. Elective surgery without transfusion: influence of preoperative hemoglobin level and blood loss on mortality. Am J Surg 1990;159:320–24.
33. Carson JL, Spence RK, Poses RM, et al. Severity of anemia and operative mortality and morbidity. Lancet 1988;2:727–9.
34. O'Brien SF, Yi QL, Fan W, et al. Current incidence and estimated residual risk of transfusion-transmitted infections in donations made to Canadian Blood Services. Transfusion 2007;47:316–25.
35. Madjdpour C, Heindl V, Spahn DR. Risks, benefits, alternatives and indications of allogeneic blood transfusions. Minerva Anestesiol 2006;72:283–98; review.
36. Rana R, Fernandez-Perez ER, Khan SA, et al. Transfusion-related acute lung injury and pulmonary edema in critically ill patients: a retrospective study. Transfusion 2006;46:1478–83.
37. Raghavan M, Marik PE. Anemia, allogeneic blood transfusion, and immunomodulation in the critically ill III. Chest 2005;127:295–307.
38. Casutt M, Seifert B, Pasch T, et al. Factors affecting the individual effects of blood transfusion on oxygen delivery and oxygen consumption. Crit Care Med 1999;27:2194–200.
39. Baele PL, De Bruyere M, Deneys V, et al. Results of the SANGUIS study in Belgium. A concerted action of the commission of the European communities IVth medical and health research programme. The Belgian SAnGUIS study group. Safe and good use of blood in surgery. Acta Chir Belg 1994;94(Suppl.):1–61.
40. Corwin HL, Parsonnet KC, Gettinger A. RBC transfusion in the ICU. Is there a reason? Chest 1995;108:767–71.
41. Corwin HL, Gettinger A, Pearl RG, et al. The CRIT study: anemia and blood transfusion in the critically ill-current clinical practice in the United States. Crit Care Med 2004;32:39–52.
42. Vincent JL, Baron JF, Reinhart K, et al. Anemia and blood transfusion. JAMA 2002;288:1499–507.
43. Walsh TS Saleh EED. Anemia during critical illness. Br J Anaesth 2006;97:278–91.
44. Carson JL, Duff A, Poses RM, et al. Effect of anemia and cardiovascular disease on surgical mortality and morbidity. Lancet 1996;348:1055–60.
45. Carson JL, Duff A, Berlin JA, et al. Perioperative blood transfusion and postoperative mortality. JAMA 1998;279:199–205.
46. Escobar JF, Jones NL, Rapaport E, et al. Ventricular performance in acute normovolemic anemia. Am J Physiol 1966;211:877–84.
47. Wei JY. Age and the cardiovascular system. N Engl J Med 1992;327:1735–9.
48. Muller G, N'tita I, Nyst M, et al. Application of blood transfusion guidelines in a major hospital of Kinshasa, Zaire [Letter]. AIDS 1992;6:431–2.
49. Carmel R, Shulman IA. Blood transfusion in medically treatable chronic anemia. Pernicious anemia as a model for transfusion overuse. Arch Path Lab Med 1989;113:995–7.
50. Weiskopf RB, Viele MK, Feiner J, et al. Human cardiovascular and metabolic response to acute, severe isovolemic anemia. JAMA 1998;279:217–21.
51. Welch HG, Meehan KR, Goodnough LT. Prudent strategies for elective red blood cell transfusion. Ann Intern Med 1992;116:393–402.
52. Hebert PC, Wells G, Tweedale M, et al. Does transfusion practice affect mortality in critically ill patients? Am J Respir Crit Care Med 1997;155:1439–44.
53. Carson JL, Terrin FB, Barton RA, et al. A pilot randomized trial comparing symptomatic vs. hemoglobin-level-driven red blood cell transfusions following hip fracture. Transfusion 1998;38:522–9.
54. Wu WC, Rathore SS, Yang Y, et al. Blood transfusion in elderly patients with acute myocardial infarction. N Engl J Med 2001;345:1230–36.
55. Linman JW. Physiologic and pathophysiologic effects of anemia. N Engl J Med 1968;279:812–8.

CHAPTER 25

Calculation of Blood Loss

Mark E. Brecher

Department of Pathology Laboratory Medicine; McLendon Clinical Laboratories; University of North Carolina, Chapel Hill, USA

Introduction

Key to the planning of a transfusion strategy or a blood-conservation intervention is an understanding of the anticipated blood loss. Attempts to anticipate the needs for autologous blood have traditionally been on the basis of red cell usage. Therefore, not surprisingly, one frequently finds the terms blood loss and red cell loss used interchangeably in the literature, albeit incorrectly.

Further complicating estimates of blood loss is that the use of an intraoperative estimated blood loss for a surgical procedure is both poorly reproducible and typically an underestimate. Attempts to carefully quantitate blood loss by the weighing of sponges and the collection of suctioned fluids in volumetric container are complicated by lavage fluids, evaporation, and blood lost on the floor. Therefore, comparison of blood loss from one institution to another or from one surgeon to another has been difficult.

Use of validated mathematical models have led to a better understanding of the limited but real "savings" attainable with acute normovolemic hemodilution, preoperative autologous donation, preoperative erythropoietin, and intraoperative hemodilution [1–8]. The mathematical models that have been derived to analyze the benefits of such blood-conservation strategies can also be applied to planning for the provision of red cells in an individual patient.

Alternatives to Blood Transfusion in Transfusion Medicine, 2nd edition. Edited by A. Maniatis, P. Van der Linden, J.-F. Hardy.

This chapter reviews the mathematical methodology by which either the anticipated red cell usage or the actual blood loss can be estimated on the basis of historical data for a given surgical procedure. In general such models are based on one-, two-, or three-variable (univariant, bivariant, or trivariant) analyses. As the models account for additional clinically significant variables, the potential for more accurate forecasting of blood needs for an individual patient is realized.

Univariant analysis (blood usage)

Initial attempts to predict the blood usage for a specific surgical procedure involved the use of a "maximum surgical blood ordering schedule" (MSBOS) [9, 10]. In these schedules the amount of blood required by patients undergoing a specific surgical procedure would be rank ordered and the number of units that would support a threshold of acceptance (typically taken as the 80th or 90th percent of patients), which would be the recommended number of units to be crossmatched for surgery. This type of mathematical manipulation of data (the calculation of the *x*th sample percentile among the values in range) is referred to as a cumulative percentage. In the case of 90% of patients not requiring any units of red blood cells (RBCs), a type and screen would be sufficient.

The use of such schedules reduces the number of units of blood crossmatched preoperatively for patients undergoing elective surgery, reduces the amount of time units spent in an assigned or crossmatched status allowing better utilization of a hospital's blood inventory with reduced outdating of units. The decreased number of crossmatches, the reduced inventory requirements, and the decreased outdating result in financial savings without compromising patient care.

A refinement of such schedules for autologous predeposit RBC collection is a schedule of optimal preoperative collection of autologous blood (SOPCAB) which includes the RBC needs for the entire hospitalization rather than the operative procedure alone [11].

The use of such schedules depends on quantifying one variable (RBC usage) alone to allow for the provision of RBCs. Unfortunately, the use of such schedules for the collection of autologous blood inevitably leads to the over collection of autologous RBCs as the average patient uses the 50th percentile of blood usage and not the 90th percentile. Such a mismatch of collection and transfusion leads to the nearly half of predeposit autologous RBCs being discarded.

Bivarant analysis

Multiple groups have described the use of stratification of the admission hematocrit or hemoglobin and the cumulative percent of red cell needs within each group as a predictor of the blood needs. For example, in a study of 332 total hip arthroplasties it was predicted that the use of a stratified SSBOS based on the admission hemoglobin would have reduced the collection of autologous RBCs 12% and would have reduced the discard rate from 53.5 to 36.7% [12]. Similarly, in radical prostatectomies at Washington University in St. Louis, an admission hematocrit of 45% required no transfusion of banked units [13].

A group from the Mayo Clinic (Rochester, Minnesota, USA) have advocated the use of algebraic models for optimizing transfusion strategies on the basis of red cell volume or mass [14, 15]. Such models deal principally with two surgical variables: (i) the volume or mass of red cells transfused and (ii) the volume or mass of red cells lost. The goal of such a mathematical approach is to determine the total red cell volume or mass that must be available before surgery.

For example, the amount of hemoglobin lost for a surgical procedure such as a primary total hip arthroplasty would be calculated as:

$$\text{PreHb} - \text{PostHb} + \text{RBCs} = \text{Hblost}$$

where PreHb = preoperative Hb (g/dL), PostHb = Hb 24 hours after the surgical procedure (g/L), RBCs = Hb (g/dL) provided by allogeneic RBC units transfused on the day of surgery (assuming 1 unit = 1 g/dL Hb), and Hb lost = Hb lost secondary to the surgical procedure (g/dL).

In the case of a primary total hip arthroplasty it was found that patients lost 3.7 ± 1.7 g/dL of Hb (with intraoperative blood salvage being routinely employed).

A surgical blood ordering equation (SBOE) is then used to calculate the number of RBC units to order for surgery.

$$\text{Hb lost} - (\text{PreHb} - \text{MinHb}) = \text{Units to order} -$$

the SBOE equation

where MinHb = minimal acceptable Hb (g/dL) considered the transfusion trigger or minimal allowable Hb, and units to order = the number of RBC units to be crossmatched for surgery.

For a patient undergoing a primary total hip arthroplasty with a blood volume of 5000 mL, whose admission Hb/hct was 10.7 g/dL/32.1%, and for whom a minimally allowable Hb was 10 g/dL the number of units to order would be:

$$3.7 - (10.7 - 10.0) = 3 \text{ units.}$$

In actual practice, the use of such equations was (a better predictor of the number of units to be crossmatched (Table 25.1).

Table 25.1 Surgical blood ordering equation.

	Number of patients (%)	
	MSBOS ($n = 29$)	SBOE ($n = 31$)
Exact match	2 (7%)	18 (58%)
Underordered RBCs	0 (0%)	7 (23%)
Overordered RBCs	27 (93%)	6 (19%)
C:T ratio	4.12	0.83

Adapted from Nuttall et al. [15].

As one might suspect, underordering was not a problem with the MSBOS, which was optimized to support 90% of patients, however, with the SBOE 23% of the patients had underordering. As the mean number value for the hemoglobin lost was used in the SBOE, it is inevitable that there would be underordering. If such an approach was used to plan for preoperative autologous collections, allowances must be made for the falling hemoglobin during the predeposit process and the total hospitalization must be analyzed, not simply during the first 24 hours following the operative procedure as was done at the Mayo Clinic.

Trivariant analysis

The algebraic approach

Mercurali and Inghilleri from the Gaetano Pini Orthopedic Institute (Milan, Italy) have also proposed the use of an algebraic approach, similar to the Mayo bivariant approach described above [16]. However, they consider the additional variable of the patients' blood volume. In this approach the "tolerated blood loss" depends upon the baseline circulating RBC mass and the circulating RBC mass that gives a value of hematocrit compatible with clinical and cardiocirculatory condition of the patient (the minimally tolerated hematocrit). Although this group talks about "blood loss," what they actually describe is the RBC loss (expressed in mL of RBCs).

The predicted "blood loss" for each surgical procedure represents the 80th percentile of distribution of the volume of estimated RBC loss during surgery and during the first five postoperative days.

The calculations employed are as follows:

$$\text{Predicted RBC loss} = \text{C-RBC-V}_{\text{presurgery}} - \text{C-RBC-V}_{\text{Day 5 postoperative}} + \text{mL of RBC transfused}$$

where C-RBC-V (circulating RBC volume) = estimated blood volume (EBV) × Hct and

$$\text{Estimated RBC loss (mL of RBCs)} = \text{EBV} \times (\text{Hct}_{\text{preoperative}} - \text{Hct}_{\text{Day 5 postoperative}}) + \text{mL of RBC transfused}$$

For example, transfusion needs for a patient with a 5000-mL EBV, a baseline Hct of 32.1%, and minimally tolerated hematocrit of 28%, who was to undergo a total hip arthroplasty and for whom a predicted RBC loss of 907 mL was to be expected would be calculated as follows:

$$\text{Tolerated RBC loss} = (5000 \times 0.321) - (5000 \times 0.28) = 1605 - 1400 = 205 \text{ mL of RBC}$$

$$\text{Transfusion needs} = 907 - 205 = 702 \text{ mL of RBC}$$

assuming that every unit of predeposit autologous blood has 180 mL of RBCs this would be equivalent to 3.9 units.

While this method further individualizes the approach to the patient it has some limitations. With such an approach one cannot account for the "savings" attributable to the use of hemodilution of patients as a means of blood conservation. For example, if one determined that a patient would require 600 mL of RBCs above that needed to maintain a minimal hematocrit, but the patient may have only an "extra" 500 mL of RBCs above his minimum hematocrit red cell volume. If the patient underwent acute hemodilution, no additional red cell volume is created, yet there is a "savings" associated with performing this procedure that would likely be sufficient to carry the patient through surgery.

In addition, the use of RBC loss rather then actual blood loss can lead to miscalculations at extremes of blood volume. If the predicted RBC loss for a specific operative procedure was 2000 mL, in patients with blood volumes of 4000 or 6500 mL, one would need a preoperative hematocrit of 50 and 31% respectively (one strategy to achieve a hematocrit of 50% would be the use of erythropoietin preoperatively). If a minimally tolerated hematocrit was 28%, the patient with a blood volume of 4000 mL and a hematocrit of 50% could tolerate a blood loss of 2319 mL while the patient with a blood volume of 6500 mL and a hematocrit of 31% could only tolerate a blood loss of 611 mL! Could this phenomenon not be explained by the fact that the volume calculated correspond in fact to the "net red blood cell" loss that is tolerable? The amounts of tolerable blood loss are quite different and are unlikely to reflect actual practice.

Not surprisingly, a variation of this approach that attempts to convert back to total blood loss has also been described from the Albert Einstein Medical Center [17]. In this method variables are defined as follows: preoperative hemoglobin (Hgb(i)), preoperative hematocrit (Hct(i)), body weight (Wt), postoperative day one morning hemoglobin (Hgb(f)) and hematocrit (Hct(f)). For each patient, the actual blood loss (ABL), i.e., the amount of blood that left the patient's body, was calculated as the average ABL(n) resulting from two computations of the following formula:

$$\mathrm{ABL}(n) = \frac{\mathrm{EBV} \times (\mathrm{H(i)} - \mathrm{H(f)})}{(\mathrm{H(i)} + \mathrm{H(f)})/2} + (500 \times \mathrm{T(u)})$$

where

1 EBV is assumed to be 70 cm^3 (or mL) /kg;

2 H(i) and H(f) represent Hgb(i) and Hgb(f) for one computation and Hct(i) and Hct(f) for the second computation, and

3 T(u) is the sum of autologous whole blood (AWB), packed red blood cells (PRBC), and cell saver (CS) units transfused.

The calculus approach

A more sophisticated approach to the estimation of the actual blood loss that employs calculus has also been described [18]. Using the differential equation originally described by Bourke and Smith in 1975 for isovolemic hemodilution [19]:

$$\frac{d\mathrm{Hct}}{dV_L} = \frac{-\mathrm{Hct}}{\mathrm{EBV}}$$

where Hct = hematocrit,,V = volume, L = loss, and EBV = estimated blood volume

which indicates that a small change in hematocrit from the initial hematocrit should equal a small change in blood volume from the initial blood volume. This equation can be integrated from time zero (0) to time final (F) to yield:

$$V_L = \mathrm{EBV} \times \ln(\mathrm{Hct}_0/\mathrm{Hct}_F)$$

This equation indicates the volume that must be lost while maintaining an isovolemic state to achieve a final Hct of Hct_F. From this equation one can create plots of the blood loss, initial hematocrit, and the transfusion trigger for a given blood volume. From such equations one can derive nomograms that can help guide the blood-conservation strategy for a specific patient (Figure 25.1) [4].

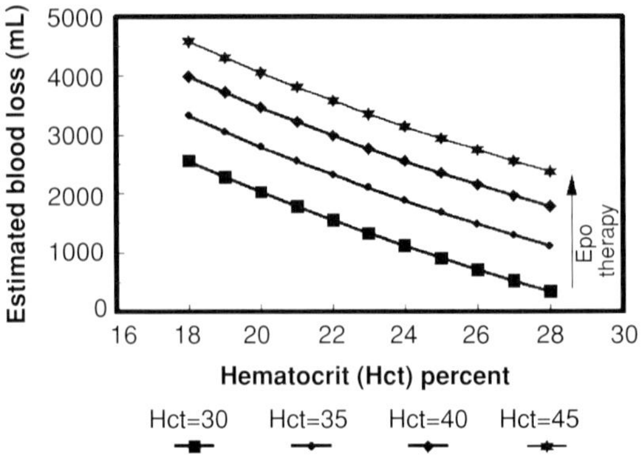

Figure 25.1 Relationship of allowable blood loss to minimally tolerated hematocrit (transfusion trigger) at various initial hematocrit levels (30, 35, 40, and 45%) in a patient with a blood volume of 5000 mL. Other blood volumes would result in proportional changes in blood loss. Through the use of an erythropoieten (EPO) intervention, one might shift a patient from a low hematocrit curve to a higher one and thereby allow greater blood loss before allogeneic red cells would be necessary. Adapted from Cohen [4].

Calculations of blood loss in specific patients

For modeling purposes a surgical procedure can be divided into three phases (Figure 25.2) [18]. Phase 1 encompasses the blood loss that occurred once surgery is started until a minimum hematocrit at which transfusion would begin is reached. Phase 2 encompassed the period after which the minimum hematocrit was reached (it was assumed that the patient would be transfused with red cells so as to maintain the minimum allowable hematocrit throughout the remainder phase 2. The third and final phase assumed hemostasis and been achieved and that a final volume equilibrium was reached (this would also include the postoperative period).

Phase 1

Phase 1 encompasses the blood loss that occurred once surgery is started until a minimum hematocrit at which transfusion would begin is reached.

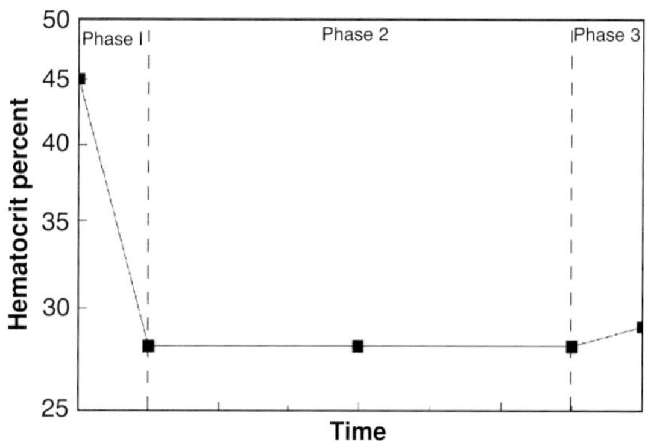

Figure 25.2 Diagramatic rendering of the hematocrit over time for a patient undergoing hospitalization for a surgical procedure. The time period is divided into three phases. Phase 1 encompasses the blood loss that occurred once surgery begins until a minimum hematocrit is reached at which transfusion would begin. Phase 2 encompassed the period after which the minimum hematocrit was reached; it was assumed that the patient would be transfused with red cells so as to maintain the minimum allowable hematocrit throughout the remainder phase 2. The third and final phase assumed hemostasis and been achieved and that a final volume equilibrium was reached. Reproduced from Nuttall et al. [14] .

Such a volume is calculated by:

$$V_L = -\mathrm{EBV} \times \ln(\mathrm{Hct}_0/\mathrm{Hct}_{\mathrm{min}})$$

where V_L = volume lost, EBV = estimated blood volume, Hct_0 = the hematocrit at the start of surgery, and $\mathrm{Hct}_{\mathrm{min}}$ = the final Hct (in this case the minimum Hct allowable or the transfusion trigger).

If acute normovolmic hemodilution is employed the starting Hct would be the Hct following the completion of the dilution or:

$$\mathrm{Hct}_F = \mathrm{Hct}_0 \times e^{(-V_{\mathrm{ANH}}/\mathrm{EBV})}$$

where in this case Hct_F = the Hct following the drawing of the ANH blood and V_{ANH} would be the volume of ANH blood drawn.

Phase 2

After the minimum hematocrit is reached it is assumed that the patient would be transfused with red cells so as to maintain the minimum allowable hematocrit and normovolemia throughout the remainder of phase 2. Actual practice may reflect some fluctuations in hematocrit or volume status. However, for the purposes of a mathematical model such assumptions are common and are unlikely to greatly effect the overall approximation.

The blood loss during this phase can be calculated as:

$$\frac{\mathrm{RBC}_T - \mathrm{RBC}_F}{\mathrm{Hct}_{\mathrm{min}}}$$

where RBC_T = the total amount of RBCs (mL) transfused during the hospitalization and RBC_F = the RBC volume given during the third phase if the hematocrit is raised above the transfusion trigger. RBC_T can represented as:

$$\mathrm{RBC}_T = \mathrm{RBC}_{\mathrm{ANH}} + \mathrm{RBC}_{\mathrm{ALLO}} + \mathrm{RBC}_{\mathrm{PAD}} + \mathrm{RBC}_{\mathrm{IBS}}$$

where $\mathrm{RBC}_{\mathrm{ANH}}$ = the volume of RBCs in the ANH blood reinfused, $\mathrm{RBC}_{\mathrm{ALLO}}$ = the volume of RBCs in the allogeneic units infused, $\mathrm{RBC}_{\mathrm{PAD}}$ = the volume of RBCs in the preoperative autologous donation (PAD) units, and $\mathrm{RBC}_{\mathrm{IBS}}$ = the volume of RBCs in the intraoperatively blood salvaged and reinfused. If postoperative salvage were employed, an additional RBC term for the postoperatively salvaged red cells could be similarly added.

For purposes of calculation, it was assumed that an allogeneic unit of RBCs had an average of 200 mL of RBC while a predeposit unit of autologous RBCs would average 180 mL [20]. Intraoperatively salvaged blood was assumed to have an average Hct of 55%. Alternative values could be employed if they differ at different institutions. Similarly, if the actual red cell volumes of the units are known these values can be substituted.

The RBC volume of the ANH blood is calculated by:

$$\mathrm{V}_{\mathrm{ANH}} \times \mathrm{Hct}_{\mathrm{ANH}}$$

where $\mathrm{Hct}_{\mathrm{ANH}}$ = the average Hct of the ANH blood drawn and calculated by:

$$\mathrm{Hct}_{\mathrm{ANH}} = (\mathrm{Hct}_0 \times \mathrm{EBV}) \times (1 - e^{-V_{\mathrm{ANH}}/\mathrm{EBV}})/V_{\mathrm{ANH}}$$

Alternatively, the RBC volume of the ANH blood can be calculated by

$$\mathrm{EBV} \times (\mathrm{Hct}_0 - \mathrm{Hct}_F)$$

where Hct_F = the posthemodilution hematocrit.

Phase 3

The third and final phase assumed hemostasis had been achieved and allows for a final volume equilibrium in the patient to occur. In some cases remaining ANH blood or salvaged blood is transfused before the patient leaving the operating room and may transiently lead to a hypervolemic state. Thus, an increase in the patient's hematocrit above the minimum allowable hematocrit may be seen. Alternatively, postoperative bleeding may decrease the hematocrit, which can also be accounted for.

$$RBC_F = (Hct_{DC} - Hct_{min}) \times EBV$$

where RBC_F = the RBC mL infused during the final phase and Hct_{DC} = the discharge hematocrit.

A straightforward example of such a calculation would be a patient with an initial Hct of 45%, an EBV of 5000 mL and a transfusion trigger and discharge hematocrit of 28% who received 2 units of allogeneic blood would be calculated as follows:

- Phase I—the blood loss from moving from a Hct of 45–28% would be:

$$5000\text{ mL} \times \ln(0.45/0.25) = 2372\text{ mL}$$

- Phase II—the transfusion of 2 units of allogeneic would have added an additional blood volume of

$$(2 \times 200\text{ mL RBCs/unit})/0.28 \text{ (the transfusion trigger)} = 1429\text{ mL}$$

- Phase III—since the discharge hematocrit equals the transfusion trigger there would be no additional blood loss.

So that the final blood loss would be:

$$2372\text{ mL} + 1429\text{ mL} = 3801\text{ mL}$$

A somewhat more complicated example would be a patient with an initial hematocrit of 45%, an EBV of 5000 mL, a transfusion trigger hematocrit of 28% who underwent 1 L of hemodilution at the beginning of the operative procedure, received two units of allogeneic blood and the ANH blood and had a discharge hematocrit of 30% would be calculated as follows:

- Phase I—the initial hemodilution and subsequent blood loss to the transfusion trigger

The 1000 mL hemodilution would result in a postdilution hematocrit of

$$45 \times e^{(-1000/5000)} = 36.8$$

the volume of RBCs contained in the ANH blood would be

$$(0.45 - 0.368) \times 5000 = 410\text{ mL}$$

The blood loss from the hematocrit of 36.8 to 28% would be calculated as

$$5000\text{ mL} \times \ln(0.36.8/0.28) = 1366\text{ mL}$$

- Phase II—the transfusion of 2 units of allogeneic would have added an additional blood volume of

$$(2 \times 200\text{ mL RBCs/unit})/0.28 \text{ (the transfusion trigger)} = 1429\text{ mL}$$

the transfusion of the ANH blood would have an additional blood volume of 410/0.28 (the transfusion trigger) = 1464 mL

- Phase III—the change in hematocrit from 28 to 30 would be the result of "tanking up" the patient. Therefore the portion of the transfused red cell mass that moved the patient from a hematocrit of 28–30% needs to be subtracted from the blood loss would be:

$(0.30 - 0.28) \times 5000 = 100$ mL of RBCs
which is the equivalent to
$100/0.28 = 357$ mL of blood loss

Therefore, the total blood loss would be equal to:

$$1366 + 1464 + 1429 - 357 = 3902\text{ mL.}$$

Had the patient had a final hematocrit of 26% instead of 30% the phase III blood loss would have been

$$\text{Phase III blood loss} = 5000 \times \ln(0.28/0.26) = 371\text{ mL}$$

So that the total blood loss would have been equal to:

$$1366 + 1464 + 1429 + 371 = 4630\text{ mL}$$

A distinct advantage of this approach is that when one calculates an actual blood loss, such modeling has the inherent flexibility to allow for the savings attributable to hemodilution.

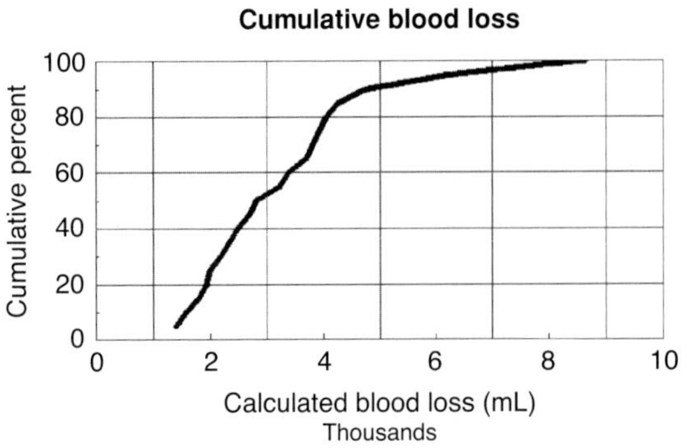

Figure 25.3 Cumulative percent blood loss graph. From a plot of this type one can decide the amount of blood loss that would encompass a given percent of the surgeons patients. In this example a 5000-mL blood loss account for 90% of patients while a 3000-mL blood loss would only account for approximately 50% of patients. Automated spreadsheet templates that allow for such rapid calculations and the creation of such a plot are available in both Lotus 123 and Microsoft Excel format.

Computer modeling

While the equations described can be calculated with a scientific calculator the use of commercially available spreadsheet application programs can greatly facilitate such calculations. Templates have been designed that given a patient's EBV; preoperative Hct, the discharge Hct, the number of units of PAD and allogeneic units infused, the milliliters of intraoperatively salvaged red cells reinfused; the volumes of ANH blood drawn and reinfused; and the minimum Hct at which transfusion would be initiated-automatically calculates an estimated blood loss. Such templates can calculate the blood loss of a larger number of cases and automatically plot a cumulative percent blood loss graph (Figure 25.3).

Validation of the calculus/computer model

Such modeling has been validated in 250 radical retropubic prostatectomy patients (Figures 25.4 and 25.5). This study found a significant relation ($p < 0.001$) between the calculated blood loss for the hospitalization and the estimated intraoperative blood loss. On average, the calculated blood loss was 2.1 times the intraoperative blood loss estimated by the anesthesiologist (median 1.9). However, the correlation coefficient ($r = 0.38$) suggested that, for any single value, there was not a good correlation.

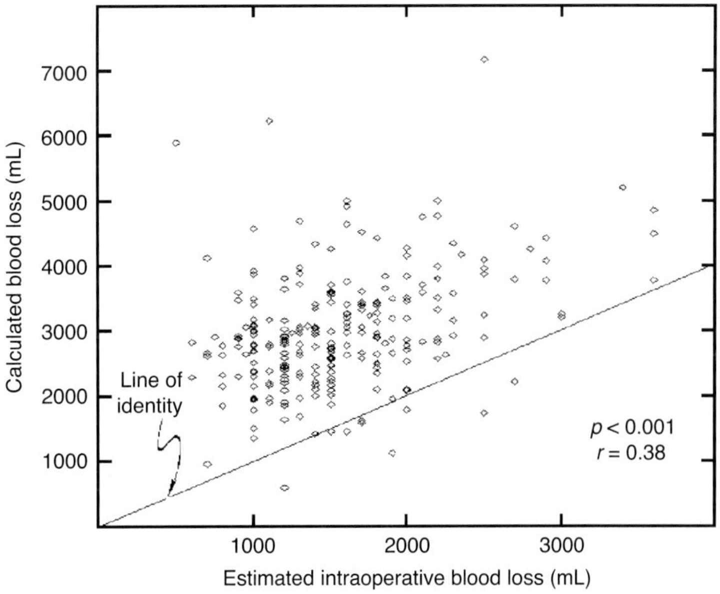

Figure 25.4 Comparison of the calculated blood loss for hospitalization with the intraoperative estimated blood loss in 250 radical retropubic prostatectomy patients. The line of identity is the line where estimated blood loss would equal calculated blood loss. Reproduced from Nuttall et al. [14].

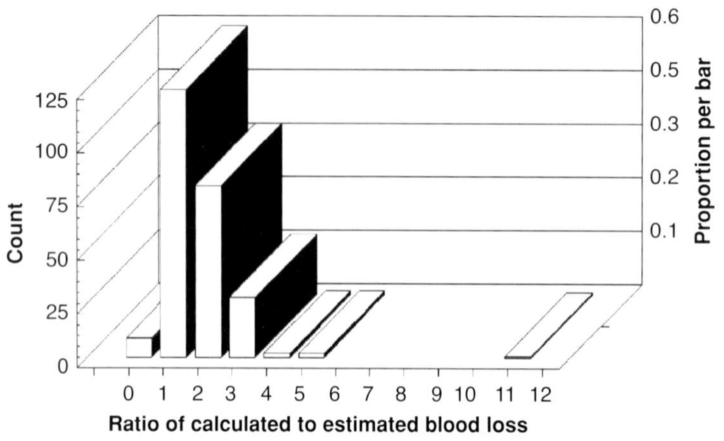

Figure 25.5 Distribution of the ratios of the calculated to the intraestimated blood loss in 250 radical retropubic prostatectomy patients. The majority of cases clustered about 2 (mean = 2.1, median = 1.9). The one extreme outlier involved a patient whose course was complicated by extensive intraperitoneal bleeding in the postoperative period following the placement of a drain. Reproduced from Nuttall et al. [14].

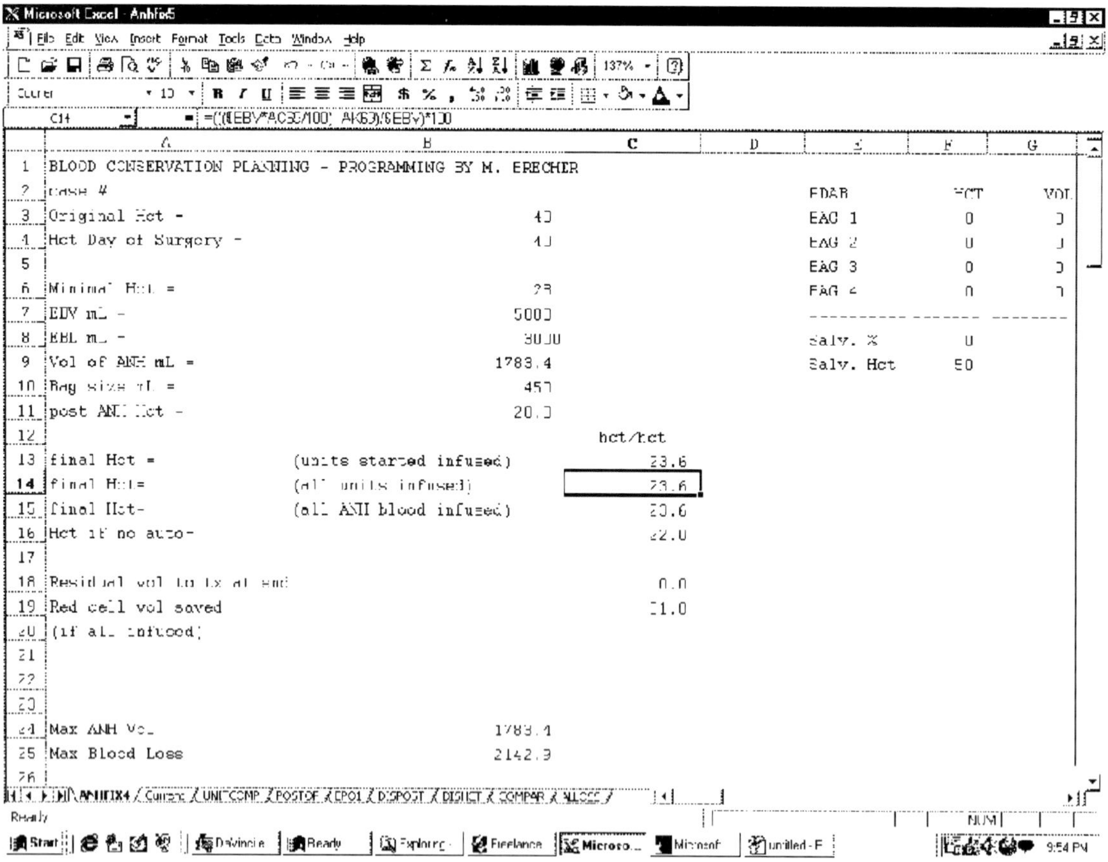

Figure 25.6 Representative screen from a Microsoft Excel template that allows the rapid evaluation of what-if scenario planning for a surgical patient. In this example the patient with an initial hematocrit of 40%, a blood volume of 5000 mL, and a minimal allowable hematocrit of 28% underwent ANH to a hematocrit of 28%, who sustains a 3000-mL blood loss would be expected to have a final hematocrit of 23.6%. Had ANH not been performed the final hematocrit would have been 22.0%.

Conclusion

Initial attempts at planning for the blood usage concentrated on assessing the blood usage that would be adequate for 80–90% of patients. Such methods, however, did not adequately address the needs of the individual patient and resulted in considerable overcollection and disposal of autologous blood. Recently, several groups have attempted to refine the art of predicting blood usage by the inclusion of additional red cell variables and an algebraic approach to red cell loss. However, such approaches fall short of actually estimating the blood loss. Other groups have been involved in a resurgence of interest in the mathematical modeling of transfusion strategies with the application of calculus methodology. Application of the mathematical principles outlined in such studies also allow for a calculated blood loss based on easily obtained data.

Given the inexpensive computing power available today, it does not take much of a leap of faith to anticipate that simulation programs will soon be readily available to surgeons as they plan for the blood needs of their patients. Such programs could even be run from palm-top computers. An example of such "what-if" type scenario planning would be a patient with an initial hematocrit of 40%, a blood volume of 5000 mL, and a minimally allowable hematocrit of 28% (the transfusion trigger), who sustains a 3000-mL blood loss. In this case, the final hematocrit following this blood loss would be 22.0%, which is below the minimum allowable hematocrit of 28%. Had the patient been given preoperative erythropoietin and the patient's hematocrit raised from 40 to 45%, following the 3000-mL blood loss, the hematocrit would be 24.7%, still not above the required minimum hematocrit of 28%. If acute normovolemic hemodilution (instead of the use of erythropoietin) were performed to a minimum hematocrit of 28% (and the ANH blood was transfused so as to maintain this hematocrit during the case and any residual ANH blood was returned at the end of the case the final hematocrit would have been 23.6%, again not above the required final hematocrit of 28% (Figure 25.6). However, if ANH and erythropoietin were combined before the 3000-mL blood loss the patient would be able to achieve a nadir hematocrit above 28% (in this case 28.2%).

The technology to apply such patient specific modeling is available today. The challenge is to use it in such a fashion that results in direct patient benefit (decreased allogeneic exposure, cost, and anemia).

The use of mathematical modeling of blood loss and "what-if" scenario planning offers the potential for more judicial and informed decisions regarding the use of blood-conservation techniques.

References

1. Brecher ME, Rosenfeld M. Mathematical and computer modeling of acute normovolemic hemodilution. Transfusion 1994;34:176–9.
2. Weiskopf RB. Mathematical analysis of isovolemic hemodilution indicates that it can decrease the need for allogeneic blood transfusion. Transfusion 1995;35:37–41.
3. Goodnough LT, Monk TG, Brecher ME. Acute normovolemic hemodilution in surgery. Hematology 1997;2:413–20.
4. Cohen JA, Brecher ME. Preoperative autologous blood donation, benefit or detriment: a mathematical analysis. Transfusion 1995;35:640–44.
5. Brecher ME, Goodnough LT, Monk T. Where does preoperative erythropoietin therapy add up? A mathematical perspective. Transfusion, in press.
6. Hay SN, Monk TG, Brecher ME. Intraoperative blood salvage: a mathematical perspective. Transfusion 2002;42:451–5.
7. Waters JH, Lee JS, Karafa MT. A mathematical model of cell salvage compared and combined with normovolemic hemodilution. Transfusion 2004;44: 1412–16.
8. Waters JH, Lee JS, Karafa MT. A mathematical model of cell salvage efficiency. Anesth Analg 2002;95:1312–17.
9. Friedman BA, Oberman HA, Chadwick AR. Kingdon KI. The maximum surgical blood order schedule and surgical blood use in the United States. Transfusion 1976;16 (4): 380–87.
10. Friedman BA. An analysis of surgical blood use in United States hospitals with application to the maximum surgical blood order schedule. Transfusion 1979;19(3):268–78.

11. Axelrod FB, Pepkowitz SH, Goldfinger D. Establishment of a schedule of optimal preoperative collection of autologous blood. Transfusion 1989;29: 677–80.
12. Bandarenko N, Brecher ME. Stratified standard surgical blood order schedule for autologous blood donation. Transfusion 1997;37(Suppl.):38S.
13. Monk TG, Goodnough LT, Brecher ME, Colberg JW, Andriole GL, Catalona WJ. A randomized trial of three blood conservation strategies for radical prostatectomy. Anesthesiology 1999;91:24–33.
14. Nuttall GA, Santrach PJ, Oliver WC, Jr, et al. The predictors of red cell transfusions in total hip arthroplasties. Transfusion 1996;36:144–9.
15. Nuttall GA, Santrach PJ, Oliver WC, et al. A prospective randomized trial of the surgical blood order equation for ordering red cells for total hip arthroplasty patients. Transfusion 1998;38:828–33.
16. Mercurali F, Inghilleri G. Proposal of an algorithm to help the choice of the best transfusion strategy. Curr Med Res Opin 1996;13:465–78.
17. McCullough TC, Roth JV, Ginsberg PC, Harkaway RC. Estimated blood loss underestimates calculated blood loss during radical retropubic prostatectomy. Urol Int 2004;72:13–16.
18. Brecher ME, Monk TG, Goodnough LT. A standardized method for the calculation of blood loss. Transfusion 1997;37:1071–4.
19. Bourke DL, Smith TC. Estimating allowable hemodilution. Anesthesiology 1974;41:609–12.
20. Goodnough LT, Bravo JR, Hsueh Y, Keating LJ, Brittenham GM. Red blood cell mass in autologous and homologous blood units. Implications for risk/benefit assessment of autologous blood crossover and directed blood transfusion. Transfusion 1989;29:821–2.

CHAPTER 26
Management of Massive Transfusion

Jean-François Hardy[1] *& Marc Samama*[2]
[1]Department of Anesthesiology, University of Montreal, Québec, Canada
[2]Hôtel-Dieu de Paris, Paris, France

Introduction

Uncontrolled hemorrhage and, as a consequence, massive transfusion (MT) is a frequent complication of trauma and surgery. MT is commonly defined as the loss of one blood mass in a period of 24 hours. However, a more dynamic definition of MT, such as the transfusion of four or more red cell concentrates within 1 hour when ongoing need is foreseeable, [1] appears preferable in the clinical setting. Massively transfused patients will show evidence of coagulopathy in a high percentage of cases.

This percentage will vary according to the clinical context: blunt versus penetrating trauma, presence of brain injury, and elective surgery [2, 3]; according to the definition of coagulopathy: clinical versus based on coagulation testing [3]; and according to the blood products administered to the massively bleeding patient: fresh whole blood, stored whole blood, "modified whole blood" (MWB—whole blood from which platelets and/or cryoprecipitate are salvaged before storage [4, 5], packed red blood cells (PRBC), concentrated red cells, etc. [6]. For example, before the era of blood fractionation, the transfusion of large volumes of stored blank blood did *not* result in hemorrhagic diatheses in young and previously healthy soldiers wounded during the Vietnam War [7]. More recently, it has been shown that abnormalities of the prothrombin time (PT) and of the activated partial thromboplastin (aPTT) time occur after the transfusion of 12 units of PRBC and that thrombocytopenia develops after the transfusion of 20 units [8]. Yet, despite several attempts at defining meaningful laboratory indicators of impending or established coagulopathy, the relationship between laboratory hemostatic abnormalities and abnormal clinical bleeding remains unclear.

Most studies of MT have been conducted in trauma patients and most are retrospective or uncontrolled observational studies [9], for obvious reasons. Given the variable and complex clinical context, the results of these studies have seldom led to definitive conclusions. Furthermore, factors other than the transfusion strategy, related to trauma itself, may have led to the observed hemostatic abnormalities [10]. Unfortunately, conventional teaching has sometimes failed to appreciate the evolution of transfusion practices and the context in which these were developed. As a result, anesthesiologists may have been led to apply transfusion strategies, e.g., those developed for trauma patients at a time when MWB was available, inappropriately to patient receiving red cell concentrates for massive bleeding during elective surgery. The situation can become even more confusing when disseminated intravascular coagulation (DIC) is associated with trauma and/or MT.

In this chapter on MT and coagulopathy, we will attempt to:

1 Identify the causes of coagulopathy in massively transfused, adult, and previously hemostatically competent patients to determine the most appropriate transfusion/treatment strategies.

Alternatives to Blood Transfusion in Transfusion Medicine, 2nd edition. Edited by A. Maniatis, P. Van der Linden, J.-F. Hardy.

2 Differentiate between the elective surgical setting and trauma, hypothesizing that recommendations derived from studies of MT in elective surgical patients may not apply in trauma patients and inversely.

Variables responsible for coagulopathy in association with MT

Platelets

Since the publication of Miller's classic study on coagulation defects associated with massive blood transfusions, thrombocytopenia resulting from hemodilution has been thought to be the most important hemostatic abnormality associated with MT [11]. This explanation is intuitively appealing: replacement of lost blood with fluids that do not contain platelets (or coagulation factors) results in a dilutional coagulopathy. However appealing, hemodilution fails to explain several observations.

In wounded (excluding burns and head trauma) young and previously healthy soldiers, platelet levels fell rapidly to about 100,000/mm^3 during rapid transfusion of stored whole blood and remained at that level after the first 6 L of stored whole blood [7]. PTs, partial thromboplastin times, and fibrinogen levels were less severely affected and, most important, significant operative bleeding was not encountered in conjunction with these mild dilutional coagulation changes [7]. On average, the platelet count fell below 100,000/mm^3 after transfusion of 18 units of blood in the study by Counts et al. [5]. Nonetheless, in that study, slightly less than half (43%) of the variation in platelet counts could be ascribed to the functional relationship between blood transfused and the platelet count. In a study conducted to determine the efficacy of prophylactic platelet administration to prevent microvascular bleeding (MVB) associated with MT, Reed et al. observed that platelet counts were not different between patients who received prophylactic platelet transfusions and those who did not [4]. Further, both groups had higher platelet counts than predicted by a standard washout equation. The implication of this finding is that platelets are being released into the circulation counteracting the effects of dilution. Sequestered platelets can be released from the spleen and the lung, in addition to the premature release of platelets from the bone marrow. Elevated stress hormones and the administration of cathecolamines, a situation more likely to occur in the trauma patient, will influence release.

As in the study by Counts, the relationship between platelet counts and units of blood transfused was significant but variability was high ($R^2 = 0.24$ for patients receiving platelets and $R^2 = 0.35$ for patients receiving fresh frozen plasma or FFP) [4], suggesting that factors other than simple dilution affect platelet count. Finally, in the study by Miller, platelet counts did not parallel the predicted platelet counts on the basis of a standard washout equation [11]. For example, the observed platelet count after the administration of 25 units of blood was of the order of 60,000/mm^3 while hemodilution predicted a platelet count of approximately 20,000/mm^3.

In patients undergoing elective surgery, the situation appears somewhat different, possibly because tissue trauma is more controlled, normovolemia is maintained, and blood losses are replaced in a timely manner. In this context, coagulopathy is primarily related to a coagulation factor deficit [3, 12]. The role of fibrinogen appears to be preponderant. The deficiency in fibrinogen concentration develops earlier than any other hemostatic abnormality when plasma-poor red cell concentrates and colloid plasma substitutes are used for the replacement of major blood loss. Approximately 90% of the variation in fibrinogen concentration is explained by blood loss and the critical level of 1.0 g/L is reached when blood losses reach 142% (95% confidence interval: 117–169%) of the calculated blood volume [12]. In the same study, thrombocytopenia (defined as a platelet count below 50,000/mm^3) was a late occurrence and, to a great extent, quite variable from patient to patient.

Murray et al. studied coagulation changes during crystalloid and PRBC replacement of major blood loss during elective surgery [13]. Four out of 12 patients presented a coagulopathy. All patients with inadequate clinical hemostasis had a low platelet count (83,000/mm^3 or below) and transfusion of platelet concentrates corrected the problem in those two who had fibrinogen concentrations above 1.0 g/L. Interestingly, platelet transfusion was ineffective in those two patients who had concurrent low fibrinogen concentrations (0.73 and 0.40 g/L). The subsequent transfusion of 2 and 4 units of FFP (respectively) normalized hemostasis. The report by Ciavarella et al. supports the association between MVB and a low platelet count (below 50,000/mm^3) or a low fibrinogen concentration (below 0.5 g/L) [14].

Primary hemostasis is characterized by the formation of the "platelet plug." The mechanism is complex and involves the presence of fibrinogen and activation of several glycoprotein receptors on platelets [15–19]. Hemostasis is initiated by injury to the vascular wall, leading to the deposition of platelets adhering to blood vessel subendothelial matrix proteins (collagen and von Willebrand factor) via interactions with platelet membrane glycoprotein receptors. Subsequently, the GP IIb/IIIa receptor is activated. This receptor has a high affinity for fibrinogen. Binding of fibrinogen to adjacent platelets results in irreversible platelet aggregation and the formation of the platelet aggregate. It appears then logical to consider that coagulopathy after MT can be a problem resulting from a combined deficit of platelets and fibrinogen. Focusing on platelet levels or concentrations of specific coagulation factors may not lead to the most appropriate therapeutic approach.

Trauma-associated coagulopathy

Disseminated intravascular coagulation often complicates the management of MT and is secondary to the systemic and excessive activation of coagulation. It may be defined by the association of hemostatic defects related to the excessive generation of thrombin and fibrin (with or without clinical signs) and the excessive consumption of platelets and coagulation factors [20].

In earlier studies of trauma patients, DIC leading to MVB was, apparently, relatively infrequent, occurring for example in 1 out of 21 patients [11] and 3 out of 27 patients [5]. In wounded, previously healthy, soldiers requiring MT, DIC was mild and was not associated with clinical bleeding [7, 11]. More recent studies, however, suggest that there is no significant correlation between the severity of impaired hemostasis and total units of blood transfused, suggesting that consumption of coagulation factors and platelets is more important than simple hemodilution [21–23].

In trauma patients, two major mechanisms are responsible for the occurrence of DIC. The first relates to shock and tissue hypoxia. The second relates to the nature and to the importance of tissue trauma. In approximately 25% of trauma patients, clinically significant coagulopathy is present on arrival in the emergency room [24]. This acute coagulopathy appears to be secondary to activation of anticoagulant (activation of protein C by the thrombin–thrombomodulin complex) and fibrinolytic (release of tissue plasminogen activator or tPA and reduction of plasminogen activator inhibitor-1 or PAI-1) pathways [25]. In the study by Cosgriff et al., in the absence of massive head injury and preexisting disease, life-threatening coagulopathy was associated with a pH of less than 7.10, a temperature of less than 34°C, an Injury Severity Score greater than 25, and a systolic blood pressure of less than 70 mmHg [23]. When all risk factors were present, the incidence of coagulopathy was 98% [23]. Brain injury is associated with a particularly high incidence of coagulopathy. In the study by Faringer et al., more than 40% of patients with penetrating or blunt trauma with associated brain injuries had abnormal coagulation tests on admission, compared with 0% in patients with blunt trauma but without brain injury [2]. After blunt brain injury, a DIC syndrome secondary to the extravasation of tissue factor can rapidly (within 1–4 hours after injury) lead to a consumptive coagulopathy that is associated with a high frequency of death [26].

Mannucci et al. studied changes in the hemostatic system in 172 patients undergoing MT for excessive bleeding during or in the early postoperative period after elective, emergent, or trauma surgery [27]. Of these, 52 (30%) suffered decompensated DIC and there was no significant relation between the number of whole blood or PRBC units transfused and the values of any variable of hemostasis measured [27]. In a series of 64 patients receiving more than 10 units of red cell concentrates (elective and urgent surgical procedures, multiple trauma), Hewson et al.'s data suggest that coagulopathy is, initially, secondary to hemodilution but that, within 3 hours, coagulopathy is related to the duration of antecedent hypotension [28]. Reading these articles, it is difficult to determine which patient population (elective or urgent operations, trauma) is most likely to sustain DIC. No patient suffered from DIC among the 32 young American Society of Anesthesiologists (ASA) physical status I or II patients undergoing posterior spinal stabilization in the study by Murray et al. [3]. Clinically increased surgical bleeding was present in 17 patients and in 14 of the 17 patients hemostasis improved after the administration of FFP (approximately 10 mL/kg). Again, these results suggest that when tissue hypoxia is avoided and surgical trauma is controlled, the occurrence of DIC may remain low despite MT.

Coagulation factors

The effects of decreased levels of coagulation factors have been dealt within the previous section since it is not possible to separate entirely the influence of coagulation factors and platelets on the development of impaired hemostasis after MT. However, it is important to realize that studies conducted at a time when fresh, stored, or modified whole blood was in common use seldom reported low levels of coagulation factors as the primary factor responsible for impaired hemostasis [4, 5, 7, 11, 14]. Since the widespread use of volume resuscitation with crystalloids, colloids and red cell solutions containing minimal amounts of plasma during the late 1980s and early 1990s, dilution or consumption of coagulation factors has become a significant issue requiring specific treatment with, primarily, FFP [3, 6, 8, 12]. Failure to recognize this important change in transfusion practice has led to the persistence of inappropriate beliefs in transfusion requirements.

In addition to the importance of tissue trauma, shock, and tissue hypoxia, three other considerations tend to confound the issue. First, as mentioned previously, impaired hemostasis is most probably multifactorial in origin. The net adverse hemostatic effect of multiple concurrent coagulation factor deficits combined with variable degrees of thrombocytopenia remains unclear [6]. Second, clinicians seldom administer "pure" blood products. PRBC contain a small amount of plasma (30–60 mL) or even no plasma, as do platelet concentrates (80 mL approximately). Therefore, it may be difficult to differentiate precisely the therapeutic effect of the different blood components transfused. Third, all coagulation testing is performed at 37°C. Thus, a test may be normal in vitro in the laboratory but abnormal in vivo in the hypothermic patient.

While numerous studies have measured changes in the PT and in the aPTT in relationship with bleeding and MT, few have examined individual hemostatic factors. In 1979, transfusing modified whole blood to patients who sustained major trauma, massive gastrointestinal hemorrhage, or aortic aneurysm rupture, Counts et al. reported that the number of units of blood transfused explained less than 20% of the variance in factors V and VIII and was not related to factor VII, X, XI, XII, and fibrinogen levels [5]. The authors concluded that it was not necessary to supplement transfusions of stored, modified whole blood with fresh blood or FFP [5]. In 1995, using plasma poor red cell concentrates, Hiippala et al. showed that a concentration of fibrinogen of 1.0 g/L was reached when the blood loss was 1.42 times the calculated blood volume and that blood losses in excess of two blood volumes caused the deficiency of prothrombin, factor V, platelets, and factor VII, in this order [12]. These observations were made in ASA physical status I or II patients undergoing elective major urologic or abdominal surgery and, obviously, may not apply to emergent operations or trauma. Nonetheless, they illustrate well the difference between earlier days when red cell solutions contained significant amounts of plasma and contemporary component therapy.

Red cells

An often-ignored effect of RBC transfusion is the improvement of hemostatic function. Transfusion of RBC shortens the bleeding time (BT) in anemic thrombocytopenic patients despite persistent thrombocytopenia [29]. Similarly, RBC shorten the BT and control the hemorrhagic diathesis of uremic patients [30]. This correlation between the BT and hematocrit levels was studied in rabbits. In nonthrombocytopenic animals, the BT varied inversely with the hematocrit, animals with hematocrit levels above 35% having shorter BTs than animals with hematocrits lower than 35% [31]. In subjects with normal renal function and platelet counts over 100,000/mm^3, there exists a modest but statistically significant inverse correlation ($r = -0.47$) between the hematocrit and the BT [32]. In 42 patients with chronic anemia, the aPTT and BT decreased significantly after transfusion, by a mean of 1.3 seconds ($p = 0.01$) and 2.6 minutes ($p < 0.01$), respectively [33]. Valeri et al. have shown that, in healthy volunteers, an acute 15% reduction in hematocrit produced a 60% increase in the BT while the BT remained normal despite a 32% reduction in platelet count [34]. All this being said, the clinical significance of these findings remains unclear since the relationship between the BT and perioperative blood loss is highly controversial [34, 35].

Erythrocytes have been shown to modulate biochemical and functional responsiveness of activated platelets, suggesting that erythrocytes contribute to thrombosis and hemostasis and supporting the concept that thrombus formation is a multicellular event [36–38]. This proaggregatory property of erythrocytes is enhanced by diabetes [39] and can be decreased by an appropriate aspirin regimen [40, 41]. In a rabbit model of cyclic arterial thrombosis and clot lysis, Ouaknine-Orlando et al. have shown that decreases in the hematocrit reduced the cyclic arterial thrombosis rate and increased the BT [42]. Interestingly, normalization of the hematocrit caused thrombosis to reappear.

Another mechanism by which erythrocytes modulate hemostasis is the rheological effect of red cells on the margination of platelets [43]. Under normal circumstances, red cell flow is maximal at the center of a vessel, tending to push platelets toward the periphery of the vessel lumen, thereby optimizing their interaction with injured endothelium and promoting hemostasis. In rabbit arterioles, platelet numbers are highest near the vessel wall [44] and platelets align themselves with their equatorial plane parallel to the vessel wall as they move closer toward the periphery of the vessel [45]. Experimental data have shown that platelets are expelled toward the red blood cell depleted marginal layer near the tube wall by mutual interaction with erythrocytes. Under these circumstances, the near-wall concentration of platelets is enhanced up to about *seven times* the average concentration [46].

The hemostatic effects of profound normovolemic hemodilution were investigated in eight patients undergoing surgical correction of idiopathic scoliosis by McLoughlin et al. [47]. Abnormal hemostasis developed before compromise of global tissue oxygenation suggesting that, in healthy anesthetized subjects, normovolemic hemodilution may be limited more by preservation of normal coagulation. In this report, reinfusion of all collected blood at the end of the procedure did not normalize the PT or the aPTT. Unfortunately, the authors did not describe if the MVB observed during hemodilution was corrected by increasing the hematocrit. Modified ultrafiltration in pediatric open-heart operations has been shown to increase the hematocrit and attenuate the dilutional coagulopathy associated with cardiopulmonary bypass in infants [48]. Use of modified ultrafiltration to increase the hematocrit to 36–42% reduced the rise in total body water and the need for donor blood in children undergoing open-heart surgery [49]. In 2004, Segal et al. reviewed a total of 42 trials comparing hemodilution to usual care or to another blood conservation method. The risk of allogeneic transfusion was similar among patients receiving acute normovolemic hemodilution and those receiving usual care (relative risk [RR], 0.96; 95% CI, 0.90–1.01), or another blood conservation method (RR, 1.11; 95% CI, 0.96–1.28). Hemodiluted patients, however, were transfused from 1 to 2 fewer units of allogeneic blood. They had less total bleeding than patients receiving usual care (91 mL; 95% CI, 25–158 mL), although more intraoperative bleeding [50].

Thus, further investigations into the role of the hemoglobin concentration or hematocrit on hemostasis in massively transfused patients appear warranted. The data presented above tend to support the concept of a minimal hematocrit for optimal hemostasis. Currently the optimal hematocrit/hemoglobin concentration to avoid/treat coagulopathy remains unknown. The experimental evidence presented above suggests that hematocrits as high as 35–36% may be required to sustain hemostasis in bleeding patients undergoing MT.

Crystalloids and colloids

Rapid hemodilution with crystalloid has been shown to induce a hypercoagulable state [51, 52]. The clinical significance of this effect, specially in trauma patients who are initially hypercoagulable [7], remains unclear. Interestingly however, crystalloid-induced hypercoagulability casts a doubt on studies describing the effects of colloids on coagulation that used crystalloids as a control [53].

Gelatins have the reputation of not influencing coagulation other than by their hemodiluting effect [54, 55]. A study comparing a 3% modified fluid gelatin to 6% hydroxyethyl starch (HES) in patients undergoing primary total hip replacement concluded that the gelatin-based plasma expander had a poorer volume effect than HES and that blood losses were less important with gelatin compared to HES [54]. Coagulation tests were similar in both groups except for the higher incidence of an abnormal BT in the HES group. In volunteers, 1L of a gelatin-based plasma substitute significantly impaired primary hemostasis and thrombin generation compared to normal saline [56]. Dilution of whole blood samples with two gelatin solutions resulted in a reduction of clot quality (less extensive fibrin mesh formation, reduced clot weight and mean shear modulus) compared to dilution with normal saline [57]. As for other colloids, the clinical significance of these findings remains unclear. Perhaps the effects on coagulation of gelatin-based plasma substitutes are not clinically important. On the contrary, they may have been underestimated, given the difficulties of studying coagulation in the uncontrolled context of trauma, MT and ongoing bleeding.

HES solutions are effective plasma expanders in common use both in Europe and in North America. It has long been known that HES solutions interfere with coagulation [58] and that the effects vary according to the dose and type of solution administered [59]. Solutions with a high molecular weight and a high degree of substitution accumulate in the plasma and the tissues and are responsible for more pronounced hemostatic effects [60]. Abnormal platelet function occurs more frequently after high molecular weight HES [61]. Conversely, HES solutions with a low molecular weight and a lesser degree of substitution are eliminated more rapidly and tend to affect measures of hemostasis less [62–64].

In addition to their effects on hemostasis, the infusion of large volumes of HES solutions will result in significant hemodilution. The resulting drop in hemoglobin and platelet concentrations may compromise primary hemostasis. In addition, Innerhofer et al. have shown that the administration of HES or modified gelatin in patients undergoing knee replacement surgery results in reduced clot strength owing to impaired fibrinogen polymerization and that reduced fibrinogen concentrations might be reached earlier than expected [65].

Adverse events associated with the use of HES solutions for the resuscitation of patients requiring MT have not been reported, inasmuch as the allowed maximal daily dose is not exceeded [55]. A large retrospective study suggested that the use of 6% high in vitro molecular weight HES in primary cardiac surgery with cardiopulmonary bypass may increase bleeding and transfusion requirements, despite the infusion of volumes smaller than the manufacturer's recommended dose [66]. Conversely, large volumes (up to 5L) have been infused without major complications [67], but the safety of this practice remains controversial [68]. In 2008, a re-analysis of pooled data from 449 patients undergoing major surgery and included in seven clinical trials suggested that HES 130/0.4 may be associated with less blood losses and transfusion requirements as compared to HES 200/0.5 [69].

The clinical significance of the effects of HES solutions on hemostasis remains unclear. It may never be possible to determine precisely the effect of volume replacement in massively transfused patients with ongoing bleeding. In these patients, hemostasis is stressed severely by numerous factors other than the type of clear fluid used for resuscitation and the underlying cause of coagulopathy is difficult to ascertain. Nonetheless, it is interesting to note that the use of colloids in trauma patients is not recommended by the American College of Surgeons [70].

Temperature

An important measure to reduce blood loss through preservation of hemostasis is the maintenance of normothermia both during and after the operation. Several animal studies conducted under hypothermic conditions have shown reversible platelet count decreases and platelet function defects, altered coagulation patterns, and an enhanced fibrinolytic response. In dogs cooled to 19°C, Yoshihara et al. [71] found a severe decrease in platelet count and collagen-induced platelet aggregability and an increase in fibrinolysis. No variations of the PT and aPTT were observed but these tests were performed in vitro at 37°C. These modifications, which could potentially increase bleeding, were not documented in the normothermic control animals. Pina-Cabral et al. [72] also observed a decrease in platelet count in hypothermic dogs. The presence of platelet clumps was detected inside the hepatic sinusoids. The authors concluded that hepatic platelet sequestration could explain the decrease in platelet count in this setting. In swine, Oung et al. [73] showed a prolongation of the BT (10.9 minutes vs 5.5 minutes in the control group), confirming the impairment of hemostasis induced by hypothermia (30°C). Prolongation of the BT has also been observed by Valeri et al. in baboons subjected to systemic hypothermia at 32°C and skin hypothermia at 27°C [74].

In humans, several laboratory studies have emphasized the role of hypothermia on bleeding during surgical procedures. Valeri et al. observed the effects of skin temperature in 33 patients undergoing CPB [75]. Local hypothermia produced an increased BT and a significant reduction in thromboxane B2 at the BT site. Local rewarming produced a significant increase in shed blood thromboxane B2. Thus, hypothermia caused a reversible platelet dysfunction and rewarming improved platelet function and reduced both BT and blood loss. These data have been confirmed by Michelson et al. [76] who demonstrated the involvement of platelet glycoprotein receptor (GP Ib and GMP 140) alterations in this hemostatic defect. Again, rewarming completely reversed the activation defect as soon as temperature returned to 37°C. Other studies have shown an important prolongation of PT and aPTT that was inversely correlated to temperature [77, 78]. This additional contribution of hypothermia to the hemorrhagic diathesis may be overlooked since coagulation testing is normally performed at 37°C [79].

The contribution of hypothermia to coagulopathy in trauma patients has been alluded to previously [23]. Hypothermia (temperature less than 34°C) occurred in 80% of nonsurvivors and 36% of survivors in the 45 trauma patients reported by Ferrara et al. [80]. Patients who were hypothermic and acidotic developed clinically significant bleeding despite adequate blood, plasma, and platelet replacement. The authors concluded that avoidance or correction of hypothermia may be critical in preventing or correcting coagulopathy in the patient receiving MT.

Monitoring of coagulopathy

Numerous attempts have been made to monitor changes to the hemostatic system in relationship to trauma, surgery, and MT. Unfortunately, results have been disappointing and, today, there is no simple, reliable, and rapid diagnostic test that allows clinicians to manage MVB in massively transfused, critically ill patients.

Usefulness of the BT to diagnose or predict coagulopathy in massively transfused patients has been investigated in a few studies. Overall, the BT increases early in the course of surgery and transfusion [81], remains elevated for several days postoperatively [82] and does not allow the differentiation between bleeding and nonbleeding patients [5]. In their critical reappraisal of the BT, Rodgers and Levin concluded that there is no evidence that abnormalities in the test occur sufficiently in advance of other indicators of bleeding to allow actions to be taken that could alter outcome favorably [83]. Consequently, the BT is of no use in the context of MT.

The platelet count has been discussed earlier. It is the only indicator of coagulation that can be obtained rapidly through the use of automated counters in contrast to conventional hemostasis testing that takes a minimum of 30 minutes since it requires centrifugation of blood samples. Reliable bedside monitors have become available to monitor the PT and aPTT [84] and this may add to the timely management of the bleeding patient. Coagulation is a multicellular event, in which platelets play an important role, obviously. Even so, a decreased platelet count is not a specific indicator of a coagulopathy. Rather, the significance of decreased platelet counts should be interpreted in the patient's specific clinical context: is platelet function expected to be normal? Is the fibrinogen concentration sufficient? Is the hemoglobin concentration adequate? Is there any evidence of a consumption coagulopathy? Answering these questions will assist in making the appropriate diagnosis of coagulopathy and help the clinician to decide if transfusion of platelet concentrates is likely to treat the hemostatic defect.

As for decreased platelet counts and prolongations of the BT, prolongations of the PT and aPTT are very common [2, 3, 5, 7, 8, 11–13, 22, 23, 27, 28, 85]. Controversy remains, however, on the proper use of coagulation screening tests to guide replacement therapy. Ciavarella et al. have shown that, in 36 massively transfused patients, marked prolongations of the PT and aPTT predicted clotting factor levels below 20% and were good predictors of bleeding as well [14]. Patients with a PT or aPTT ratio greater or equal to 1.8 had an 80–85% chance of exhibiting MVB. Lesser prolongations of the PT or aPTT ratio are poorer predictors of bleeding in massively transfused patients [5]. The PT and aPTT are expected to become elevated when levels of Factor V, VIII, and IX are less than 50% of values found in a control patient population [86]. In trauma patients, when massive blood loss was replaced with MWB, factor V and VIII levels $\leq$30% have been cited as indications for coagulation factors replacement [4, 14]. When the fibrinogen level is adequate, a PT or aPTT ratio greater or equal to 1.8 reliably predicts that factor V and VIII levels are less than 30% [14]. In the presence of a decreased fibrinogen concentration (less than 0.75 g/L), a PT or aPTT ratio greater than 1.5 is associated with Factors V and VIII of less than 20% [13]. Another argument against the indiscriminate interpretation of abnormal PT and aPTT results is the finding that coagulation factor concentrations do not vary as expected on the basis of dilution. Factor levels are much higher than expected by dilution and, in fact, most of their variation is explained by influences other than transfused blood, whether patients are transfused with MWB [5] or PRBC [13]. In summary, only *marked* prolongations of the PT or aPTT are likely to be significant from a clinical perspective. As for platelets, prolongations should be interpreted in light of the concomitant fibrinogen and platelet concentrations.

Other instruments have been developed to study coagulation at the bedside, using whole blood. While their use in the context of MT appeared promising, results have, unfortunately, been disappointing. The best known is the thromboelastograph, a device that measures the viscoelastic properties of the clot during its formation and subsequent lysis. In general surgical patients, thromboelastography analysis showed a trend toward increased coagulability with progressive blood loss and contributed to the identification of two patients who required treatment of a coagulopathy [87]. Thromboelastography has a high negative predictive value (82%) for bleeding after routine cardiac surgery, allowing the differentiation between surgical bleeding and coagulopathy. Unfortunately, the positive predictive value of the test is low (41%) [88]. Thromboelastography has been used to evaluate the hemostatic effects of administering a transfusion package to massively bleeding patients [89] and showed that none of the patients remained hypocoagulable after transfusion of up to 7 transfusion packages. On the contrary, a MEDLINE search (January 2008) on the use of thromboelastography to orient transfusion therapy during massive bleeding and MT failed to retrieve any relevant references.

Another instrument measures an ex vivo BT in the presence of different agonists: the PFA-100. This device has been used extensively for the diagnosis of hereditary coagulation disorders, particularly von Willebrand's disease. In patients undergoing routine cardiac operations, the PFA-100 was not correlated with mediastinal chest drainage [90, 91]. Again, a MEDLINE search (January 2008) on the use of the PFA-100 during MT failed to retrieve any relevant references. The reader is referred to Chapter 21 devoted to Monitoring of Hemostasis in the Perioperative Setting by S. Kozek-Langenecker for more detailed information on currently available monitors.

Treatment of coagulopathy

Elective surgery

The treatment of coagulopathy associated with MT is not simple. The causal diagnosis of MVB remains elusive and the clinician must intervene rapidly if the patient is to survive. The situation is further complicated by the increased risks associated with transfusion, mandating that patients receive the smallest number of blood products possible. As a general principle, especially in the context of elective surgery, it should be mentioned that hemostatic blood components should be transfused only to treat a *clinical* coagulopathy. No prophylactic regimen involving the administration of FFP and/or platelet concentrates has been shown to be effective [5, 27]. The prophylactic administration of (potentially) unnecessary transfusions exposes patients to multiple donors and increases the risks to the patient [92,93]. Nonetheless, given the delay required to prepare and/or obtain blood products, MT associated with evidence of an evolving laboratory coagulopathy may warrant ordering of blood components that will, then, be readily available to treat MVB should it occur.

The figure by Erber et al. summarizes well the use of blood and nonblood products involved in the resuscitation of a bleeding patient undergoing elective surgery (Figure 26.1) [94]. Initially, crystalloids or colloids are infused to maintain

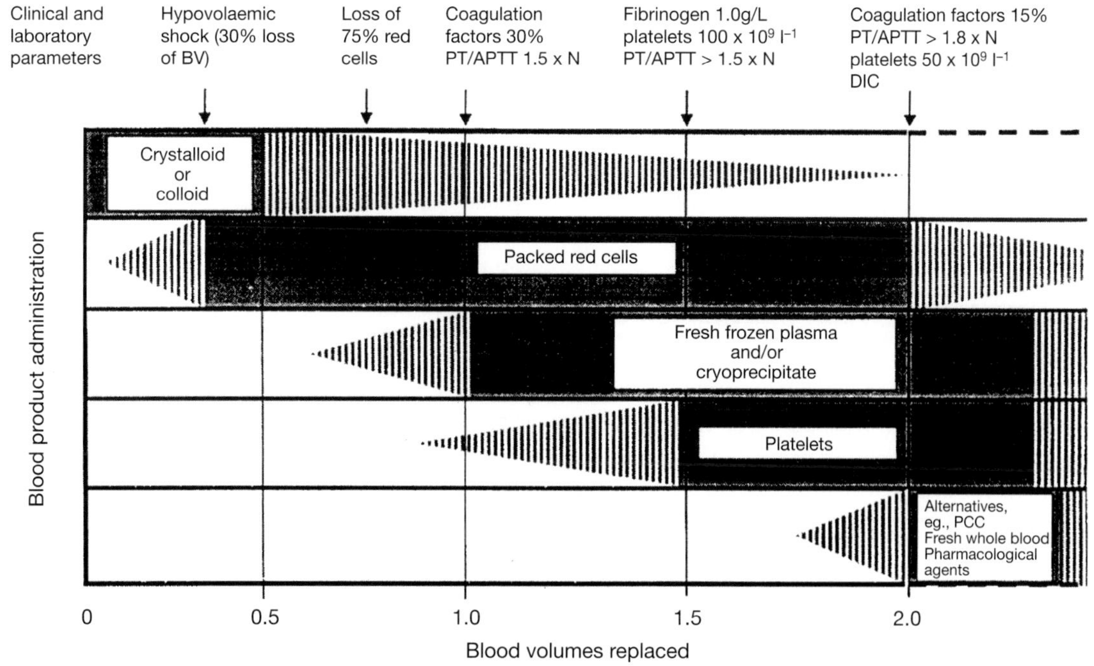

Figure 26.1 Fluid resuscitation and administration of blood products/alternatives as a function of blood volumes replaced. Reproduced from Erber et al. [94] with permission from Elsevier.

normovolemia. As the percentage of blood volume lost and replaced increases, PRBC, FFP, and platelets will be required, in that order, guided by clinical and laboratory variables. Pharmacological agents are administered late in the process.

Basic recommendations include the maintenance of normothermia and correction of a low hemoglobin concentration. Maintaining a normal body temperature is probably one of the simplest and most effective strategies of blood conservation. When a hypothermic patient bleeds without an apparent surgical cause, temperature should be restored to normal before administering any blood product. Correction of the hypothermia-induced hemostatic defect can be expected as soon as the patient is rewarmed. Surgery under normothermic conditions may help prevent bleeding complications and decrease the intraoperative use of transfusions [95].

A low hemoglobin concentration should be corrected before administration of hemostatic blood products, in view of normalizing hemostasis. If the circumstances allow, allogeneic red blood cells should be transfused one unit at a time and the effects of transfusion on hemostasis monitored before administering supplemental units. The optimal hematocrit/hemoglobin concentration to sustain hemostasis in the context of MT remains unknown but is probably higher than that required for oxygen transport and delivery.

In the bleeding patient, the use of platelets and/or FFP should depend on clinical judgment and the results of coagulation testing. A markedly prolonged PT and aPTT suggests a coagulation factor deficiency and is best treated with FFP. Decreased levels of fibrinogen will also require treatment with FFP or, when available, with fibrinogen concentrate. It is not clear now if coagulation factor concentrates are as effective as FFP but, clearly, this is a developing field in transfusion medicine.

FFP should be administered in doses large enough to increase coagulation factor levels and maintain them above critical levels. Doses ranging from 5 to 20 mL/kg have been recommended. In the average adult, 4 units of FFP (800–1000 mL) should suffice initially but additional bolus doses should be administered according to ongoing blood losses and transfusions [6].

Platelets should be administered only to correct a clinical coagulopathy associated with a decreased platelet count and/or platelet function. Clinicians must remember that platelet counts will decrease in a majority of massively transfused patients but that not all patients will bleed excessively as a result of thrombocytopenia. Other hemostatic anomalies may warrant a more urgent (a marked prolongation of the PT and aPTT) or concurrent (a decreased fibrinogen level) correction. From the time PRBC have replaced whole blood, there is laboratory and clinical evidence in the literature that FFP may be required before platelet concentrates to treat a coagulopathy [3, 6, 8, 13].

Trauma

In the context of trauma, recent evidence suggests that the management of massive bleeding should be more aggressive. While the escalating scheme suggested by Erber is appealing and applicable in the elective surgical setting where bleeding is usually progressive and coagulopathy can be monitored and anticipated [94], the situation can be quite different in the traumatized patient. In the interval between injury and arrival to the hospital, the patient has lost an undefined amount of blood that has been replaced, in part, by crystalloids or colloids. Tissue trauma, shock, tissue anoxia, and hypothermia contribute to the development of coagulopathy and the results of coagulation testing are not immediately available. Clinicians are called upon to intervene rapidly in a very unclear and unstable situation.

Two older studies have shown that survival in massively transfused trauma patients is associated with the increased transfusion of platelet concentrates [23, 96]. In the context of trauma and massive bleeding, several recent case series suggest that survival is improved by the administration of RBC, FFP, and platelets in a 1:1:1 ratio [97–101]. Most of these come from the military but 1:1:1 ratios of RBC, FFP, and platelets have also been shown to improve outcomes in civilian trauma [102–104]. Although interesting and promising, these data are retrospective, remain somewhat controversial

[105] and will require confirmation by properly conducted prospective trials.

One may postulate that a more aggressive control of coagulopathy could be beneficial in traumatized, massively bleeding patients. Unfortunately, today, no physiologic monitor (of coagulation or other) allows clinicians to identify which patient is likely to benefit from the increased transfusion of hemostatic blood components.

Recombinant activated factor VII in trauma

The reader is referred to Chapter 23 devoted to rFVIIa for a complete review of the efficacy and safety of rFVIIa administered to prevent or to treat excessive bleeding associated with a variety of medical and surgical conditions.

The article by Boffard et al. reports the results of two parallel randomized, placebo-controlled, double-blind clinical trials on the use of rFVIIa as adjunctive therapy to control bleeding in severely injured trauma patients [106]. Patients received either rFVIIa (three doses for a total of 400 μg/kg) or an equal volume of placebo and were stratified to blunt or penetrating injury, hence the two trials. The primary end point was the total number of RBC units transfused from start of treatment to 48 hours. Secondary end points included requirement for other transfusion products (FFP, platelets, and cryoprecipitates), mortality, days on the ventilator, and days in the intensive care unit. Safety outcomes included frequency and timing of adverse events, and changes in coagulation laboratory variables. In addition, the authors studied a composite end point of death and critical complications [multiple organ failure (MOF) and acute respiratory distress syndrome (ARDS)].

The study enrolled 301 trauma victims, mostly young, coagulopathic, acidotic, and hypothermic young males, from 32 centers in eight countries. Most penetrating trauma resulted from gunshot and stab wounds (68 and 30% of 134 subjects analyzed, respectively) while blunt trauma resulted from motor vehicle accidents (77% of 143 subjects analyzed). Baseline characteristics were similar in both groups when stratified for penetrating and blunt trauma.

When all patients are considered (intent-to-treat analysis), total RBC transfusions during the first 48 hours after first dose of trial drug were not different between placebo and treatment groups for the two trials. No significant differences were observed in either of the trauma population regarding the administration of hemostatic blood products. Mortality at 48 hours and 30 days was similar in both groups for the two trials. The composite end point of mortality, MOF, and ARDS was not different between placebo and treatment groups for the two trials.

In patients with penetrating trauma alive at 48 hours (subgroup analysis), transfusion of RBC was not different between groups (estimated reduction of 1.0 RBC unit with rFVIIa; $p = 0.10$). MT (>20 U of RBC) occurred in 19% of patients receiving placebo versus 7% of patients treated with rFVIIa ($p = 0.08$).

In patients with blunt trauma, a significant decrease in the number of RBC transfusions was observed in patients alive at 48 hours receiving rFVIIa (estimated reduction 2.6 RBC units; $p = 0.02$). MT occurred in 33% of patients receiving placebo versus 14% of patients treated with rFVIIa ($p = 0.03$).

Twelve thromboembolic events were reported and there was no difference between rFVIIa and placebo (six in each treatment group). Finally, rFVIIa did not increase the incidence of adverse events and showed a potential to reduce complications such as MOF and ARDS. In the penetrating trauma group, the incidence of MOF was 3% with rFVIIa versus 11% for placebo ($p = 0.09$); in the blunt trauma group, the incidence of ARDS was 4% with rFVIIa versus 16% for placebo ($p = 0.03$).

Overall, the results of these first randomized, placebo-controlled studies in severely injured trauma patients are disappointing. They suggest that rFVIIa may have the potential to reduce blood transfusion requirements and complications in this critically ill patient population. Unfortunately, a confirmatory study (ClinicalTrials.gov identifier NCT00184548) initiated in 2005 was terminated after enrolling 576 patients because a futility analysis conducted by the Data Monitoring Committee predicted a low likelihood of obtaining a positive trial outcome with the planned study population. Thus, today, the use of rFVIIa to control massive bleeding in trauma patients cannot be recommended.

Conclusions

The answer to our first objective ("Identify the causes of coagulopathy in massively transfused adult patients in order to determine the most appropriate transfusion/treatment strategies") is complex. The "classic" view that thrombocytopenia is responsible for the majority of bleeding complications in massively transfused patients should be abandoned. In view of the current literature, decreased levels of platelets and coagulation factors cannot be predicted by dilution alone. In the trauma patient, coagulopathy secondary to tissue injury and hypoxia often complicates the management of MT. As a result, it is often difficult to ascertain the exact cause of MVB. Coagulopathy associated with MT and surgery is an intricate, multicellular, and multifactorial event. While the interaction between platelets, fibrinogen, and red cells is particularly important, the contribution of anemia, fluid replacement therapy, hypothermia, and acidosis should not be overlooked.

The answer to our second objective ("Differentiate between the elective surgical setting and trauma, hypothesizing that recommendations derived from studies of MT in elective surgical patients may not apply in trauma patients") is clearer. In the elective surgical situation, tissue trauma is controlled, normovolemia can usually be maintained, tissue hypoxia is avoided and there is more time to monitor coagulation variables and anticipate deficits. In this context, coagulopathy is more often related to decreased coagulation factors and best treated initially with FFP. In trauma patients, tissue trauma is, by definition, uncontrolled, hypovolemia and tissue hypoxia are nearly always present, there is little or no time to monitor coagulation variables, and the precise pathological mechanisms responsible for the observed coagulopathy remain unclear. In the context of trauma, the aggressive management of these patients with RBC, FFP, and platelets in a 1:1:1 ratio appears to improve outcomes, but requires further confirmation with well-designed prospective trials.

Whether for elective surgery or for the management of trauma patients, reliable bedside monitors of hemostasis are needed urgently. By assisting clinicians in making the correct diagnosis in a timely manner, monitors will contribute to the optimal use of blood products.

Times have changed, blood products have changed, and so has the management of the bleeding patient. Therapy should take into account *all* the factors known to affect hemostasis in these patients. Ideally, transfusion of blood components should be based on appropriate hematological testing and initiated only in those patients who bleed actively. Nevertheless, a laboratory-based management of MVB may not always be possible in massively bleeding patients, especially in the context of trauma.

Finally, anesthesiologists tend to focus on hemorrhage and MT that occur as an immediate consequence of trauma or surgery. Yet, in the postoperative period, many of these patients will experience thrombotic complications related to the consumption of coagulation factors (especially antithrombin) associated with coagulopathy. Once the initial, hemorrhagic, phase of coagulopathy is controlled, efforts should be directed toward the prevention of later, potentially disastrous thrombotic complications. Only then will the management of coagulopathy associated with MT be complete.

References

1. Crosson JT. Massive transfusion. Clin Lab Med 1996;16(4):873–82.
2. Faringer PD, Mullins RJ, Johnson RL, Trunkey DD. Blood component supplementation during massive transfusion of AS-1 red cells in trauma patients. J Trauma 1993;34(4):481–5.
3. Murray DJ, Pennell BJ, Weinstein SL, Olson JD. Packed red cells in acute blood loss: dilutional coagulopathy as a cause of surgical bleeding. Anesth Analg 1995;80(2):336–42.
4. Reed RL, 2nd, Ciavarella D, Heimbach DM, et al. Prophylactic platelet administration during massive

transfusion. A prospective, randomized, double-blind clinical study. Ann Surg 1986;203(1):40–48.
5. Counts RB, Haisch C, Simon TL, Maxwell NG, Heimbach DM, Carrico CJ. Hemostasis in massively transfused trauma patients. Ann Surg 1979;190(1):91–9.
6. Hiippala S. Replacement of massive blood loss. Vox Sang 1998;74(Suppl. 2):399–407.
7. Simmons RL, Collins JA, Heisterkamp CA, Mills DE, Andren R, Phillips LL. Coagulation disorders in combat casualties. I. Acute changes after wounding. II. Effects of massive transfusion. 3. Post-resuscitative changes. Ann Surg 1969;169(4):455–82.
8. Leslie SD, Toy PT. Laboratory hemostatic abnormalities in massively transfused patients given red blood cells and crystalloid. Am J Clin Pathol 1991;96(6):770–73.
9. Stainsby D, MacLennan S, Hamilton PJ. Management of massive blood loss: a template guideline. Br J Anaesth 2000;85(3):487–91.
10. Guay J, Ozier Y, de Moerloose P, Samana CM, Belisle S, Hardy JF. Polytrauma and hemostatic anomalies. Can J Anaesth 1998;45(7):683–91.
11. Miller RD, Robbins TO, Tong MJ, Barton SL. Coagulation defects associated with massive blood transfusions. Ann Surg 1971;174(5):794–801.
12. Hiippala ST, Myllyla GJ, Vahtera EM. Hemostatic factors and replacement of major blood loss with plasma-poor red cell concentrates. Anesth Analg 1995;81(2):360–65.
13. Murray DJ, Olson J, Strauss R, Tinker JH. Coagulation changes during packed red cell replacement of major blood loss. Anesthesiology 1988;69:839–45.
14. Ciavarella D, Reed RL, Counts RB, et al. Clotting factor levels and the risk of diffuse microvascular bleeding in the massively transfused patient. Br J Haematol 1987;67(3):365–8.
15. Triplett DA. Coagulation and bleeding disorders: review and update. Clin Chem 2000;46(8 Pt 2):1260–69.
16. Fitzgerald DJ. Vascular biology of thrombosis: the role of platelet-vessel wall adhesion. Neurology 2001;57(5 Suppl. 2):S1–4.
17. Fuss C, Palmaz JC, Sprague EA. Fibrinogen: structure, function, and surface interactions. J Vasc Interv Radiol 2001;12(6):677–82.
18. Nurden AT, Nurden P. A review of the role of platelet membrane glycoproteins in the platelet-vessel wall interaction. Baillieres Clin Haematol 1993;6(3):653–90.
19. Calvete JJ. On the structure and function of platelet integrin alpha IIb beta 3, the fibrinogen receptor. Proc Soc Exp Biol Med 1995;208(4):346–60.
20. Hardy JF, De Moerloose P, Samama M. Massive transfusion and coagulopathy: pathophysiology and implications for clinical management. Can J Anaesth 2004;51(4):293–310.
21. Harke H, Rahman S. Haemostatic disorders in massive transfusion. Bibl Haematol 1980;46:179–88.
22. Harvey MP, Greenfield TP, Sugrue ME, Rosenfeld D. Massive blood transfusion in a tertiary referral hospital. Clinical outcomes and haemostatic complications [see comments]. Med J Aust 1995;163(7):356–9.
23. Cosgriff N, Moore EE, Sauaia A, Kenny-Moynihan M, Burch JM, Galloway B. Predicting life-threatening coagulopathy in the massively transfused trauma patient: hypothermia and acidoses revisited. J Trauma 1997;42(5):857–61.
24. Brohi K, Singh J, Heron M, Coats T. Acute traumatic coagulopathy. J Trauma 2003;54(6):1127–30.
25. Brohi K, Cohen MJ, Davenport RA. Acute coagulopathy of trauma: mechanism, identification and effect. Curr Opin Crit Care 2007;13(6):680–85.
26. Hulka F, Mullins RJ, Frank EH. Blunt brain injury activates the coagulation process. Arch Surg 1996;131(9):923–7.
27. Mannucci PM, Federici AB, Sirchia G. Hemostasis testing during massive blood replacement. A study of 172 cases. Vox Sang 1982;42(3):113–23.
28. Hewson JR, Neame PB, Kumar N, et al. Coagulopathy related to dilution and hypotension during massive transfusion. Crit Care Med 1985;13(5):387–91.
29. Escolar G, Garrido M, Mazzara R, Castillo R, Ordinas A. Experimental basis for the use of red cell transfusion in the management of anemic-thrombocytopenic patients. Transfusion 1988;28(5):406–11.
30. Livio M, Benigni A, Remuzzi G. Coagulation abnormalities in uremia. Semin Nephrol 1985;5(2):82–90.
31. Blajchman MA, Bordin JO, Bardossy L, Heddle NM. The contribution of the haematocrit to thrombocytopenic bleeding in experimental animals. Br J Haematol 1994 Feb; 86(2):347–50.
32. Small M, Lowe GD, Cameron E, Forbes CD. Contribution of the haematocrit to the bleeding time. Haemostasis 1983;13(6):379–84.
33. Ho CH. The hemostatic effect of packed red cell transfusion in patients with anemia. Transfusion 1998;38(11–12):1011–14.
34. Valeri CR, Cassidy G, Pivacek LE, et al. Anemia-induced increase in the bleeding time: implications

for treatment of nonsurgical blood loss. Transfusion 2001;41(8):977–83.

35. Khuri SF, Wolfe JA, Josa M, et al. Hematologic changes during and after cardiopulmonary bypass and their relationship to the bleeding time and nonsurgical blood loss. J Thorac Cardiovasc Surg 1992;104(1):94–107.
36. Valles J, Santos MT, Aznar J, et al. Erythrocytes metabolically enhance collagen-induced platelet responsiveness via increased thromboxane production, adenosine diphosphate release, and recruitment. Blood 1991;78(1):154–62.
37. Santos MT, Valles J, Marcus AJ, et al. Enhancement of platelet reactivity and modulation of eicosanoid production by intact erythrocytes. A new approach to platelet activation and recruitment. J Clin Invest 1991;87(2):571–80.
38. Valles J, Santos MT, Aznar J, et al. Platelet-erythrocyte interactions enhance alpha(IIb)beta(3) integrin receptor activation and P-selectin expression during platelet recruitment: down-regulation by aspirin ex vivo. Blood 2002;99(11):3978–84.
39. Valles J, Santos MT, Aznar J, Velert M, Barbera G, Carmena R. Modulatory effect of erythrocytes on the platelet reactivity to collagen in IDDM patients. Diabetes 1997;46(6):1047–53.
40. Valles J, Santos MT, Aznar J, et al. Erythrocyte promotion of platelet reactivity decreases the effectiveness of aspirin as an antithrombotic therapeutic modality: the effect of low-dose aspirin is less than optimal in patients with vascular disease due to prothrombotic effects of erythrocytes on platelet reactivity. Circulation 1998;97(4):350–55.
41. Santos MT, Valles J, Aznar J, Marcus AJ, Broekman MJ, Safier LB. Prothrombotic effects of erythrocytes on platelet reactivity. Reduction by aspirin [see comments]. Circulation 1997;95(1):63–8.
42. Ouaknine-Orlando B, Samama CM, Riou B, et al. Role of the hematocrit in a rabbit model of arterial thrombosis and bleeding. Anesthesiology 1999;90(5):1454–61.
43. Eberst ME, Berkowitz LR. Hemostasis in renal disease: pathophysiology and management. Am J Med 1994;96(2):168–79.
44. Tangelder GJ, Teirlinck HC, Slaaf DW, Reneman RS. Distribution of blood platelets flowing in arterioles. Am J Physiol 1985;248(3 Pt 2):H318–23.
45. Teirlinck HC, Tangelder GJ, Slaaf DW, Muijtjens AM, Arts T, Reneman RS. Orientation and diameter distribution of rabbit blood platelets flowing in small arterioles. Biorheology 1984;21(3):317–31.
46. Uijttewaal WS, Nijhof EJ, Bronkhorst PJ, Den Hartog E, Heethaar RM. Near-wall excess of platelets induced by lateral migration of erythrocytes in flowing blood. Am J Physiol 1993;264(4 Pt 2): H1239–44.
47. McLoughlin TM, Fontana JL, Alving B, Mongan PD, Bunger R. Profound normovolemic hemodilution: hemostatic effects in patients and in a porcine model. Anesth Analg 1996;83(3):459–65.
48. Friesen RH, Campbell DN, Clarke DR, Tornabene MA. Modified ultrafiltration attenuates dilutional coagulopathy in pediatric open heart operations. Ann Thorac Surg 1997;64(6):1787–9.
49. Naik SK, Knight A, Elliott M. A prospective randomized study of a modified technique of ultrafiltration during pediatric open-heart surgery. Circulation 1991;84(Suppl. 5):III422–31.
50. Segal JB, Blasco-Colmenares E, Norris EJ, Guallar E. Preoperative acute normovolemic hemodilution: a meta-analysis. Transfusion 2004;44(5): 632–44.
51. Ng KF, Lam CC, Chan LC. In vivo effect of haemodilution with saline on coagulation: a randomized controlled trial. Br J Anaesth 2002;88(4):475–80.
52. Ruttmann TG, James MF, Finlayson J. Effects on coagulation of intravenous crystalloid or colloid in patients undergoing peripheral vascular surgery. Br J Anaesth 2002;89(2):226–30.
53. Ruttmann TG. Haemodilution enhances coagulation. Br J Anaesth 2002;88(4):470–72.
54. Mortelmans YJ, Vermaut G, Verbruggen AM, et al. Effects of 6% hydroxyethyl starch and 3% modified fluid gelatin on intravascular volume and coagulation during intraoperative hemodilution. Anesth Analg 1995;81(6):1235–42.
55. Samama CM. Traumatic emergencies and hemostasis. Cah Anesthesiol 1995;43(5):479–82.
56. de Jonge E, Levi M, Berends F, Van Der Ende AE, ten Cate JW, Stoutenbeek CP. Impaired haemostasis by intravenous administration of a gelatin-based plasma expander in human subjects. Thromb Haemost 1998;79(2):286–90.
57. Mardel SN, Saunders FM, Allen H, et al. Reduced quality of clot formation with gelatin-based plasma substitutes. Br J Anaesth 1998;80(2):204–7.
58. Strauss RG. Review of the effects of hydroxyethyl starch on the blood coagulation system. Transfusion 1981;21(3):299–302.
59. Traylor RJ, Pearl RG. Crystalloid versus colloid versus colloid: all colloids are not created equal. Anesth Analg 1996;83(2):209–12.

60. de Jonge E, Levi M. Effects of different plasma substitutes on blood coagulation: a comparative review. Crit Care Med 2001;29(6):1261–7.
61. Boldt J, Muller M, Heesen M, Heyn O, Hempelmann G. Influence of different volume therapies on platelet function in the critically ill. Intensive Care Med 1996;22(10):1075–81.
62. Boldt J, Haisch G, Suttner S, Kumle B, Schellhaass A. Effects of a new modified, balanced hydroxyethyl starch preparation (Hextend) on measures of coagulation. Br J Anaesth 2002;89(5):722–8.
63. Strauss RG, Pennell BJ, Stump DC. A randomized, blinded trial comparing the hemostatic effects of pentastarch versus hetastarch. Transfusion 2002;42(1):27–36.
64. Langeron O, Doelberg M, Ang ET, Bonnet F, Capdevila X, Coriat P. Voluven, a lower substituted novel hydroxyethyl starch (HES 130/0.4), causes fewer effects on coagulation in major orthopedic surgery than HES 200/0.5. Anesth Analg 2001;92(4):855–62.
65. Innerhofer P, Fries D, Margreiter J, et al. The effects of perioperatively administered colloids and crystalloids on primary platelet-mediated hemostasis and clot formation. Anesth Analg 2002;95(4):858–65.
66. Knutson JE, Deering JA, Hall FW, et al. Does intraoperative hetastarch administration increase blood loss and transfusion requirements after cardiac surgery? Anesth Analg 2000;90(4):801–7.
67. Gan TJ, Bennett-Guerrero E, Phillips-Bute B, et al. Hextend, a physiologically balanced plasma expander for large volume use in major surgery: a randomized phase III clinical trial. Hextend Study Group. Anesth Analg 1999;88(5):992–8.
68. Haynes GR, Bailey MK. Excessive use of hetastarch: An iatrogenic cause of bleeding and hypocalcemia? Anesth Analg 2000;90(6):1455–6.
69. Kozek-Langenecker SA, Jungheinrich C, Sauermann W, Van Der Linden P. The effects of hydroxyethyl starch 130/0.4 (6%) on blood loss and use of blood products in major surgery: a pooled analysis of randomized clinical trials. Anesth Analg 2008;107(2):382–90.
70. American College of Surgeons. *Advanced Trauma Life Support Course Manual.* American College of Surgeons, Chicago, Illinois, 1997, pp. 103–12.
71. Yoshihara H, Yamamoto T, Mihara H. Changes in coagulation and fibrinolysis occurring in dogs during hypothermia. Thromb Res 1985;37:503–12.
72. Pina-Cabral JM, Ribeiro-da-Silva A, Almeida-Dias A. Platelet sequestration during hypothermia in dogs treated with sulphinpyrazone and ticlopidine – reversibility accelerated after intra-abdominal rewarming. Thromb Haemost 1985;54:838–41.
73. Oung CM, Li MS, Shum-Tim D, Chiu RCJ, Hinchey EJ. In vivo study of bleeding time and arterial hemorrhage in hypothermic versus normothermic animals. J Trauma 1993;35:251–4.
74. Valeri CR, Feingold H, Cassidy G, Ragno G, Khuri SF, Altschule MD. Hypothermia-induced reversible platelet dysfunction. Ann Surg 1987;205: 175–81.
75. Valeri CR, Khabbaz K, Khuri SF, et al. Effect of skin temperature on platelet function in patients undergoing extracorporeal bypass. J Thorac Cardiovasc Surg 1992;104:108–16.
76. Michelson AD, MacGregor H, Barnard MR, Kestin AS, Rohrer MJ, Valeri CR. Reversible inhibition of human platelet activation by hypothermia in vivo and in vitro. Thromb Haemost 1994;71:633–40.
77. Rohrer MJ, Natale AM. Effect of hypothermia on the coagulation cascade. Crit Care Med 1992;20:1402–5.
78. Reed RL, 2nd, Johnson TD, Hudson JD, Fischer RP. The disparity between hypothermic coagulopathy and clotting studies. J Trauma 1992;33(3): 465–70.
79. Douning LK, Ramsay MA, Swygert TH, et al. Temperature corrected thrombelastography in hypothermic patients. Anesth Analg 1995;81(3): 608–11.
80. Ferrara A, MacArthur JD, Wright HK, Modlin IM, McMillen MA. Hypothermia and acidosis worsen coagulopathy in the patient requiring massive transfusion. Am J Surg 1990;160(5):515–18.
81. Harrigan C, Lucas CE, Ledgerwood AM, Mammen EF. Primary hemostasis after massive transfusion for injury. Am Surg 1982;48(8):393–6.
82. Harrigan C, Lucas CE, Ledgerwood AM, Walz DA, Mammen EF. Serial changes in primary hemostasis after massive transfusion. Surgery 1985;98(4): 836–44.
83. Rodgers RP, Levin J. A critical reappraisal of the bleeding time. Semin Thromb Hemost 1990;16(1): 1–20.
84. Samama CM, Quezada R, Riou B, et al. Intraoperative measurement of activated partial thromboplastin time and prothrombin time with a new compact monitor. Acta Anaesthesiol Scand 1994;38(3): 232–7.
85. Lucas CE, Ledgerwood AM. Clinical significance of altered coagulation tests after massive transfusion for trauma. Am Surg 1981;47(3):125–30.

86. Turi DC, Peerschke EI. Sensitivity of three activated partial thromboplastin time reagents to coagulation factor deficiencies. Am J Clin Pathol 1986;85(1): 43–9.
87. Tuman KJ, Spiess BD, McCarthy RJ, Ivankovich AD. Effects of progressive blood loss on coagulation as measured by thrombelastography. Anesth Analg 1987;66(9):856–63.
88. Cammerer U, Dietrich W, Rampf T, Braun SL, Richter JA. The predictive value of modified computerized thromboelastography and platelet function analysis for postoperative blood loss in routine cardiac surgery. Anesth Analg 2003;96(1):51–7.
89. Johansson PI, Bochsen L, Stensballe J, Secher NH. Transfusion packages for massively bleeding patients: the effect on clot formation and stability as evaluated by Thrombelastograph (TEG). Transfus Apheresis Sci 2008;39(1):3–8.
90. Forestier F, Coiffic A, Mouton C, Ekouevi D, Chene G, Janvier G. Platelet function point-of-care tests in post-bypass cardiac surgery: are they relevant? Br J Anaesth 2002;89(5):715–21.
91. Lasne D, Fiemeyer A, Chatellier G, Chammas C, Baron JF, Aiach M. A study of platelet functions with a new analyzer using high shear stress (PFA 100) in patients undergoing coronary artery bypass graft. Thromb Haemost 2000;84(5):794–9.
92. Blumberg N, Laczin J, McMican A, Heal J, Arvan D. A critical survey of fresh-frozen plasma use. Transfusion 1986;26(6):511–13.
93. Guideline for the use of fresh-frozen plasma. Medical Directors Advisory Committee, National Blood Transfusion Council. S Afr Med J 1998;88(10): 1344–7.
94. Erber WN. Massive blood transfusion in the elective surgical setting. Transfus Apheresis Sci 2002;27(1):83–92.
95. Schmied H, Kurz A, Sessler DI, Kozek S, Reiter A. Mild hypothermia increases blood loss and transfusion requirements during total hip arthroplasty. Lancet 1996;347(8997):289–92.
96. Cinat ME, Wallace WC, Nastanski F, et al. Improved survival following massive transfusion in patients who have undergone trauma. Arch Surg 1999;134(9):964–8.
97. Duchesne JC, Hunt JP, Wahl G, et al. Review of current blood transfusions strategies in a mature level I trauma center: were we wrong for the last 60 years? J Trauma 2008;65(2):272–6; discussion 6–8.
98. Gonzalez EA, Moore FA, Holcomb JB, et al. Fresh frozen plasma should be given earlier to patients requiring massive transfusion. J Trauma 2007;62(1): 112–9.
99. Kashuk JL, Moore EE, Johnson JL, et al. Postinjury life threatening coagulopathy: is 1:1 fresh frozen plasma:packed red blood cells the answer? J Trauma 2008;65(2):261–70; discussion 70–71.
100. Sperry JL, Ochoa JB, Gunn SR, et al. An FFP:PRBC transfusion ratio $\geq$ 1:1.5 is associated with a lower risk of mortality after massive transfusion. J Trauma 2008;65(5):986–93.
101. Stinger HK, Spinella PC, Perkins JG, et al. The ratio of fibrinogen to red cells transfused affects survival in casualties receiving massive transfusions at an army combat support hospital. J Trauma 2008;64(Suppl. 2):S79–85; discussion S.
102. Holcomb JB, Wade CE, Michalek JE, et al. Increased plasma and platelet to red blood cell ratios improves outcome in 466 massively transfused civilian trauma patients. Ann Surg 2008;248(3):447–58.
103. Moore FA, Nelson T, McKinley BA, et al. Is there a role for aggressive use of fresh frozen plasma in massive transfusion of civilian trauma patients? Am J Surg 2008;196(6):948–58; discussion 58–60.
104. Maegele M, Lefering R, Paffrath T, Tjardes T, Simanski C, Bouillon B. Red-blood-cell to plasma ratios transfused during massive transfusion are associated with mortality in severe multiple injury: a retrospective analysis from the Trauma Registry of the Deutsche Gesellschaft fur Unfallchirurgie. Vox Sang 2008;95(2):112–19.
105. Scalea TM, Bochicchio KM, Lumpkins K, et al. Early aggressive use of fresh frozen plasma does not improve outcome in critically injured trauma patients. Ann Surg 2008;248(4):578–84.
106. Boffard KD, Riou B, Warren B, et al. Recombinant factor VIIa as adjunctive therapy for bleeding control in severely injured trauma patients: two parallel randomized, placebo-controlled, double-blind clinical trials. J Trauma 2005;59(1):8–15; discussion-8.

PART 7

Alternatives to Allogeneic Blood Transfusion

SECTION 1
Pharmaceutical Approaches

CHAPTER 27

Iron Deficiency: Causes, Diagnosis, and Management

Manuel Muñoz[1], *José Antonio García-Erce*[2] *& Elvira Bisbe*[3]
[1]GIEMSA, Transfusion Medicine, University of Málaga, Málaga, Spain
[2]Department of Hematology, University Hospital Miguel Servet, Zaragoza, Spain
[3]Department of Anesthesiology, University Hospital Mar-Esperanza, Barcelona, Spain

Introduction

Iron deficiency in the developing world is frequent and is mainly the result of poor nutrition. In the developed world, iron deficiency has been reported to be in 5% of the general population. The frequency of anemia in the older people is of the order of 10% and is the result of iron deficiency due to chronic blood loss from gastrointestinal lesions, but also chronic inflammatory diseases and decreased renal function leading to functional iron deficiency (FID) (1). It is this population that often presents for elective surgical procedures with preoperative anemia or even with iron deficiency without anemia (2, 3). At the time of preoperative assessment, one study evaluated the prevalence of anemia and iron deficiency in 715 patients scheduled for major elective orthopedic surgery. According to WHO criteria, the prevalence of anemia was 10.5% (65/715), and it increased with age, with no gender-related difference. Prevalence of iron deficiency was 30% in anemic patients and 18% in nonanemic patients (3). In this regard, it is important to investigate the cause of iron deficiency, which is frequently due to gastrointestinal blood losses (e.g., chronic NSAID intake or colon adenocarcinoma) (4). In fact, iron deficiency is found in approximately 50% of the patients scheduled for colon adenocarcinoma resection (5). In addition, preoperative anemia is one of the major predictive factors for perioperative blood transfusion in surgical procedures with moderate–high perioperative blood loss (6–8). Thus, timely diagnosis of iron deficiency preoperatively has dual benefits. It decreases the need for perioperative blood transfusions and decreases morbidity and mortality in these patients. Perioperative stimulation of erythropoiesis with the administration of iron with or without erythropoiesis stimulating agents may correct the anemia.

Therefore, according to a recent NATA guideline, whenever clinically feasible, patients undergoing elective surgery with a high risk of severe postoperative anemia should have hemoglobin (Hb) level and iron status tested a minimum of 30 days before the scheduled surgical procedure (9). For patients older than 60 years, vitamin B12 and folic acid should also be measured (9, 10). In this chapter we will focus on the iron homeostasis in humans, the diagnosis of iron deficiency, and the efficacy and safety of iron administration for the treatment of anemic patients in different clinical contexts.

Iron homeostasis

Most of the iron in the body is distributed within red blood cell hemoglobin (70%). Approximately 10% is present in muscle fibers (in myoglobin) and other tissues (in enzymes and cytochromes). The remaining body iron is stored in the liver

Alternatives to Blood Transfusion in Transfusion Medicine, 2nd edition. Edited by A. Maniatis, P. Van der Linden, J.-F. Hardy.

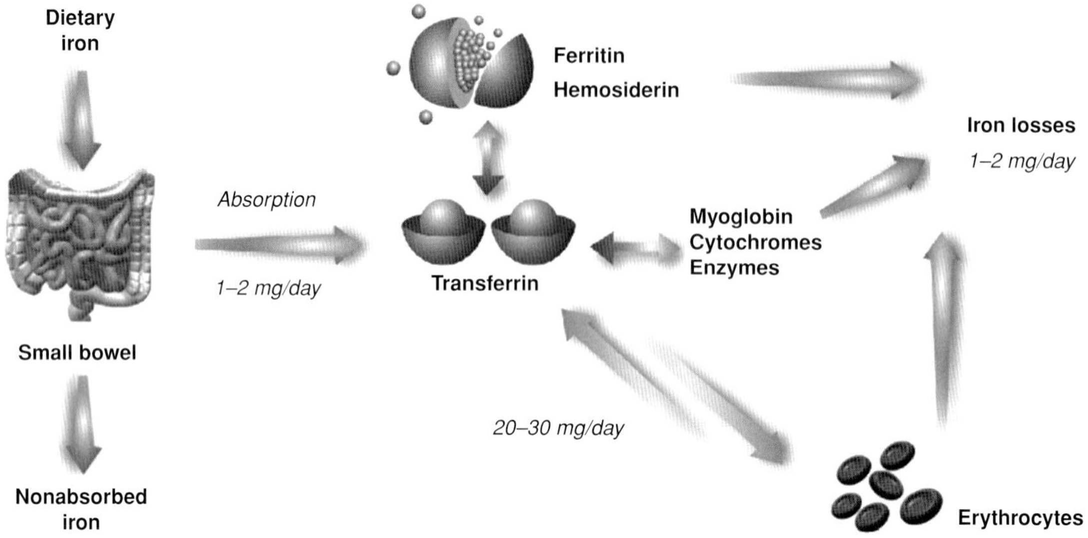

Figure 27.1 Iron turn-over under physiological conditions. Modified from Muñoz et al. [12].

and macrophages of the reticuloendothelial system (RES). The body absorbs 1–2 mg of dietary iron a day and this is balanced with losses via sloughed intestinal mucosal cells, menstruation, and other blood losses. Therefore, internal turnover of iron is essential to meet the bone marrow requirements for erythropoiesis (20–30 mg/day, and up to 50 mg/day during recovery from bleeding or treatment with erythropoiesis stimulating agents) (Figure 27.1) (11, 12). On the other hand, the body has no effective means of excreting iron and thus the regulation of absorption of dietary iron from the duodenum plays a critical role in iron homeostasis in the body (13). This is extremely important as iron is essential for cellular metabolism and aerobic respiration, while cellular iron overload leads to toxicity and cell death via free radical formation and lipid peroxidation and thus, iron homeostasis requires tight regulation (11).

Iron absorption

Nearly all absorption of dietary iron occurs at the apical surface of duodenal enterocytes via different mechanisms (Figure 27.2). Dietary nonhem iron primarily exists in an oxidized (Fe^{3+}) form that is not bioavailable and must first be reduced to the Fe^{2+} form before it is transported across the intestinal epithelium cell by a transporter called *divalent metal transporter 1* (DMT1), which also traffics other metal ions such as zinc, copper, and cobalt by a proton coupled mechanism. Hem iron is absorbed into the enterocyte by a different, as yet unidentified, *hem receptor*. Once internalized in the enterocyte, iron is released from hem by hem oxygenase and then either stored or transported out of the enterocyte across the basolateral membrane via mechanisms similar to that of ionic iron (14, 15). *Ferroportin 1* (Ireg1) is the only putative iron exporter identified to date. Ferrous iron once exported across the basal membrane by Ireg1, is then oxidized by a multi-copper oxidase protein called *hefastin* (similar to plasma ceruloplasmin) before being bound by plasma *transferrin*. Ferroportin1 is also the putative iron exporter in macrophages and hepatocytes (Figure 27.2) (13, 16).

Iron distribution

Iron released into the circulation binds to *transferrin* and is transported to sites of use and storage (Figure 27.2). Transferrin has two binding sites binding one iron atom each. About 30–40% of these sites are occupied in normal physiological conditions. Transferrin-bound iron (TBI) enters target cells—mainly erythroid cells, but also immune and

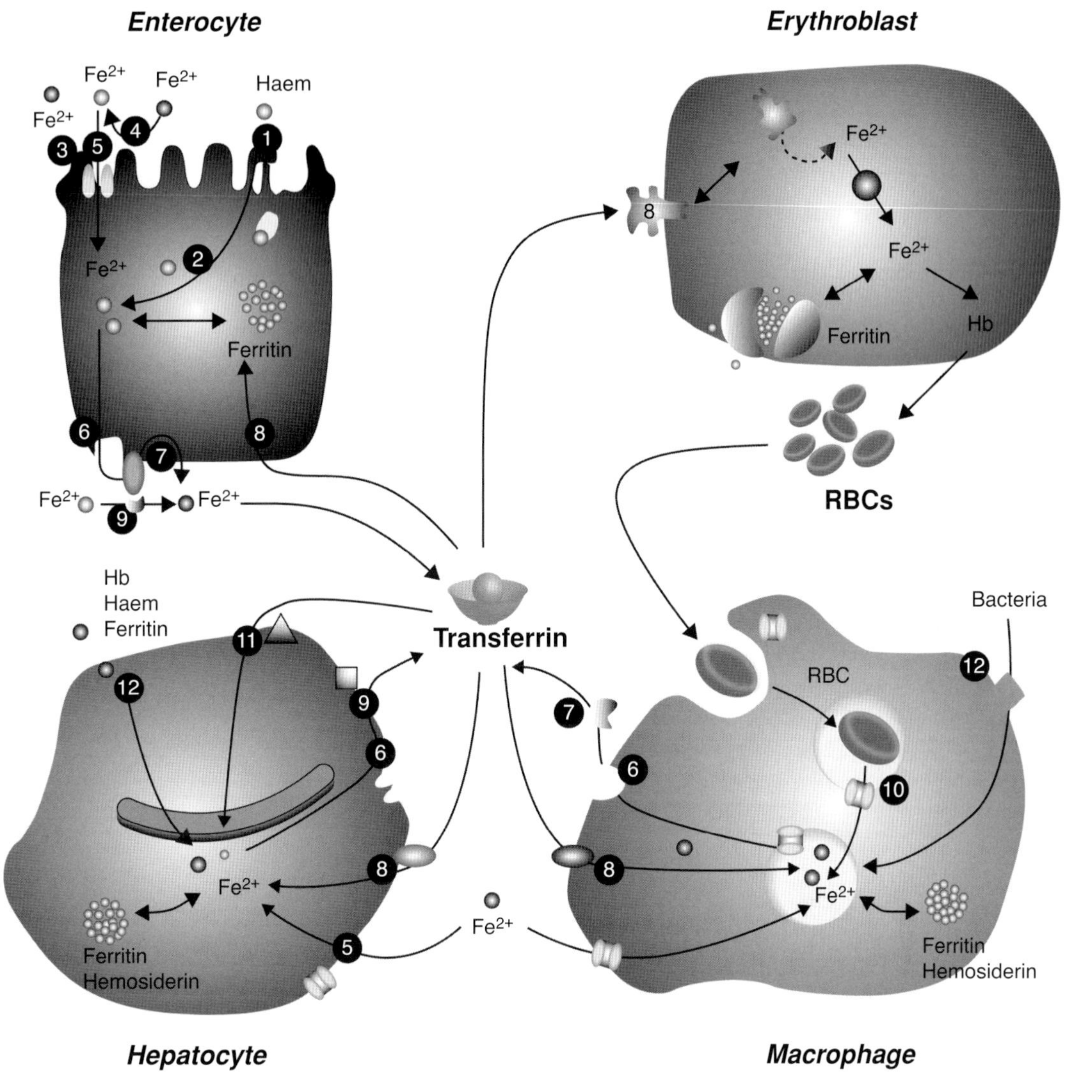

Figure 27.2 Mean pathways of iron homeostasis Modified from Muñoz et al. [12]. Keys: 1. Hem receptor; 2. Hem oxygenase; 3. Mobilferrin-β_3-integrin complex; 4. Ferrireductase; 5. Divalent metal transporter (DMT-1); 6. Ferroportin 1; 7. Hefastin; 8. Transferrin receptor-1 (TfR1); 9. Ceruloplasmin; 10. Natural resistance macrophage protein (Nramp-2); 11. Transferrin receptor-2 (TfR2); 12. Others: bacteria, lactoferrin, Hb-haptoglobin, Hem-haemopexin, Hb, hem, ferritin, etc.

hepatic cells—through the interaction of transferrin with specific surface receptors (Transferrin receptor 1, TfR1) and endocytosis of the transferrin–receptor complex. Production of Hb by the erythron accounts for most iron use. High-level expression of TfR1 in erythroid precursors ensures the uptake of iron into this compartment.

A truncated form of the transferrin receptor can be detected in human serum. The serum concentration of this *soluble form of transferrin receptor* (sTfR; normal median concentration: 1.2–3.0 mg/dL, depending on the assessment kit used) is proportional to the total amount of surface transferrin receptor. Increased sTfR concentrations indicate iron deficiency even during the anemia of chronic disease (ACD), as well as increased erythropoietic activity without iron deficiency (17, 18).

Iron storage

As stated above, Hb iron has substantial turnover, as senescent erythrocytes undergo phagocytosis by RES macrophages (Figure 27.2). Iron export from macrophages is accomplished primarily by ferroportin 1, the same iron-export protein expressed in the duodenal enterocyte (12–16). The liver is the main storage organ for iron, where it is sequestered predominantly in the form of ferritin or hemosiderin. The uptake of TBI by the liver from plasma is mediated by TfR1 and TfR2.

As transferrin becomes saturated in iron overload states, excess iron is also found as nontransferrin-bound iron (NTBI), which is transported across the hepatocyte membrane via a carrier-mediated process consistent with DMT1. Besides the blood erythrocyte mass, the hepatocyte may also store iron from ferritin, hemoglobin–haptoglobin complexes, and hem–hemopexin complexes. In contrast, once again, ferroportin 1 is likely to be the only protein mediating the transport of iron out of hepatocytes, which is then oxidized by ceruloplasmin and bound to transferrin (12–16).

Regulation

The absorption of iron is dependent on the body's iron stores, hypoxia, and rate of erythropoiesis, and is mainly regulated by hepcidin. Liver *hepcidin* is a 25 amino acid cysteine rich peptide with antimicrobial properties, which is regulated by a number of factors such as liver iron levels, inflammation, hypoxia, and anemia The *hepcidin model* proposes that hepcidin is secreted into the blood and interacts with villous enterocytes to regulate the rate of iron absorption by controlling the expression of ferroportin at their basolateral membranes. Hepcidin binds to cell-surface ferroportin, triggering its phosphorylation, internalization, and ubiquitin-mediated degradation in lysosomes. By removing ferroportin from plasma membrane, hepcidin shuts off cellular iron export (18). Ferroportin molecules present in macrophages and liver is also target for hepcidin.

Thus it is hypothesized that when hepcidin levels are increased in noncongenital iron overload (by the uptake of transferrin bound iron via TfR1/HFE and TfR2) or inflammation (via IL-6), iron release from intestinal crypt cells, liver, and macrophages is reduced. In contrast, when hepcidin levels are reduced, as in iron deficiency, anemia, or hypoxia, it is likely that Ireg1 expression and iron release from intestinal cells, liver, and RES cells are increased (14, 15).

In the erythroid precursors, the expression of TfR1, DMT-1, and ferritin are reciprocally regulated through iron-responding proteins (IRP)1 and IRP2, which act on the iron-responding elements (IRE) present in their RNA. Thus, when an increased iron uptake is needed, the expression of TfR1 and DMT-1 is increased, whereas the synthesis of ferritin is halted (19). In addition, there is evidence that erythropoietin (EPO) activates IRP-1, leading to an upregulation of TfR1 expression in the erythroid precursors which is maintained along the differentiation process (13). There are also data indicating that EPO may downregulated DMT-1 and upregulate ferroportin in macrophages, thus increasing iron supply to the bone marrow (20).

In iron overload, TfR1 is downregulated in hepatocytes, whereas TfR2 lacks an iron response element and thus is not reciprocally regulated in response to the level of plasma iron. Instead, TfR2 protein expression is regulated by transferrin saturation, and is upregulated in iron overload. In normal and iron loaded conditions, expression of TfR2 exceeds that of TfR1 suggesting that TfR2 plays an important role in hepatic iron loading in hemochromatosis (10).

Effects of inflammation on iron homeostasis

In addition to blood loss, hemolysis, hepatic or endocrine disorders, and nutritional deficiencies, iron homeostasis can be disturbed by inflammation (Figure 27.3). Activation of the immune and inflammatory system results in pathologic iron homeostasis due to increased DMT-1 (IFNγ; lipopolysaccharide, LPS) and TfR (IL-10) expression in macrophages, reduced Ireg-1 expression (IFNγ, LPS, and LPS- or IL-6-induced hepcidin) in enterocytes (inhibition

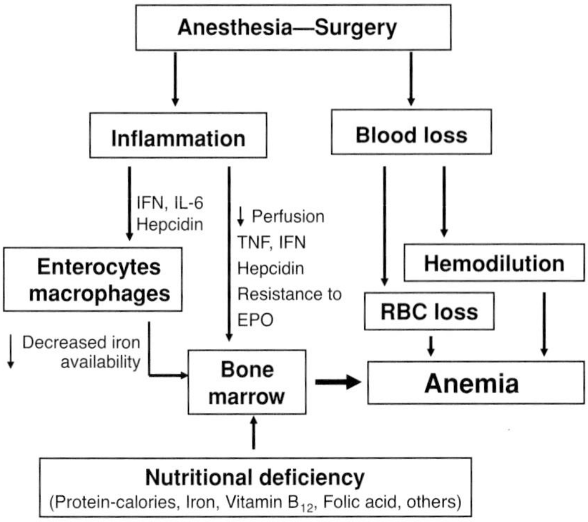

Figure 27.3 Main pathophysiological mechanisms involved in perioperative anemia.

of iron absorption) and macrophages (inhibition of iron recirculation), and increased ferritin synthesis (TNFα, IL-1β, IL-6, IL-10) (increased iron storage). All these lead to hypoferremia, iron-restricted erythropoiesis, and finally mild–moderate anemia (21–24).

Thus, at least three major immunity-driven mechanisms contribute to the development of *ACD*: (1) inflammation-induced disturbances of iron homeostasis (FID or decrease iron availability); (2) cytokines, like TNFα, IFNγ, and IL-1β exert a negative impact on the proliferation and differentiation of erythroid progenitor cells and can induce apoptosis; and (3) patients with ACD display a blunted secretion of endogenous EPO and an impaired response of erythroid progenitor cells to EPO (19).

However, the pathophysiology of *acute event-related anemia* (AERA, e.g., trauma, surgery) is somehow different. In this setting, inflammatory responses are mediated mainly by IL-6 and IL-8 (with transient contribution of TNFα and IL-1β in some visceral surgeries, such as colonic or cardiac procedures), whereas IFNγ plasma levels are undetectable or within the normal range (21–23). Therefore, in most of these conditions, the two major mechanisms leading to anemia are perioperative or traumatic blood loss and blunted erythropoiesis due to decreased iron availability, whereas EPO levels are normal or near-to-normal.

The anemia associated to chronic or acute inflammatory diseases is typically mild to moderate, and erythrocytes may not show any stigmata of iron deficiency. But the underlying iron etiology is evident: macrophages that normally recycle iron are found to sequester it, intestinal iron absorption is interrupted, and erythroid precursors respond very rapidly when iron-transferrin is made available, especially by the administration of intravenous (i.v.) iron preparations. In contrast, congenital, iron-refractory, iron-deficiency anemia (IRIDA), which is also caused by inappropriately high hepcidin expression, is associated with severe microcytosis whereas the ACD is typically normocytic. Therefore, it can be speculated that the normocytic RBCs result from the combination of iron insufficiency and an as-yet-unexplained tendency to macrocytocis (e.g., alterations in folates or B12 metabolism in response to inflammation) (13).

Diagnosis of iron deficiency

Iron deficiency without anemia

Normal Hb level does not exclude ID, because individual with normal body iron stores must lose a large portion of body iron before the Hb falls below the various laboratory definitions of anemia (24). Isolated or uncomplicated ID in the absence of other diseases that influence measurements of iron status is seen most often in infants and preschool children (because of rapid growth), in pregnant women (because of the iron demands of the fetus), and in patients with excessive uterine or gastrointestinal blood loss (24).

In nonanemic patients, the most important clinical clue of ID is the symptom of chronic fatigue. However, it is of little screening value because clinicians rarely consider the diagnosis of ID in patients who are not anemic, and therefore ID is invariably diagnosed in the laboratory (24). A normal Hb level with a mean corpuscular hemoglobin (MCH) in the lower limit of normality (28–35 pg) or an increased red cell distribution width (RDW) point to mild ID without anemia, but the main laboratory finding is a ferritin level <30 ng/mL in the absence of inflammation (normal serum concentrations of C-reactive protein [CRP]; <0.5 mg/dL).

On the other hand, nonanemic patients with a serum ferritin level <100 ng/mL (or ferritin 100–300 ng/mL and transferrin saturation <20%) undergoing surgical procedures with an expected blood loss >1500 mL (Hb drop of 3–5 g/dL) may be considered for preoperative oral or i.v. iron administration, depending on the presence of comorbidities and on the timescale before surgery, as they may not have enough stored iron to replenish their perioperative Hb loss and maintain normal iron stores (serum ferritin ≥30 ng/mL) (25).

Iron deficiency anemia

Patients should be considered to suffer from iron deficiency anemia (IDA) when they are presented with low Hb (men, <13 g/dL and women, <12 g/dL), TfS (<20%), and ferritin concentrations (<30 ng/mL) but no signs of inflammation (26) (Figure 27.4). The mean corpuscular haemoglobin (MCH) rather than mean corpuscular volume (MCV) became the most important red-cell marker for detecting IDE in circulating red blood cells. MCV is a reliable and widely available measurement but is a relatively late indicator in patients who are not actively bleeding. Thalassemia must be considered in the differential diagnosis of a low MCV, but the distinction between IDE and thalassemia is seldom difficult (24), although RDW may help with diagnosis. Gastrointestinal evaluation for potential malignancy or peptic ulcer is recommended for any patient with IDA, except possibly menstruating women or when the source of blood loss is readily apparent (27). Patients with IDA may benefit from oral or i.v. iron replacement therapy. If after a few weeks of iron therapy, a normal Hb level has not been attained, treatment with erythropoiesis stimulating agents (ESAs: epoetin, darbepoetin) might be considered (Figure 27.4).

Anemia of chronic disease

Patients should be considered to suffer from ACD when they have the following: (1) a chronic infection or inflammation, autoimmune disease, or malignancy (high CRP level); (2) a Hb concentration <13 g/dL for men and <12 g/dL for women; and (3) a low transferrin saturation (TfS < 20%), but normal or increased serum ferritin concentration (>100 ng/mL) or low serum ferritin concentration (30–100 ng/mL) and a sTfR/log ferritin ratio <1 (19, 28) (Figure 27.4). Measurement of reticulocyte counts, endogenous EPO secretion (ratio of

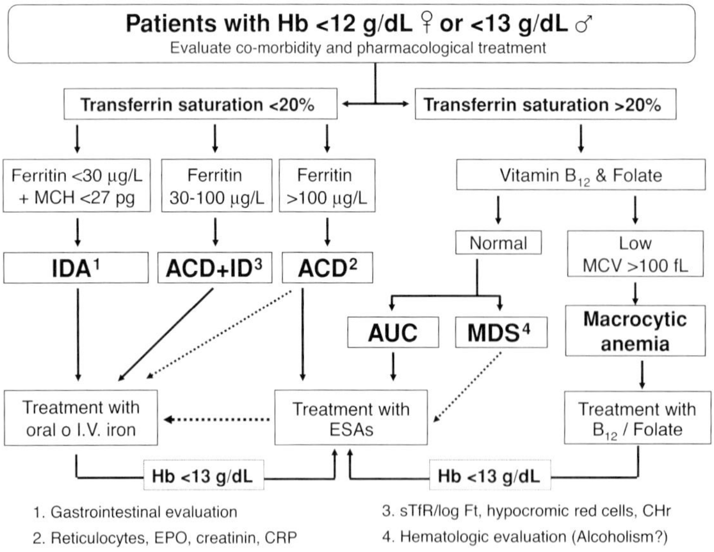

Figure 27.4 A simplified algorithm for anemia management. ACD, anemia of chronic disease; ACD + ID, ACD with true iron deficiency; AUC, anemia of unknown cause; CRP, C-reactive protein; CHr, reticulocyte hemoglobin content; EPO, erythropoietin; ESA, erythropoiesis stimulating agent; Ft, ferritin; Hb, hemoglobin; IDA, iron deficiency anemia; MCV, mean corpuscular volume; MCH, mean corpuscular hemoglobin; MDS, myelodysplastic syndrome; sTfR, serum transferrin receptor.

observed EPO to expected EPO) (29), and serum creatinin (glomerular filtration), will be helpful in defining the cause of ACD. Although patients with ACD benefit from treatment with ESAs, some of them respond to i.v. iron. Nevertheless, i.v. iron replacement therapy should always be considered in patients receiving ESAs (Figure 27.4).

ACD with true iron deficiency

Patients should be considered to have ACD with true iron deficiency (ACD + ID) when they have the following: (1) a chronic infection or inflammation, autoimmune disease, or malignancy (high CRP level); (2) a Hb concentration <13 g/dL for men and <12 g/dL for women; and (3) low transferrin saturation (TfS < 20%), a serum ferritin concentration <100 ng/mL and a sTfR/log ferritin ratio >2 (19, 28) (Figure 27.4). There are two important hematologic indices that may also help in the diagnosis of ID in ATC: reticulocyte hemoglobin content (CHr) and hypochromic red blood cells (HYPO). In nonferropenic patients, the 2.5 percentile values were 28 pg for CHr and 5% for HYPO (15). However, these hematologic indices are only available in specific hematology analyzers. The Advia 120 hematology analyzer determined CHr and erythrocyte hemoglobin content (CH; ≥ 27 pg), whereas the Sysmex XE-2100 hematology analyzer determines RET-Y, which can be considered as the reticulocyte hemoglobin equivalent (RET-He), as well as RBC-Y, which can be considered as the erythrocyte hemoglobin equivalent (30, 31). These hematologic indices (CHr, CH, and HYPO) are direct indicators of FID in contrast to the majority of biochemical markers, which measure FID indirectly via iron-deficient erythropoiesis and demonstrate weaknesses in the diagnosis of functional ID as defined by hematologic indices (15). Although patients with ACD + ID benefit from treatment with ESAs, most of them may initially respond to i.v. iron or even oral iron (26) (Figure 27.4).

Noniron deficiency anemia

As shown in Figure 27.4, in patients presenting with anemia and TfS >20%, vitamin B12 and folate levels should be investigated. If low and accompanied of a MCV >100 fL, macrocytic anemia should be suspected and the patient should be referred to the hematologist for further evaluation. However, up to one third of older patients may present with vitamin B12 or folate deficiency and without macrocytosis, especially when coexisting ID. Nevertheless, when vitamin B12 or folate levels are normal, the diagnosis of a myelodisplastic syndrome (MDS) or an anemia of unknown cause (AUC) should be considered and patient should be referred to the hematologist for further evaluation. In this regard, it has been recently reported that both AUC and B12/folate deficiency anemia in elderly patients are characterized by low levels of inflammatory markers (CRP) and low endogenous EPO secretion (32). Therefore, patients with AUC and those with B12/folate deficiency not responding to vitamin supplementation might benefit from treatment with ESAs (Figure 27.4). Two important considerations should be taken: first, after starting with the specific treatment (intramuscular [i.m.] or high oral dose), patients with vitamin B12 deficiency should receive oral iron to avoid iron-restricted erythropoiesis; second, no older patient should receive folic acid without vitamin B12 (unless vitamin B12 deficiency has been ruled out) to avoid further complications as transverse myelitis.

Iron therapy

When body iron stores are depleted, iron supplementation seems beneficial, although the optimal route of administration remains a controversial. Oral iron supplementation is adequate in some clinical conditions. Administration of oral iron, in the absence of inflammation or significant ongoing blood loss, can correct the anemia, provided significant doses (200 mg) can be tolerated. However, although conventional wisdom "says" that up to 200 mg of elemental iron per day is required to correct IDA, this is probably incorrect. As a maximum of 10 mg of iron can be absorbed per day, higher doses are questionable. Early studies indicated that the coadministration of iron with ascorbic acid (vitamin C) might be of benefit in enhancing iron absorption, since, in theory, more ferrous iron is maintained in solution. However, reports indicated that such coadministration could induce severe toxicity in the gastrointestinal tract. Moreover, intake independent of meals is recommended for increasing iron absorption but increases digestive intolerance and, therefore, decreases compliance. The absorption of oral iron can be diminished by coadministration of tretracyclines, proton pump inhibitor and anti-acid medication, phytates (high fiber diets), calcium, and phenolic compounds (coffee, tea).

On the other hand, nonabsorbed iron salts may produce a variety of highly reactive oxygen species including hypochlorous acid, superoxides, and peroxides that may lead to digestive intolerance, causing nausea, flatulence, abdominal pain, diarrhea or constipation, and black or tarry stools, and perhaps could activate relapsed inflammatory bowel disease (IBD). To avoid the risk of poisoning, other compounds (such as iron polymaltose, which has very low toxicity and meets the requirements for a food supplement) might be used instead of ferrous salt preparations. In addition, lower doses of iron compounds (e.g., 50–100 mg of elemental iron) should be recommended, especially in patients with IBD (33).

Total iron deficit (TID) can be calculated using the Ganzoni's formula: TID (mg) = Weight (kg) × [Ideal Hb − Actual Hb] (g/dL) × 0.24 + depot iron (500 mg). According to this formula, a person weighing 70 kg with an Hb level of 9 g/dL would have a body iron deficit of about 1400 mg (34). Following the administration of oral iron in the preoperative period, it takes 2–2.5 weeks for the Hb to start rising, 2 months for it to return to normal levels, and 6 months for iron stores to be repleted (35). Although preoperative oral iron plus a restrictive transfusion protocol reduces transfusion requirements in patients scheduled for knee arthroplasty (36) or colorectal cancer resection (37), in ACD (e.g., rheumatoid arthritis, Crohn's disease, chronic renal or heart failure, cancer, etc.), as well as in that associated with acute inflammation (e.g., trauma, postoperative period, etc.), the utility of oral iron administration is rather limited, since absorption is downregulated, and the small amount of iron absorbed is directed to the RES, where it is sequestered. Currently available evidence does not support the efficacy of postoperative oral iron supplementation: in five randomized controlled trials (RCTs) (four after orthopedic surgery and one after cardiac surgery), postoperative administration of oral iron failed to increase hemoglobin levels (9).

In these situations, i.v. iron has emerged as a safe and effective alternative for perioperative anemia management. This takes into consideration factors such as intolerance of or contraindications to oral iron, short time to surgery, severe preoperative anemia (especially if accompanied by significant ongoing bleeding), or the use of erythropoiesis-stimulating agents (9). As i.v. iron can allow up to a fivefold erythropoietic response to significant blood-loss anemia in normal individuals (38), Hb starts rising in a few days, the percentage of responding patients is higher and iron stores are repleted. Boosting iron stores is an advantage, particularly for patients receiving ESAs (34).

Intravenous iron agents

All i.v. iron agents are colloids with spheroidal iron–carbohydrate nanoparticles. Each particle consists of an iron-oxyhydroxide core (Fe [III]) and a carbohydrate shell that stabilizes the iron-oxyhydroxide core. Differences in core size and carbohydrate chemistry determine pharmacological and biologic differences between the different iron complexes, including clearance after injection, iron release in vitro, early evidence of iron bioactivity in vivo, and maximum tolerated dose and rate of infusion (39, 40). Complexes can generally be classified as labile or robust (kinetic variability), and as week or strong (thermodynamic variability), with all possible intermediates. Four different products are principally used in clinical practice: iron gluconate, iron sucrose, iron dextran, and iron polycarboxymaltose (41–43) (Table 27.1).

Iron gluconate, which has a core tightly bound to gluconate and weakly associated with sucrose (molecular weight 38 kD), is a type III iron complex (labile and weak) with fast degradation kinetics and direct release to plasma proteins (apotransferrin, apoferritin, and others). The potential for acute adverse reactions related to labile iron release after i.v. injection, which is caused by oversaturation of the transferrin binding capacity, is higher with iron

Table 27.1 Some characteristics of the different intravenous iron formulations.

	Iron gluconate	Iron sucrose	Iron dextran (LMWID)	Ferric carboxymaltose
Preparations	Ferrlecit®	Venofer®	Cosmofer® InFeD®	Ferinject® Injectafer®
Complex type	Type III Labile and weak	Type II Semi-robust and moderately strong	Type I Robust and strong	Type I Robust and strong
Molecular weight (kD)	38	43	73	150
Initial distribution volume (L)	6	3.4	3.5	3.5
Plasma half-life (hours)	1	6	30	16
Labile iron release	+++	±*	—	—
Direct iron donation to transferrin (% injected dose)	5–6	4–5	1–2	1–2
Test dose required	No	No	Yes	No
Maximal single dose (mg)	125	300	TDI	1000
Premedication	No	No	TDI only	No
Life-threatening ADE† ($\times 10^6$ doses)	0.9	0.6	11.3	??
Death rate ($\times 10^6$ doses)†	0.25	0.11	0.78	??

ADE, adverse drug events; LMWID, low molecular weight iron dextran; TDI, total dose infusion.
*If the infusion speed >4 mg Fe^{3+}/min or dose >7 mg Fe^{3+}/kg.
†Data from patients with chronic kidney disease.

gluconate compared to the other available i.v. iron preparations. Nontransferrin bound labile iron may induce acute endothelial cell injury and a transient capillary leak syndrome. Clinical symptoms of iron acute toxicity include nausea, hypotension, tachycardia, chest pain, dyspnea (lung edema), and bilateral edema of the hands and feet, and should not be misread as anaphylaxis (39). To avoid these side effects, maximum recommended dose is 125 mg, whereas the administration of total dose is not recommended. The use of iron gluconate for iron deficiency in patients on dialysis has been found to be efficacious and safe (39, 40).

Iron sucrose, which has a core tightly bound to sucrose (molecular weight 43 kDa), is a partially stable type with medium degradation kinetics and partial uptake of released iron by plasma proteins such as (apo)-transferrin but also by the RES (Type II: semirobust and moderately strong). Its half-life is relatively short (5–6 hours) and the amount of iron transported by transferrin, calculated using the Michaelis–Menten model for a single dose containing 100 mg of iron, is around 30 mg Fe/24 hours (44). Following a single i.v. injection of 100 mg iron sucrose administered to anemic patients, up to 95% of the injected iron was utilized within 2–4 weeks. During the last few years, experience of using iron sucrose in various forms of ID has evolved. Single dose of 100–200 mg as an i.v. injection (45) or up to 500 mg over an infusion time of 3.5 hours seems to be safe (46). The maximal recommended dosage is 600 mg/week (200 mg iron as iron sucrose injected or infused intravenously no more than 3 times a week) but this amount exceeds the physiological needs of the proliferating erythroblast. If the infusion speed is too fast (above 4 mg Fe^{3+}/minute) or the single total iron dose too high (above 7 mg Fe^{3+}/kg, with a maximum of 500 mg), nontransferrin bound labile iron may cause transient hypotension, tachycardia, and dyspnea, as described for iron gluconate. Overall, iron sucrose is currently considered as the safest i.v. iron preparation (47).

Low molecular weight iron dextran (LMWID) is a stable parenteral iron product with a molecular weight of 73 kDa. This type I iron complex (robust and strong) shows high structural homogeneity and only slow and competitive delivery to endogenous iron binding proteins. Complexes are actively phagocyted by macrophages of the RES before they are released and become available for hemoglobin synthesis. Although plasma half-life is 30 hours (3 days for high molecular weight iron dextran, HMWID), the full process of iron release from dextran complex in the RES, storage in ferritin, and delivery as TBI to the bone marrow or other tissues may take several months (48). Iron dextran can be administered as i.m. or i.v. injections and as i.v. infusion. The stability of the dextran complex allows administration of high single doses (so-called "total dose infusion" which may be given for over 4–6 hours). In contrast, the bioavailability of iron following i.m. administration has not been studied extensively. There seems to be a risk of incomplete and variable absorption of the iron from the injection site, and considerable amount (30–50%) of iron can remain at the i.m. injection site for many months. Therefore i.m. injections are no longer recommended (49). However, these iron complexes may cause well know dextran-induced anaphylactic reactions, especially in patients receiving high molecular weight iron dextran (not commercially available in Europe and considered as an obsolete i.v. iron agent). Although the exact mechanism of the anaphylactic reaction to iron dextran has not been clarified yet, it seems to be related to the antibody-mediated release of mediators by mast cells.

Ferric carboxymaltose (FCM) is another stable parenteral iron product with a molecular weight of 150 kDa very similar to iron dextran in terms of stability and structure (Type I, robust and strong). The pharmacokinetics characteristics of FCM are similar but not identical to iron dextran. The distribution volume of both preparations corresponds nearly to that of plasma, but half-life is approximately 16 hours for FCM as compared with 30 hours for LMWID. It seems that the FCM is broken down more rapidly than iron dextran because a-amylase does no affect to dextran, or acts at a very slow rate (43). A study using positron emission tomography has shown that the iron from FCM accumulates in the liver, spleen, and bone marrow and substantial amounts were found in these organs within minutes. In addition, FCM is able to exchange iron rapidly with transferrin (50). As a result, the utilization of iron for RBC increased rapidly up to day 6–9, after which the utilization increased at a much lower rate. Patients with IDA showed over 90% iron utilization after 24 days compared with 60–80% utilization for patients with renal anemia (50). FCM is designed to mimic physiologically occurring ferritin, provide high iron utilization, and eliminate disadvantageous characteristics associated with iron dextran (anaphylaxis) and iron sucrose (high pH, high osmolarity, dosage limitations, and the long duration of administration). Up to 100–200 mg FCM can be administered as i.v. injection and up to 1000 mg iron can be infused in at least 15 minutes and test dose is not required.

Efficacy of parenteral iron agents

FID is frequent and neglected in the perioperative setting. Serum ferritin < 100 g/L, TSAT < 20%, increase in% HYPO, and low CHr values have been proposed as the most indicative parameters for the assessment of FID outside the context of CKD. The early detection and treatment of FID is essential to assure an adequate iron supply to the bone marrow, particularly in patients receiving EPO therapy.

Experience with the use of i.v. iron therapy is extensive in different clinical settings over the last 60 years. In the late 1980s, the introduction of rHuEPO led to a revitalized interest in the use of iron therapy, either in combination with rHuEPO therapy, or alone. Intravenous iron therapy can be used in a variety of clinical settings, as long as iron parameters are carefully monitored. In a number of studies, i.v. iron was shown to be clearly superior to oral iron for the treatment of anemia associated with CKD, IBD, chronic inflammatory arthritis, congestive cardiac failure, pregnancy, and postpartum, or cancer (35, 51, 52). In the settings of CKD or cancer related anemia, the use of i.v. iron resulted not only in a more rapid and complete response to rHuEPO, but also in a reduction of rHuEPO dose, and probably in a reduction of rHuEPO side effects, such as thrombosis (53–55).

Only recently, i.v. iron therapy has been used in patients undergoing orthopedic, cardiac and gynecological surgical procedures (35, 51, 52), whereas the information regarding the use of i.v. in critically ill patients is even more scant (56, 57).

Safety of parenteral iron agents

Nausea, abdominal pain, constipation, diarrhea, injection site reactions (pain, superficial phlebitis), metallic taste, headache, dizziness, and rash may occur with all i.v. preparations, and were observed in clinical trial with an incidence of 1–3%. However, the incidence of adverse drug events (ADEs) associated with parenteral iron is much smaller.

Allergic and anaphylactic reactions

The numbers of non-CKD patients receiving i.v. iron are not large enough to draw definitive conclusions regarding the safety of i.v. iron agents in these clinical settings. Therefore, we will focus on ADEs associated with parenteral iron in CKD patients, as they are the largest collective receiving these drugs. According to data from the United States Food and Drug Administration (FDA) on ADEs attributed to the provision of four formulations of intravenous iron (HMWID, LMWID, iron gluconate, and iron sucrose) during 2001–2003, including, the total number of reported parenteral iron-related ADEs was 1141 among approximately 30 million doses administered (approximately 38 ADEs per million), with 11 deaths (7 iron dextran, 3 iron gluconate, 1 iron sucrose) (47). Relative to lower molecular weight iron dextran, total and life-threatening ADEs were significantly more frequent among recipients of higher molecular weight iron dextran and significantly less frequent among recipients of sodium ferric gluconate complex and iron sucrose. The absolute rates of life-threatening ADEs were 0.6, 0.9, 3.3, and 11.3 per million for iron sucrose, sodium ferric gluconate complex, lower molecular weight iron dextran, and higher molecular weight iron dextran, respectively, whereas absolute rates of death were 0.11, 0.25, 0.75, and 0.78 per million, respectively (Table 27.1). However, there were no significant differences in mortality rates between LMWID and iron gluconate (OR 0.3, 95% CI 0.1–1.3) or iron sucrose (OR 0.2, 95% CI 0.1–1.0), and there are no data available regarding the safety of iron carboxymaltose. As for FCM, since 2007 the use of Ferinject corresponds to over 17,000 patient-years (one patient corresponds to 2000 mg iron). Up to September 2008, no anaphylactoid reactions or death have been reported, confirming the good safety profile of FCM (43).

Therefore, the frequency of intravenous iron-related ADEs reported to the FDA has decreased, and overall, the rates are extremely low (Table 27.1). In addition, the rates of ADES associated with i.v. iron, including iron-related deaths, are much lower than that of ABT-related severe side effects (10 per million) and ABT-related deaths (4 per million) (58).

Intravenous iron and infection

Current information on the relationship between i.v. iron and infection, and between i.v. iron and oxidative stress deserves special consideration. Elemental iron is an essential growth factor for bacteria with many species expressing iron transport proteins that compete with transferrin, and it has long been suggested that patients with iron overload are at increased risk of infection (59). In contrast, in the peritoneal dialysis population, no increased risk of peritonitis was found in patients receiving with respect to those not receiving i.v. iron (60). In addition, a meta-analysis of 6 observational studies (807 patients) revealed that the administration of i.v. iron to patients undergoing major orthopedic surgery led to a significant decrease in both transfusion rate (RR: 0.60; 95% confidence interval [CI]: 0.50–0.72; $p < 0.001$) and infection rate (RR: 0.45; 95%CI: 0.32–0.63; $p < 0.001$) (61). Nevertheless, despite this absence of definitive clinical data, it seems sensible to avoid i.v. iron administration in the setting of acute infection, and to withhold i.v. iron in patients with pretreatment ferritin values >500 ng/mL (43).

Intravenous iron and oxidant damage

Biologically active iron, which is released by all i.v. iron agents, also plays a role in inflammation, oxidant stress, and the propensity for accelerated atherosclerosis. Persistent oxidative stress in CKD patients promotes inflammation and, in turn, atherogenesis, and increased cardiovascular morbidity and mortality. However, available evidence relating i.v. iron administration to atherogenesis is indirect, and there is little evidence that i.v. iron adversely affects survival in patients with dialysis-dependent CKD. Nevertheless, the evidence argues for caution, not complacency, in prescribing i.v. iron (43).

Intravenous iron and cancer development

The association between iron overload with cancer risk in humans has been under increased scrutiny in recent decades, although epidemiological studies on the association of iron with cancer remain inconclusive. The concerns are mostly focused on a possible risk associated with dietary iron in colorectal cancer, the increased risk of developing hepatocellular carcinoma in hereditary hemochromatosis and related hepatic iron overload and cirrhosis, and association between occupational exposure to iron and kidney, lung, and stomach cancers. The risk of iron-induced sarcoma by repeated intramuscular injections of iron dextran has also been raised. However, i.v. iron therapy has not been associated with a tumor incidence increase (62).

General good practice points

Based on the clinical experience of the expert panel members of the Consensus Statement on the use of i.v. iron for the treatment of perioperative anemia, the following points might be considered as good clinical practice for surgical patients (9):

- Patients at risk of receiving perioperative transfusions should be identified on the basis of patient's RBC mass, the transfusion trigger, and the expected blood loss (e.g., using Mercuriali's algorithm).
- Whenever clinically feasible, patients undergoing elective surgery with a high risk of severe postoperative anemia should have Hb level and iron status (serum iron, ferritin, and transferrin saturation index) tested preferably 30 days before the scheduled surgical procedure. For patients older than 60 years, vitamin B12 and folic acid should also be measured.
- Patients with preoperative anemia due to iron deficiency or chronic diseases may receive preoperative treatment with i.v. iron, with or without rHuEPO. In addition, i.v. iron should be given to improve the response to rHuEPO and might allow for a reduction in the total dose of rHuEPO.
- Unexplained anemia should always be considered as secondary to some other process and, therefore, elective surgery should be deferred until an appropriate diagnosis has been made.
- Nonanemic patients with ferritin <100 ng/mL and scheduled for surgical procedures with an expected blood loss >1500 mL (Hb drop of 30–50 g/L) might benefit from preoperative oral or i.v. iron administration, as they may not have enough stored iron to reconstitute their perioperative Hb loss and to keep a normal iron store (ferritin ≥ 30 ng/mL).
- The administration of i.v. iron should be avoided in patients with pretreatment ferritin values >500 ng/mL. Nevertheless, as all i.v. iron agents have the potential to release biologically active iron, i.v. iron should not be given to patient with ongoing bacteremia.

Acknowledgments

The authors gratefully acknowledge the critical review of the manuscript by Prof. Alice Maniatis (Athens, Greece), Prof. Antonio Herrera (Zaragoza, Spain), and Dr. Jorge Cuenca (Zaragoza, Spain).

References

1. Guralnik JM, Eisenstaedt RS, Ferrucci L, Klein HG, Woodman RC. The prevalence of anemia in persons aged 65 and older in the United States: evidence for a high rate of unexplained anemia. Blood 2004; 104:2263–8.
2. Shander A, Knight K, Thurer R, Adamson J, Spence R. Prevalence and outcomes of anemia in surgery: a systematic review of the literature. Am J Med 2004; 116:58S–69.

3. Bisbe E, Castillo J, Saez M, Santiveri X, Nomen N, Muñoz M. Prevalence of preoperative anemia and hematinic deficiencies in patients scheduled for elective major orthopedic surgery. TATM 2008;10: 166–73.
4. Semba RD, Guralnik JM, Chaves P, Ricks MO, Fried LP. Women's health and aging studies. Iron status and anemia in a population-based study of women with and without disability living in the community: the women's health and aging studies. Haematologica 2004;89:357–8.
5. Muñoz M, Campos A, Garcia-Erce JA. Intravenous iron in colorectal cancer surgery. Semin Hematol 2006;43 (Suppl. 6): S36–8.
6. Rosencher N, Kerkkamp HE, Macheras G, et al. Orthopedic surgery transfusion hemoglobin European overview (OSTHEO) study: blood management in elective knee and hip arthroplasty in Europe. Transfusion 2003;43:459–69.
7. García-Erce JA, Cuenca J, Solano VM. Factores predictivos de la necesidad de transfusión en la fractura subcapital de cadera en pacientes mayores de 65años. Med Clin (Barc) 2003;120:161–6.
8. Scottish Intercollegiate Guidelines Network. Perioperative blood transfusion for elective surgery. A national clinical guideline. www.sign.ac.uk, 2001 (update in 2009; last accessed February 2010).
9. Beris P, Muñoz M, García-Erce JA, Thomas D, Maniatis A, Van Der Linden P. Perioperative anaemia management: consensus statement on the role of intravenous iron. Br J Anaesth 2008;100:599–604.
10. Clarke R, Grimley Evans J, Schneede J, et al. Vitamin B12 and folate deficiency in later life. Age Ageing 2004;33:34–41.
11. Siah CW, Ombiga J, Adams LA, Trinder D, Olynyk JK. Normal iron metabolism and the physiopathology of iron overload disorders. Clin Biochem Rev 2006; 27:5–16.
12. Muñoz M, Molero S, García-Erce JA. Fisiopatología del metabolismo del hierro y sus implicaciones en la anemia perioperatoria. Anemia 2008;1:47–60.
13. Andrews NC. Forging a field: the golden age of iron biology. Blood 2008;112:219–30.
14. Fleming RE, Bacon BR. Orchestration of iron homeostasis. N Engl J Med 2005;352:1741–4.
15. Nemeth E, Ganz T. Hepcidin and iron loading anemias. Haematologica 2006;91:727–32.
16. Muñoz M, Campos A, García-Erce JA, Ramírez G. Fisiopatología del metabolismo del hierro: implicaciones diagnósticas y terapéuticas. Nefrología 2005; 25:9–19.
17. Thomas C, Thomas L. Biochemical markers and hematologic indices in the diagnosis of functional iron deficiency. Clin Chem 2002;48:1066–76.
18. Thomas C, Krischbaum A, Boehm D, Thomas L. The diagnostic plot. Med Oncol 2006;23:23–36.
19. Weiss G, Goodnough LT. Anemia of chronic disease. N Engl J Med 2005;352:1011–23.
20. King WN, Zhao SE, Duan XL, Yang Z, Qian ZM, Chang YZ. Decreased DMTI and increased ferroportin I expression in the mechanisms of reduced iron retention in macrophages by erythropoietin in rats. J Cell Biochem 2008;104:629–41.
21. Franke A, Lante W, Fackeldey V, et al. Proinflammatory cytokines after different kinds of cardio-thoracic surgical procedures: is what we see what we know? Eur J Cardiothorac Surg 2005;28: 569–75.
22. Muñoz M, García-Vallejo JJ, Sempere JM, Romero R, Olalla E, Sebastián C. Acute phase response and cytokine release in patients undergoing lumbar spinal surgery: modulation by perioperative treatment with naproxen and famotidine. Eur Spine J 2004; 13:367–73.
23. Van Iperen CE, Kraaijenahgen RJ, Biesma DH, Beguin Y, Marx JJM, van de Wiel A. Iron metabolism and erythropoiesis after surgery. Br J Surg 1998;85:41–5.
24. Cook JD. Diagnosis and management of iron-deficiency anaemia. Best Pract Res Clin Haematol 2005;18:319–32.
25. García-Erce JA, Cuenca J, Martínez F, Cardona R, Pérez-Serrano L, Muñoz M. Perioperative intravenous iron may transfusion requirements and hasten the recovery from postoperative anaemia after knee replacement surgery. Transf Med 2006;16: 335–41.
26. Theurl I, Aigner E, Theurl M, et al. Regulation of iron homeostasis in anemia of chronic disease and iron deficiency anemia: diagnostic and therapeutic implications. Blood 2009;113:5277–86.
27. Goodnough LT, Shander A, Spivak JL, et al. Detection, evaluation, and management of anemia in the elective surgical patient. Anesth Analg 2005;101: 1858–61.
28. Punnonen K, Irjala K, Rajamaki A. Serum transferrin receptor and its ratio to serum ferritin in the diagnosis of iron deficiency. Blood 1997;89:1052–7.
29. Beguin Y, Clemons GK, Pootrakul P, Fillet G. Quantitative assessment of erythropoiesis and functional classification of anemia based on measurements of serum transferring receptors and erythropoietin. Blood 1993;81:1067–76.

30. Thomas L, Franck S, Messinger M, Linssen J, Thomas M, Thomas C. Reticulocyte hemoglobin measurement–comparison of two methods in the diagnosis of iron-restricted erythropoiesis. Clin Chem Lab Med 2005;43:1193–202.
31. Brugnara C, Schiller B, Moran J. Reticulocyte hemoglobin equivalent (RetHe) and assessment of iron-deficient states. Clin Lab Haematol 2006;28: 303–8.
32. Ferrucci L, Guralnik JM, Bandinelli S, et al. Unexplained anaemia in older persons is characterised by low erythropoietin and low levels of pro-inflammatory markers. Br J Haematol 2007;136: 849–55.
33. Gisbert JP, Gomollón F. Common misconceptions in the diagnosis and management of anemia in inflammatory bowel disease. Am J Gastroenterol 2008; 103:1299–307.
34. Briges KR. Prevention of iron deficiency in surgical women. In: *Transfusion Medicine and Alternatives to Blood Transfusion*. R & J Éditions Médicales, Paris, 2000, pp. 251–8.
35. Maniatis A. The role of iron in anaemia management: can intravenous iron contribute to blood conservation? ISBT Sci Ser 2008;3:139–43.
36. Cuenca J, García-Erce JA, Martínez F, Cardona R, Pérez-Serrano L, Muñoz M. Preoperative haematinics and transfusion protocol reduce the need for transfusion after total knee replacement. Int J Surg 2007; 5:89–94.
37. Okuyama M, Ikeda K, Shibata T, Tsukahara Y, Kitada M, Shimano T. Preoperative iron supplementation and intraoperative transfusion during colorectal cancer surgery. Surg Today 2005;35:36–40.
38. Goodnough LT, Skikne B, Brugnara C. Erythropoietin, iron, and erythropoiesis. Blood 2000;96:823–33.
39. Aronoff GR. Safety of intravenous iron in clinical practice: implications for anemia management protocols. J Am Soc Nephrol 2004;15:S99–106.
40. Van Wyck DB. Labile iron: manifestations and clinical implications. J Am Soc Nephrol 2004;15 (Suppl. 2): S107–11.
41. Fishbane S, Kowalski EA. The comparative safety of intravenous iron dextran, iron saccharate, and sodium ferric gluconate. Semin Dial 2000;13:381–4.
42. Silverstein SB, Rodgers GM. Parenteral iron therapy options. Am J Hematol 2004;76:74–8.
43. Crichton RR, Danielsson BG, Geisser P. *Iron Therapy With Special Emphasis On Intravenous Administration*. UNI-Med Verlag AG, Bremen, 2008.
44. Danielson BG. Structure, chemistry, and pharmacokinetics of intravenous iron agents. J Am Soc Nephrol 2004;15:S93–8.
45. Madougall. Experience with intravenous iron en nephrology. Semin Hematol 2006;43 (Suppl. 6): S9–12.
46. Schroder O, Mickisck O, Seidler U, et al. Intravenous iron sucrose versus oral iron supplementation for the treatment of iron deficiency anemia in patients with inflammatory bowel disease – a randomized, controlled, open-label, multicenter study. Am J Gastroenterol 2005;100:2503–9.
47. Chertow GM, Mason PD, Vaaga-Nilsen O, Ahlmén J. Update on adverse drug events associated with parenteral iron. Nephrol Dial Transplant 2006; 21:378–82.
48. Grau PW. Intravenous iron therapy. In: Beaumont C, Beris P, Beuzard Y, Brugnara C (eds) *Disorders of Iron Homeostasis, Erythrocytes, Erythropoiesis*. European School of Haematology, Paris, 2006, pp. 420–34.
49. Auerbach M, Ballard H, Glaspy J. Clinical update: intravenous iron for anaemia. Lancet 2007;369: 1502–4.
50. Beshara S, Sörensen J, Lubberink M, et al. Pharmacokinetics and red cell utilization of 52Fe/59Fe-labelled iron polymaltose in anaemic patients using positron emission tomography. Br J Haematol 2003;120:853–9.
51. Muñoz M, Breymann C, García-Erce JA, Gómez-Ramírez S, Comin J, Bisbe E. Efficacy and safety of intravenous iron therapy as an alternative/ adjunct to allogeneic blood transfusion. Vox Sang 2008;94:172–83.
52. Auerbach M, Goodnough LT, Picard D, Maniatis A. The role of intravenous iron in anemia management and transfusion avoidance. Transfusion 2008;48:988–1000.
53. Streja E, Kovesdy CP, Greenland S, et al. Erythropoietin, iron depletion, and relative thrombocytosis: a possible explanation for hemoglobin-survival paradox in hemodialysis. Am J Kidney Dis 2008;52: 727–36.
54. Kapoian T, O'Mara NB, Singh AK, et al. Ferric gluconate reduces epoetin requirements in hemodialysis patients with elevated ferritin. J Am Soc Nephrol 2008;19:372–9.
55. Dahl NV, Henry DH, Auerbach M. Is thromboembolism in cancer patients treated with erythropoietic stimulating agents related to thrombocytosis and iron restricted erythropoiesis?. Blood (ASH Annual Meeting Abstracts) 2007;110:1625 [Abstract].

56. Van Iperen CE, Gaillard CA, Kraaijenhagen RJ, Braam BG, Marx JJ, Van de Wiel A. Response of erythropoiesis and iron metabolism to recombinant human erythropoietin in intensive care unit patients. Crit Care Med 2000;28:2773–8.
57. Georgopoulos D, Matamos D, Routsi C, et al. Recombinant human erythropoietin therapy in critically ill patients: a dose-response study. Crit Care 2005;9:R508–15.
58. Stainsby D, Jones H, Asher D, et al. Serious hazards of transfusion: a decade of hemovigilance in the UK. Transfus Med Rev 2006;20:273–82.
59. Weiss G. Iron and immunity: a double-edged sword. Eur J Clin Invest 2003;32 (Suppl. 1): 70–8.
60. Vychytil A, Haag-Weber M. Iron status and iron supplementation in peritoneal dialysis patients. Kidney Int 1999;55 (Suppl.): S71–8.
61. García-Erce JA, Cuenca J, Gómez-Ramírez S, Villar I, Herrera A, Muñoz M. Posibilidades de tratamiento de la anemia perioperatoria en cirugía ortopédica y traumatología. Anemia 2009;2:17–27.
62. Huang X. Iron overload and its association with cancer risk in humans: evidence for iron as a carcinogenic metal. Mutat Res 2003;533:153–71.

CHAPTER 28

Current Status of Perisurgical Erythropoietin Therapy

Lawrence T. Goodnough
Departments of Medicine and Pathology, Stanford University School of Medicine, Stanford, CA, USA

Introduction

Recombinant human erythropoietin (EPO) therapy has been approved for use in patients undergoing autologous blood donation (ABD) in Japan, the European Union, and Canada since 1993, 1994, and 1996 respectively, and is also approved for perisurgical adjuvant therapy in Canada, Australia, the United States, and the European Union [1]. Emerging strategies to improve the dose–response relationship between EPO therapy and red cell production include low dose EPO and intravenous iron therapy, which are to be addressed in this chapter.

Current status of ABD

Since 1992, the percentages of blood collected and transfused nationally that are autologous have declined substantially (Table 28.1). A recent national, multicenter study audited current autologous blood predonation activity and transfusion outcomes for patients undergoing total joint replacement surgery [9]. Forty-seven to 65% of patients predonate, on average, 1.6–2.1 autologous blood units before procedures ranging from unilateral knee to bilateral knee arthroplasty or hip revision. Twenty-nine to 55% of these autologous units collected are wasted. Allogeneic transfusion outcomes are detailed in Table 28.2. The benefit of autologous blood predonation can be seen to reduce the likelihood of allogeneic blood exposure by approximately two-thirds for patients who are nonanemic and by approximately one-third in patients with baseline anemia (Hct < 39%), when compared to patients who do not predonate autologous blood before total joint arthroplasty.

Alternatives to Blood Transfusion in Transfusion Medicine, 2nd edition. Edited by A. Maniatis, P. Van der Linden, J.-F. Hardy.

Clinical trials of EPO therapy

Patients donating autologous blood under standard conditions (i.e., one blood unit weekly [4, 5] have an inadequate response of endogenous EPO to blood loss anemia, suggesting a role for EPO therapy in facilitating ABD. This was confirmed [6, 7] in a study comparing aggressive ABD (up to six units over a 3-week preoperative interval) with EPO therapy in patients undergoing orthopedic surgery. However, a subsequent clinical trial [8] in orthopedic patients demonstrated that for autologous blood donors who were not anemic (hematocrit > 39%) at first donation, no clinical benefit (defined as reduced allogeneic blood exposure) was seen with EPO therapy when compared to aggressive autologous phlebotomy alone. Thus, for nonanemic patients, ABD remains an option if they can tolerate aggressive blood phlebotomy (i.e., up to six units over for 3 weeks) and thereby achieve stimulation of erythropoiesis via their endogenous EPO response [9].

For anemic (hematocrit ≤ 39%) autologous blood donors, a European clinical trial demonstrated that EPO therapy (300 or 600 U/kg i.v. in six

Table 28.1 Approval of status of recombinant human erythropoietin therapy in surgical anemia.

	United States	Canada	European Union*	Australia	Japan
Autologous blood donation	1996	1994	1996	1993	
Surgery	1996†	1996	1998‡	1996	Under review

*Approval dates for France, Germany, Italy, and the United Kingdom are the same as for other countries of the European Union.
†Non-cardiac, non-vascular surgery.
‡Orthopedic surgery.

doses) reduced exposure to allogeneic blood during orthopedic surgery when compared to placebo-treated patients [10]. However, this result was only achieved with concurrent administration of both intravenous and oral supplemental iron. A subsequent US trial with supplemental oral iron and EPO therapy (600 U/kg i.v. in six doses) could not demonstrate reduced allogeneic blood transfusions when compared to placebo-treated patients [11] largely because a substantial percentage of the patients were either severely anemic (hematocrit < 33%) or were iron deficient upon entry into the clinical trial.

Several studies have evaluated perisurgical EPO therapy in nonanemic orthopedic surgical patients without autologous blood procurement. Both a Canadian [12] and two US studies [13, 14] were able to show that EPO-treated (300 U/kg s.q. × 14 days, beginning nine days preoperatively) patients had one half the rate of exposure (approximately 25%) to allogeneic blood as the placebo-treated patients (approximately 50%), despite mean initial hemoglobin levels that exceeded 130 g/L for patients in both studies. On the basis of these clinical trials, EPO therapy was approved for perisurgical use in Canada and the United States in 1996.

EPO therapy and erythropoietic response

An analysis of the relationship between EPO dose and the response in red blood cell production [15] has demonstrated a good correlation [Figure 28.1]. EPO-stimulated erythropoiesis is independent of age and gender [16], and the variability in response among patients is partly due to iron-restricted erythropoiesis [17]. There is no evidence that surgery or EPO therapy affects the endogenous EPO response to anemia or the erythropoietic response to EPO [18].

Red blood cell expansion is seen with an increase in reticulocyte count by day 3 of treatment in nonanemic patients treated with EPO who are iron-replete [4]. As illustrated in [Figure 28.2], the equivalent of one blood unit is produced by day 7 and the equivalent of five blood units produced over 28 days [5]. If three to five blood units are

Table 28.2 Collection and transfusion of autologous blood in the United States.

Source	1980	1986	1989	1992	1994	1997
Transfused antologous, 1000s (% of total)	n/a	n/a	369 (3.1)	566 (5.0)	482 (4.3)	421 (3.7)
Total	9,934	12,159	12,059	11,307	11,107	11,476
Collected antologous, 1000s (% of total)	28 (0.25)	206 (1.5)	655 (4.8)	1,117 (8.5)	1,013 (7.8)	611 (4.9)
Total	11,174	13,807	13,554	13,169	12,908	12,550

*Modified from Goodnough et al. NEJM 1999;340:439 with permission.

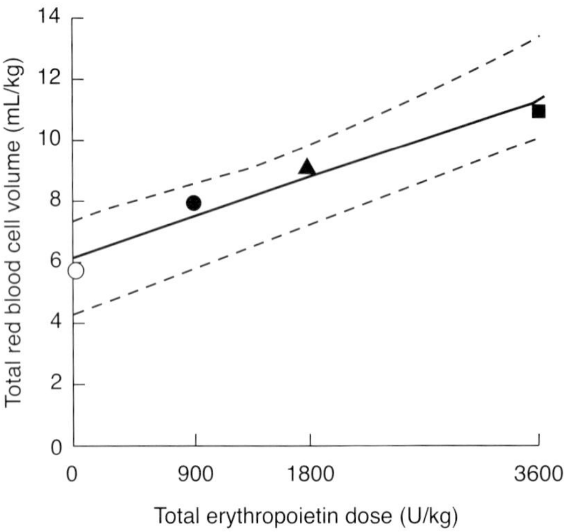

Figure 28.1 The dose and response relationship between total (cumulative) amount of erythropoietin (EPO) administered (units per kg body weight for six treatments over 3 weeks) and the red blood cell volume increase (ml per kg body weight) during the preoperative interval for patients treated intravenously with placebo, 150 U/kg, 300 U/kg, and 600 U/kg. Doses of erythropoietin are given in total (cumulative) units per kilogram of body weight for all six treatments combined over a period of 3 weeks; increases in red cell volume are given in milliliters per kilogram of body weight. The dotted lines indicate the 95 percent confidence interval. Reproduced from Goodnough et al. J Amer Coll Surg 1994;179:171–176 [15] with permission from Elsevier.

necessary to minimize allogeneic blood exposure in patients undergoing complex procedures such as orthopedic joint replacement surgery, the preoperative interval necessary for EPO-stimulated erythropoiesis can be estimated to be 3–4 weeks.

Normal individuals have been shown to have difficulty providing sufficient iron to support rates of erythropoiesis that are greater than three times basal [19]. A recent study confirmed that the maximum erythropoietic response in the acute setting, seen in EPO-treated patients with measurable storage iron, is approximately four times basal marrow RBC production [17]. Previous investigators have shown that conditions associated with enhanced plasma iron and transferrin saturation are necessary to produce a greater marrow response, such as in patients with hemochromatosis [20], or in patients supplemented with intravenous iron administration [21]. In hemochromatosis, marrow response has been estimated to increase by six to eightfold over baseline RBC production with aggressive phlebotomy [20]. The term "relative iron deficiency" has thus been termed by Finch [22] to occur in individuals when the iron stores are normal but the increased erythron iron requirements exceed the available supply of iron.

A previous study demonstrated with ferrokinetic studies that iron supplementation with at least 100 mg elemental iron per day taken with food, can cover the increased iron needs from exogenous EPO in autologous blood donors [23]. For all patients, initial storage iron status was not a clinically important limitation for red blood cell production in the presence of oral iron supplementation [17]. For iron-replete patients, however, there was a significant relationship between storage iron and marrow response in patients receiving EPO therapy [Figure 28.3]. These results suggest that storage iron is important for maintaining sufficient plasma transferrin saturation for optimal erythropoiesis.

Iron therapy

In circumstances with significant ongoing iron losses, oral iron does not provide enough iron to correct the iron-deficient erythropoiesis, and intravenous iron therapy should be considered. Renal dialysis patients have such blood losses, and the role of intravenous iron therapy has been best defined in clinical trials achieving target hematocrit levels in this setting. Addressing iron deficiency with intravenous iron therapy allows correction of anemia along with utilization of lower EPO dosage [24]. Another role for intravenous iron therapy is in the arena of bloodless medicine and bloodless surgery programs for patients who refuse blood transfusions on the basis of religious beliefs [25]. Common clinical settings here include pregnancy [26] and patients with dysfunctional uterine bleeding who are scheduled for hysterectomy [27].

Currently there are four commercially available preparations. Intravenous iron therapy has been closely scrutinized for risks and adverse events.

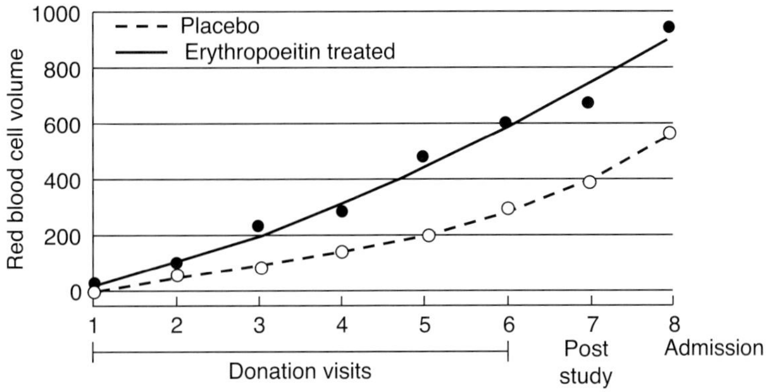

Figure 28.2 Red cell (RBC) production during autologous blood donation, in 23 placebo treated (white circles) and 21 erythropoietin-treated (black circles) patients. Data points represent calculated RBC production (mL) at donation visit 1 through 6, the post study visit, and hospital admission. RBC production is indicated by polynomial regression curve for each treatment group ($n = 44$ at each point). The rate of RBC production can be derived for any preoperative interval. The mean cumulative interval since donation visit 1 was 3.5 days to visit 2, 7.2 days to visit 3, 10.6 days to visit 4, 14.2 days to visit 5, 17.6 days to visit 6, 20.9 days to visit 7 (poststudy visit) and 26.3 days to visit 8 (hospital admission). Reproduced from Goodnough LT et al. Transfusion 1992; 32:441–445 [6] with permission from Blackwell Publishing Ltd.

Imferon (Iron Dextran BP) is an iron preparation previously associated with a 0.6% risk of life threatening anaphylactoid reactions and 1.7% risk of severe, delayed reactions that were serum sickness-like and characterized by fever, arthragias, and myalgias [28]. An increased incidence of delayed reactions of up to 30% and severe reactions of 5.3% was subsequently described [29]; this product was eventually withdrawn from use.

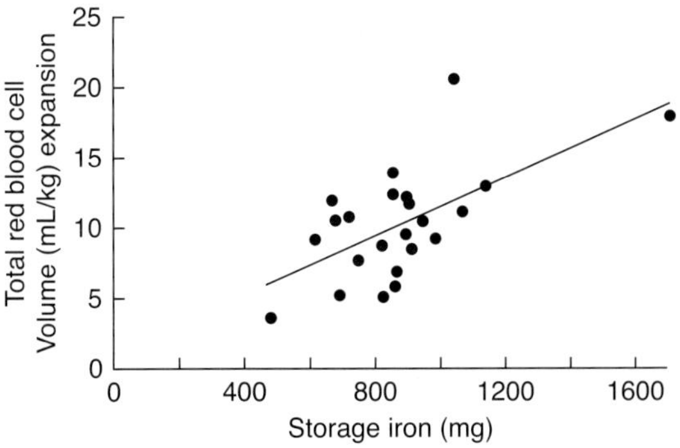

Figure 28.3 The relationship between initial storage iron (mg) and red blood cell volume expansion (ml/kg) in patients who received erythropoietin therapy. Linear regression analysis demonstrated a significant correlation ($r = 0.6$, $p = 0.02$). Reproduced from Goodnough et al. [17] with permission from Blackwell Publishing Ltd.

InFed (Iron Dextran USP, Schein Pharm Corp., Florham Park, NJ) is currently approved for parenteral (intramuscular or intravenous) use, with widespread experience in intravenous administration in renal dialysis patients. Clinical studies have shown that InFed administered intravenously during the dialysis procedure was associated with clinically significant adverse reactions in 4.7% of patients, of which 0.7% were serious or life-threatening, and another 1.75% were characterized as anaphylactyoid reactions [30]. The prevalence of these reactions does not appear to differ among patients receiving low-dose (100 mg) or higher-dose (250–500 mg) infusions [31]. A recent review reported 196 allergic/anaphylaxis cases with the use of iron dextran in the United States between 1976 and 1996, of which 31 (15.8%) were fatal [32].

Safety aspects of parenteral iron in patients with end-stage renal disease for iron dextran, ferric gluconate, and iron saccharate have been scrutinized [33]. Iron saccharate is a preparation available in

Europe but not in the United States, in which allergic reactions are very rare. Possible adverse effects include a metallic taste, arthralgia, chest pain, or brochospasm [33–35]. Ferric gluconate (Ferrlecit, Schein Pharm Corp., Florham Park, NJ) was approved for use in the United States in February 1999 as an intravenous iron preparation in renal dialysis patients. Dosage of Ferrlecit is limited to 125 mg over a 1-hour infusion at each administration [36]. The rate of allergic reactions (3.3 episodes per million doses) appears lower than iron dextran (8.7 episodes per million doses) and the safety profile of iron gluconate is substantially better; among 74 adverse events reported as severe reported with its use from 1976 to 1996, there were no deaths [32].

Adverse events that have been reported associated with ferric gluconate include hypotension, rash, chest, or abdominal pain, with an incidence of less than 5% [37]. Another potential adverse effect of intravenous iron therapy is a clinical syndrome of acute iron toxicity (nausea, facial reddening, and hypotension), which has been attributed to oversaturation (>100%) of transferrin. This has been described with rapid infusion of ferric gluconate (62.5–125 mg within 30 minutes) in a study of 20 dialysis patients [38]. However, a recent report disputed the existence of this effect (i.e., oversaturation of transferrin) by demonstrating that two laboratory assays for measurement of serum iron yield misleading results for transferrin saturation if performed within 24 hours after infusion [39]. Serious reactions (including one hypotensive event) were reported in only three (1.3%) of 226 patients undergoing renal dialysis while treated with ferric gluconate in one European study [40].

The clinical setting for which intravenous iron is to be used should determine which preparation is chosen [41]. For total dose infusion, iron dextran is required because the iron salts cause dose-dependent gastrointestinal or vasoactive reactions at doses above 200–400 mg [42]. The preferred dextran is the LMW preparation as the HMW preparation is associated with a significantly higher incidence of serious acute events [43, 44]. For patients receiving cyclical therapies, such as cancer chemotherapy or dialysis, the iron salts, or LMW ID, can be used as short 100- to 400-mg infusions [42, 45, 46]. However, settings such as the preoperative period, pregnancy, menometrorrhagia, gastric bypass, and uncomplicated iron deficiency in those intolerant to oral iron, a total dose infusion of LMW iron dextran is more convenient, equally efficacious, and far less expensive. Three studies comparing LMW ID with the two salts show no difference in efficacy or toxicity among the three products, but demonstrate considerable savings and increased convenience with LMLW ID [47–49].

Previous studies [50] have shown that the increased erythropoietic effect (4.5–5.5 times basal) of intravenous iron dextran (with an estimated half-life of 60 hours) is transient and lasts 7–10 days, after which the iron is sequestered in the reticuloendothelial system, and erythropoiesis returns to 2.5–3.5 times normal [51]. A dose–response relationship of EPO and erythropoiesis that is affected favorably by intravenous iron, even in iron replete individuals, has important implications for EPO dosage [52], especially if the cost of therapy is taken into account. Current recommended EPO dosage to be administered in patients scheduled for elective surgery range from 1800 U/kg [53] to 4200 U/kg total dosage [13, 54], which for a 70-kg patient would cost $1300–3000 [55]. However, an economic analysis of EPO therapy in patients undergoing orthopedic surgery concluded that even with the lower currently recommended (1800 U/kg) total dosage, EPO therapy is not cost-effective [56]. Intravenous iron may potentiate the erythropoietic response in the setting of EPO therapy by improving iron-restricted erythropoiesis induced by EPO therapy.

Economic considerations

The costs associated with EPO therapy and the potential impact of reimbursement policies are important issues in the setting of surgical anemia, as has been the case in medical anemia [55]. Costs associated with EPO therapy may be lowered by strategies that improve the dose and response relationship. One study [54] demonstrated that four weekly injections of subcutaneous EPO (600 U/kg)

Table 28.3 Allogeneic blood transfusion outcomes in patients undergoing total joint replacement: USA 1996–1997.

Procedure	Autologous blood predonated No ($n = 3741$)	Yes ($n = 5741$) Non-anemic	Anemic (Hct < 39%)
Knee			
Unilateral	18	6	11
Revision	30	11	18
Bilateral	57	16	21
Hip			
Unilateral	32	9	14
Bilateral	59	21	33

*Modified, from Bierbaum et al. J bone J Surgery 1999;81A:2–10.
†Data shown represent (%) of patients receiving allogenic blood.

was less costly but was just as effective as a daily dose of EPO (300 units per kilogram for 14 doses). A similar regimen (300 U/kg × 6 for over 3 weeks) was recently recommended for administration of EPO in surgery [57]. However, an economic analysis of EPO therapy in orthopedic surgery concluded that with these doses, EPO therapy was not cost-effective [56]. One report demonstrated erythropoietic responses with EPO dosage as low as 100 U/kg s.q. administered weekly, although not clinical outcomes were studied [56]. These regimens [12–14] remain expensive, and when unaccompanied by autologous blood procurement, are still associated with an allogeneic exposure rate of 16–25%. The costs of EPO therapy ($0.01/unit [51]) for a 70-kg patient in selected clinical trials is summarized in Table 28.3.

A review of randomized trials concluded that the optimal dose of perioperative EPO therapy remains to be established [59]. Nevertheless, the superiority of EPO therapy when compared to ABD in reducing allogeneic blood exposure during total joint replacement procedures was reaffirmed in a recent multicenter study [60].

Safety considerations

A randomized, controlled study (SPINE) evaluated 681 patients undergoing spinal surgery who received either epoetin alfa and standard of care (SOC) or SOC alone. These patients did not receive prophylactic anticoagulation. Preliminary analysis showed a higher incidence of deep vein thrombosis in the epoetin alfa group than the SOC cohort (4.7% vs 2.1%) [61]. Twelve patients in the epoetin alfa group and 7 in the SOC had additional thrombotic vascular events. These findings have resulted in a black box warning for perisurgical use of epoetin alfa in the United States, in which, "Antithrombotic prophylaxis should be strongly considered when Procrit is used to reduce allogeneic red blood cell transfusions."

Conclusion

The use of EPO therapy in the perisurgical setting, as well as in oncology, is undergoing re-evaluation in light of recent safety concerns. Supplementation with intravenous iron therapy may improve the dose–response relationship between EPO therapy and erythropoiesis therapy addressing some of the safety concerns. Clinical studies are needed to address these issues.

References

1. Goodnough LT, Monk TG, Andriole GL. Erythropoietin therapy. N Engl J Med 1997;336:933–8.
2. Goodnough LT, Brecher ME, Kanter Mh, AuBuchon JP. Transfusion medicine, part I: blood transfusion. N Engl J Med 1999;340:439–47.

3. Bierbaum BE, Callaghan JJ, Galante EJ, et al. An analysis of blood management in patients having total hip or knee arthroplasty. J Bone Joint Surg 1999;81A:2–10.
4. Goodnough LT, Brittenham G. Limitations of the erythropoietic response to serial phlebotomy: implications for autologous blood donor programs. J Lab Clin Med 1990;115:28–35.
5. Kickler TS, Spivak JL. Effect of repeated whole blood donations on serum immunoreactive erythropoietin levels in autologous donors. JAMA 1988;260:65–7.
6. Goodnough LT, Rudick S, Price TH, et al. Increased collection of autologous blood preoperatively with recombinant human erythropoietin therapy. N Engl J Med 1989;321:1163–7.
7. Goodnough LT, Price TH, Rudnick S. Preoperative red blood cell production in patients undergoing aggressive autologous blood phlebotomy with and without erythropoietin therapy. Transfusion 1992;32:441–5.
8. Goodnough LT, Price TH, EPO Study Group. A phase III trial of recombinant human erythropoietin therapy in non-anemic orthopaedic patients subjected to aggressive autologous blood phlebotomy: dose, response, toxicity, and efficacy. Transfusion 1994;34:66–71.
9. Goodnough LT, Brecher ME, Kanter MH, AuBuchon JB. Autologous blood procurement: transfusion medicine, part II. Blood conservation. N Engl J Med 1999;340:525–33.
10. Mercuriali F, Zanella A, Barosi G, et al. Use erythropoietin to increase the volume of autologous blood donated by orthopaedic patients. Transfusion 1993;33:55.
11. Price TH, Goodnough LT, Vogler W, et al. The effect of recombinant erythropoietin administration on the efficacy of autologous blood donation in patients with low hematocrits. Transfusion 1996;36:29–36.
12. Canadian Orthopedic Perioperative Erythropoietin Study Group. Effectiveness of perioperative recombinant human erythropoietin in elective hip replacement. Lancet 1993;341:1227–32.
13. Faris PM, Ritter MA, Abels RI. The effects of recombinant human erythropoietin on perioperative transfusion requirements in patients undergoing major orthopaedic operation. J Bone Joint Surg 1996;78-A:62–72.
14. de Andrade JR, Jove M, Landon G, Frei D, Guilfoyle M, Young DC. Baseline hemoglobin as a predictor of risk of transfusion and response to epoietin alpha in orthopedic surgery patients. Am J Orthop 1996;25:533–42.
15. Goodnough LT, Verbrugge D, Marcus RE, Goldberg V. The effect of patient size and dose of recombinant human erythropoietin therapy on red blood cell expansion. J Am Coll Surg 1994;179:171–6.
16. Goodnough LT, Price TH, Parvin CA. The endogenous erythropoietin response and the erythropoietic response to blood loss anemia: the effects of age and gender. J Lab Clin Med 1995;126:57–64.
17. Goodnough LT, Marcus RE. Erythropoiesis in patients stimulated with erythropoietin: the relevance of storage iron. Vox Sang 1998;75:128–33.
18. Goodnough LT, Price TH, Parvin CA, et al. Erythropoietin response to anaemia is not altered by surgery or recombinant human erythropoietin therapy. Br J Haematol 1994;87:695–9.
19. Coleman PH, Stevens AR, Dodge HT, Finch CA. Rate of blood regeneration after blood loss. Arch Intern Med 1953;92:341–8.
20. Crosby WH. Treatment of hemochromatosis by energetic phlebotomy. One patient's response to getting 55 liters of blood in 11 months. Br J Haematol 1958;4:82–8.
21. Goodnough LT, Merkel K. The use of parenteral iron and recombinant human erythropoietin therapy to stimulate erythropoiesis in patients undergoing repair of hip fracture. Int J Hematol 1996;1:163–6.
22. Finch CA. Erythropoiesis, erythropoietin, and iron. Blood 1982;60:1241–6.
23. Goodnough LT, Skikne B, Brugnara C. Erythropoietin, iron, and erythropoiesis. Blood 2000;96:823–33.
24. KDOQI clinical practice guidelines and clinical practice recommendations for anemia in chronic kidney disease. Am J Kid Dis 2006;47:511–145.
25. Goodnough LT, Spence R, Shander A. Bloodless medicine:clinical care without allogeneic blood transfusion. Transfusion 2003;43:668–76.
26. Kaisi M, Ngwalle EWK, Runyoro DE, Rogers J. Evaluation and tolerance of response to iron dextran (Imferon) administered by total dose infusion to pregnant women with iron deficiency anemia. Int J Gynecol Obstet 1988;26:235.
27. Mays T, Mays T. Intravenous iron dextran therapy in the treatment of anemia occurring in surgical, gynecologic, and obstetric patients. Surg Gynecol Obstet 1976;143:381.
28. Hamstra RD, Block MH, Schocket AL. Intravenous iron dextran in clinical medicine. JAMA 1980;243:1726.
29. Woodman J, Shaw RJ, Shipman AJ, Edwards AM. A surveillance program on a long-established product: Imferon (Iron Dextran BP). Pharm Med 1987;1:289.

30. Fishbane S, Ungureanu VD, Maeska JK, et al. The safety of intravenous iron dextran in hemodialysis patients. Am J Kidney Dis 1996;28:529–34.
31. Auerbach M, Winchester J, Wahab A, et al. A randomized trial of three iron dextran infusion methods for anemia in EPO-treated dialysis patients. Am J Kidney Dis 1998;31:81.
32. Faich G, Strobos J. Sodium ferric gluconate complex in sucrose: safer intravenous iron therapy than iron dextran. Am J Kidney Dis 1999;33:464.
33. Sunder-Plassmann G, Horl WH. Safety aspects of parenteral iron in patients with end stage renal disease. Drug Saf 1997;17:241.
34. Silverberg DS, Blum M, Peer G, Kaplan E, Iaina A. Intravenous ferric saccharate as an iron supplementation in dialysis patients. Nephron 1996;72:413.
35. Sunder-Plassmann G, Horl WH. Importance of iron supply for erythropoietin therapy. Nephrol Dial Transplant 1995;10:2070.
36. Nissenson AR, Lindsay RM, Swan S, Sellgman P, Strobos J. Sodium ferric gluconate complex in sucrose is safe and effective in hemodialysis patients: North American Trial. Am J Kidney Dis 1999;33: 471.
37. Calvar C, Mata D, Alonso C, Ramos B, Lopez de Novales E. Intravenous administration of iron gluconate during haemodialysis. Nephrol Dial Transplant 1997;12:574.
38. Zanen AL, Adriaansen HJ, Van Bommel EFH, Posthuma R, Th. de Jong GM. "Over saturation" of transferrin after intravenous ferric glucomate (Ferrlecit) in haemodialysis patients. Nephrol Dial Transplant 1996;11:820.
39. Seligman PA, Schleicher RB. Comparison of methods used to measure serum iron in the presence of iron gluconate or iron dextran. Clin Chem 1999;45: 898.
40. Pascual J, Teruel JL, Liano F, Sureda A, Ortuna J. Serious adverse reactions after intravenous ferric gluconate. Nephrol Dial Transplant 1992;7:271.
41. Auerbach M, Goodnough LT, Picard D, Maniatis A. The role of intravenous iron in anemia management and transfusion avoidance. Transfusion, in press.
42. Chertow GM, Mason PD, Vaage-Nilsen O, Ahlmen J. Update on adverse drug events associated with parenteral iron. Nephrol Dial Transplant 2006;21 (2): 378–82.
43. Chandler G, Harchowal J, Macdougall IC. Intravenous iron sucrose: establishing a safe dose. Am J Kidney Dis 2001;38 (5): 988–91.
44. Mamula P, Piccoli DA, Peck SN, Markowitz JE, Baldassano RN. Total dose intravenous infusion of iron dextran for iron-deficiency anemia in children with inflammatory bowel disease. J Pediatr Gastroenterol Nutr 2002;34 (3): 286–90.
45. Fishbane S, Frei GL, Maesaka J. Reduction in recombinant human erythropoietin doses by the use of chronic intravenous iron supplementation. Am J Kidney Dis 1995;26 (1): 41–6.
46. Macdougall IC, Roche A. Administration of intravenous iron sucrose as a 2-minute push to CKD patients: a prospective evaluation of 2,297 injections. Am J Kidney Dis 2005;46 (2): 283–9.
47. Critchley J, Dundar Y. Adverse events associated with intravenous iron infusion (low-molecular-weight iron dextran and iron sucrose): a systematic review. Transfus Altern Transfus Med 2007;9:8–36.
48. Moniem KA, Bhaandari S. Tolerability and efficacy of parenteral iron therapy in hemodialysis patients, a comparison of preparations. Transfus Altern Transfus Med 2007;9:37–42.
49. Sav T, Togoz B, Sipahioglu MH, et al. Is there a difference between the allergic potencies of the iron sucrose and low molecular weight iron dextran? Ren Fail 2007;29 (4): 423–6.
50. Hillman RS, Henderson PA. Control of marrow production by the level of iron supply. J Clin Invest 1969;48:454.
51. Henderson PA, Hillman RS. Characteristics of iron dextran utilization in man. Blood 1969;34:357.
52. Goodnough LT, Monk TG, Andriole GL. Erythropoietin therapy. N Engl J Med 1997;336:933.
53. Messmer K. Consensus statement: using epoietin alfa to decrease the risk of allogeneic blood transfusion in the surgical setting. Semin Hematol 1996;33:73.
54. Goldberg MA, McCutchen JW, Jove M, et al. A safety and efficacy comparison study of two dosing regiments of erythropoietin alfa in patients undergoing major orthopedic surgery. Am J Orthop 1996;25:544–52.
55. Doolittle RF. Biotechnology – the enormous cost of success. N Engl J Med 1991;324:1360–62.
56. Coyle D, Lee KM, Ferguson DA, Laupacis A. Economic analysis of erythropoietin use in orthopaedic surgery. Transfus Med 1999;9:21–39.
57. Messmer K. Consensus statement: using epoietin alfa to decrease the risk of allogeneic blood transfusion in the surgical setting. Semin Hematol 1966;33:73–80.
58. Sans T, Bofill C, Joven J, et al. Effectiveness of very low doses of subcutaneous recombinant

human erythropoietin in facilitating autologous blood donation before orthopedic surgery. Transfusion 1996;36:822–6.

59. Laupacis A, Fergusson D. Erythropoietin to minimize perioperative blood transfusion: a systematic review of randomized trials. Transfus Med 1998;8:309–17.

60. Stowell CP, Chandler H, Jove M, Guilfoyle M, Wacholtz MC. An open-label, randomized study to compare the safety and efficacy of perioperative epoietin alpha with preoperative autologous blood donation in total joint arthoplasty. Orthopedics 1999;22:S105–112.

61. Stowell CP, Jones SC, Enny C, Langholff W, Leitz G. An open-label, randomized, parallel-group study of perioperative epoetin alfa versus standard of care for blood conservation in major elective spinal surgery: safety analysis. Spine 2009;34:2479–85.

CHAPTER 29

Erythropoietin and Iron Therapy in Patients with Renal Failure

Lucia Del Vecchio & Francesco Locatelli
Department of Nephrology, Dialysis, and Renal Transplantation, Alessandro Manzoni Hospital, Lecco, Italy

Introduction

Anemia is a common complication of chronic kidney disease (CKD). It is characterized by a reduced ability of the damaged kidney to produce erythropoietin (EPO), the hormone involved in proliferation and maturation of red blood cells in the bone marrow. Left untreated, anemia may significantly impair quality of life, increase cardiovascular risk, and reduce long-term survival.

Previously, treatment options were essentially limited to blood transfusions; however, since the late 1980s, the availability of recombinant human erythropoietin (rHuEPO) has revolutionized the management of anemia in CKD patients. Today, erythropoiesis-stimulating agents (ESAs) are the main tool for anemia correction in CKD patients.

Treatment indications

Anemia develops early in the course of CKD and it affects nearly all patients with CKD stage 5; treatment with ESAs is a well-established practice that is able to reduce symptoms and complications of anemia. ESA therapy should be given to treat anemia to all CKD patients with a hemoglobin (Hb) level persistently below 11 g/dL after having ruled out all other causes of anemia. This applies to all CKD stages, from the early phases to patients receiving renal replacement therapy [1, 2]. Letting Hb levels fall too much before starting treatment exposes patients to reduced quality of life and increased morbidity. Moreover, patients starting ESA with very low Hb levels need higher ESA doses than those with milder anemia. In order to anticipate Hb decreases, anemia workup should be started before Hb levels are below 11 g/dL (<13.5 g/dL in adult males, <12.0 g/dL in adult females [2].

Aim of treatment: hemoglobin target

A number of observational studies have described a clear relationship between anemia and mortality in CKD patients [3–5]. This is probably due to the impact of chronic anemia on cardiac function, as it causes vasodilatation, cardiac dilation, and increased cardiac output, leading to left ventricular dilation and compensatory hypertrophy.

Starting from this clear association, the availability of an effective therapy to treat renal anemia raised the question whether correcting anemia may improve patient outcome. Several intervention studies have been performed to test this hypothesis. Many of them were also aimed at verifying whether complete rather than partial correction of renal anemia through rHuEPO administration would lead to the best results in terms of survival or surrogate end points (left ventricular mass, quality of life, and CKD progression). This is also important in pharmacoeconomic terms: heading

Alternatives to Blood Transfusion in Transfusion Medicine, 2nd edition. Edited by A. Maniatis, P. Van der Linden, J.-F. Hardy.

to higher Hb targets implies higher ESA doses. Currently, randomized clinical trials [6–9] and meta-analyses [10, 11] do not suggest any major effect of complete anemia correction on hard, intermediate, or surrogate end points, except for quality of life. Considering these findings, there is wide international agreement that today the most reasonable Hb target should be of 11–12 g/dL [12].

The effect of Hb target on progression of kidney disease in patients not on dialysis is unclear. Individual trials showed either prolongation of kidney survival, acceleration of progression to kidney failure, or no effect, but many of the trials were underpowered to detect potentially relevant effects in either direction. For this reason, this aspect is not currently taken into account by international guidelines for the definition of the optimal Hb target.

Types of ESAs

Erythropoietin is a hydrophobic protein of 165 amino acids stabilized by three N-glycans and one O-linked sugar chain; the carbohydrate content is essential to stability and plays some important roles in the activity and biosynthesis of the molecule. The sialic acid-containing carbohydrate content of the molecule is directly related to its serum half-life and in vivo biological activity but is inversely related to its receptor binding affinity. Currently, five different types of ESAs are available in the market: epoetin alfa, epoetin beta, epoetin omega (only in Central and Eastern Europe), darbepoetin alfa, and continuous erythropoiesis receptor activator (CERA). Mean half-life of ESAs are summarized in Table 29.1.

Epoetin alfa and epoetin beta are both synthesized in Chinese hamster ovary cells and share the same amino acid sequence as endogenous EPO; but differences in the manufacturing process between the two glycoproteins translate into slight differences in their carbohydrate moieties [13] as well as their pharmacokinetic and pharmacodynamic properties [14]. Epoetin omega is synthesized in baby hamster kidney cells [15]. It differs from epoetin alfa and epoetin beta in the proportion of O-glycosylation [16]. Epoetin delta shares the same amino acid sequence as endogenous EPO but is synthesized in human cells [17, 18]. This process circumvents problems arising from species-dependent differences in protein folding or posttranslational modification. It has been retired from the market recently.

Darbepoetin alfa is a hyperglycosylated EPO analog designed for prolonged survival in the circulation and thus greater biological activity. Like epoetin alfa and epoetin beta, darbepoetin alfa is produced in Chinese hamster ovary cells. Darbepoetin alfa differs from EPO in the amino acid sequence at five positions and contains five N-linked carbohydrate chains instead of three [19]. As a result, it has increased molecular weight (37,100 Da compared to 30,400 Da), sialic acid content (22 compared to 14 sialic acid residues) and negative charge compared with EPO. In Sprague–Dawley rats, darbepoetin alfa given intravenously had greater in vivo efficacy than rHuEPO. This increased biological activity was due to an increase in the circulating

Table 29.1 Mean half-life ± SD of ESA expressed in hours according to administration route.

	Intravenous	Subcutaneous
Epoetin alfa [14]	6.8 ± 2.7	19.4 ± 10.7
Epoetin beta [14]	8.8 ± 2.2	24.2 ± 11.2
Epoetin omega	ND	ND
Epoetin delta [68]	9.9 (SD not available)	33.1 (SD not available)
Darbepoetin alfa [69]	25.3 ± 7.3	48.8 ± 12.7
CERA [70]	134 ± 19*	139 ± 20†

*CERA dosage of 0.4 μg/kg.
†CERA dosage of 0.8 μg/kg.
CERA, continuous erythropoiesis receptor activator.

half-life, which counterbalanced a lower relative affinity for the EPO receptor than that of rHuEPO. On the basis of the peptide mass, 200 IU of epoetin alfa is equivalent to 1 μg of darbepoetin alfa.

CERA is a large molecule, approximately twice the size of EPO that was created by integrating a single polymer chain into the erythropoietin molecule. In vitro, CERA dissociates faster from the soluble erythropoietin receptor than epoetin beta. It has been suggested that the binding of CERA to the EPO receptor is too brief for internalization, resulting in repeated cycles of receptor binding, stimulation, and dissociation, and consequent increased erythropoietic activity [20]. In 2007, the European Commission approved its use to treat anemia associated with CKD and its entering the market at the beginning of 2009.

In addition to these molecules, new agents are under clinical development. Hematide, a synthetic, dimeric, pegylated peptide derived from original research on the EPO mimetics, is undergoing Phase II and III of its clinical trial program [21]. Its primary amino acid sequence is unrelated to that of rHuEPO. In 28 healthy male volunteers, hematide showed a dose-dependent increase in reticulocytes; the 0.1 mg/kg dose seemed to be the most effective with sustained activity for longer than 1 month [21].

Clinical use of ESAs

All ESAs are effective in correcting renal anemia and increasing Hb levels. However, ESAs differ in amino acid sequence, carbohydrate content, charge, and molecular weight. These characteristics influence their half-life and biological activity and thus their clinical use. Moreover, their pharmacokinetic and pharmacodynamic properties vary according to the route of administration. This is to be chosen not only according to ESA characteristics and economical considerations but also after taking into account CKD stage and the type of renal replacement therapy. In general, the intravenous route is more convenient for hemodialysis patients, whereas the subcutaneous one is preferable in all other CKD patients.

ESA dose requirements are rarely predictable in the individual patient and thus need to be titrated according to Hb increases. In general, predialysis patients are likely to need smaller doses than patients with CKD Stage 5. As a rule, during the correction phase, ESA requirements are 20–30% higher than during the maintenance phase. In order to avoid side effects and/or adverse events (hypertension, seizures, vascular access thrombosis), Hb should be increased slowly during the correction phase, by no more than 1–2 g/dL per month. In general, dose adjustment should not be made in the first month after the start of treatment, and not more often than every 2 weeks thereafter, as time is needed before significant Hb changes following dose or schedule modifications will be observed. These modifications should be determined by the rate of increase in Hb levels during the correction phase, their stability during the maintenance phase, and the frequency of Hb testing (at least monthly) [2]. When Hb levels exceed the target, it is warranted to decrease ESA dose, but preferably not to interrupt treatment. Indeed, this may cause Hb to decrease too much, requiring new ESA treatment at higher doses, eventually leading to excessive Hb cycling. Hb cycling has recently been cited as a risk factor for increased mortality in hemodialysis patients [22].

Epoetin alfa

Epoetin alfa is administered two or three times weekly either intravenously or subcutaneously. Frequency of administration can reasonably be set at once per week in stable HD patients with low dose requirements or in predialysis patients. However, this practice is not supported by clinical trials. In 2002, following the upsurge of pure red cell aplasia (PRCA) cases, its administration by the subcutaneous route was no longer licensed for treatment of CKD patients in many countries. Currently, the subcutaneous use of Eprex® has been readmitted when the vascular access is not available in conjunction with an extensive pharmacovigilance plan.

Generic formulations of epoetin alfa have been approved by European Medicines Agency and entered the European Union market.

Epoetin beta

Dose requirements to maintain target Hb levels are significantly lower when epoetin beta is administered subcutaneously compared with intravenously [23]; current treatment guidelines recommend the subcutaneous route of administration of epoetin beta in order to minimize treatment costs [1, 2]. Like epoetin alfa, epoetin beta has been administered two to three times weekly. However, studies evaluating less frequent administration regimens have demonstrated that once weekly subcutaneous administration during the maintenance phase has the same efficacy as the three-times-weekly regimen [24, 25].

Darbepoetin alfa

Given its longer half-life than rHuEPO, darbepoetin alfa can be administered once a week [26–28] or once every other week [29]. According to the label, the drug can be administered also once a month. In dialysis patients, this may require higher doses to achieve a given Hb target compared with more frequent administration. Data from secondary analyses [27, 28] and from one prospective, randomized crossover, study [30] suggest that dose requirements are independent of the administration route. In other words, patients given the drug intravenously need the same dose as that given subcutaneously.

Continuous erythropoietin receptor activator

Phase II [31, 32] and III [33, 34] studies indicate that CERA corrects anemia and maintains Hb levels within guideline targets when administered up to once monthly in predialysis and dialysis patients. The most suitable starting dose seems to be 0.60 μg/kg given twice monthly.

Dialysis adequacy and response to ESAs

A clear relationship among Hb levels, ESA dose and increase in dialysis dose has been pointed out by a number of prospective or retrospective studies [35, 36]. This is particularly true in patients receiving inadequate dialysis [35]. Increasing attention has also been paid to the relationship between dialysis, increased inflammatory stimulus, and ESA response, as dialysate contamination and low-compatible treatments may increase cytokine production and consequently inhibit erythropoiesis. The biocompatibility of dialysis membranes and flux are other important factors. However, in highly selected, adequately dialyzed patients without iron or vitamin depletion, the effect of these treatment modalities on anemia seems to be smaller than expected [37]. The role of online treatments is still controversial, given that it is still difficult to discriminate between the effect of online hemodiafiltration per se from that of an increased dialysis dose [38].

Failure to respond to treatment

Dose requirements to achieve anemia correction are quite variable and poorly predictable in the individual patient. However, a number of patients need a greater than usual ESA dose and are defined as hyporesponsives. According to the last revision of the European Best Practice Guidelines (EBPG) [1], resistance to ESA treatment is defined as a continued need for >20,000 IU/week (300 IU/kg/week) of rHuEPO administered subcutaneously or 1.5 μg/kg of darbepoetin alfa (greater than 100 μg/week); this means that resistant patients require more than 2.5 times the average ESA dose. The true incidence of ESA hyporesponsiveness is still a matter of study, and probably differs from country to country (in the United States it is likely to be higher than in Europe). According to the definition above, the prevalence of resistance to ESA was only of 2.4% in a recent cross-sectional study of 550 Italian hemodialysis patients [39]. Conversely, the prevalence of hyporesponsiveness to ESA was much greater in a cohort from a large dialysis organization (DaVita) in the United States (43% of the patients received more than 18,000 IU/week of rHuEPO) [22]. In this population of nearly 60,000 subjects, requiring higher ESA doses was a marker of higher death risk. Hyporesponsiveness also occurs in predialysis patients [40].

Causes of incomplete response to ESAs are summarized in Table 29.2. The most common one is iron deficiency—absolute or functional. According to an Italian cross-sectional study [39], 16% of the patients had a transferrin saturation (TSAT) of less than 15%, which is considerably below that recommended in the EBPG and the National Kidney Foundation-Kidney Disease Outcomes Quality Initiative (KDOQI) guidelines. Occult blood loss, infection, inflammation, and inadequate dialysis are also important causes. In recent years, increasing attention has been paid to the relationship between dialysis, increased inflammatory stimulus, malnutrition, and ESA response [39, 41]. Angiotensin-converting enzyme (ACE) inhibitors and angiotensin II receptor antagonists may also play a role. Compliance should be checked in patients self-administering an ESA.

Pure red cell aplasia

Antibody-mediated PRCA is a serious adverse event related to ESA therapy. In this disease, epoetin-induced antibodies neutralize all the exogenous rHuEPO and cross-react with endogenous EPO. As a result, serum EPO levels are undetectable and erythropoiesis becomes ineffective. Despite the widespread use of rHuEPO, PRCA remained a very rare complication for many years. Since 1998, the number of reported cases has increased dramatically [42]; the majority of the cases were observed in patients treated with subcutaneous Eprex® (Janssen-Cilag BV, Tilburg, the Netherlands), the epoetin alfa produced outside the United States. The upsurge coincided with the substitution of human serum albumin by polysorbate 80 in the Eprex formulation. Polysorbate 80 may elicit the formation of epoetin-containing micelles that could be immunogenic. Alternatively, leachates released by uncoated rubber stoppers of prefilled syringes may interact with polysorbate 80 and act as an adjuvant of the immune reaction. After December 2002, the subcutaneous use of Eprex in CKD patients was contraindicated in Europe by regulatory authorities and was strongly discouraged in Canada and Australia. Starting from 2003, the number of reported cases dramatically dropped. This may have been caused by the shift in administration route, reinforcement of product cold chain, or elimination of uncoated rubber syringe stoppers. Interestingly,

Table 29.2 Main causes of resistance to treatment with ESA.

	Chronic kidney disease	
	Related	Unrelated
Iron deficiency	√	√
Chronic blood loss	√	√
Chronic infections and inflammation		√
Malnutrition	√	√
Hyperparathyroidism/osteitis fibrosa	√	
Aluminum toxicity	√	
Malignancies		√
Multiple myeloma, myelofibrosis		√
Hemoglobinopathies		√
Hemolysis	√	√
Vitamin deficiencies (e.g., folate or vitamin B_{12})	√	√
Dialysis-related carnitine deficiency	√	
Inadequate dialysis	√	
Cytotoxic and immunosuppressive agents		√
ACE inhibitors or ARBs		√
Pure red cell aplasia	√	

ACE, angiotensin-converting enzyme; ARB, angiotensin receptor blocker.

despite of the large use of rHuEPO in oncology, cases were identified only in CKD patients.

The number of reported cases of PRCA has decreased sharply since 2003 and with no more cases reported in 2007. This may be due to a change in the route of administration, the reinforcement of the product cold chain or the elimination of uncoated rubber syringe stoppers.

Other complications of ESA treatment

Despite their widespread use, ESAs are effective and safe products. Nevertheless, a number of complications are described (Table 29.3).

Hypertension

A number of pathophysiological mechanisms may explain ESA-induced rise in blood pressure [43]. The increase in blood viscosity secondary to anemia correction appears to be the most obvious one. This is particularly true when anemia correction is achieved too rapidly or higher Hb targets are reached [11]. However, blood pressure changes are often not clearly related to achieved Hb levels. Moreover, even single dose administrations of ESA are capable of inducing hypertension in some patients. Enhanced vascular reactivity and vasoconstrictor responses have been suggested to play a role.

Seizure

Seizure was first reported in early clinical trials in patients who developed severe hypertension in association with a rapid increase in hematocrit [44]. Nowadays, this side effect is quite rare.

Table 29.3 Most common side effects of ESA therapy.

Hypertension
Seizure
Diabetic retinopathy
Thrombotic complications
Vascular access thrombosis
Metabolic disturbances
Headache
Injection-site pain
Pure red cell aplasia

Thrombotic complications

An association of ESA therapy with vascular thrombotic events has been suggested. This complication is more likely when Hb is increased too fast or when it largely exceeds the target, especially in patients with diabetes or already established cardiovascular disease [6, 7]. According to a recent meta-analysis of 9 clinical trials [11], the risk of arteriovenous access thrombosis is significantly higher in patients randomized to near-to-normal Hb levels than in patients randomized to a lower target.

Headache

Clinical trials have noted a 15–17% frequency of headaches in patients receiving ESA [45]. However, the role of ESA is unclear, as end-stage renal disease patients not receiving ESA have a similar rate for headache [45]. Headache is generally mild and usually does not preclude treatment.

Diabetic retinopathy

Erythropoietin increases proliferation of vascular endothelial cells and is a potential retinal angiogenic factor. Experimental data suggest that the binding of EPO to its receptor leads to activation of the mitogen-activated protein kinase pathway; this pathway may elicit angiogenesis in diabetic retinopathy [46]. Today, there is no clinical evidence indicating that ESA is the cause of proliferative retinopathy.

Iron therapy

In CKD patients, iron therapy is not only aimed at correcting iron deficiency, but is also an adjuvant therapy in patients receiving ESA to achieve and maintain the Hb target. In these patients, iron stores may be nearly normal, but during ESA treatment, there may be insufficient immediately available iron to optimize ESA therapy. In this context, iron therapy significantly reduces ESA dose requirements.

Iron status

According to clinical needs, iron status testing should be made every 1–3 months [1,2]. This information should then be weighted together with Hb level, ESA dose, and their trend over time to elucidate the status of both external iron balance (gain or losses) and internal iron balance (distribution of iron in stores and erythrocytes) [2].

Traditional and more widely used iron tests are serum ferritin and TSAT levels. However, these are not optimal tests, as they lack accuracy and stability. Indeed, they are influenced greatly by inflammation and malnutrition, two conditions often affecting CKD patients. For this reason, there has been interest in developing other iron status tests for use in patients with CKD. Two of these, the percentage of hypochromic red blood cells (%HRBC) and the reticulocyte hemoglobin content (CHr), are the most reliable, providing direct insight into bone marrow iron supply and utilization. According to the data by Tessitore et al. [47] a %HRBC level greater than 6% is the single most accurate predictor of response to intravenous iron treatment in hemodialysis patients. Unfortunately, %HRBC is affected by inflammation and is positively influenced by erythropoietic activity, as reticulocytes are considered hypochromic by cell counters. CHr has been found to be an early predictor of response to iron therapy in hemodialysis patients [48]. However, the cutoff of this marker to discriminate iron deficiency still needs to be fully clarified [49]. Currently, neither test is as easy to use, cost-effective, and widely available as the traditional tests, such as serum ferritin and TSAT.

The reticulocyte hemoglobin equivalent (RET-He), recently introduced to determine the forward scatter of fluorescence-labeled reticulocytes, seems to be a sensitive indicator of iron-deficiency anemia. Compared with CHr, the value of 30.5 pg for RET-He appears to be the best cutoff point with a very good sensitivity and specificity to determine patients needing iron supplementation [50]. Combined use of CHr and high-fluorescence reticulocyte count is very accurate in predicting response to intravenous iron therapy in hemodialysis patients [51].

Soluble transferrin receptor is not affected by acute inflammation; however, it reflects ongoing erythropoiesis and not iron availability [52]. Zinc protoporphyrin (ZPP) concentration has also been suggested as an indicator of functional iron deficiency. In cases of iron deficiency, zinc replaces iron in newly formed protoporphyrin IX to form ZPP. However, ZPP is an inferior measure of iron availability and ESA response compared with %HRBC and CHr [1].

An ideal marker of functional iron deficiency should be independent of erythropoietic activity. New cell counters are able to determine cell volume and Hb concentration separately on reticulocytes and mature erythrocytes. According to Bovy et al. [53], overall RBC was not significantly different from RBC assessed only in mature erythrocytes.

Targets of iron therapy

For patients on hemodialysis, the last available international guideline on anemia [2] recommends the following iron targets in hemodialysis patients:

- serum ferritin—200–500 ng/mL
- TSAT—>20% or CHr >29 pg/cell

Support for the guideline comes from several interventional trials [54–57]. The upper limit of serum ferritin of 500 ng/mL was chosen in order minimize the risks of iron overload, without denying iron therapy to inflamed patients who may have high ferritin levels but functional iron deficit.

Evidence for iron target in CKD patients not on dialysis and in patients on peritoneal dialysis (PD) is poorer. In these patients, lower serum ferritin levels are probably adequate to ensure effective erythropoiesis with ESA treatment, with a suggested target of 100–500 ng/mL [2].

Iron administration

There is wide consensus that the preferred route of iron administration is intravenous in hemodialysis patients; in PD patients and CKD patients not on dialysis, the route of iron administration can be either intravenous or oral [1,2].

Oral iron is absorbed best when given without food; constipation, diarrhea, nausea, or abdominal pain limit compliance.

Iron dextran, ferric gluconate, and iron sucrose are available for intravenous administration. They differ in pharmacokinetics, maximum dose size, maximum rate of infusion [58], and in the rate of adverse reactions [59, 60]. In particular, anaphylactic reactions have been mainly described following administration of iron dextran [61]. This is particularly true for the high-molecular weight formulation; ferric gluconate and iron sucrose are associated with lower rates of serious adverse events [62, 63]. The safety and the efficacy of ferumoxytol, a semisynthetic carbohydrate-coated iron oxide, is undergoing phase III clinical trials [64].

There are two main approaches to i.v. iron administration, both valuable and widely used. The first is the episodic administration of a series of i.v. doses when iron tests go below the target; the second is the regular administration of smaller doses to maintain stable iron levels [65]. No randomized clinical trial so far has compared the efficacy and safety of these two approaches.

Some worries persist on possible long-term complications of i.v. iron therapy. An increased risk of infection has been suggested to be associated with iron overload and iron administration [66]. In addition, iron therapy may cause in vitro and in vivo oxidation of lipids and proteins, leading to oxidative damage [67]. Their clinical relevance is still to be elucidated.

References

1. Locatelli F, Aljama P, Barany P, et al. Revised European best practice guidelines for the management of anaemia in patients with chronic renal failure. Nephrol Dial Transplant 2004;19(Suppl. 2):ii1–47.
2. KDOQI clinical practice guidelines and clinical practice recommendations for anemia in chronic kidney disease. Am J Kidney Dis 2006;47:S11–145.
3. Collins AJ, Li S, St Peter W, et al. Death, hospitalization, and economic associations among incident hemodialysis patients with hematocrit values of 36 to 39%. J Am Soc Nephrol 2001;12:2465–73.
4. Locatelli F, Pisoni RL, Combe C, et al. Anaemia in haemodialysis patients of five European countries: association with morbidity and mortality in the Dialysis Outcomes and Practice Patterns Study (DOPPS). Nephrol Dial Transplant 2004;19:121–32.
5. Volkova N, Arab L. Evidence-based systematic literature review of hemoglobin/hematocrit and all-cause mortality in dialysis patients. Am J Kidney Dis 2006;47:24–36.
6. Besarab A, Bolton WK, Browne JK, et al. The effects of normal as compared with low hematocrit values in patients with cardiac disease who are receiving hemodialysis and epoetin. N Engl J Med 1998;339: 584–90.
7. Parfrey PS, Foley RN, Wittreich BH, et al. Double-blind comparison of full and partial anemia correction in incident hemodialysis patients without symptomatic heart disease. J Am Soc Nephrol 2005;16: 2180–89.
8. Drueke TB, Locatelli F, Clyne N, et al. Normalization of hemoglobin level in patients with chronic kidney disease and anemia. N Engl J Med 2006;355:2071–84.
9. Singh AK, Szczech L, Tang KL, et al. Correction of anemia with epoetin alfa in chronic kidney disease. N Engl J Med 2006;355:2085–98.
10. Strippoli GF, Craig JC, Manno C, Schena FP. Hemoglobin targets for the anemia of chronic kidney disease: a meta-analysis of randomized, controlled trials. J Am Soc Nephrol 2004;15:3154–65.
11. Phrommintikul A, Haas SJ, Elsik M, Krum H. Mortality and target haemoglobin concentrations in anaemic patients with chronic kidney disease treated with erythropoietin: a meta-analysis. Lancet 2007;369: 381–8.
12. KDOQI clinical practice guideline and clinical practice recommendations for anemia in chronic kidney disease: 2007 update of hemoglobin target. Am J Kidney Dis 2007;50:471–530.
13. Storring PL, Tiplady RJ, Gaines Das RE, et al. Epoetin alfa and beta differ in their erythropoietin isoform compositions and biological properties. Br J Haematol 1998;100:79–89.
14. Halstenson CE, Macres M, Katz SA, et al. Comparative pharmacokinetics and pharmacodynamics of epoetin alfa and epoetin beta. Clin Pharmacol Ther 1991;50:702–12.
15. Powell JS, Berkner KL, Lebo RV, Adamson JW. Human erythropoietin gene: high level expression in stably transfected mammalian cells and chromosome localization. Proc Natl Acad Sci USA 1986;83:6465–9.
16. Nimtz M, Martin W, Wray V, et al. Structures of sialylated oligosaccharides of human erythropoietin expressed in recombinant BHK-21 cells. Eur J Biochem 1993;213:39–56.

17. Deicher R, Horl WH. Differentiating factors between erythropoiesis-stimulating agents: a guide to selection for anaemia of chronic kidney disease. Drugs 2004;64:499–509.
18. Kwan JT, Pratt RD. Epoetin delta, erythropoietin produced in a human cell line, in the management of anaemia in predialysis chronic kidney disease patients. Curr Med Res Opin 2007;23:307–11.
19. Egrie JC, Browne JK. Development and characterization of novel erythropoiesis stimulating protein (NESP). Nephrol Dial Transplant 2001;16(Suppl. 3):3–13.
20. Macdougall IC. CERA (Continuous Erythropoietin Receptor Activator): a new erythropoiesis-stimulating agent for the treatment of anemia. Curr Hematol Rep 2005;4:436–40.
21. Stead RB, Lambert J, Wessels D, et al. Evaluation of the safety and pharmacodynamics of Hematide, a novel erythropoietic agent, in a phase 1, double-blind, placebo-controlled, dose-escalation study in healthy volunteers. Blood 2006;108:1830–34.
22. Regidor DL, Kopple JD, Kovesdy CP, et al. Associations between changes in hemoglobin and administered erythropoiesis-stimulating agent and survival in hemodialysis patients. J Am Soc Nephrol 2006;17:1181–91.
23. Kaufman JS, Reda DJ, Fye CL, et al. Subcutaneous compared with intravenous epoetin in patients receiving hemodialysis. Department of Veterans Affairs Cooperative Study Group on Erythropoietin in Hemodialysis Patients. N Engl J Med 1998;339:578–83.
24. Weiss LG, Clyne N, Divino Fihlho J, et al. The efficacy of once weekly compared with two or three times weekly subcutaneous epoetin beta: results from a randomized controlled multicentre trial. Swedish Study Group. Nephrol Dial Transplant 2000;15:2014–19.
25. Locatelli F, Baldamus CA, Villa G, et al. Once-weekly compared with three-times-weekly subcutaneous epoetin beta: results from a randomized, multicenter, therapeutic-equivalence study. Am J Kidney Dis 2002;40:119–25.
26. Locatelli F, Olivares J, Walker R, et al. Novel erythropoiesis stimulating protein for treatment of anemia in chronic renal insufficiency. Kidney Int 2001;60:741–7.
27. Locatelli F, Canaud B, Giacardy F, et al. Treatment of anaemia in dialysis patients with unit dosing of darbepoetin alfa at a reduced dose frequency relative to recombinant human erythropoietin (rHuEpo). Nephrol Dial Transplant 2003;18:362–9.
28. Vanrenterghem Y, Barany P, Mann JF, et al. Randomized trial of darbepoetin alfa for treatment of renal anemia at a reduced dose frequency compared with rHuEPO in dialysis patients. Kidney Int 2002;62:2167–75.
29. Mann J, Kessler M, Villa G, et al. Darbepoetin alfa once every 2 weeks for treatment of anemia in dialysis patients: a combined analysis of eight multicenter trials. Clin Nephrol 2007;67:140–48.
30. Aarup M, Bryndum J, Dieperink H, Joffe P. Clinical implications of converting stable haemodialysis patients from subcutaneous to intravenous administration of darbepoetin alfa. Nephrol Dial Transplant 2006;21:1312–16.
31. de Francisco AL, Sulowicz W, Klinger M, et al. Continuous Erythropoietin Receptor Activator (C.E.R.A.) administered at extended administration intervals corrects anaemia in patients with chronic kidney disease on dialysis: a randomised, multicentre, multiple-dose, phase II study. Int J Clin Pract 2006;60: 1687–96.
32. Provenzano R, Besarab A, Macdougall IC, et al. The continuous erythropoietin receptor activator (C.E.R.A.) corrects anemia at extended administration intervals in patients with chronic kidney disease not on dialysis: results of a phase II study. Clin Nephrol 2007;67:306–17.
33. Levin NW, Fishbane S, Cañedo FV, et al. MAXIMA study investigators. Intravenous methoxy polyethylene glycol-epoetin beta for haemoglobin control in patients with chronic kidney disease who are on dialysis: a randomised non-inferiority trial (MAXIMA). Lancet 2007;370(9596):1415–21.
34. Macdougall IC, Walker R, Provenzano R, et al. ARCTOS Study Investigators. C.E.R.A. corrects anemia in patients with chronic kidney disease not on dialysis: results of a randomized clinical trial. Clin J Am Soc Nephrol 2008;3(2):337–47.
35. Ifudu O, Feldman J, Friedman EA. The intensity of hemodialysis and the response to erythropoietin in patients with end-stage renal disease. N Engl J Med 1996;334:420–25.
36. Coladonato JA, Frankenfield DL, Reddan DN, et al. Trends in anemia management among US hemodialysis patients. J Am Soc Nephrol 2002;13:1288–95.
37. Locatelli F, Andrulli S, Pecchini F, et al. Effect of high-flux dialysis on the anaemia of haemodialysis patients. Nephrol Dial Transplant 2000;15:1399–409.
38. Bonforte G, Grillo P, Zerbi S, Surian M. Improvement of anemia in hemodialysis patients treated

by hemodiafiltration with high-volume on-line-prepared substitution fluid. Blood Purif 2002;20:357–63.
39. Locatelli F, Andrulli S, Memoli B, et al. Nutritional-inflammation status and resistance to erythropoietin therapy in haemodialysis patients. Nephrol Dial Transplant 2006;21:991–8.
40. Rossert J, Gassmann-Mayer C, Frei D, McClellan W. Prevalence and predictors of epoetin hyporesponsiveness in chronic kidney disease patients. Nephrol Dial Transplant 2007;22:794–800.
41. Kalantar-Zadeh K, McAllister CJ, Lehn RS, et al. Effect of malnutrition-inflammation complex syndrome on EPO hyporesponsiveness in maintenance hemodialysis patients. Am J Kidney Dis 2003;42:761–73.
42. Gershon SK, Luksenburg H, Cote TR, Braun MM. Pure red-cell aplasia and recombinant erythropoietin. N Engl J Med 2002;346:1584–6; author reply-6.
43. Zhu X, Perazella MA. Nonhematologic complications of erythropoietin therapy. Semin Dial 2006;19:279–84.
44. Edmunds ME, Walls J, Tucker B, et al. Seizures in haemodialysis patients treated with recombinant human erythropoietin. Nephrol Dial Transplant 1989;4:1065–9.
45. Eschbach JW, Abdulhadi MH, Browne JK, et al. Recombinant human erythropoietin in anemic patients with end-stage renal disease. Results of a phase III multicenter clinical trial. Ann Intern Med 1989;111:992–1000.
46. Watanabe D, Suzuma K, Matsui S, et al. Erythropoietin as a retinal angiogenic factor in proliferative diabetic retinopathy. N Engl J Med 2005;353:782–92.
47. Tessitore N, Solero GP, Lippi G, et al. The role of iron status markers in predicting response to intravenous iron in haemodialysis patients on maintenance erythropoietin. Nephrol Dial Transplant 2001;16:1416–23.
48. Fishbane S, Galgano C, Langley RC, Jr, et al. Reticulocyte hemoglobin content in the evaluation of iron status of hemodialysis patients. Kidney Int 1997;52:217–22.
49. Horl WH. Clinical aspects of iron use in the anemia of kidney disease. J Am Soc Nephrol 2007;18:382–93.
50. Garzia M, Di Mario A, Ferraro E, et al. Reticulocyte hemoglobin equivalent: an indicator of reduced iron availability in chronic kidney diseases during erythropoietin therapy. Lab Hematol 2007;13:6–11.
51. Chuang CL, Liu RS, Wei YH, et al. Early prediction of response to intravenous iron supplementation by reticulocyte haemoglobin content and high-fluorescence reticulocyte count in haemodialysis patients. Nephrol Dial Transplant 2003;18:370–77.
52. Brugnara C. Iron deficiency and erythropoiesis: new diagnostic approaches. Clin Chem 2003;49:1573–8.
53. Bovy C, Gothot A, Delanaye P, et al. Mature erythrocyte parameters as new markers of functional iron deficiency in haemodialysis: sensitivity and specificity. Nephrol Dial Transplant 2007;22:1156–62.
54. Besarab A, Amin N, Ahsan M, et al. Optimization of epoetin therapy with intravenous iron therapy in hemodialysis patients. J Am Soc Nephrol 2000;11:530–38.
55. DeVita MV, Frumkin D, Mittal S, et al. Targeting higher ferritin concentrations with intravenous iron dextran lowers erythropoietin requirement in hemodialysis patients. Clin Nephrol 2003;60:335–40.
56. Fishbane S, Shapiro W, Dutka P, et al. A randomized trial of iron deficiency testing strategies in hemodialysis patients. Kidney Int 2001;60:2406–11.
57. Kaneko Y, Miyazaki S, Hirasawa Y, et al. Transferrin saturation versus reticulocyte hemoglobin content for iron deficiency in Japanese hemodialysis patients. Kidney Int 2003;63:1086–93.
58. Danielson BG. Structure, chemistry, and pharmacokinetics of intravenous iron agents. J Am Soc Nephrol 2004;15(Suppl. 2):S93–8.
59. Charytan C, Levin N, Al-Saloum M, et al. Efficacy and safety of iron sucrose for iron deficiency in patients with dialysis-associated anemia: North American clinical trial. Am J Kidney Dis 2001;37:300–307.
60. Michael B, Coyne DW, Fishbane S, et al. Sodium ferric gluconate complex in hemodialysis patients: adverse reactions compared to placebo and iron dextran. Kidney Int 2002;61:1830–39.
61. Walters BA, Van Wyck DB. Benchmarking iron dextran sensitivity: reactions requiring resuscitative medication in incident and prevalent patients. Nephrol Dial Transplant 2005;20:1438–42.
62. Chertow GM, Mason PD, Vaage-Nilsen O, Ahlmén J. Update on adverse drug events associated with parenteral iron. Nephrol Dial Transplant 2006;21(2):378–82.
63. Auerbach M, Rodgers GM. Intravenous iron. N Engl J Med 2007;357(1):93–4.
64. Spinowitz BS, Kausz AT, Baptista J, et al. Ferumoxytol for treating iron deficiency anemia in CKD. J Am Soc Nephrol 2008;19(8):1599–605.
65. Schiesser D, Binet I, Tsinalis D, et al. Weekly low-dose treatment with intravenous iron sucrose maintains iron status and decreases epoetin requirement

in iron-replete haemodialysis patients. Nephrol Dial Transplant 2006;21:2841–5.
66. Brewster UC, Perazella MA. Intravenous iron and the risk of infection in end-stage renal disease patients. Semin Dial 2004;17:57–60.
67. Pai AB, Boyd AV, McQuade CR, et al. Comparison of oxidative stress markers after intravenous administration of iron dextran, sodium ferric gluconate, and iron sucrose in patients undergoing hemodialysis. Pharmacotherapy 2007;27:343–50.
68. Smith WB, Dowell JA, Pratt RD. Pharmacokinetics and pharmacodynamics of epoetin delta in two studies in healthy volunteers and two studies in patients with chronic kidney disease. Clin Ther 2007;29:1368–80.
69. Macdougall IC, Gray SJ, Elston O, et al. Pharmacokinetics of novel erythropoiesis stimulating protein compared with epoetin alfa in dialysis patients. J Am Soc Nephrol 1999;10:2392–5.
70. Macdougall IC, Robson R, Opatrna S, et al. Pharmacokinetics and pharmacodynamics of intravenous and subcutaneous continuous erythropoietin receptor activator (C.E.R.A.) in patients with chronic kidney disease. Clin J Am Soc Nephrol 2006;1:1211–15.

CHAPTER 30
Hemoglobin-based Blood Substitutes

G. Deby-Dupont[1], *Bernadette Remy*[2] *& Maurice Lamy*[2]
[1]Centre of Oxygen Research and Development, University of Liege, Liege, Belgium
[2]Department of Anaesthesia and Intensive Care Medicine, University Hospital, Domaine universitaire du Sart Tilman, Liège, Beligum

The risk of transmission of viral diseases and the difficulty to perform correct donor screenings in some countries created the mistrust in the hospital practice of allogeneic blood transfusion, what, together with the increase in blood request and military interest, boosted the development of blood substitutes. Different solutions have been proposed [1–4], but this review only deals with hemoglobin (Hb)-based solutions of the first and second generations, which have reached the stage of large clinical assays, are still under development or have entered clinical trials [5, 6].

First attempts to replace blood with free Hb solutions

The first attempts to replace blood in human were done in the nineteenth century with solutions of lysed erythrocytes. Side effects were described such as fever, chills, headache, and nausea [7, 8]. Further studies reported toxic effects, which were attributed to the presence of residual fragments of erythrocyte membranes and lipids. But, despite careful purification to obtain stroma-free Hb (SFH), the administration of a free Hb solution remained an "at risk" intervention, mainly for its hypertensive effect and rapid catabolism leading to renal toxicity [7–10].

Hb toxicity is linked to the structure of the molecule, the presence of the ferrous (Fe^{2+}) iron, and the binding of oxygen (O_2). Hb is a tetrameric molecule, with 2α and 2β hemic (Fe^{2+}) monomers, linked by a weak bound between the identical monomers and a tight bound between the α and β monomers. Free Hb is rapidly broken into dimers, which are taken up by plasma proteins and discarded from the circulation. When the binding capacity of plasma proteins is overwhelmed, the tetramers and dimers reach the kidney causing hemoglobinuria and nephrotoxicity. The tetramers also cross the endothelium and extravasate into the interstitial spaces ("jaundice-like" syndrome).

Hb in erythrocytes is under the form of oxyhemoglobin (high affinity for O_2) and deoxyhemoglobin (low affinity for O_2) [11]. The affinity for O_2 depends on the partial pressure of O_2 (pO_2) and the pH (Bohr effect) of the blood. The arterial pO_2 corresponding to 50% saturation of the Hb molecule (P_{50}) is 26–27 mmHg. The transition from oxy- to deoxyhemoglobin is regulated by allosteric effectors like 2,3 diphosphoglycerate (2,3-DPG). In the deoxygenated Hb molecule, a slight modification of the monomer structure renders the Fe^{2+} atom more sensitive to oxidation into Fe^{3+} generating methemoglobin (metHb) and producing reactive oxygen species.

Definition of the ideal Hb-based blood substitute

Solutions of free Hb cannot replace the red blood cells in all their functions, since Hb is obtained by the lysis of the erythrocytes and further

Alternatives to Blood Transfusion in Transfusion Medicine, 2nd edition. Edited by A. Maniatis, P. Van der Linden, J.-F. Hardy.

Table 30.1 Sources and techniques used to obtain the free Hb molecule, and short description of advantages and problems for each type of Hb.

Source of Hb	Technical way of obtention	Advantages	Problems
Human blood	Hb extraction from outdated donor blood and modification of Hb molecule	Cheap source	Number of blood donors is decreasing, improvement of blood storage diminishes waste blood
Cow blood	Hb extraction from slaughterhoused cow blood	Cheap and abundant. No need of Hb modification	Possible effects on immune system. Transmission of disease
Micro-organisms (genetic engineering)	Genetic modification of bacteria, fungi, or plants to produce Hb	Unlimited source of pure Hb. No ethical or culture objection	Difficulty and cost of large-scale production
Transgenic animals	Introduction of human genes producing Hb in animal fetus and production by mature individuals	Unlimited source and large volumes	Ethical objections. Need of complex Hb extraction.

purified: the numerous components included in the red blood cell are lost. The term blood substitute is thus misleading: these solutions are developed primarily with the function of carrying O_2 to tissues, and it is thus more accurate to design them by the terms "cell-free oxygen carriers," "Hb-based oxygen carriers (HBOCs)" or "oxygen therapeutics." Together with the property of carrying O_2, a red blood substitute must be free of the problems presented by donated human blood and must have all the following properties [4, 6, 7]:

- Free of toxicity and side effects (no chemical reaction, physiological values of pH, viscosity, and oncotic pressure);
- Adequate O_2 uptake in the lungs and adequate delivery to tissues;
- Sufficient half-life time in the circulation to avoid repeated administrations
- Harmful and rapid excretion;
- Stable at room temperature, easy to store, and easy to use;
- Easy to sterilize (to assure the absence of pathogens and viruses transmission);
- Cheap to manufacture;
- Widely applicable by no need of crossmatching or compatibility tests.

First generation of HBOCs

The HBOCs of the first generation are prepared with free Hb of different sources, after a careful purification [12]. Two problems to overcome are the Hb dissociation and the excessive affinity of free Hb for O_2 due to the absence of 2,3-DPG: chemical modifications of the Hb molecule and its encapsulation try to solve these problems.

Sources of free Hb

The sources of Hb molecules used in the first-generation HBOCs are summarized in Table 30.1.

Free human Hb is obtained from lysis of the erythrocytes from outdated banked blood and carefully purified to eliminate stromal remnants, considered as responsible for undesirable effects, like vasomotor effects, activation of the complement, kinin and coagulation systems, nephrotoxicity, interference with macrophage function, antigenic effects, histamine release, and iron deposits. Free human Hb has an increased affinity for O_2 (P_{50}: 12–14 mmHg) compared with intracellular Hb, because it lacks the allosteric inhibitor 2,3-DPG [13], and thus delivers less O_2 to the tissues. Human Hb solutions have a high colloid oncotic pressure, which limits Hb concentration to 7 g/dL, and must be stored in an anaerobic environment to avoid the oxidation into metHb.

The bovine source is particularly interesting for easy and cheap access. Bovine free Hb is obtained by procedures similar to those applied for human Hb, but does not require 2,3-DPG to control its affinity for O_2. It has a P_{50} of approximately 30 mmHg, favoring O_2 delivery to the tissues. But its use is limited by the risk of transmission of bovine spongiform encephalopathy, difficulties with purification causing persistence of membrane fragments, and the possible production of antibodies due to infusion of large quantities of bovine proteins.

Recombinant technology has produced a hybrid Hb product, a synthetic heme bound to recombinant human albumin, with a P_{50} value similar to that of human erythrocytes and an intravascular life greater than 36 hours in rats [14]. A recombinant human Hb has been produced in *Escherichia coli*, of which the genome is designed to produce the native human Hb [15], a di-α-globin molecule in which the 2 α chains are fused and cannot dissociate in plasma [16] or the Presbyterian Hb with a mutation on β chains resulting in changes in the allosteric control mechanism and a lower affinity for O_2 [17]. This Hb variant (Optro®, Somatogen) has a P_{50} higher (30–33 mmHg) than the natural Hb with an improved O_2 delivery, a plasma half-life 4 times greater than free Hb, and an indefinite storage life when frozen. Recombinant Hb is also developed in yeast and transgenic plants [3, 18], but for large scale production, the recombinant molecule has to be produced at a high yield, with a high level of gene expression, correct protein folding and assembly, and purification from the other products of microorganism or the plant while maintaining reasonable cost.

Attempts are made to produce recombinant Hb in transgenic animal (pigs, mice), but the red cells of the transgenic animals contain human Hb, animal Hb, and a hybrid: techniques of isolation and purification of the human Hb and to scale up the production are still to improve.

Chemical modifications of Hb molecule

The following modifications have been tried: internal stabilization of the tetrameric molecule by cross-linking of dimers, pyridoxylation, surface modification by conjugation with large molecules, polymerization, and encapsulation in synthetic liposomes [7, 19].

The intramolecular cross-linking is obtained with polyanionic molecules (often diacids) reacting at specific cationic binding loci. A chemical bond between the α monomers is obtained by acetylation of Hb at physiologic pH by acetylsalicylic acid (aspirin), or by bis (3,5 dibromosalicyl) fumarate (DBBF), the diester of dibromo actelylsalicylic acid [20]. Diaspirin Cross-Linked Hb (DCLHb) is a typical example of an α–α cross-linked Hb prepared by reaction with DBBF. A β–β cross-linking is obtained by reaction with bis-pyridoxal-5-phosphate, an analog of 2,3-DPG. Intramolecular cross-linking is also obtained with dialdehydes derived from the oxidation of the cyclic structure of sugar (o-raffinose) or open ring-adenosine triphosphate (o-ATP) [21]. These cross-linked Hb have a circulation half-time varying from a few to 30 hours (depending on the dose administered) and are characterized by a P_{50} of 30–35 mmHg.

The intermolecular cross-linking of intramolecularly cross-linked Hb is obtained by reaction with macromolecules [hydroxyethyl starch, polyethyleneglycol (PEG), Dextran 20] or artificial support ("nanocrystalline" beads). It aims at increasing the stability and modifying the surface electric charges of Hb, what will reduce the extravasation of Hb, and increase its plasma half-life. Polymerization is obtained with cross-linkers (cyanate or glutaraldehyde reagents) that react on surface amino groups and link adjacent molecules. External cross-linked and polymerized Hbs have molecular weight ranging from 64,000 to 400,000 Da, what increases the risk of immunogenicity but decreases the renal toxicity, increases the lifetime in blood, and allows the administration of important concentrations without increase of the oncotic pressure. They correctly deliver O_2 to tissues even when infused at low doses. Pyridoxalated Hb polyoxyethylene (PHP) is an example of human Hb internally cross-linked with pyridoxal phosphate to lower its affinity for O2, and conjugated with polyoxyethylene. PolyHeme® is a glutaraldehyde polymerized human Hb, and HemoLink® a cross-linked human Hb further polymerized with ring-opened raffinose (o-raffinose). Hemopure® is prepared from bovine hemoglobin polymerized with glutaraldehyde [8].

Encapsulation of Hb

In red blood cells, Hb is "encapsulated" into the cell membrane with many other compounds, especially antioxidant systems and enzymes to prevent the oxidation into MetHb. Polymerized Hb can be cross-linked to catalase and superoxide dismutase (Poly-Hb-SOD-CAT) to avoid the oxidation by reactive oxygen species in pathological conditions such as ischemia reperfusion [22,23]. Modified Hb is also encapsulated into synthetic, nonantigenic vesicles prepared from synthetic lipids, which do not activate the platelets (the "Hb-vesicles") [24]. A coencapsulation of protective and regulatory molecules is possible to mimic the erythrocytes and form "artificial red blood cells" [23]. The encapsulation and coencapsulation techniques attenuate the vasoactive effects, and yield a P_{50} of 30 mmHg, with a convenient kinetics of O_2 binding and delivery. But artificial red blood cells have a short circulation time due to a rapid phagocytosis and uptake by reticuloendothelium system, with hepatic overload in relation with the infused volume. Modifications of the surface properties by addition of polysaccharides modestly change the circulation time, but increase the size of the microcapsules (1–5 μm). Another possibility is the encapsulation in lipid membrane liposomes and PEG-lipid vesicles, what increases the circulation lifetime [23].

Current status of first-generation HBOCs

The benefits of the HBOCs include universal compatibility, immediate availability, and long-term storage. Their main functions are to carry O_2 and to restore adequate volume in a large range of clinical situations with important blood loss such as cardiac surgery [4, 25] and trauma [26]. Several HBOCs reached phase II and III clinical trials (Table 30.2).

Table 30.2 Hemoglobin-based blood substitutes (or Hb-based oxygen carriers) in clinical trials.

Product name	Company	Characteristics	Clinical trial
HemAssist™	Baxter Healthcare Corp. (Boulder, CO, USA)	Cross-linked (α–α)Hb	Discontinued; safety (increased mortality)
Optro®	Somatogen, Inc. And Baxter Healthcare Corp. (Boulder, CO, USA)	Human recombinant Hb (rHb 1-1 and rHb 2-0) (α-–α bond; amino acid substitution)	Discontinued; safety (hypertension)
PolyHeme®	Northfield Laboratories Inc. (Evanston, IL, USA)	Polymerized human Hb (glutaraldehyde, pyridoxal)	Phase III (trauma, surgery)
Hemopure® (HBOC-201)	Biopure Corp. (Cambridge, MA, USA)	Polymerized bovine Hb (glutaraldehyde)	Phase II (USA) on hold
HemoLink®	Hemosol Inc. (Mississauga, Canada)	Polymerized cross-linked human Hb (o-raffinose)	Discontinued; safety (myocardial infarction)
PHP	Apex Bioscience	Conjugated human Hb (PEG, pyridoxal)	Phase III septic shock
PEG-Hemoglobin	Enzon	Conjugated bovine Hb (PEG)	Discontinued
Hemospan®	Sangart Inc. (San Diego, CA, USA)	Conjugated human Hb (PEG)	Entering phase III

PHP: pyridoxalated Hb polyoxyethylene; PEG: polyethylene glycol.

Table 30.3 Problems encountered with Hb-based blood substitutes in clinical trials [4, 6].

Type of problem	Possible cause of the problem
Vasoconstriction (increase in systemic and pulmonary arterial pressure and vascular resistance)	NO scavenging, activation of endothelin production, direct stimulation of alpha adrenergic receptors
"Jaundice-like" syndrome	Hb extravasation (endothelial cells, tissues)
Nephrotoxicity (oliguria, hematuria)	Direct toxicity leading to kidney dysfunction (tubular obstruction and necrosis)*
Increase in blood levels of metHb (production of reactive oxygen species)	Hb autoxidation (during storage or in vivo?)
Bilirubinemia	Hb destruction (short lifetime in circulation) and overload of Hb elimination capacity of plasma
Cardiovascular events (myocardial infarction)	NO scavenging? Direct toxicity on organ?
Neurotoxicity	Direct toxicity on organ?
Gastrointestinal symptoms (abdominal discomfort, pain, nausea, vomiting)	Binding of NO? direct toxicity on intestine?
Elevation of blood levels of liver enzymes	Direct toxicity leading to organ dysfunction?
Elevation of blood levels of pancreatic enzymes	Direct toxicity leading to organ dysfunction?
Increased bacterial virulence (in septic patients)	Iron supply
Interference with macrophage function	Blocking of macrophage functions by binding of Hb-haptoglobin complexes to receptors?
Activation of complement, kinin, and coagulation cascades	NO scavenging leading to platelet aggregation?
Immunogenicity	Xenogeneic Hb, important chemical modification of Hb (polymerization)
Interference with laboratory tests	"Hemolysis-like" effect

*Cross-linked Hb passes across renal peritubular capillaries and is found in renal hilar lymph [27].

But they have a short intravascular life-time, thus unlikely to use in the treatment of chronic anemia, and carry many side effects, with variable consequences (Table 30.3) [4, 6, 27]. Therefore, several manufacturers stopped the clinical trials and the production of HBOCs.

HBOCs for which clinical assays are stopped or on hold

HemAssist™ (DCLHb; Baxter Healthcare Corp.) reached phase II and III clinical trials in orthopedic surgery, abdominal aortic repair surgery, major abdominal surgery, and cardiac surgery. In surgery patients, modest results in allogeneic blood cell transfusion avoidance, increased adverse events (including hypertension, yellowing of the skin, hemoglobinuria, and pancreatic suffering) and short plasma persistence of DCLHb (±24 hours) did not support the routine use for transfusion avoidance [25, 28]. A phase III clinical study in noncardiac surgery was stopped early for safety concerns [29]. In the European "on-scene" multicenter study in trauma patients with severe hemorrhagic shock, the mortality was not significantly different in the treated group (44%) versus the standard treatment group (37%). But adverse events were increased (not significantly: 90% versus 76%), and 10% of the patients in the treated group developed pancreatitis. The study was prematurely arrested for lack of efficacy [30]. In a similar phase III study in the USA in patients with severe traumatic hemorrhagic shock, an increased mortality was observed [31]. Subsequently, ongoing clinical trials were arrested and Baxter stopped the development of DCLHb.

After successful safety trial in volunteers [32], the phase II clinical study with the recombinant Hb (Optro®, Somatogen Inc.) was also stopped for hypertension, pyrogenicity, and other adverse events [33, 34]. A recombinant Hb molecule designed with a reengineered heme pocket to reduce the affinity for nitric oxide (reducing so vasopressor effect) seems not to have reached human trial despite encouraging results in animal trauma model [35].

Hemolink® (Hemosol Inc.) was in phase II and III clinical trials in high-blood-loss surgery a few years ago and the results were soon expected, but the trials were discontinued for safety problems [5], and the production of Hemolink has been terminated [36].

Hb lipid vesicles were tried with success in preclinical animal studies, but it seems that there are no ongoing clinical trials with these products.

HBOCs still in clinical assays

Two Hb-based blood substitutes of the first generation are still in advanced clinical development: Hemopure® (Biopure Corp.) and PolyHeme® (Northfields Laboratories). Hemopure® (HBOC-201) was used in cardiac surgery with a reduction of allogeneic blood transfusion in the intraoperative period, but not during the entire hospitalization period [37]. In a phase III orthopedic surgery study, Hemopure® was used with doses ranging from 65 g (±1 RBC unit) to 325 g (±10 RBC units). The results indicate that HBOC-201 reduced the need for allogeneic transfusion, but with more adverse and serious adverse effects: gastrointestinal events, elevated plasma levels of amylase and lipase, and clearly hypertensive properties mainly in elderly patients [38, 39]. The company announced that a phase III study in Europe and South Africa demonstrated that Hemopure® reduced the need of red blood cells transfusion in general surgery patients, and that a phase II study is ongoing in Europe to reduce myocardial necrosis during cardiopulmonary bypass [4]. Hemopure® is approved for sale in South Africa to treat acutely anemic surgical patients: more than 250 postclinical trial applications would have been performed. Biopure has applied in the United Kingdom for regulatory approval of a proposed indication of Hemopure® in orthopedic surgical anemia. The company is participating to the US Navy's efforts to conduct a phase II clinical trial in trauma patients (the "Restore Effective SUrvival in Shock" or RESUS), which is under consideration by the FDA since 2005 [4]. A veterinary product, Oxyglobin® (HBOC-301) is approved in United States and Europe for the treatment of anemia in dogs, and around 100,000 animals have already been treated. On October 2007 [40], the company announced that new phase II trials are proposed and being designed for 2008: Hemopure® will be used as "potential cardioprotector" in myocardial infarction or major heart attack patients, for its erythropoietic effect in chemotherapy patients, and for palliative treatment in terminally ill patients. The company is also interested in trauma trials, but they are actually on clinical hold. At the end of 2006, Hemopure® was still not approved by the FDA.

PolyHeme® was used with success in several animal studies, but a trial of resuscitation after blood bleeding in rats did not prove a better survival with PolyHeme® and failed to improve metabolic acidosis [41].

In clinical trials, PolyHeme® was administered without safety problems in phase I and II studies. It was administered with success to trauma and emergency surgery (aneurysm rupture) patients in a phase III clinical trials with up to 1000 g in 10 L: the results demonstrated a conservation of total Hb concentration, 50% reduction of blood transfusion, and did not report major concerns [42, 43]. The study was halted on late 2001, before completion, and Northfield Laboratories filed for FDA approval in August 2001 [44]. In the beginning of 2006, an online article of the Wall Street Journal revealed that adverse events were observed in this phase III study, which were not disclosed: 10 out of 81 patients receiving PolyHeme® had heart attack within 7 days after administration (compared to 0/71 patients who received red blood cells). The heart attacks were attributed by the company to an excess of total fluids given to PolyHeme® patients, and not to the product itself [44–46].

A multicenter phase III nonconsent trial with PolyHeme® in trauma patients with severe blood loss started in January 2004 with the approval of the FDA and enrolled 714 patients (350 patients with PolyHeme® in the ambulance and until 12 hours of hospital stay, versus 364 patients receiving saline in the ambulance and allogeneic blood at hospital). The enrolment was completed in July 2006, and criticisms were rapidly formulated on the ethical aspect of the study and in relation with the Wall Street Journal revelation on the previous phase III study in aneurysm surgery patients [46]. The results were published in the beginning of 2009: a blood transfusion avoidance was observed in the PolyHeme group with no difference in survival at 30 days, but adverse events (coagulopathy, hypertension, myocardial infarction) were higher compared to control group ($p < 0.05$), and severe adverse events were more frequent although not statistically different between the two groups [47, 48].

Second-generation HBOCs

The second generation of HBOCs is developed on the basis of the observations collected from the numerous animal and human studies performed with the first-generation HBOCs, which pointed out vasoconstriction, and the gastrointestinal symptoms.

Oxygen therapeutics

A hypothesis suggests that hypertension observed with HBOCs is the consequence not only of NO trapping, but also of an arteriolar vasoconstriction in response to O_2 delivery [49, 50]. To counteract this autoregulatory response, the group of Winslow [8, 49, 51] has modified the surface of human Hb with polyethylene glycol to increase the molecular volume, the affinity for O_2, the viscosity, and the oncotic pressure: the main properties of this new Hb molecule (MP4) are compared to HBOCS of the first generation in Table 30.4. Animal studies performed with MP4 do not show hypertension by avoiding autoregulatory vasoconstriction [52]; MP4 supports life in rats with no detectable erythrocytes [53]. It is safe and without hemodynamics effects when administered as an exchange transfusion of 30% of blood volume in monkeys, but a transient elevation of hepatic enzymes and the presence of foamy macrophages in the bone marrow and spleen are reported [54].

For clinical use, MP4 (Hemospan®, Sangart Inc.) is designed as an O_2-carrying plasma expander for administration in patients with elective surgery, to deliver O_2 to hypoxic tissues. It is an "oxygen therapeutics" more than a blood substitute and is administered in solution at low concentration [50]. When administered to human volunteers (phase I single blind clinical study) at the doses of 50 or 100 mg/kg, Hemospan® does not increase the blood pressure, reduce the heart rate, or cause any detectable organ dysfunction [55]. The results

Table 30.4 Comparison of main properties of Hb-based blood substitutes of the first and second generation.

Property	First-generation Hb-based blood substitutes	Second-generation Hb-based blood substitutes-do these characteristics correspond to Hemospan?
O_2 binding: P_{50}	28–50 mmHg	6 ± 2 mmHg
Viscosity	± 1 cP	2.5 ± 1.0 cP
Oncotic pressure	± 15 mmHg	55 ± 20 mmHg
Hb concentration	± 15 g/dL	4.2 ± 0.2 g/dL
Plasma half-life	12 to 24 hours	$\pm$ 24 hours
Proposed clinical use	Red blood cell substitute	O_2 transport agent: is the term "plasma expander with O_2 carrying properties" not more adequate?

P_{50}: oxygen partial pressure producing 50% saturation of Hb molecule with O_2, reflecting the affinity of the modified Hb for O_2.

of a phase Ib/II study with dose escalation (from 200 mL up to 1000 mL Hemospan) in patients receiving spinal anesthesia for elective orthopedic surgery suggested that the highest dose may have been slightly less well-tolerated, but did not prevent from continuing clinical trials [56]. A phase II clinical study is achieved with 250 mL or 500 mL of Hemospan® in elderly patients undergoing elective hip arthroplasty under spinal anesthesia [8, 57]. No serious event can be attributed to the blood substitute, and no significant hypertension is observed, but the hypotension linked to the type of anesthesia is reduced in the patients treated with the highest dose. The heart rate is significantly lower in the treatment groups starting with infusion and during the surgery period. Increases of blood levels of hepatic enzymes, amylase, and lipase are observed, but only significant for lipase. The half-life of Hemospan® is around 20 hours, with a metHb concentration of 1 g/dL at the same moment. A phase II study in elective prostatectomy patients has been completed, but the results are not yet published. From these phase II studies, Hemospan® appears safe, but the doses are low (around 42 g for the highest one), and despite these low doses, bradycardia and elevation of hepatic and pancreatic enzymes are observed (this was also observed with the first-generation blood substitutes). Questions remain concerning the half-time life of Hemospan® in plasma and the metHb production. Studies with larger doses are expected before the innocuity (and the utility) of this new generation blood substitute can be firmly assured. Two phase III studies have been recently completed in Europe on the efficacy and safety of Hemospan for prevention or treatment of perioperative hypotension in patients undergoing primary hip arthroplasty with spinal anesthesia. The efficacy endpoints seem to have been reached and no statistically significant imbalances in the incidence of serious adverse events were identified as reported in May 2009 [58], but the publications of the detailed results are expected.

Biodegradable nanocapsules

A new approach is to encapsulate Hb in biodegradable nanocapsules (less than 0.2 μm) of polylactide, a polymer of lactic acid, which is degraded in vivo into water and carbon dioxide [23, 59]. A nanocapsule solution containing around 11 g bovine Hb/dL has O_2 carrying and delivery properties similar to that of free bovine Hb, and the degradation of the nanocapsules does not accumulate polylactic acid in the reticuloendothelial system or overload the daily lactic acid elimination capacity of the body [23]. The enzyme of the red blood cells can be coencapsulated: carbonic anhydrase and enzymes (superoxide dismutase, catalase, metHb reductase), which protect Hb from oxidation into MetHb. The nanocapsules are permeable (owing to their membrane thickness of 5–15 nm) which allows the diffusion of glucose and small hydrophilic molecules (reducing agents) needed for a "metabolic activity" and a correct function of the encapsulated enzymes. The circulation lifetime of the nanocapsules can be increased when they are made with PEG-polyactide copolymers. Infusions of nanocapsule solutions in rats (one-third of their blood volume) showed no vasopressor effect and a lifetime around 40 hours [60, 61].

A meta-analysis: the deathblow for Hb-based blood substitutes?

In almost all the clinical trials with HBOC, a common observation is an increase in adverse effects (reaching statistical significance) and severe adverse effects in the HBOC group, mainly hypertension and myocardial infarction. The RBC transfusion avoidance when HBOCs are used is also a common point, but there is no benefit in patient survival. A recent meta-analysis uses as outcome variables the data on deaths and myocardial infarctions of 16 randomized controlled trials involving 3711 surgical, stroke, and trauma patients, with 5 Hb-based blood substitutes (HemAssist, Hemopure, Hemolink, Polyheme, and Hemospan) [62]. A statistically significant increase in the risk of death and the risk of myocardial infarction is observed in the HBOC-treated group. The authors also underline that the results of the clinical trials with HBOC are generally made public with an important delay, and that a prompt meta-analyses of the trials would have demonstrated the risks as soon as the year 2000.

From this meta-analysis and taking into account the well-demonstrated toxicity of Hb out of the erythrocyte (particularly its ability to cross the endothelial barrier, to produce oxidant species, and to induce renal toxicity) [21,63–66], the use of HBOC cannot be recommended especially in fragile (elderly and severe hemorrhagic) patients. Some hope remains for Hemospan, but this HBOC is an oxygen therapeutics and not a substitute of RBC [50].

Conclusion

In clinical trials, the HBOCs of the first generation have encountered an increase of severe side effects (hypertension, renal toxicity) compared with classical treatment, together with a limited success in avoiding red blood cell transfusion, no significant results in improving survival, a short intravascular lifetime, and some risk of antibody formation with repeated administrations. Only two HBOCs, Hemopure® and PolyHeme®, remain in phase III clinical trials, but there is a questionable lack of published results, even partial ones. Hemospan®, a new generation modified Hb solutions has reached the step of clinical trial, but is more an oxygen therapeutics than an universal blood substitute.

Projects are on the way to obtain human Hb from microorganisms (*E. coli* and *Aspergillus niger*) or from worms, which have a polymeric Hb molecule (around 50 times the human Hb), thus not needing chemical modification for sufficient stability in bloodstream, with no breakdown and no kidney damage. It seems that successful preclinical assays were made in mice with a correct O_2 transport and no allergy. But technical problems of extraction remain to solve, and there is no knowledge on the effects of worm Hb on blood pressure and on its sensibility to oxidation [3].

An universal use-blood substitute remains necessary for urgent transfusion at the site of severe traumatic injuries, where typing and crossmatching of donated blood is not possible, and in conditions where there is severe shortage of blood donors or high potential for contaminated donor blood. It is important to carry out more basic research for solving the problem of free Hb toxicity by oxidation and metHb formation, either by engineering the Hb molecule to obtain a more stable and less vasoactive compound, or by using antioxidants or antioxidant enzymes to control the Hb oxidative side reactions. The technique of biodegradable nanoparticles carrying natural Hb or a synthetic Hb in an environment mimicking that inside the erythrocyte is a promising step in this way.

But a more promising way is the in vitro erythroid cell generation. Important progress has been made in the last decade in the field of stem cell cultures: starting from human hematopoietic stem cells, conditions have been established for producing mature red blood cells after around 18 days of culture [67, 68]. Two important problems remain to be solved now: the technical conditions for large scale cultures in bioreactors [69] and the control of the membrane expression of blood group systems ABO and Rh [70]. A delay of 5–10 years appears reasonable to reach these targets, taking into account that clinical interest persists and economical conditions are good.

References

1. Remy B, Deby-Dupont G, Lamy M. Red blood cell substitutes: fluorocarbon emulsions and haemoglobin solutions. Br Med Bull 1999;1:277–98.
2. Spahn DR, Kocian R. Artificial O_2 carriers: status in 2005. Curr Pharm Des 2005;11:4099–114.
3. Lowe KC. Blood substitutes: from chemistry to clinic. J Mater Chem 2006;16:4189–96.
4. Ness P, Cushing M. Oxygen therapeutics. Pursuit of an alternative to the donor red blood cell. Arch Pathol Lab Med 2007;131:734–41.
5. Winslow RM. Current status of oxygen carriers ("blood substitutes"): 2006. Vox Sang 2006;91:102–10.
6. Jahr JS, Walker V, Manoochehri K. Blood substitutes as pharmacotherapies in clinical practice. Curr Opin Anaesthesiol 2007;20:325–30.
7. Deby-Dupont G, Remy B, Lamy M. Oxygen carriers: hemoglobin-based solutions. In: *Transfusion Medicine and Alternatives to Blood Transfusion- NATA (Network for Advancement of Transfusion Alternatives)*. R&J Editions Médicales, Paris, 2000, pp. 298–311.

8. Winslow RM. Red blood cell substitutes. Semin Hematol 2007;44:51–9.
9. Rabiner SF, O'Brien K, Peskin GW, Friedman LH. Further studies with stroma-free hemoglobin solution. Ann Surg 1970;171:615–22.
10. Savitsky JP, Doczi J, Black J, Arnold JD. A clinical safety trial of stroma-free hemoglobin. Clin Pharmacol Ther 1978;23:73–80.
11. Perutz MF. Stereochemistry of cooperative effects in haemoglobin. Nature 1970;228:726–39.
12. Feola M, Simoni J, Tran R, Canizaro P. Mechanisms of toxicity of hemoglobin solutions. Biomater Artif Cells Artif Organs 1988;16:217–26.
13. Benesch R, Benesch RE. Intracellular organic phosphates as regulators of oxygen release by haemoglobin. Nature 1969;221:618–22.
14. Tsuchida E, Komatsu T, Hamamatsu K, et al. Exchange transfusion with albumin-heme as an artificial O_2-infusion into anesthetized rats: physiological response, O_2-delivery, and reduction of the oxidized hemin sites by red blood cells. Bioconjug Chem 2000; 11:46–50.
15. Hoffman SJ, Looker D, Roehrich JM, et al. Expression of fully functional human hemoglobin in *Escherichia Coli*. Proc Natl Acad Sci USA 1990;87:8521–5.
16. Looker D, Abbott-Brown D, Cozart P, et al. A human recombinant haemoglobin designed for use as a blood substitute. Nature 1992;356:258–60.
17. Gottfried DS, Manjula BN, Malavalli A, et al. Probing the diphosphoglycerate binding pocket of HbA and HbPresbyterian (beta 108Asn –> Lys). Biochemistry 1999;38:11307–15.
18. Dieryck W, Pagnier J, Poyart C, et al. Human haemoglobin from transgenic tobacco. Nature 1997; 386:29–30.
19. Riess JG. Oxygen carriers ("blood substitutes")–raison d'être, chemistry, and some physiology. Chem Rev 2001;101:2797–920.
20. Walder JA, Zangg RH, Walder RY, et al. Diaspirins that cross-link beta chains of hemoglobin: bis (3,5 dibromosalicyl) succinate and bis (3,5 dibromosalicyl) fumarate. Biochemistry 1979;18:4265–70.
21. Simoni J, Simoni G, Hartsell A, Feola M. An improved blood substitute. In vivo evaluation of its renal effects. ASAIO J 1997;43:M714–25.
22. D'Agnillo F, Chang TMS. Poly-Hb-superoxide dismutase-catalase as a blood substitute with antioxidant properties. Nat Biotechnol 1998;16:667–71.
23. Chang TMS. Blood substitutes based on nanobiotechnology. Trends Biotechnol 2006;24:372–7.
24. Sakai H, Sou K, Horinouchi H, Kobayashi K, Tsuchida E. Haemoglobin-vesicles as artificial oxygen carriers: present situation and future visions. J Intern Med 2008;263:4–15.
25. Larbuisson R, Deby-Dupont G, Lamy M. Oxygen carriers in cardiac surgery. TATM 2005;7:42–57.
26. Shirley PJ. Fluids as oxygen carriers and the potential role in trauma resuscitation. Trauma 2008;10:139–47.
27. Matheson B, Kwansa H, Bucci E, et al. Appearance of dissociable and cross-linked hemoglobins in the renal hilar lymph. J Lab Clin Med 2000;135:459–64.
28. Lamy ML, Daily EK, Brichant JF, et al. Randomized trial of diaspirin cross-linked hemoglobin solution as an alternative to blood transfusion after cardiac surgery. The DCLHb Cardiac Surgery Trial Collaborative Group. Anesthesiology 2000;92:646–56.
29. Schubert A, Przybelski RJ, Eidt JF, et al. Diaspirin-crosslinked hemoglobin reduces blood transfusion in noncardiac surgery: a multicenter, randomized, controlled, double-blinded trial. Anesth Analg 2003;97: 323–32.
30. Kerner T, Ahlers O, Veit S, et al. DCL-Hb for trauma patients with severe hemorrhagic shock: the European "On-Scene" Multicenter Study. Intensive Care Med 2003;29:378–85.
31. Sloan EP, Koenigsberg M, Gens D, et al. Diaspirin cross-linked hemoglobin (DCLHb) in the treatment of severe traumatic hemorrhagic shock: a randomized controlled efficacy trial. JAMA 1999;282:1857–64.
32. Viele MK, Weiskopf RB, Fisher D. Recombinant human hemoglobin does not affect renal function in humans: analysis of safety and phamacokinetics. Anesthesiology 1997;86:848–858.
33. Shoemaker S, Gerber M, Evans G, et al. Initial clinical experience with a rationally designed genetically engineered recombinant human hemoglobin. Artif Cells Blood Substit Immobil Biotechnol 1994;22:457–65.
34. Hayes JK, Stanley TH, Lind GH, et al. A double-blind study to evaluate the safety of recombinant human haemoglobin in surgical patients during general anesthesia. J Cardiothorac Vasc Anesth 2001;15:593–602.
35. Malhotra AK, Kelley ME, Miller PR, Hartman JC, Fabian TC, Proctor KG. Resuscitation with a novel hemoglobin based oxygen carrier in a swine model of uncontrolled peri-operative hemorrhage. J Trauma 2003;54:925–29.
36. Greenburg AG, Kim HW. Hemoglobin-based oxygen carriers. Crit Care 2004;8(Suppl 2):S61–4.
37. Sprung J, Kindscher JD, Wahr JA, et al. The use of bovine hemoglobin glutamer-250 (Hemopure) in

surgical patients: results of a multicenter, randomized, single-blind trial. Anesth Analg 2002;94:799–808.
38. Jahr JS, Mackenzie C, Pearce LB, Pitman A, Greenburg AG. HBOC-201 as an alternative to blood transfusion: efficacy and safety evaluation in a multicenter phase III trial in elective orthopedic surgery. J Trauma 2008;64:1484–97.
39. Freilich D, Pearce LB, Pitman A, et al. HBOC-201vasoactivity in a phase III clinical trial in orthopedic surgery subjects—extrapolation of potential risk for acute trauma trials. J Trauma 2009;66(2):365–76.
40. Biopure announces expanded clinical program to target anemia. News Release 10/15/2007. www.biopure.com.
41. Handrigan MT, Bentley BB, Oliver JD, et al. Choice of fluid influences outcome in prolonged hypotensive resuscitation after hemorrhage in awake rats. Shock 2005;23:337–43.
42. Gould SA, Moore EE, Hoyt DB, et al. The first randomized trial of human polymerized hemoglobin as a blood substitute in acute trauma and emergent surgery. J Am Coll Surg 1998;187:113–20.
43. Gould SA, Moore E, Hoyt DB, et al. The life-sustaining capacity of human polymerized hemoglobin when red cells might be unavailable. J Am Coll Surg 2002; 195:445–52.
44. Jahr JS, Varma N. PolyHeme. Northfield Laboratories. Idrugs 2004;7:478–82.
45. Thomas M. Burton, The Wall Street Journal on line, February 22, 2006. http://online.wsj.com/article/SB114057765651379801.html?mod=home_page_one_us.
46. Thomas M. Burton, The Wall Street Journal on line, March 10, 2006. http://www.mindfully.org/Health/2006/PolyHeme-OHRP-Criticized10mar06.html.
47. Moore EE, Moore FA, Fabian TC, et al. PolyHeme Study Group. Human polymerized hemoglobin for the treatment of hemorrhagic shock when blood is unavailable: the USA multicenter trial. J Am Coll Surg 2009;208(1):1–13.
48. Moore EE, Johnson JL, Moore FA, Moore HB. The USA multicenter prehosptial hemoglobin-based oxygen carrier resuscitation trial: scientific rationale, study design, and results. Crit Care Clin 2009;25(2): 325–56.
49. Intaglietta M. Microvascular transport factors in the design of effective blood substitutes. In: Messmer K, Burhop KE, Hutter J (eds) *Microcirculatory Effects of Hemoglobin Solutions*. Vol. 25: *Progress in Applied Microcirculation,*. Karger, Basel, 2004, pp. 8–15.
50. Winslow RM. Cell-free oxygen carriers: scientific foundations, clinical development, and new directions. Biochim Biophys Acta 2008;1784(10):1382–6.
51. Vandegriff KD, Malavalli A, Wooldridge J, et al. MP4, a new non-vasoactive polyethytlene glycol-hemoglobin conjugate. Transfusion 2003;43:509–16.
52. Winslow RM. Current status of blood substitute research: toward a new paradigm. J Intern Med 2003; 253:508–17.
53. Winslow RM, Lohman J, Malavalli A, Vandegriff KD. Comparison of PEG-modified albumin and hemoglobin in extreme hemodilution in the rat. J Appl Physiol 2004;97:1527–34.
54. Young MA, Malavalli A, Winslow N, et al. Toxicity and hemodynamic effects after single dose administration of MalPEG-hemoglobin (MP4) in rhesus monkeys. Transl Res 2007;149:333–42.
55. Björkholm M, Fagrell B, Przybelski R, et al. A phase I single blind clinical trial of a new oxygen transport agent (MP4), human hemoglobin modified with maleimide-activated polyethylene glycol. Haematologica 2005;90:505–15.
56. Olofsson C, Nygards EB, Ponzer S, et al. A randomized, single blind, increasing dose safety trial of an oxygen-carrying plasma expander (Hemospan®) administered to orthopedic surgery patients with spinal anesthesia. Transfus Med 2008;18:28–39.
57. Olofsson C, Ahl T, Johansson T, et al. A multicenter clinical study of the safety and activity of maleimide-polyethylene glycol–modified hemoglobin (Hemospan®) in patients undergoing major orthopedic surgery. Anesthesiology 2006;105:1153–63.
58. http://www.sangart.com/hemospan/clinical-trials.php (accessed on 5 May 2009).
59. Chang TMS. Evolution of artificial cells using nanobiotechnology of hemoglobin based RBC. Blood substitute as an example. Artif Cells Blood Substit Biotechnol 2006;34:551–66.
60. Yu WP, Chang TMS. Submicron polymer membrane hemoglobin nanocapsules as blood substitutes: preparation and characterization. Artif Cells Blood Substit Immobil Biotechnol 1996;24(3):169–83.
61. Chang TMS, D'Agnillo F, Yu WP, Razack S. Two future generations of blood substitutes based on polyhemoglobin-SOD-catalase and nanoencapsulation. Adv Drug Deliv Rev 2000;40:213–18.
62. Natanson C, Kern SJ, Lurie P, Banks SM, Wolfe SM. Cell-free hemoglobin-based blood substitutes and risk of myocardial infarction and death. JAMA 2008; 299:2304–12.

63. Reeder BJ, Svistunenko DA, Cooper CE, Wilson MT. The radical and redox chemistry of myoglobin and hemoglobin. Antioxid Redox Signal 2004;6:954–66.
64. Balla J, Jacob HS, Balla G, et al. Endothelial cell heme uptake from heme proteins: induction of senstitization and desensitization to oxidant damage. Proc Natl Acad Sci U S A 1993;90:9285–9.
65. Everse J, Hsia N. The toxicities of native and modified hemoglobins. Free Radic Biol Med 1997;22:1075–99.
66. Nagababu E, Ramasamy S, Rifkind JM, Alayash AI. Site-specific crosslinking of human and bovine hemoglobins differentially alters oxygen binding and redox side reactions producing rhombic heme and heme degradation. Biochemistry 2002;41:7407–15.
67. Douay L, Andreu G. Ex vivo production of human red blood cells from hematopoietic stem cells: what is the future in transfusion? Transfus Med Rev 2007;21:91–100.
68. Lu SJ, Feng Q, Park JS, et al. Biological properties and enucleation of red blood cells from human embryonic stem cells. Blood 2008;112:4475–84.
69. Harding FJ, Cameron CM, Hu WS, Kaufman DS. Scaleable production of hematopoietic cells suitable for transfusion from human embryonic stem cells in a stirred bioreactor system. Blood (ASH Annual Meeting Abstracts) Nov 2006;108:728.
70. Douay L. Cell culture for transfusion purposes: the concept of "cultured red blood cells". Transfus Clin Biol 2009;16:134–7.

CHAPTER 31
Perfluorocarbon Emulsions

Pedro Cabrales
La Jolla Bioengineering Institute, La Jolla, CA, USA

An oxygen-carrying fluid that sustains life in the absence of blood would have many benefits. Possible applications include emergency resuscitation, angioplasty, tumor therapy, and organ preservation. Although an oxygen carrier is not available yet, recent progress in biotechnology, however, could make development of these solutions an unprecedented medical achievement of the twentieth century. Perfluorocarbons are derived from hydrocarbons by replacing all the hydrogen atoms by fluorine atoms. A loose but common definition includes highly fluorinated molecules containing occasional hydrogen, oxygen, or nitrogen atoms and halogens other than fluorine [1, 2].

Perfluorocarbons offer unique combinations of high oxygen and the capacity to dissolve other gases, low water, and lipid solubility, and has exceptional chemical and biological inertness. Gas solubility reflects the very low intermolecular interactions (fluorine's low polarizability translates into low van der Waals forces) within the perfluorocarbon. The basic difference in how oxygen is transported between perfluorocarbons and hemoglobin (Hb) is that perfluorocarbons dissolve whereas Hb binds oxygen. In the case of Hb, a strong bond is established between the oxygen and the heme. In the case of perfluorocarbons, there is only physical solubility of oxygen because of their loose nondirectional van der Waals interactions. The difference in the nature of how Hb and perfluorocarbon interact is clearly reflected by the differences in profiles of the oxygen content curves as a function of pO_2, i.e., sigmoidal for Hb versus linear for PFC emulsions (Figure 31.1). With perfluorocarbons, there is no saturation and no possibility for chemical binding and as the oxygen is released, carbon dioxide (CO_2) comes in. Oxygen dissolved in PFC is immediately available to tissues; furthermore, oxygen dissolution and release to tissues can increase when temperature decreases.

Perfluorocarbons are hydrophobic, and are therefore not miscible with water, and thus, have to be emulsified for intravenous use. With sophisticated technology, it is possible to generate a stable perfluorocarbon emulsion with exceptionally small particles (median diameter <0.2 μm) [3]. Perfluorocarbons, as opposed to Hb, are among the most inert organic materials chemists have ever invented. Their initial industrial development was for handling the extremely corrosive uranium fluorides. They are not subject to oxidation, and there is no indication that any sort of chemical modification occurs under the conditions of processing, storage, and use. PFCs can typically be heated to 300°C and higher for several days without detectable changes [2]. Appropriately formulated PFC emulsions can be terminally heat-sterilized at the standard temperature of 121°C [4].

The risks and side effects of allogenic blood transfusions include transfusion reactions, alloimmunization, transmission of infectious agents, and immunosuppression resulting in an increased incidence of postoperative infections with prolonged hospitalization, higher costs, and probably a shorter period of recurrence-free survival after surgery [5–7]. The development of a safe and effective erythrocyte substitute for oxygen delivery has been the focus of considerable effort. Hb-based

Alternatives to Blood Transfusion in Transfusion Medicine, 2nd edition. Edited by A. Maniatis, P. Van der Linden, J.-F. Hardy.

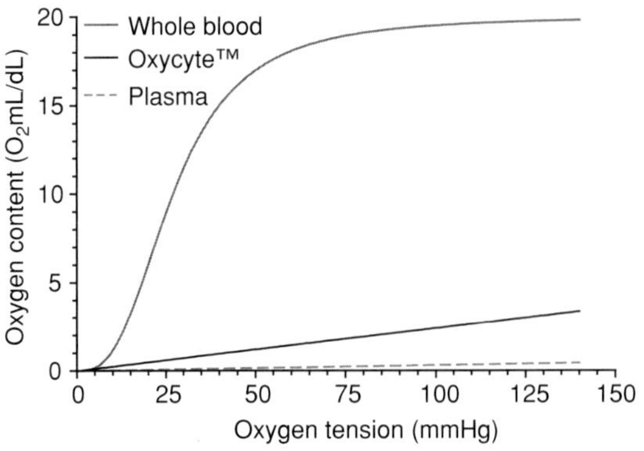

Figure 31.1 Oxygen content for whole blood, Oxycyte^{TM} (Synthetic Blood International, Inc. Costa Mesa, CA) and plasma as a function of oxygen partial pressure.

oxygen carriers (HBOCs) and PFCs are two types of products that have been extensively evaluated and are currently in clinical trials [8]. The interest in use of temporary oxygen carriers as "blood substitutes" is expected to increase as a means to reduce requirements for allogeneic blood [9, 10]. Preliminary results of clinical trials with HBOC and PFC based blood substitute have been reported and Phase I and II trials of two oxygen carriers are ongoing [11, 12]. One is a polyethylene glycol conjugated Hb from Sangart Inc. (San Diego, CA) [12], the other, a PFC-based oxygen carrier, Perflubron emulsion from Alliance Pharmaceutical Corp. (San Diego, CA) [11].

PFCs are based on an oxygen carrier that is synthetic, and in principle available in very large quantities at modest costs. This has been tempting to investigators and business enterprises, since it could in principle lead to a convenient, largely available, economic, pathogen-free, and storable oxygen carrier. However, fluorocarbons only became water soluble when emulsified in phospholipids (derived from egg yolk), which make them, not truly, synthetic. Furthermore, while Hb-based products carry oxygen via a reversible chemical reaction, PFCs carry oxygen as a function of the solubility of oxygen in these compounds. PFC emulsion's oxygen carrying capacity is about twice that of plasma, and about 10 times less than that of Hb. The low oxygen carrying capacity of PFCs can be significantly increased by exposing them to higher fractions of inspired oxygen (FiO_2). The effects due to superposition of hyperoxia on the changes of circulating fluid composition, present an additional variable in the analysis of the effectiveness of PFCs.

Fluorocarbon emulsions

Perfluorocarbon are insoluble in water, thus, PFCs are formulated into emulsions for parenteral administration. The PFC droplets size is less than 0.5 μm and is coated with a surfactant that serves as emulsifier and stabilizes the suspension. PFC emulsion are produced at different concentrations from 20 to 120% weight/volume, because perfluorocarbons specific gravity is ~2. Currently, PFC emulsions use egg yolk phospholipids as the emulsifier. Therefore, these emulsions have a definite similarity to the lipid emulsions used for parenteral nutrition. Osmolarity of the suspension media is independent of PFC concentration and is adjusted by the addition of tonicity agents. The principal challenges in the development of an injectable PFC include the following: selecting the appropriate perfluorocarbon (easily eliminable, highly pure, and easy to emulsify); preparing stable emulsions (small-sized, heat-sterilizable, and well-tolerated surfactant); and counteracting molecular diffusion, which is responsible for particle size growth over time.

Few perfluorocarbons are acceptable for parenteral use, because of their slow excretion and stability of the final emulsions. It has been determined that in vivo perfluorocarbons excretion is mostly determined by their molecular weight, and lower rapid excretion. On the other hand, emulsion stability requires perfluorocarbons with higher molecular weights. These two conditions are clearly difficult to satisfy, simultaneously. Additionally, vapor pressure, which also depends on molecular weight, is an important parameter, which can favor retention of air in the alveoli, resulting in increased pulmonary residual volume (also known as pulmonary gas trapping). In order to avoid this phenomenon, the vapor pressure of the final PFC phase at body temperature should probably not exceed about 10 mmHg [2, 13, 14].

Biologic interactions of PFC with macrophages, which might impair microvascular perfusion, have been discarded because observed activation of intravascular leukocytes during perioperative hemodilution has been related to the interaction of PFC with the colloids clinically applied as plasma expanders. Incompatible interactions of PFC with only Dextran 60 kDa were established by Nolte D. et al. [15], and other studies have been performed with hydroxyl ethyl starch (HES) [3, 16, 17].

Gas solubility by PFC

Fluorocarbons are passive gas carriers; they physically dissolve the gases following Henry's law, and are directly proportional to the partial pressure of the gas, or the concentration gradient. No chemical bonding is involved and there is no saturation. Oxygen solubility in a given PFC depends on the solubility coefficient of the PFC for that gas. Oxygen content can be adjusted by simply controlling oxygen tension. The principles that underlie gas transport by PFC emulsions are basically the same as those that operate for plasma. In both cases, dissolution is proportional to a concentration gradient; simply, the solubility of inert gases in PFCs is typically 10–20 times larger than that for the plasma. Gas solubility of the pure perfluorocarbon is reduced during the emulsification process, although the effective area for the gas exchange with the PFC is increased.

Off-loading of gases from PFCs to tissues is not subordinated to any change in conformation and does not require the assistance of an allosteric effector. In the case of oxygen, the van der Waals interactions between oxygen and PFC molecules are an order of magnitude lower than Hb and oxygen reactions, resulting in higher extraction rates and ratios [18]. Oxygen in normal condition, central arterial pO_2 of 100 mmHg and venous pO_2 of 35 mmHg, PFC emulsion can release 65% of the oxygen, as compared with about 30% for Hb in the RBCs. Oxygen release from PFCs is effective at any physiologically relevant partial pressure, rendering a cooperativity-like effect unnecessary. Likewise, oxygen release by PFCs is not dependent on pH and is not adversely affected by temperature [19]. Since PFCs undergo no oxidation or other modification over time, their oxygen uptake and release characteristics are not affected by storage or during circulation. Introducing a PFC emulsion into the circulation is akin to increasing the oxygen solubility of the plasma compartment of blood. When Hb and a PFC are present in the circulation simultaneously, the PFC will always release its oxygen load first, thus conserving the oxygen bound to the Hb until it is released to the hypoxic tissues [17]. A valuable consequence of PFC's following Henry's law is that the oxygen content of a PFC emulsion can be increased severalfold by just increasing the FiO_2, which is a simple thing to do in a rescue vehicle critical care or surgical setting.

Facilitated oxygen diffusion by PFC

Diffusion of oxygen from the RBCs into the tissues is driven by the pO_2 gradient that exists between the blood and these tissues [20]. Thus, the rates of both oxygenation and deoxygenation of an Hb solution are limited by diffusion and governed by the oxygen gradient between internal and external spaces [21]. Diffusion should be facilitated when the RBC membrane is absent and when numerous small size (as compared with RBCs), highly mobile oxygen reservoirs are present in the circulation. Cell free plasma layers between RBC column and the endothelium are particularly large during anemic or is hemodiluted states. Cell free Hb molecules, Hb-loaded liposomes, and PFC droplets, fill these gaps in large numbers, increase oxygen content and potentially facilitate oxygen diffusion by providing "stepping stones" or dynamic chains of particles over which oxygen can travel. As circulating PFC droplets are more than RBCs by several orders of magnitude, the area for gas exchange provided by PFC is also significantly larger. In the larger vessels, a near-wall excess of the smaller particles is likely to develop, as RBCs would tend to migrate nearer the lower shear central axis of the vessel.

Likewise, the large pO_2 gradients set in place at the high FiO_2 at which PFC emulsions are utilized provide a strong driving force for oxygen diffusion from the PFC droplets to the tissues. The movement of emulsion microdroplets in the blood stream was proposed to create dynamic chains of particles and hence, channels which would help transfer oxygen from the RBCs to tissues. Numerous studies in the literature indicated erroneously that PFC emulsions can facilitate oxygen diffusion. The postulated theory of augmented oxygen delivery through very narrow microvascular channels that are more readily perfused with the tiny PFC particles (<0.2 μm in diameter) than relatively large red blood cells (7–8 μm in diameter) [3, 16, 22, 23], is completely discarded. Concurrent study of systemic and microvascular oxygen exchange presented that the increase on FiO_2 with PFC increases DO_2 to the tissue, although most of the oxygen was transported by the Hb. The logical explanation may be PFC allows RBC to remain partially oxygenated when they arrive to the tissue [17].

PFC oxygen transport capacity was investigated in the hamster window chamber model microcirculation during extreme hemodilution [17]. Pentaspan, (10%, B. Brown, Medical, Irvine, CA, HES, 200 kDa MW) was used as a plasma expander to reduce Hct to 18% by two isovolemic hemodilution steps. A third step reducing the Hct to 11% and was completed with either HES or Oxycyte™ (Synthetic Blood International, Inc. Costa Mesa, CA). Comparisons of HES only hemodiluted animals versus animals that received 4.2 g/kg of emulsion were made at normoxia ($FiO_2 = 0.21$) and hyperoxia ($FiO_2 = 1.0$). Systemic and microvascular oxygen delivery for PFC was 25% (normoxia) and 400% (hyperoxia) higher than for HES. The combination of PFCs and hyperoxic ventilation delivered oxygen to the tissue without causing vasoconstriction or impairing microvascular perfusion. Positive acid base balance, restoration of mean arterial pressure, and cardiac output suggested correspondence between microvascular and systemic events. PFC and increased FiO_2 increased systemic oxygen delivery and extraction, when compared to a plasma expander, because of higher plasma oxygen content when PFC is present. In the microcirculation, oxygen delivery was also increased by PFC, again the oxygen was mostly released from the Hb in the RBCs [17].

Transport of carbon dioxide

Intravascular CO_2 transport relies on several mechanisms including physical dissolution in plasma, carbonic anhydrase induced transformation into bicarbonate, and chemical binding consequent to reaction with the Hb. About 25% of total CO_2 transport uses Hb, this transport is also affected by the Bohr effects since hydration of CO_2 and the formation of bicarbonate depend on pH, acid base balance equation. As for any gas, PFCs transports CO_2 in the dissolved form. PFC CO_2 solubilities are typically in the 3–5 times higher than for oxygen [24]. There is no indication that transport of CO_2 by PFCs interferes with CO_2 transport mechanisms by Hb and plasma. However, clinical and experimental result had shown a tendency to faster recovery of acid balance when PFCs are in circulation [3, 17, 22, 25].

Transport of other gases

The capacity for PFCs to dissolve nitrogen (and air) may find applications in the treatment of decompression sickness and for protection from neurologic damage caused by air microemboli during cardiopulmonary bypass (CPB) surgery [26, 27]. The solubility of xenon in PFCs can be exploited for magnetic resonance imaging (MRI). Both Hb and PFCs transport Nitric oxide (NO) but by different mechanisms, which changes the availability of the gas [28, 29].

During CPB, volatile anaesthetics can be added to the oxygenator to provide anesthesia, regulate systemic vascular resistance and reduce hormonal responses to CPB. The rate of washin and washout of volatile anesthetics via oxygenators depends on their solubility in blood. Two important factors affect the solubility of volatile anesthetics: hypothermia increases solubility and crystalloid hemodilution decreases it. PFC unique physicochemical characteristics, chemically inert with high solubility, provide the ideal media to dissolve larger quantities of gases. Volatile anesthetics also have a higher solubility in perfluorodecalin, the main component of Fluosol™ (Alpha Therapeutic Corp., Los Angeles, CA), a first-generation emulsion [30].

The question therefore arises whether clinically relevant volumes of PFC might significantly increase the blood solubility of volatile anesthetics. More recently, studies on the solubility of desflurane, sevoflurane, and isoflurane were performed using human blood in vitro mixed with clinical concentrations of perflubron emulsion Oxygent™ (Alliance Pharmaceutical Corp., San Diego [3], which has three times greater concentration than Fluosol (30% vs 10% by volume) [31]. This study showed that perflubron concentrations equivalent to in vivo doses of 1.8–5.4 g/kg, increased the amount of gas carried by blood ranging from 0.9 (desflurane) to 2.6 (sevoflurane) times the normal value. However it was concluded that this finding lacked apparent clinical implications.

NO is enzymatically produced by various types of cells and represents a central mediator within the cardiovascular system. As a free radical, NO is highly unstable in vivo. Its primary targets include heme proteins such as guanylyl cyclase and free radical species. NO is readily oxidized by oxygen in an aqueous media and mainly converted into nitrite anion. The partition coefficient of NO for PFC emulsion is defined as the ratio of the equilibrium concentrations between the aqueous and PFC phases. Partition coefficient of NO for Perftoran was found to be ~200 [32]. The sequestration of NO by PFC emulsion without the presence of oxygen to account for oxidation was very significant. Thus, the partition coefficient indicates that PFC micelle can increase micellar concentrations of NO to a higher level than an aqueous solution, and readily collect NO from regions with overproduction.

The use of PFC emulsions as oxygen carriers has been suggested to have several advantageous properties in the microcirculation [17, 33, 34]. However, these studies mostly deal with conditions of extreme hemodilution, hemorrhagic shock, and 100% oxygen inhalation. Therefore, more subtle effects due to loading and unloading of other circulatory gases are often masked. The NO preferential partition coefficient of PFC emulsion allows the droplets to absorb NO from the aqueous phase, greatly accelerating NO oxidation and S-nitrosothiols formation under aerobic conditions. The reaction of NO and O_2 with thiols results in thiol nitrosalation through the intermediary dinitrogen trioxide (N_2O_3) formed from the combination of NO with NO_2 [32]. In the presence of PFC (hydrophobic compartments), NO should be quickly sequestrated by PFC micelles. The high local concentration of NO within the hydrophobic compartment leads to the acceleration of NO oxidation and the formation of nitrosative N_2O_3 from the combination of NO with NO_2 [32]. According to the theory of micellar catalysis [35], the rate of NO oxidation and S-nitrosothiols formation depends on the volume of the hydrophobic phase. Larger or smaller amounts of PFC could be progressively less effective as a tool for modulating plasma NO bioavailability [32]. Consistently, thiols are in excess relative to NO, and a large fraction of NO_2 should react with thiols rather than NO itself. However, it remains unclear whether intrinsic plasma NO or S-nitrosothiols play a significant role in cardiovascular processes. Notably, the administration of a large dose of PFC caused vasoconstriction, reduction of erythrocyte velocity in post-capillary venules, and increased venular leukocyte sticking, which is probably due to rapid sequestration of NO [32, 35].

PFC emulsions have been extensively evaluated as substitute oxygen carriers to reduce allogeneic blood transfusion and improve circulatory oxygen carrying capacity and tissue oxygenation in acute hemodilution after trauma or surgery and in ischemia [36]. Although PFCs are tolerated in animals and humans, pulmonary and systemic hemodynamic effects have limited their clinical use [37]. Higher doses of PFC have been associated with progressive hypertension and decreased heart rate [38], and also with beneficial anti-inflammatory and antithrombotic effects [34,39] that could not be explained solely by the ability of PFCs to transport oxygen. They could be explained by the findings of the present study, which indicates that PFC are NO scavengers, but different from heme molecules. In the case of PFC, the NO scavenged remains partially available in the form of S-nitrosothiols.

Developments of PFC

First commercial development efforts were Fluosol-DA in Japan, Perftoran® in the Soviet Union, Emulsion No. II in China. They had in common the use of F-decafin as principal perfluorocarbon and of a poloxamer (Pluronic, F68) as the primary emulsifier. The main limitations of these emulsions was the presence of large amounts, >30%, of a heavy perfluorocarbons which reduced molecular diffusion increasing organ retention half-life to several months, as well a poor stability [2, 4]. Pluronic F68 also caused complement activation-type side effects.

Fluosol-DA came as a frozen emulsion concentrate that needed to be thawed and mixed with two annex solutions before administration; it then had to be used within few hours. These constraints certainly had a part in Fluosol's commercial failure. Oxypherol-ET was 25% weight/volume emulsion of perfluorotributylamine, was stable but not intended for human use due to excessively long retention time. A ready-to-use Perfloran has been licensed for use in Russia; recent experimental work with Perftoran includes microvascular gas embolism clearance studies following emulsion administration [40].

Oxygent™ AF0144 (Alliance Pharmaceutical Corp., San Diego, CA) overcame the retentions and stability limitations. It was a 60% weight/volume emulsion, primarily of perfluorooctyl bromide. It was an average micelle size of 0.16 μm after heat sterilization, and a viscosity around 5 cp. It was stable for over 2 years at 5–10°C, without excessive organ retention. These properties were obtained by adding perfluorodecyl bromide.

A randomized, multicenter, European Phase III clinical evaluation of Oxygent in general surgery patients established its ability to significantly reduce and avoid red blood cell transfusion. The trial was conducted using an augmented acute normovolemic hemodilution with PFC emulsion protocol. In the protocol-defined target population (330 subjects with blood loss >20 mL/kg body weight), significantly greater avoidance of any blood cell transfusion, as compared to controls, was maintained through day 21 or day of hospital discharge. There was also a significant reduction in the number of units of blood transfused [41]. However, the voluntary suspension of a CPB surgery trial with Oxygent, because of side effects assigned to an inadequate clinical protocol that resulted in overly aggressive autologous blood harvesting in the treatment group prior to bypass, was a setback in the development of this emulsion.

Clinical development is now being resumed by Double-Crane Pharmaceutical, China. The clinical supplies are used in the Phase 2 Proof of Concept trial that will be conducted in Europe and by Alliance's partner in China, Beijing Double-Crane Pharmaceutical Co. Ltd. (Double-Crane), for its Investigational New Drug application to the State Food and Drug Administration, China. On December 18, 2006, Alliance announced that the French Competent Authority (regulatory agency) approved the start of the Phase 2 clinical trial for Oxygent to prevent post-op ileus resulting from hypoxia during major surgery trial. Double-Crane will initiate the clinical development program for Oxygent in China, starting with its Phase 1 safety study. Double-Crane will be pursuing transfusion avoidance with a new protocol design based on knowledge gained by Alliance from previous clinical trials conducted in the United States and in Europe.

Recent experimental work with Oxygent has demonstrated significant improvement of cerebral oxygenation and mitochondrial function after traumatic brain injury [42]. Resuscitation with Oxygent was superior to stored blood or a plasma expander with respect to restoration of hepatocellular energy metabolism [33]. Proper oxygenation of the gastrointestinal system was preserved in cardiac surgical patients administered with the emulsion, demonstrating the potential for Oxygent to prevent perioperative tissue hypoxia [43]. Postdive intravenous treatment with the emulsion decreased the incidence of decompression sickness [44].

Oxyfluor, HemaGen, St. Louis, MO, selected perfluorodichlorooctane at 40% volume/volume, using egg yoke phospholipid (EYP) as emulsifier.

Oxyfluor was halted after having reached Phase II clinical trials. Several other egg yolk phospholipid based perfluorocarbon emulsions have been reported. *Therox*, a concentrated emulsion 48% v/v with a particle size of 0.25 m, was developed by DuPont for research purposes [45]. Adamantech, Inc. (Marcus Hook, PA) locked onto a mixture of cyclic perfluorocarbons obtained to produce *Addox*, a 40% w/v PFC [46]. Both *Therox* and *Addox* were had a shelf life of 1 year at 4°C [2], the tissue residence half-life of more than 50 days was deemed unacceptable, and these PFC projects were halted. Oxycyte, (Synthetic Blood International; Costa Mesa, CA) consisted of a perfluoronated C-10, cyclohexane compound, 60% w/v emulsion, has completed Phase I clinical trials. In general, the properties of PFCs appear to be progressively improving, their applicability in conjunction with hyperoxia is better understood, and the origin and nature of their side effects are presently well documented [17].

PFC microbubbles

Stable PFC microbubbles developed by Lundgren et al. [47, 48] are reported to dissolve clinically relevant amounts of oxygen when administered in dosages that are about 1/500 of the usual quantities in which PFCs are administered to provide oxygen-carrying capacity [47, 48]. The presence of gas bubbles in the circulation is generally considered medical anathema; however, based on theoretical calculations, it has been proposed that these intravascular bubbles will remain subcapillary in size and transport significant amounts of oxygen. Intravascular microbubbles volume-stabilized by dodecafluoropentane gas are formed when a dodecafluoropentane-emulsion is injected into the circulation at normothermic conditions. The dodecafluoropentane has a boiling point of 29°C at atmospheric pressure and the particles in this emulsion undergo phase shift and form bubbles when warmed in the bloodstream. Initial bubble size depends on the size of the emulsion particles and theoretically, the bubbles undergo size variations as they exchange oxygen, nitrogen, and carbon dioxide by diffusion in the lungs and the tissues [47–49].

Further research objective is to prolong the intravascular persistence, reduce phagocytosis by macrophages, increase stability, and surface-modified PFCs. Substantial efforts are currently being devoted to investigating targeted PFCs for the purpose of molecular imaging, i.e., detection of molecular markers, such as proteins and other cell-surface receptors, characteristic of a given pathology [50]. Such emulsions also have potential for site-directed drug delivery and monitoring of therapy. Important potential target pathologies include inflammation, atherosclerosis, tumor-related angiogenesis, and thrombi. PFC remains very interesting as a gas carrier because its large gas solubility is not restricted to oxygen.

Acknowledgments

This work was supported by Bioengineering Research Partnership grant R24-HL64395 and grants R01-HL62354, R01-HL62318, and R01-HL76182 to Marcos Intaglietta and Amy G. Tsai.

References

1. Riess JG. Understanding the fundamentals of perfluorocarbons and perfluorocarbon emulsions relevant to in vivo oxygen delivery. Artif Cells Blood Substit Immobil Biotechnol 2005;33(1):47–63.
2. Riess JG. Oxygen carriers ("blood substitutes")–raison d'etre, chemistry, and some physiology. Chem Rev 2001;101(9):2797–920.
3. Spahn DR, van Brempt R, Theilmeier G, et al. Perflubron emulsion delays blood transfusions in orthopedic surgery. European perflubron emulsion study group. Anesthesiology 1999;91(5):1195–208.
4. Riess JG. Fluorocarbon-based in vivo oxygen transport and delivery systems. Vox Sang 1991;61(4):225–39.
5. Goodnough LT, Brecher ME, Kanter MH, AuBuchon JP. Blood transfusion. N Engl J Med 1999;340(6):438–47.
6. Berezina TL, Zaets SB, Morgan C, et al. Influence of storage on red blood cell rheological properties. J Surg Res 2002;102(1):6–12.

7. Practice strategies for elective red blood cell transfusion. American College of Physicians. Ann Intern Med 1992;116(5):403–6.
8. Winslow RM. New transfusion strategies: red cell substitutes. Annu Rev Med 1999;50:337–53.
9. Sullivan MT, Cotten R, Read EJ, Wallace EL. Blood collection and transfusion in the United States in 2001. Transfusion 2007;47(3):385–94.
10. Hogman CF, Meryman HT. Red blood cells intended for transfusion: quality criteria revisited. Transfusion 2006;46(1):137–42.
11. Hill SE, Leone BJ, Faithfull NS, Flaim KE, Keipert PE, Newman MF. Perflubron emulsion (AF0144) augments harvesting of autologous blood: a phase II study in cardiac surgery. J Cardiothorac Vasc Anesth 2002;16(5):555–60.
12. Olofsson C, Ahl T, Johansson T, et al. A multicenter clinical study of the safety and activity of maleimide-polyethylene glycol-modified Hemoglobin (Hemospan) in patients undergoing major orthopedic surgery. Anesthesiology 2006;105(6):1153–63.
13. Clark LC, Jr, Wesseler EP, Miller ML, Kaplan S. Ring versus straight chain perfluorocarbon emulsions for perfusion media. Microvasc Res 1974;8(3):320–40.
14. Clark LC, Jr, Wesseler EP, Kaplan S, et al. Emulsions of perfluorinated solvents for intravascular gas transport. Fed Proc 1975;34(6):1468–77.
15. Nolte D, Pickelmann S, Lang M, Keipert P, Messmer K. Compatibility of different colloid plasma expanders with perflubron emulsion: an intravital microscopic study in the hamster. Anesthesiology 2000;93(5):1261–70.
16. Habler OP, Kleen MS, Hutter JW, et al. Hemodilution and intravenous perflubron emulsion as an alternative to blood transfusion: effects on tissue oxygenation during profound hemodilution in anesthetized dogs. Transfusion 1998;38:145–55.
17. Cabrales P, Tsai AG, Frangos JA, Briceno JC, Intaglietta M. Oxygen delivery and consumption in the microcirculation after extreme hemodilution with perfluorocarbons. Am J Physiol 2004;287(1): H320–30.
18. Lowe KC. Perfluorocarbons as oxygen-transport fluids. Comp Biochem Physiol A 1987;87(4):825–38.
19. Ignarro LJ, Byrns RE, Buga GM, Wood KS. Endothelium-derived relaxing factor from pulmonary artery and vein possesses pharmacologic and chemical properties identical to those of nitric oxide radical. Circ Res 1987;61(6):866–79.
20. Tsai AG, Johnson PC, Intaglietta M. Oxygen gradients in the microcirculation. Physiol Rev 2003;83:933–63.
21. McCarthy MR, Vandegriff KD, Winslow RM. The role of facilitated diffusion in oxygen transport by cell-free hemoglobins: implications for the design of hemoglobin-based oxygen carriers. Biophys Chem 2001;92:103–17.
22. Habler O, Kleen M, Hutter J, et al. IV perflubron emulsion versus autologous transfusion in severe normovolemic anemia: effects on left ventricular perfusion and function. Res Exp Med (Berl) 1998;197 (6):301–18.
23. Cernaianu AC, Spence RK, Vassilidze TV, et al. Improvement in circulatory and oxygenation status by perflubron emulsion (Oxygent HT) in a canine model of surgical hemodilution. Artif Cells Blood Substit Immobil Biotechnol 1994;22(4):965–77.
24. Braun RD, Linsenmeier RA, Goldstick TK. New perfluorocarbon emulsion improves tissue oxygenation in cat retina. J Appl Physiol 1992;72(5):1960–68.
25. Keipert PE. Use of Oxygent, a perfluorochemical-based oxygen carrier, as an alternative to intraoperative blood transfusion. Artif Cells Blood Substit Immobil Biotechnol 1995;23(3):381–94.
26. Lutz J, Herrmann G. Perfluorochemicals as a treatment of decompression sickness in rats. Pflugers Arch 1984;401(2):174–7.
27. Spiess BD, Cochran RP. Perfluorocarbon emulsions and cardiopulmonary bypass: a technique for the future. J Cardiothorac Vasc Anesth 1996;10(1):83–9; quiz 9–90.
28. Venkatesh AK, Zhao L, Balamore D, Jolesz FA, Albert MS. Evaluation of carrier agents for hyperpolarized xenon MRI. NMR Biomed 2000;13(4):245–52.
29. Pollack GL, Kennan RP, Holm GT. Solubility of inert gases in PFC blood substitute, blood plasma, and mixtures. Biomater Artif Cells Immobilization Biotechnol 1992;20(2–4):1101–4.
30. Tremper KK, Zaccari J, Cullen BF, Hufstedler SM. Liquid-gas partition coefficients of halothane and isoflurane in perfluorodecalin, fluosol-DA, and blood/fluosol-DA mixtures. Anesth Analg 1984;63 (7):690–92.
31. Cuignet OY, Baele PM, Van Obbergh LJ. A second-generation blood substitute (perflubron emulsion) increases the blood solubility of modern volatile anesthetics in vitro. Anesth Analg 2002;95(2):368–72, table of contents.
32. Rafikova O, Sokolova E, Rafikov R, Nudler E. Control of plasma nitric oxide bioactivity by perfluorocarbons: physiological mechanisms and clinical implications. Circulation 2004;110(23):3573–80.

33. Paxian M, Rensing H, Geckeis K, et al. Perflubron emulsion in prolonged hemorrhagic shock: influence on hepatocellular energy metabolism and oxygen-dependent gene expression. Anesthesiology 2003;98(6):1391–9.
34. Heard SO, Puyana JC. The anti-inflammatory effects of perfluorocarbons: let's get physical. Crit Care Med 2000;28(4):1241–2.
35. Rafikova O, Rafikov R, Nudler E. Catalysis of S-nitrosothiols formation by serum albumin: the mechanism and implication in vascular control. Proc Natl Acad Sci U S A. 2002;99(9):5913–8.
36. Lowe KC. Perfluorinated blood substitutes and artificial oxygen carriers. Blood Rev 1999;13(3): 171–84.
37. Faithfull NS, King CE, Cain SM. Peripheral vascular responses to fluorocarbon administration. Microvasc Res 1987;33(2):183–93.
38. Johnson EC, Erickson BK, Podolsky A, et al. Effects of a perfluorocarbon emulsion for enhanced O2 solubility on hemodynamics and O2 transport in dogs. J Appl Physiol 1995;79(5):1777–86.
39. Paxian M, Keller SA, Huynh TT, Clemens MG. Perflubron emulsion improves hepatic microvascular integrity and mitochondrial redox state after hemorrhagic shock. Shock 2003;20(5):449–57.
40. Eckmann DM, Lomivorotov VN. Microvascular gas embolization clearance following perfluorocarbon administration. J Appl Physiol 2003;94(3):860–68.
41. Spahn DR, Waschke KF, Standl T, et al. Use of perflubron emulsion to decrease allogeneic blood transfusion in high-blood-loss non-cardiac surgery: results of a European phase 3 study. Anesthesiology 2002;97(6):1338–49.
42. Daugherty WP, Levasseur JE, Sun D, Spiess BD, Bullock MR. Perfluorocarbon emulsion improves cerebral oxygenation and mitochondrial function after fluid percussion brain injury in rats. Neurosurgery 2004;54(5):1223– 30; discussion 30.
43. Koch CJ, Oprysko PR, Shuman AL, Jenkins WT, Brandt G, Evans SM. Radiosensitization of hypoxic tumor cells by dodecafluoropentane: a gas-phase perfluorochemical emulsion. Cancer Res 2002;62(13): 3626–9.
44. Dromsky DM, Spiess BD, Fahlman A. Treatment of decompression sickness in swine with intravenous perfluorocarbon emulsion. Aviat Space Environ Med 2004;75(4):301–5.
45. Thoolen MJ, Rasbach DE, Shaw JH, Raynolds S, Timmermans PB. Preservation of regional and global left ventricular function by intracoronary infusion with oxygenated fluorocarbon emulsion Therox in dogs. Biomater Artif Cells Immobilization Biotechnol 1993;21(1):53–62.
46. Busch OR, Hop WC, Hoynck van Papendrecht MA, Marquet RL, Jeekel J. Blood transfusions and prognosis in colorectal cancer. N Engl J Med 1993; 328(19):1372–6.
47. Lundgren CE, Bergoe GW, Tyssebotn IM. Intravascular fluorocarbon-stabilized microbubbles protect against fatal anemia in rats. Artif Cells Blood Substit Immobil Biotechnol 2006;34(5):473–86.
48. Lundgren CE, Bergoe GW, Tyssebotn I. The theory and application of intravascular microbubbles as an ultra-effective means of transporting oxygen and other gases. Undersea Hyperb Med 2004;31(1):105–6.
49. Lundgren C, Bergoe G, Olszowka A, Tyssebotn I. Tissue nitrogen elimination in oxygen-breathing pigs is enhanced by fluorocarbon-derived intravascular micro-bubbles. Undersea Hyperb Med 2005;32(4): 215–26.
50. Lanza GM, Wickline SA. Targeted ultrasonic contrast agents for molecular imaging and therapy. Prog Cardiovasc Dis 2001;44(1):13–31.

SECTION 2
Surgical Techniques

CHAPTER 32

Minimally Invasive Cardiac Surgery: Impact on Blood Loss and Transfusion

He Tao & Fraser Rubens
Division of Cardiac Surgery, University of Ottawa Heart Institute, Ottawa, Ontario, Canada

Introduction

To a degree greater than any other surgical specialty, the evolution of cardiac surgery has been intimately dependent upon blood banking resources and transfusion practice. Cardiac surgery has always been, and likely always will be a major consumer of blood products [1, 2]. With standard surgical techniques, this dependence appears to be increasing as surgeons are exposed to older, sicker patients with a greater incidence of comorbidities. Although many patients receive no transfusions, these sicker patients are obviously at higher risk, comprising the 10–20% of the patients who consume about 80% of the total transfusions in cardiac surgery [3]. During the next 30 years, it is predicted that the proportion of the population over the age of 65 will increase. This trend is expected to increase the number of patients needing a transfusion despite the fact that there is a concomitant decreasing pool of eligible donors [4].

Transfusion incidence is now becoming a marker of quality of care released on the public domain (http//:www.ccn.on.ca). This Canadian data like other studies [5] emphasizes the significant variability in practice with transfusion risks of 22–55%, despite little variability in other patient demographics between institutions.

Surgeons are also now recognizing that transfusion after cardiac surgery is a double-edged sword that may harm more patients than previously anticipated. Most surgeons in practice today were not exposed at the level of undergraduate medicine to the myriad of complications that are now being taught with regards to transfusion of allogeneic blood, other than the obvious risks related to blood incompatibility errors and viral transmission. As a consequence many surgeons continue to be influenced by a philosophy of transfusion practice involving critical hemoglobin thresholds as targets.

Numerous robust observational studies have strongly demonstrated that transfusion after cardiac surgery is associated with an increased incidence of wound and other infections even when adjusted for case severity [6–8]. Such wound problems are particularly devastating in the presence of a median sternotomy with potential devascularization with one or both internal thoracic arteries utilized for bypass conduits. Transfusion has also been associated with an increased incidence of postoperative AF after cardiac surgery [9], perioperative myocardial infarction [10], and low-output heart failure as compared to patients treated with a conservative transfusion strategy [11]. Other documented end-organ injury seen commonly in cardiac surgery patients that may be related to transfusions includes pulmonary insufficiency in the form of transfusion related lung injury and acute renal insufficiency [12].

In an effort to address these concerns, cardiac surgeons and anesthetists have embraced the concept of blood conservation and have worked together to establish the feasibility of the various technologies available to minimize transfusion,

Alternatives to Blood Transfusion in Transfusion Medicine, 2nd edition. Edited by A. Maniatis, P. Van der Linden, J.-F. Hardy.

such as retrograde autologous priming, antifibrinolytics, and cell salvage [13]. However, it has fallen into the surgeon's purview alone to consider what could be done in the operative field on our "side" of the ether screen, with novel strategies and modifications in approach that may minimize bleeding and thus transfusion. Though not originally intended to impact transfusion, the broad field of minimally invasive surgery and its expanding applications has accomplished many of these goals.

What is minimally invasive cardiac surgery?

As a general principle, this concept refers to operations that cause minimal injury to the patient, yet achieve all their surgical goals. There are several potential technical "targets" that may be modified to accomplish these needs. These include the length of the incision, the extent of retraction during exposure, the use of electrocautery, but most significantly the elimination of the traditional median sternotomy in some form, and/or the avoidance of cardiopulmonary bypass (CPB) or minimization of its effect. Many innovative techniques and technologies have been developed that allow cardiac procedures to be performed through small incisions with or without CPB. Collectively this group of techniques and technologies has been termed minimally invasive; its development fueled by industry's recognition of the strong consumer support for smaller incisions and patients' perception that these approaches are associated with improved outcomes. Most patient concerns and demands for less-invasive surgery are focused on comfort, cosmesis, and rehabilitation that are all related to the degree of invasiveness. In this chapter, we try to distinguish between "fashionable" strategies and those that are truly revolutionary as investments in the future [14].

In terms of blood conservation, minimally invasive cardiac surgery may have an impact through two primary mechanisms [4]; by avoiding the inflammatory and hemostatic defects associated with CPB and/or minimizing surgical trauma by modification of the approach and the incision. We have categorized these approaches into three major groups of minimally invasive cardiac surgery.

1 Minimally invasive coronary surgery
- **1.1** Sternotomy—off-pump
- **1.2** MIDCAB
- **1.3** Videoscopic and robotic-assisted nonsternotomy approaches

2 Minimally invasive valve surgery
- **2.1** Partial sternotomy and parasternal approaches
- **2.2** Right mini-thoracotomy
- **2.3** Total port-access—robotic

3 Minimized extra-corporeal circulation (MECC)

What are the mechanisms by which smaller incisions would decrease bleeding and transfusion?

It is intuitive for surgeons to understand that the systemic effects of surgery are proportional to the size and invasiveness of the incision. The median sternotomy itself, though superb for cardiac exposure, results in an extensive raw bone surface, contributing to bleeding and sometimes necessitating additional hemostatic maneuvers such as the use of bone wax. The impact of the length of an incision to the magnitude of the systemic changes has been infrequently characterized experimentally; however, in one clinical trial, Gu et al. [15] compared the magnitude of inflammation activation with lateral minithoracotomy and median sternotomy during off-pump surgery. Postoperatively, interleukin-6 production was greater in the median sternotomy group than the lateral group ($p < 0.05$), supporting a more pronounced inflammatory response to a larger chest incision.

What are the mechanisms by which avoiding bypass would decrease bleeding?

CPB is well-known to cause numerous derangements in platelet function and coagulation.

Through a series of interacting cascades, blood reacts to minimize the unnatural threat resulting from the exposure to the synthetic surface of the bypass device. The most immediate event within nanoseconds of contact of the blood involves protein adsorption [16]. These contact proteins (Factors XI and XII, prekallikrein, and high molecular weight kininogen) may become activated with the generation of thrombin, kallikrein which contributes to fibrinolysis [17] and bradykinin, a potent pro-inflammatory agent which also leads to tissue plasminogen activator release from endothelial cells [18]. Fibrinogen is also adsorbed and this may serve as a nidus for adhesion and accumulation of platelets [19].

Platelets also become activated during CPB [20] by various agonists including thrombin, adenosine diphosphate (ADP), and plasmin. Plasmin also significantly modifies surface platelet receptors [21].Once activated, platelet microparticles are generated which are highly thrombogenic [22]. These changes are reflected by a drop in the platelet count by up to 50%, not just due to adhesion/accumulation, but also from hemodilution and platelet aggregate formation. The resulting platelet dysfunction with CPB is quite predictable [23] and the subsequent increased bleeding time is proportional to the blood loss [24].

The mandatory use of heparin, though decreasing thrombin generation, magnifies the impact on coagulation and this drug may affect platelet function directly [25] also acting as a profibrinolytic agent [26]. Further, despite heparin, one sees subclinical ongoing thrombin generation [27] resulting in coagulation factor consumption, which compounds the effect of hemodilution of these factors [28].

Another significant factor that contributes to derangements in hemostasis includes the use of the cardiotomy suction to scavenge blood that wells in the mediastinum during CPB. This has been identified as the greatest contributor to blood activation and thrombin generation during CPB likely secondary to the extensive contact of blood to the nonendothelialized surfaces rich in tissue factor and the rapid sequestration of heparin from this blood [29, 30].

In summary, multiple surface-contact related mechanisms for coagulation and platelet dysfunction exist which when coupled with activation of fibrinolysis, compound the bleeding diathesis associated with CPB.

What is "off-pump surgery"?

Off-pump coronary bypass (OPCAB) is perhaps the most frequently performed and most accepted variant of minimally invasive cardiac surgery. This procedure utilizes a standard median sternotomy (a vertical incision through the sternum) for cardiac exposure. However, coronary bypass is accomplished without the use of CPB. The avoidance of CPB not only eliminates the systemic pro-inflammatory and thrombotic derangements but it also removes the need for arterial cannulation (normally through the ascending aorta) thus minimizing the risk of embolization of atherosclerotic debris.

Traditional on-pump techniques provide technical comfort as the heart is still and the operative target is bloodless affording ideal accuracy. The current technology for off-pump surgery uses novel means to provide these goals in a facile manner. The target epicardial vessels can be isolated with "feet" that stabilize either with direct compression or with suction devices (Figure 32.1). The heart can also be remarkably manipulated to bring the target region into view using either complex pericardial retraction sutures or, more commonly, with large suction devices which can be attached to the cardiac apex (Figure 32.1). Though difficult, with these techniques even obtuse marginal vessels may be approached off-pump and with experience, the degree of revascularization with this technique approaches that of standard on-pump strategies.

This option is particularly useful in patients with ascending aortic atherosclerosis and cerebral vascular disease, and many authors have recommended its use in patients with other comorbidities such as renal insufficiency and chronic obstructive lung disease [31]. However, there are limitations to this approach. Notably, the procedure is contraindicated in patients with moderate or greater mitral

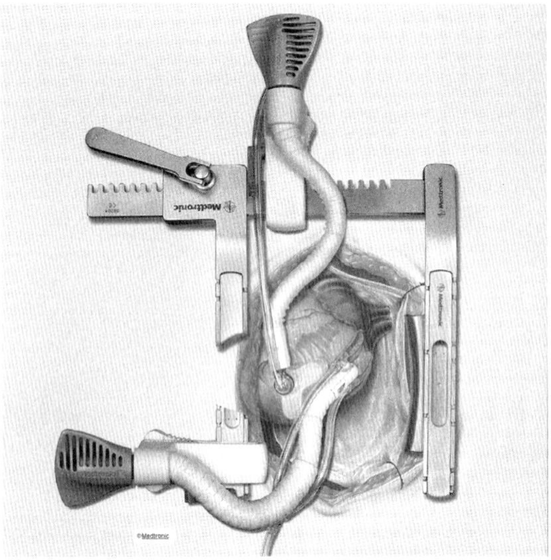

Figure 32.1 Octopus^{TM} and Starfish^{TM} (Medtronics Inc., Minneapolis, MN) suction devices used to stabilize the target epicardial regions and rotate the apex of the heart respectively. The distraction and rotation of the heart allows for full exposure to the target regions and the epicardial vessels may be controlled with atraumatic snares of intraluminal shunts (picture courtesy of Medtronics Inc., Minneapolis, MN).

insfufficiency, diffuse coronary disease, intramyocardial vessels, and coronary calcification, and thus many patients who would benefit best from this technique cannot be candidates for off-pump procedures.

As off-pump surgery obviates the pathophysiologic brunt of CPB, it is not entirely surprising that it would have an impact on the incidence of bleeding, transfusion, and reopening. Decreased transfusion may, in fact, be one of the mechanisms by which this technique may be associated with improved outcomes as excessive postoperative bleeding plays a key role as an important cause of morbidity and mortality after CPB. Surgical reexploration of the mediastinum (reopening or rethoracotomy) resulting from postoperative hemorrhage occurs in 3–5% of patients in traditional surgery, and thus any intervention that could minimize this rate should improve outcomes and expense.

A critical evaluation of current options of minimally invasive cardiac surgery to impact blood loss

Minimally invasive coronary surgery

OPCAB—median sternotomy approach

We have identified a limited number of RCTs and observational trials since 2000, in which we were able to compare blood loss, reexploration rate, and homologous transfusion after OPCAB as compared to conventional CABG (Table 32.1). The majority of clinical trials have supported the concept that off-pump coronary artery bypass grafting (CABG) through a median sternotomy is associated with decreased bleeding, and thus a decrease in the risk of transfusion as compared to conventional surgery.

Other reviewers in this area have also concluded that an off-pump approach is associated with a decreased risk of transfusion as compared to conventional surgery [32]. This question has been addressed using meta-analyses in two publications. Cheng et al. [33], in a review of 37 clinical trials, demonstrated a significant benefit of off-pump surgery to decrease the incidence of transfusion (OR 0.43; 95% CI, 0.29–0.65). On the contrary, there was no significant difference in the need for re-thoracotomy for bleeding. The transfusion effect of off-pump surgery in clinical surgery was also shown to be decreased in a random effects model analyzed by Guru et al. (OR 0.47; 95% CI, 0.32–0.59) [34].

Other factors showing benefit of this approach over conventional surgery include lower myocardial enzyme release, decreased stroke rate, lesser renal insufficiency, and perhaps a decreased incidence in atrial fibrillation [35, 36]. As there appears to be consensus on this outcome of improved hemostasis as well, why has this procedure not achieved universal appeal and acceptance? [35, 37] Many surgical teams still recognize the limitations of off-pump surgery and recent reports suggesting that this procedure may be associated with a compromise in long-term patency [38] incomplete revascularization and an increased risk of late repeat revascularization [36] have tempered their

Table 32.1 RCT trials comparing off-pump and on-pump for bleeding and transfusion.

	Number of patients		Blood loss	Reexploration rate	Homologous transfusion	
Author	OPCAB	CCABG	OPCAB/ CCABG	OPCAB/CCABG	OPCAB/CCABG Number (%)	OPCAB/CCABG Amount transfused (mL)*
Sajja et al. [65]	56	60	360/542†	NP	NP	193/470.1†
Kobayashi et al. [66]	81	86	503/560	NP	16(20%)/39(45%)†	NP
Gerola et al. [67]	80	80	678.6/680.5	NP	36(45%)/35(43.7%)	NP
Wan et al. [68]	18	19	701/748	0/0	NA	110/278‡
Wehlin et al. [69]	21	16	720/610	NP	7(33.3%)/2(12.5%)	NP
Straka et al. [70]	204	184	560/680†	4/2	49(24%)/51(28%)	NP
Khan et al. [38]	54	49	1031/898	0/2(4%)	20(37%)/32(65%)†,§	NP
Puskas et al. [71]	98	99	NA	1(1%)/2(2%)	25(26%)/44(44%)†	NP
Muneretto et al. [72]	88	88	385/514†	NP	29(32.9%)/50(56.9%)†	NP
Lee et al. [73]	30	30	789/1389†	NP	NP	300/975†
Angelini et al. [74]	200	201	41/62†,‖	6(3%)/10(5%)	35(17.5%)/97(48%)†	NP
Ascione et al. [75]	100	100	687/943.19†	2(2%)/8(8%)	23(23%)/52(52%)†	NP
van Dijk et al. [76]	142	139	500/400†(12 h)	7(4%)/3(2%)	40(28%)/40(29%)	NP
Observational cohort trials comparing off-pump and on-pump for bleeding and transfusion						
Potger et al. [77]	610	433	NP	NP	NP	NP
Frankel et al. [78]	3646	5197	NP	75(2.1%)/146(2.8%)†	NP	656/874†
Scott et al. [79]	865	881	NP	15(1.7%)/29(3.3%)†	49%/74%†	375/825†
Mack et al. [31]	7283	10118	NP	79(1.7%)/169(3.2%)†	1503(33%)/3156(41%)†	NP
Berson et al. [80]	360	1080	NP	NP	NP	90/260†
Nuttall et al. [81]	100	100	(24 h)950/808	NP	89%/94%	0/250†,¶
Scott et al. [82]	554	681	NP	1.9%/3.6%	253(46%)/491(73%)†	400/850†,#
Ishida et al. [83]	95	63	480/720†	NP	NP	300/1230†
Zamvar et al. [84]	120	247	NP	NP	40%/90%†	NP
Kirk et al. [85]	86	117	NP	NP	30(35%)/67(57%)†	275/600†,**
Petro et al. [86]	840	5528	NP	1.3%/2.2%	40%/59%†	NP
Yokoyama et al. [87]	242	483	NP	3(1.2%)/17(3.5%)	46(19%)/218(45%)†	NP

Abbreviations: OPCAB, off-pump coronary artery bypass; CCABG, conventional on-pump coronary artery bypass; NS, nonsignificant; NP, not provided; RBC, red blood cells; FFP, fresh frozen plasma; RCT, randomized controlled trial.

*Determined using conversion of one unit = 250 mL.

†$p < 0.05$.

‡OPCAB/CABG blood(units) 0.4 ± 0.9 vs 1.1 ± 1.4, NS; FFP 0.2 ± 0.5 vs 1.7 ± 0.7, NS; Platelets 0.3 ± 0.8 vs 2.3 ± 1.6, $p < 0.01$.

§RBC transfusion OPCAB/CCABG (20(37%)/32(65%), $p = 0.004$) or FFP (2(4%)/14(29%), $p = 0.002$).

‖Number of patients with blood loss >1000 mL.

¶OPCAB/CCABG intraop: Median RBC 0 mL vs 250 mL, $p = 0.001$; FFP 2% vs 6%, NS; platelets: 1%/9%, $p = 0.018$; cryoprecipitate: 0%/1%, NS Postop: RBC 575 mL/600 mL, NS.

#OPCAB/CCABG. RBC/patient (units) 1.6 ± 0.2 vs 3.4 ± 0.3, $p < 0.001$; FFP/patient (units) 0.4 ± 0.1 vs 1.2 ± 0.2, $p < 0.001$; Platelets/patient (units) 0.3 ± 0.1 vs 0.5 ± 0.1, $p < 0.001$.

**OPCAB/CABG PRBC:(units) 1.1 ± 1.8 vs 2.4 ± 3.2, $p < 0.05$; FFP 0.3 ± 0.9 vs 0.2 ± 0.9, NS; Platelets 0.1 ± 0.3 vs 0.1 ± 0.3, NS.

confidence in this strategy. Further, despite its theoretical advantages, the procedure has never been able to conclusively demonstrate a benefit in terms of the incidence of postoperative neurocognitive dysfunction [39, 40]. Therefore, larger randomized clinical trials are still necessary to clearly elucidate the specific indications for this approach in the cardiac surgery population. Recognizing its limitations in terms of the degree of successful revascularization, it may still be an option in patients in whom transfusion is particularly an issue and we believe it is an essential tool in a surgical team's armamentarium to provide cardiovascular services particularly for high-risk patients.

Minimally invasive direct coronary artery bypass

Minimally invasive direct coronary artery bypass (MIDCAB) was introduced as an attempt to combine the beneficial approach of coronary revascularization without the use of CPB, with an alternative nonsternotomy incision. Although most authors equate the term MIDCAB to reflect a left anterior mini-thoracotomy (Figure 32.2) used for revascularization of the left anterior descending with the left internal thoracic artery, this latter approach is sometimes referred to as a left anterior small thoracotomy (i.e., a type of MIDCAB) with a lower-end sternal splitting as the second type of MIDCAB. These approaches have shown improved recovery rates, reduced morbidity, costs, and length of hospital stay without compromising the quality of the surgical procedure as compared to conventional CABG completed through a sternotomy [41]. Of note, this section refers to surgery of this nature done without additional technical support such as videoscopic assistance (described below).

There are several observational trials describing results with these approaches and most studies have shown quite good outcomes with essentially no risk of mortality, stroke or myocardial infarction and in two series including our own, no transfusion required in 68 patients [42, 43]. Good results have also been achieved with this incision for multiple grafts (multi-vessel small thoracotomy (MVST) but as yet there is little clinical data on the effect of this technique to decrease bleeding.

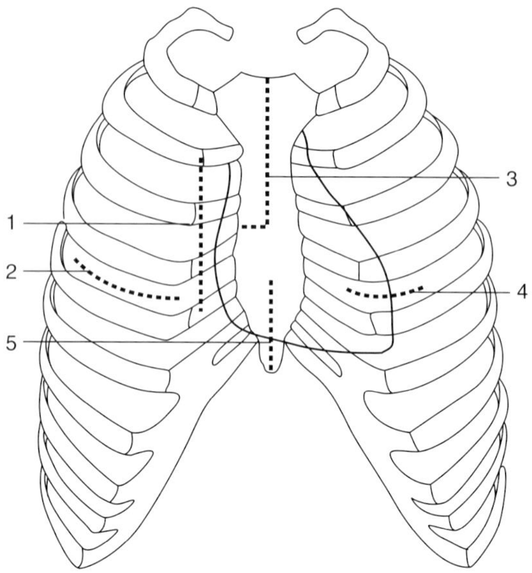

Figure 32.2 Common thoracic incisions used for minimally invasive cardiac surgery: (1) right parasternal; (2) right anterior mini-thoracotomy; (3) upper "J" mini-sternotomy; (4) left anterior mini-thoractomy; (5) lower end sternal splitting.

With the MIDCAB approach, there is a risk of conversion to sternotomy and the need for CPB, but if this is done expeditiously and liberally, there is minimal incremental risk and no patients were transfused who crossed over [42]. These outcomes are not, however, generalizable and poor outcomes have been reported in some trials [41] as in some cases re-operation for bleeding has been required [44]. As the procedure is technically challenging, it is an option not in isolation employed as a strategy primarily to decrease transfusions.

Videoscopic and robotic-assisted nonsternotomy approaches

There has been a progressive evolution in coronary revascularization through nonsternotomy approaches with the utilization of advanced technology with videoscopic equipment, and recently through the introduction of robotic assistance. Scopes introduced through thoracic ports can be utilized to harvest the internal thoracic arteries and the anastomosis can be performed on the beating heart either through a small anterior thoracotomy

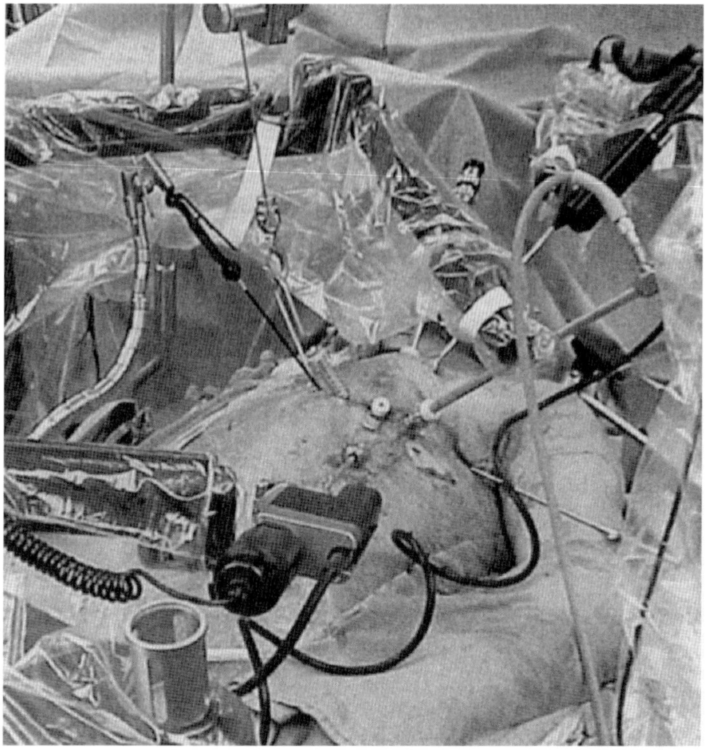

Figure 32.3 Totally endoscopic CABG setup. Data from Boyd et al. [89].

with limited rib spreading [45] or using robotic arms that can be introduced through separate ports to stabilize the target region and perform the anastomoses on the beating heart in a completely endoscopic manner (Figure 32.3). Meticulous planning is required in terms of the choice of conduits, the type of anastomoses, and the order of revascularization in cases of multiple grafts [46]. These strategies embody the fundamental premise of minimally invasive cardiac surgery by both the complete avoidance of CPB and the sternotomy with the added benefit of limited rib spreading [47]. Most case series (Table 32.2) support that these techniques are associated with minimal blood loss [48] infrequent re-operations for bleeding (2.8% [46] and infrequent transfusions as compared to conventional approaches (10% [46]).

Some centers have proposed a similar approach for completely endoscopic bypass with robotic assistance but with CPB support [49]. Bonatti et al. reported 40 patients who received robotically assisted totally endoscopic left internal thoracic artery grafts to the left anterior descending coronary artery system with the da Vinci telemanipulation device (Intuitive Surgical Inc.). All patients underwent remote access CPB perfusion through groin access, and all anastomoses were performed on the arrested heart. There were bleeding complications which included bleeding from a port hole in 3 (8%) and bleeding from the anastomosis in 4 (10%) necessitating transfusion and revision. Further, the bypass and cross-clamp times were not insignificant, thus rendering this a less-supported goal of minimally invasive surgery in terms of its capacity to minimize transfusion.

Finally, these minimally invasive approaches which capitalize on the importance of the performance of the left internal thoracic artery—left anterior descending artery bypass, can be used in collaboration with the interventionalist by revascularization of other vessels with percutaneous coronary intervention. To date, there are limited re-

Table 32.2 Video/robotic-assisted CABG; effect on reoperation and transfusion.

Author	Number	Reoperations for bleeding	Transfusion
Nesher et al. [48]	146		
Turner et al. [47]	70	2(2.8%)	7(10%)
Srivastava et al. [88]	150	5(3.3%)	19(13%)
Bonatti et al. [49]	40(20/20)*	1(5%)/6(30%), $p = 0.037$*	0/5 U, $p = 0.001$
Subramanian et al. [45]	30	2	
Boyd et al. [89]	84†	2	
Torracca et al. [44]	12	1	
Damiano et al. [90]	32	3	
Boyd et al. [91]	15	0	
Falk et al. [92]	66	1	

*Comparison of patients with (20) and without (20) technical difficulties during performance of totally endoscopic CABG.
†Report included case series from multicenter review of 215 patients with incidence of transfusion 6%.

ports and certainly none comparing this approach to conventional surgery in terms of transfusion risk. In fact, these procedures may compound bleeding as current stent placement mandates the use of potent antiplatelet and antithrombotic medications that have been shown to increase perioperative bleeding and reopening [50].

Valve surgery

General overview

Valvular surgery, by its very nature, mandates opening the cardiac chambers, thus the circulatory and respiratory functions of the heart and lungs must be circumvented with CPB. Although this particular goal of minimally invasive surgery (i.e., avoidance of CPB) cannot be achieved, groups have explored alternative nonsternotomy incisions for cardiac exposure for valve surgery (Table 32.3). Many teams have been successful in using these approaches and patient outcomes have been excellent, with documented decreases in bleeding and transfusion as compared to historical cohorts [51]. The approaches have been further supported by cosmetic benefits and lessened pain, which has translated into shorter hospital stays and, thus, decreased cost [51].

Mini-sternotomy and parasternal approaches

The aortic valve in particular can be approached successfully with a mini-sternotomy (Figure 32.2) through the upper, middle, or inferior portions. As opposed to an anterior thoracotomy, access to the great vessels is relatively easy through a ministernotomy, which renders central cannulation possible. Ministernotomy in mitral valve surgery has been progressively abandoned owing to facility of right anterior small thoracotomy with video assistance for the latter pathology (see below). Ministernotomy is also used in congenital heart surgery and in selective cases of coronary bypass, particularly in the presence of patent bypass grafts in reoperative surgery [52, 53].

Aside from pain and cosmesis, the partial nature of the mini-sternotomy may contribute to enhanced sternal stability, which may also decrease the incidence of wound infection. In terms of hemostasis, eliminating a full sternotomy decreases sternal bleeding. Bakir et al. [54] compared a ministernotomy group to a historical cohort and they demonstrated reduced CPB times compared with conventional surgery. Mean blood loss was also lower with a ministernotomy ($p < 0.05$) [54]. They described the use of this approach for minimally invasive aortic root replacement in 35 patients (mean age 51 ± 15 years) through a partial upper J-sternotomy. Revision for bleeding was necessary in 1 (2.9%) patient. [54]. Byrne et al. also reported a series of 137 aortic root replacements in which 37 (27%) were accomplished through a 5- to 8-cm minimally invasive upper hemi-sternotomy incision. There was one (3%)

Table 32.3 Robotic and video-assisted valve surgery—impact on bleeding and transfusion.

	Patient number			Blood transfusion			Blood loss (mL)
Author	Robotic	Conv.	Operation	Number(%) Robotic/Conv.	Units Robotic/Conv.	Reexploration	Robotic/Conv.
Woo, [93]	25	39	RAMV repair		2.8 ± 0.6 U/5.0 ± 1.0 U*		
Folliguet et al. [94]	25	25	RAMV repair	2(8%)/4(16%)		1(4%)/2(8%)	477 ± 213/566 ± 201
Bolotin [58]	38	33	Re-do MV surgery		2.9 ± 0.6 U/5.5 ± 0.7 U*		
Mishra et al. [95]	221	220	MV surgery			0	332 ± 104/440 ± 92
Chitwood [96]	31	100	MV surgery		2.1 ± 0.2 U/3.6 ± 0.4 U*	0/4(4%)*	623 ± 99/716 ± 86
Observational studies about video/robotic-assisted valve surgery for bleeding and transfusion							
Nifong [97]	112		RAMV repair	19(17%)†		3	
Tatooles et al. [98]	25		RAMV repair	11(44%)		0	
Sobieski et al. [99]	25		RAMV repair	6(24%)		0	
Nifong [100]	38*		RAMV repair	6(16%)		1	

Abbreviations: RAMV, robotic-assisted mitral valve; Conv., conventional; AVR, aortic valve replacement; MV, mitral valve.
*$p < 0.05$.
†Of 19 patients transfused, required average of 2.5 ± 0.9 U, 5 patients received 2.6 ± 1.1 U FFP, 6 patients with 4.0 ± 2.6 U platelets.

re-operation for bleeding and 13 patients (35%) required blood transfusions. They emphasized that minimally invasive aortic root replacement is feasible for a broad range of aortic valve pathology with acceptable morbidity and mortality. However, the operation takes longer through the smaller incision and therefore requires more careful attention to myocardial protection [55].

Other groups, particularly the surgeons at the Brigham Hospital [51] have advocated the use of parasternal incisions (Figure 32.2). This latter approach does require femoral cannulation and thus a separate groin incision. With experience, these techniques have been associated with a low incidence of reopening for bleeding [56] but not consistently any difference in transfusion rates.Most of these trials have been observational in nature with historical cohorts used, thus the lack of appropriate controls and surgeon-specific outcomes may not be generalizable.

Therefore in summary, observational trials have demonstrated the potential of the mini-sternotomy and the parasternal incision to decrease bleeding and thus transfusion; however, this premise has not be confirmed with appropriate randomized controlled trials with strict transfusion guidelines, and thus these approaches cannot be recommended definitively as blood-conserving strategies.

Right mini-thoracotomy

The primary alternative nonsternotomy minimally invasive approach for mitral surgery involves a right anterior thoracotomy in the fourth intercostal space (Figure 32.2). Central cannulation is possible; however, the cannula placement can be difficult and they may also compromise surgical exposure. Thus groin cannulation is currently preferred. This approach may also be beneficial for the repair of an atrial septal defect as for this problem, minimal rib spreading is necessary. Further, it is of particular value in cases of re-operative mitral valve surgery in which it is anticipated that there are dense pericardial adhesions which may jeopardize patient safety. In series comparing standard approaches to right anterior thoractomy, there was a significant reduction in blood loss (277 ± 152 mL thoracotomy vs 651 ± 504 mL sternotomy, $p < 0.05$) and blood transfused (2.0 ± 1.7 units thoracotomy vs 6.5 ± 3.3 units sternotomy, $p < 0.01$) [57]. Similar findings were demonstrated by Bolotin et al. who recorded that blood transfusion requirements were also reduced (2.9 ± 0.6 vs 5.5 ± 0.7 units; $p = 0.001$) [58].

Port-access—robotics in valve surgery

Port-access cardiac surgery was developed by Heartport Incorporated (Redwood City, CA) in an effort to combine the safety and support of CPB with cardioplegic arrest with limited incisions in situations in which a median sternotomy is not used. To date, well over a hundred centers in the United States and Europe are using the technology, with the indications extending to multivessel bypass, multivalve surgery, and surgery for congenital heart disease (Figure 32.4). The procedure remains technically challenging and the endoclamp (a trans-femoral intraluminal balloon used to occlude the aorta) has been associated with some complications in series with MV surgery with as many as 30% needing conversion to trans-thoracic clamping [59]. The literature supports that this approach is certainly more complicated thus it may be associated with an increased risk of bleeding and vascular damage [60].

The introduction of videoscopic and robotic assistance expanded the indications of right minithoracotomy approaches to primary surgery of mitral valve repair and replacement [61]. Excellent exposure of the mitral valve can be achieved. Initially this approach was dependent upon Heart-Port technology; however, a feasible alternative to the transthoracic aortic clamp was introduced by Chitwood et al. [62, 63]. This has provided a technical improvement related to facilitated control of the aorta for cross-clampling and cardioplegia administration. This strategy still requires groin cannulation for vascular access.

There are numerous international reports comprising large case series with this approach for mitral valve surgery. However, a convincing decrease in blood loss as compared to historical conventional controls has not been seen. This is likely related to the relatively long procedure times as compared to conventional approaches. The benefit of this approach has been mostly cosmetic but patients also experience less pain and they are able to mobilize more rapidly. In experienced hands, this approach is not associated with an increased rate of reopening.

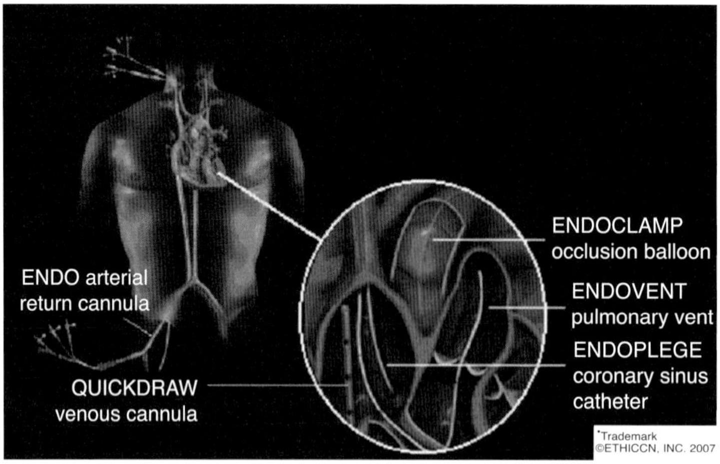

Figure 32.4 CardioVations. The arterial and venous cannulae are inserted through the groins and the aorta is occluded with an intra-aortic occlusion balloon. The jugular access is used to insert a pulmonary artery vent and a cannula to reside in the coronary sinus to administer cardioplegia (picture courtesy of CardioVations).

In summary, videoscopic and robotic assistance can be successfully used to safely accomplish many types of mitral valve surgery, however, as yet the data does not support that these approaches can consistently minimize blood loss and transfusion.

Minimized extracorporeal circulation

In an effort to minimize the systemic effects of CPB, biomedical teams have remodeled bypass circuits to address the key components thought to contribute to the pathophysiology of CPB. These novel CPB systems, referred to as MECC aim to limit the disturbance of the patient's homeostasis by designs with low-prime, closed volume, and hemocompatible extracorporeal circuits. In particular, these modified circuits have been designed with minimized surface area in the oxygenator with integrated heat exchangers, all coated tip-to-tip with biocompatible surfaces, to lessen the blood-biomaterial impact. Tubing and related cannulae are minimized in length and diameter to markedly lessen the prime volume, thus impacting significantly on the degree of hemodilution. Steps have been taken as well to remove all possible areas of blood–air interface by using a closed reservoir and eliminating the cardiotomy reservoir with routine cell salvage of all collected blood from the mediastinal field as well as all vent blood from the left heart, necessary for most procedures but particularly for valve operations. The smaller cannulae necessitate the use of vacuum-assisted venous drainage to ensure adequate flows. But with these modifications, total priming volume of 500 mL can be expected as compared to conventional volumes of 1.4–1.8 L. Owing to markedly decreased hemodilution, less intraop anemia results, and consistently trials have shown a decrease in the need for intraoperative transfusion [64].

To date, these trials have had limited impact in current practice patterns as they have been small sample sizes of mediocre design. Further, it is virtually impossible to blind the participants due to the technical nature of the intervention. Finally, as in many cardiac surgery trials, the transfusion guidelines are often poorly established and compliance to the guidelines is not often achievable.

On contrary, the magnitude of the difference in hemodilution between conventional circuits and MECC is so profound in most trials that it is not unreasonable to assume that this will translate into a significant improvement in transfusion outcomes. Several recent clinical studies have been listed in Table 32.4 that have demonstrated the value of this procedure in both valve and coronary surgery. Several authors have shown a marked decrease in the amount of shed mediastinal blood postoperatively, but most importantly, the majority of trials have demonstrated a decrease in the percentage of patients who require transfusion.

Conclusions

Minimally invasive strategies are likely here to stay in the cardiac surgical repertoire and it is probable that new technologies will continue to be implemented at a rapid pace. Few of the technologies described above were designed with blood conservation as a primary goal as this target had not yet reached critical recognition on the radar maps of cardiac surgeons. Luckily however, as a secondary outcome, many approaches such as off-pump bypass clearly have shown a benefit in terms of transfusion risk and one can recommend their implementation in high-risk patients for this reason alone.

We currently recognize that for most of these technologies, surgical teams must balance the cosmetic benefits of a smaller incision with the detrimental systemic effects of the longer bypass time that is often necessary to achieve the same surgical goals, such as seen with robotic mitral valve surgery. However, promising work with minimization of bypass circuits may provide an ideal means to overcome these limitations such that both goals can be aligned. We in fact believe that these smaller circuits will revolutionize the field of cardiac surgery such that hemodilution will be avoided in many cases, and by extension, patient outcomes will be improved dramatically. The clinical groundwork has been set to support well-designed clinical trials in this area and as accountability for transfusion rates between institutions grows, the

Table 32.4 Minimized extra-corporeal circulation (MECC); effect on bleeding, reopening, and transfusion.

Author	Number of patients		Blood loss (mL)	Reopening	Transfusion	
CABG	MECC	Conventional	MECC/Conventional	MECC/ Conventional	Units MECC/ Conventional	Percent transfused MECC/ Conventional
Perthel [101] RCT	30	30	$302 \pm 532/786 \pm 1000^*$	NP	$0.5 \pm 0.9/1.3 \pm 1.9^{*,\dagger}$	27%/43%*
Huybregts [102] RCT	25	24	$727 \pm 77/954 \pm 113^*$	NP	$0.9 \pm 0.4/1.4 \pm 0.3^*$	NP
Gerritsen [103]	93	97	$679 \pm 290/819 \pm 557^*$	NP	$0.5 \pm 0.9/0.9 \pm 1.6^{\ddagger}$	28%/34%*
Remadi [104]	200	200	NP	NP	NP	6%/13%*
Beghi [105] RCT	30	30	NP	0/1	NP	10%/26%
Beholz [106]	40	40	$373 \pm 119/501 \pm 272^*$	NP	0.2/1.3*	10%/35%*
Wiesenack [107]	485	485	$765 \pm 606/817 \pm 619$	1/15*	NP	39%/79%*,§
van Boven [108]	60	60	780/NA	NP	0.3/0.8*	13%/37%*
Vaislic [109]	40	40	$312 \pm 141/721 \pm 619^*$	1/1	NP	0/5%*
Folliguet [110]	40	40	530/575(24 h)	NP	NP	34%/30%
AVR						
Castiglioni [64] RCT	17	23	$217 \pm 62/420 \pm 219^{*,\|}$	0/1	NP	5%/43%*

Abbreviations: CABG, coronary artery bypass grafting; MECC, minimal extracorporeal circulation; AVR, aortic valve replacement; RCT, randomized controlled trial; PRBC, red blood cells; NP, not provided.

* $p < 0.05$.

† MECC:Conventional: RBC 0.5 ± 0.9 U/1.3 ± 1.9 U, $p < 0.05$; FFP 0/3 U; $p < 0.001$.

‡ MECC:Conventional: RBC 0.5± 0.9 U/0.9 ± 1.6 U, $p < 0.05$; FFP 0.3 ± 0.9 U/0.5 ± 1.0 U; $p > 0.05$; platelets : 0.01 ± 0.01 U/0.13 ± 0.40 U, $p > 0.05$.

§ RBC: 42(8.6%)/150(31%), $p < 0.05$; total: 190(39%)/383(79%), $p < 0.05$; FFP 86(17%)/80(16%).

‖ Platelet count was significantly higher in MECC (140 ± 29 × 10(9)/L vs 119 ± 37 × 10(9)/L, $p < 0.05$).

implementation of these technology will become commonplace.

References

1. Stamou SC, White T, Barnett S, et al. Comparisons of cardiac surgery outcomes in Jehovah's versus non-Jehovah's witnesses. Am J Cardiol 2006;98:1223–5.
2. Dalrymple-Hay MJ, Dawkins S, Pack L, et al. Autotransfusion decreases blood usage following cardiac surgery—a prospective randomized trial. Cardiovasc Surg 2001;9:184–7.
3. Ferraris VA, Ferraris SP. Limiting excessive postoperative blood transfusion after cardiac procedures. A review. Tex Heart Inst J 1995;22:216–30.
4. Thurer RL. Blood transfusion in cardiac surgery. Can J Anaesth 2001;48:S6–12.
5. Stover EP, Siegel LC, Parks R, et al. Variability in transfusion practice for coronary artery bypass surgery persists despite national consensus guidelines. Anesthesiology 1998;88:327–33.
6. Banbury MK, Brizzio ME, Rajeswaran J, Lytle BW, Blackstone EH. Transfusion increases the risk of postoperative infection after cardiovascular surgery. J Am Coll Surg 2006;202:131–8.
7. Leal-Noval SR, Rincon-Ferrari MD, Garcia-Curiel A, et al. Transfusion of blood components and postoperative infection in patients undergoing cardiac surgery. Chest 2001;119:1461–8.
8. Chelemer SB, Prato BS, Cox PM, Jr, O'Connor GT, Morton JR. Association of bacterial infection and red blood cell transfusion after coronary artery bypass surgery. Ann Thorac Surg 2002;73:138–42.
9. Koch CG, Li L, Van Wagoner DR, et al. Red cell transfusion is associated with an increased risk for

postoperative atrial fibrillation. Ann Thorac Surg 2006;82:1747–56.
10. Spiess BD, Ley C, Body SC, et al. Hematocrit value on intensive care unit entry influences the frequency of q-wave myocardial infarction after coronary artery bypass grafting. J Thorac Cardiovasc Surg 1998;116:460–67.
11. Surgenor SD, DeFoe GR, Fillinger MP, et al. Intraoperative red blood cell transfusion during coronary artery bypass graft surgery increases the risk of postoperative low-output heart failure. Circulation 2006;114:I43–8.
12. Habib RH, Zacharias A, Schwann TA, et al. Role of hemodilutional anemia and transfusion during cardiopulmonary bypass in renal injury after coronary revascularization: implications on operative outcome. Crit Care Med 2005;33:1749–56.
13. Ferraris VA, Ferraris SP, Saha SP, et al. Perioperative blood transfusion and blood conservation in cardiac surgery: the society of thoracic surgeons and the society of cardiovascular anesthesiologists clinical practice guideline. Ann Thorac Surg 2007;83:S27–86.
14. Vanermen H. What is minimally invasive cardiac surgery? J Card Surg 1998;13:268–74.
15. Gu YJ, Mariani MA, Boonstra PW, Grandjean JG, van Oeveren W. Complement activation in coronary artery bypass grafting patients without cardiopulmonary bypass. The role of tissue injury by surgical incision. Chest 1999;116:892–8.
16. Brash JL, Scott CF, ten Hove P, Wojciechowski P, Colman RW. Mechanism of transient adsorption of fibrinogen from plasma to solid surfaces: role of the contact and fibrinolytic systems. Blood 1988;71:932–9.
17. Ichinose A, Kisiel W, Fujikawa K. Proteolytic activation of tissue plasminogen activator by plasma and tissue enzymes. FEBS Lett 1984;175: 412–18.
18. Kitaguchi H, Hijikata A, Hirata M. Effect of thrombin on plasminogen activator release from isolated perfused dog leg. Thromb Res 1979;16: 407–15.
19. Sheppeck RA, Bentz M, Dickson C, et al. Examination of the roles of glycoprotein Ib and glycoprotein IIb/IIIa in platelet deposition on an artificial surface using clinical antiplatelet agents and monoclonal antibody blockade. Blood 1991;78:673–80.
20. Mazer CD, Hornstein A, Freedman J. Platelet activation in warm and cold heart surgery. Ann Thorac Surg 1995;59:1481–6.
21. Lu H, Soria C, Cramer EM, et al. Temperature dependence of plasmin-induced activation or inhibition of human platelets. Blood 1991;77:996–1005.
22. Nieuwland R, Berckmans RJ, Rotteveel-Eijkman RC, et al. Cell-derived microparticles generated in patients during cardiopulmonary bypass are highly procoagulant. Circulation 1997;96:3534–41.
23. Harker LA, Malpass TW, Branson HE, Hessel EA, Slichter SJ. Mechanism of abnormal bleeding in patients undergoing cardiopulmonary bypass: acquired transient platelet dysfunction associated with selective alpha-granule release. Blood 1980;56:824–34.
24. Khuri SF, Wolfe JA, Josa M, et al. Hematologic changes during and after cardiopulmonary bypass and their relationship to the bleeding time and nonsurgical blood loss. J Thorac Cardiovasc Surg 1992;104:94–107.
25. Muriithi EW, Belcher PR, Day SP, Menys VC, Wheatley DJ. Heparin-induced platelet dysfunction and cardiopulmonary bypass. Ann Thorac Surg 2000;69:1827–32.
26. Khuri S, Valeri CR, Loscalzo J, et al. Heparin causes platelet dysfunction and induces fibrinolysis before cardiopulmonary bypass. Ann Thorac Surg 1995;60:1008–14.
27. Pappalardo F, Della VP, Crescenzi G, et al. Phosphorylcholine coating may limit thrombin formation during high-risk cardiac surgery: a randomized controlled trial. Ann Thorac Surg 2006;81:886–91.
28. Despotis GJ, Avidan MS, Hogue CW, Jr. Mechanisms and attenuation of hemostatic activation during extracorporeal circulation. Ann Thorac Surg 2001;72:S1821–31.
29. Aldea GS, Soltow LO, Chandler WL, et al. Limitation of thrombin generation, platelet activation, and inflammation by elimination of cardiotomy suction in patients undergoing coronary artery bypass grafting treated with heparin-bonded circuits. J Thorac Cardiovasc Surg 2002;123:742–55.
30. De Somer F, Van Belleghem Y, Caes F, et al. Tissue factor as the main activator of the coagulation system during cardiopulmonary bypass. J Thorac Cardiovasc Surg 2002;123:951–8.
31. Mack MJ, Pfister A, Bachand D, et al. Comparison of coronary bypass surgery with and without cardiopulmonary bypass in patients with multivessel disease. J Thorac Cardiovasc Surg 2004;127:167–73.
32. Raja SG, Dreyfus GD. Impact of off-pump coronary artery bypass surgery on postoperative bleeding: current best available evidence. J Card Surg 2006;21:35–41.

33. Bainbridge D, Cheng D, Martin J, Novick R. Does off-pump or minimally invasive coronary artery bypass reduce mortality, morbidity, and resource utilization when compared with percutaneous coronary intervention? A meta-analysis of randomized trials. J Thorac Cardiovasc Surg 2007;133:623–31.
34. Guru V, Fremes SE. Impact of off-pump coronary artery bypass surgery on postoperativ bleeding: current best available evidence. J Card Surg 2006;21:42–3.
35. Sellke FW, DiMaio JM, Caplan LR, et al. Comparing on-pump and off-pump coronary artery bypass grafting: numerous studies but few conclusions: a scientific statement from the American Heart Association council on cardiovascular surgery and anesthesia in collaboration with the interdisciplinary working group on quality of care and outcomes research. Circulation 2005;111:2858–64.
36. Wijeysundera DN, Beattie WS, Djaiani G, et al. Off-pump coronary artery surgery for reducing mortality and morbidity: meta-analysis of randomized and observational studies. J Am Coll Cardiol 2005;46:872–82.
37. Guru V, Glasgow KW, Fremes SE, et al. The real-world outcomes of off-pump coronary artery bypass surgery in a public health care system. Can J Cardiol 2007;23:281–6.
38. Khan NE, De Souza A, Mister R, et al. A randomized comparison of off-pump and on-pump multivessel coronary-artery bypass surgery. N Engl J Med 2004;350:21–8.
39. Keizer AM, Hijman R, Van Dijk D, Kalkman CJ, Kahn RS. Cognitive self-assessment one year after on-pump and off-pump coronary artery bypass grafting. Ann Thorac Surg 2003;75:835–8.
40. Ernest CS, Worcester MU, Tatoulis J, et al. Neurocognitive outcomes in off-pump versus on-pump bypass surgery: a randomized controlled trial. Ann Thorac Surg 2006;81:2105–14.
41. Kettering K, Dapunt O, Baer FM. Minimally invasive direct coronary artery bypass grafting: a systematic review. J Cardiovasc Surg (Torino) 2004;45:255–64.
42. Boodhwani M, Ruel M, Mesana TG, Rubens FD. Minimally invasive direct coronary artery bypass for the treatment of isolated disease of the left anterior descending coronary artery. Can J Surg 2005;48:307–10.
43. Niinami H, Ogasawara H, Suda Y, Takeuchi Y. Single-vessel revascularization with minimally invasive direct coronary artery bypass: minithoracotomy or ministernotomy? Chest 2005;127:47–52.
44. Torracca L, Ismeno G, Franze V, Alfieri O. The use of robotic technology in the LAST operation. Ital Heart J 2001;2:900–903.
45. Subramanian VA, Patel NU, Patel NC, Loulmet DF. Robotic assisted multivessel minimally invasive direct coronary artery bypass with port-access stabilization and cardiac positioning: paving the way for outpatient coronary surgery? Ann Thorac Surg 2005;79:1590–96.
46. Lapierre H, Chan V, Ruel M. Off-pump coronary surgery through mini-incisions: is it reasonable? Curr Opin Cardiol 2006;21:578–83.
47. Turner WF, Jr, Sloan JH. Robotic-assisted coronary artery bypass on a beating heart: initial experience and implications for the future. Ann Thorac Surg 2006;82:790–94.
48. Nesher N, Bakir I, Casselman F, et al. Robotically enhanced minimally invasive direct coronary artery bypass surgery: a winning strategy? J Cardiovasc Surg (Torino) 2007;48:333–8.
49. Bonatti J, Schachner T, Bonaros N, et al. Technical challenges in totally endoscopic robotic coronary artery bypass grafting. J Thorac Cardiovasc Surg 2006;131:146–53.
50. Cannon CP, Mehta SR, Aranki SF. Balancing the benefit and risk of oral antiplatelet agents in coronary artery bypass surgery. Ann Thorac Surg 2005;80:768–79.
51. Cohn LH, Adams DH, Couper GS, et al. Minimally invasive cardiac valve surgery improves patient satisfaction while reducing costs of cardiac valve replacement and repair. Ann Surg 1997;226:421–6.
52. Farhat F, Metton O, Jegaden O. Benefits and complications of total sternotomy and ministernotomy in cardiac surgery. Surg Technol Int 2004;13:199–205.
53. Lee S, Chang BC, Lim SH, et al. Clinical results of minimally invasive open-heart surgery in patients with mitral valve disease: comparison of parasternal and low-sternal approach. Yonsei Med J 2006;47:230–36.
54. Bakir I, Casselman FP, Wellens F, et al. Minimally invasive versus standard approach aortic valve replacement: a study in 506 patients. Ann Thorac Surg 2006;81:1599–604.
55. Byrne JG, Adams DH, Couper GS, et al. Minimally-invasive aortic root replacement. Heart Surg Forum 1999;2:326–9.
56. Cohn LH. Minimally invasive aortic valve surgery: technical considerations and results with the parasternal approach. J Card Surg 1998;13:302–5.

57. Braxton JH, Higgins RS, Schwann TA, et al. Reoperative mitral valve surgery via right thoracotomy: decreased blood loss and improved hemodynamics. J Heart Valve Dis 1996;5:169–73.
58. Bolotin G, Kypson AP, Reade CC, et al. Should a video-assisted mini-thoracotomy be the approach of choice for reoperative mitral valve surgery? J Heart Valve Dis 2004;13:155–8.
59. Dogan S, Aybek T, Risteski PS, et al. Minimally invasive port access versus conventional mitral valve surgery: prospective randomized study. Ann Thorac Surg 2005;79:492–8.
60. Reichenspurner H, Detter C, Deuse T, et al. Video and robotic-assisted minimally invasive mitral valve surgery: a comparison of the port-access and transthoracic clamp techniques. Ann Thorac Surg 2005;79:485–90.
61. Walther T, Falk V, Mohr FW. Minimally invasive surgery for valve disease. Curr Probl Cardiol 2006;31:399–437.
62. Chitwood WR, Jr, Nifong LW. Minimally invasive videoscopic mitral valve surgery: the current role of surgical robotics. J Card Surg 2000;15:61–75.
63. Chitwood WR, Jr. Video-assisted and robotic mitral valve surgery: toward an endoscopic surgery. Semin Thorac Cardiovasc Surg 1999;11:194–205.
64. Castiglioni A, Verzini A, Pappalardo F, et al. Minimally invasive closed circuit versus standard extracorporeal circulation for aortic valve replacement. Ann Thorac Surg 2007;83:586–91.
65. Sajja LR, Mannam G, Chakravarthi RM, et al. Coronary artery bypass grafting with or without cardiopulmonary bypass in patients with preoperative non-dialysis dependent renal insufficiency: a randomized study. J Thorac Cardiovasc Surg 2007;133:378–88.
66. Kobayashi J, Tashiro T, Ochi M, et al. Early outcome of a randomized comparison of off-pump and on-pump multiple arterial coronary revascularization. Circulation 2005;112:I338–43.
67. Gerola LR, Buffolo E, Jasbik W, et al. Off-pump versus on-pump myocardial revascularization in low-risk patients with one or two vessel disease: perioperative results in a multicenter randomized controlled trial. Ann Thorac Surg 2004;77:569–73.
68. Wan IY, Arifi AA, Wan S, et al. Beating heart revascularization with or without cardiopulmonary bypass: evaluation of inflammatory response in a prospective randomized study. J Thorac Cardiovasc Surg 2004;127:1624–31.
69. Wehlin L, Vedin J, Vaage J, Lundahl J. Activation of complement and leukocyte receptors during on- and off pump coronary artery bypass surgery. Eur J Cardiothorac Surg 2004;25:35–42.
70. Straka Z, Widimsky P, Jirasek K, et al. Off-pump versus on-pump coronary surgery: final results from a prospective randomized study PRAGUE-4. Ann Thorac Surg 2004;77:789–93.
71. Puskas JD, Williams WH, Duke PG, et al. Off-pump coronary artery bypass grafting provides complete revascularization with reduced myocardial injury, transfusion requirements, and length of stay: a prospective randomized comparison of two hundred unselected patients undergoing off-pump versus conventional coronary artery bypass grafting. J Thorac Cardiovasc Surg 2003;125:797–808.
72. Muneretto C, Bisleri G, Negri A, et al. Off-pump coronary artery bypass surgery technique for total arterial myocardial revascularization: a prospective randomized study. Ann Thorac Surg 2003;76:778–82.
73. Lee JD, Lee SJ, Tsushima WT, et al. Benefits of off-pump bypass on neurologic and clinical morbidity: a prospective randomized trial. Ann Thorac Surg 2003;76:18–25.
74. Angelini GD, Taylor FC, Reeves BC, Ascione R. Early and midterm outcome after off-pump and on-pump surgery in beating heart against cardioplegic arrest studies (BHACAS 1 and 2): a pooled analysis of two randomised controlled trials. Lancet 2002;359:1194–9.
75. Ascione R, Williams S, Lloyd CT, et al. Reduced postoperative blood loss and transfusion requirement after beating-heart coronary operations: a prospective randomized study. J Thorac Cardiovasc Surg 2001;121:689–96.
76. Van Dijk D, Nierich AP, Jansen EW, et al. Early outcome after off-pump versus on-pump coronary bypass surgery: results from a randomized study. Circulation 2001;104:1761–6.
77. Potger KC, McMillan D, Southwell J, et al. Transfusion and bleeding in coronary artery bypass grafting: an on-pump versus off-pump comparison. J Extra Corpor Technol 2007;39:24–30.
78. Frankel TL, Stamou SC, Lowery RC, et al. Risk factors for hemorrhage-related reexploration and blood transfusion after conventional versus coronary revascularization without cardiopulmonary bypass. Eur J Cardiothorac Surg 2005;27:494–500.
79. Scott BH, Seifert FC, Grimson R, Glass PS. Resource utilization in on- and off-pump coronary artery

surgery: factors influencing postoperative length of stay—an experience of 1,746 consecutive patients undergoing fast-track cardiac anesthesia. J Cardiothorac Vasc Anesth 2005;19:26–31.
80. Berson AJ, Smith JM, Woods SE, Hasselfeld KA, Hiratzka LF. Off-pump versus on-pump coronary artery bypass surgery: does the pump influence outcome? J Am Coll Surg 2004;199:102–8.
81. Nuttall GA, Erchul DT, Haight TJ, et al. A comparison of bleeding and transfusion in patients who undergo coronary artery bypass grafting via sternotomy with and without cardiopulmonary bypass. J Cardiothorac Vasc Anesth 2003;17:447–51.
82. Scott BH, Seifert FC, Glass PS, Grimson R. Blood use in patients undergoing coronary artery bypass surgery: impact of cardiopulmonary bypass pump, hematocrit, gender, age, and body weight. Anesth Analg 2003;97:958–63, table.
83. Ishida M, Kobayashi J, Tagusari O, et al. Perioperative advantages of off-pump coronary artery bypass grafting. Circ J 2002;66:795–9.
84. Zamvar VY, Khan NU, Madhavan A, Nihal Kulatilake NK, Butchart EG. Clinical outcomes in coronary artery bypass graft surgery: comparison of off-pump and on-pump techniques. Heart Surg Forum 2002;5:109–13.
85. Kirk KC, Aldridge RA, Sistino JJ, et al. Coronary artery bypass grafting with and without cardiopulmonary bypass: a comparison analysis. J Extra Corpor Technol 2001;33:86–90.
86. Petro KR, Dullum MK, Garcia JM, et al. Minimally invasive coronary revascularization in women: a safe approach for a high-risk group. Heart Surg Forum 2000;3:41–6.
87. Yokoyama T, Baumgartner FJ, Gheissari A, et al. Off-pump versus on-pump coronary bypass in high-risk subgroups. Ann Thorac Surg 2000;70:1546–50.
88. Srivastava S, Gadasalli S, Agusala M, et al. Use of bilateral internal thoracic arteries in CABG through lateral thoracotomy with robotic assistance in 150 patients. Ann Thorac Surg 2006;81:800–806.
89. Boyd WD, Kodera K, Stahl KD, Rayman R. Current status and future directions in computer-enhanced video- and robotic-assisted coronary bypass surgery. Semin Thorac Cardiovasc Surg 2002;14:101–9.
90. Damiano RJ, Jr, Tabaie HA, Mack MJ, et al. Initial prospective multicenter clinical trial of robotically-assisted coronary artery bypass grafting. Ann Thorac Surg 2001;72:1263–8.
91. Boyd WD, Kiaii B, Novick RJ, et al. RAVECAB: improving outcome in off-pump minimal access surgery with robotic assistance and video enhancement. Can J Surg 2001;44:45–50.
92. Falk V, Diegeler A, Walther T, et al. Total endoscopic computer enhanced coronary artery bypass grafting. Eur J Cardiothorac Surg 2000;17:38–45.
93. Woo YJ, Nacke EA. Robotic minimally invasive mitral valve reconstruction yields less blood product transfusion and shorter length of stay. Surgery 2006;140:263–7.
94. Folliguet T, Vanhuyse F, Constantino X, Realli M, Laborde F. Mitral valve repair robotic versus sternotomy. Eur J Cardiothorac Surg 2006;29:362–6.
95. Mishra Y, Sharma M, Bapna R, et al. Minimally invasive mitral valve surgery. Indian Heart J 2002;54:279–83.
96. Chitwood WR, Jr, Wixon CL, Elbeery JR, et al. Video-assisted minimally invasive mitral valve surgery. J Thorac Cardiovasc Surg 1997;114:773–80.
97. Nifong LW, Chitwood WR, Pappas PS, et al. Robotic mitral valve surgery: a United States multicenter trial. J Thorac Cardiovasc Surg 2005;129:1395–404.
98. Tatooles AJ, Pappas PS, Gordon PJ, Slaughter MS. Minimally invasive mitral valve repair using the da Vinci robotic system. Ann Thorac Surg 2004;77:1978–82.
99. Sobieski MA, Slaughter MS, Hart DE, Pappas PS, Tatooles AJ. Peripheral cardiopulmonary bypass with modified assisted venous drainage and transthoracic aortic crossclamp: optimal management for robotic mitral valve repair. Perfusion 2003;18:307–11.
100. Nifong LW, Chu VF, Bailey BM, et al. Robotic mitral valve repair: experience with the da Vinci system. Ann Thorac Surg 2003;75:438–42.
101. Perthel M, El Ayoubi L, Bendisch A, Laas J, Gerigk M. Clinical advantages of using mini-bypass systems in terms of blood product use, postoperative bleeding and air entrainment: an in vivo clinical perspective. Eur J Cardiothorac Surg 2007;31:1070–75.
102. Huybregts RA, Morariu AM, Rakhorst G, et al. Attenuated renal and intestinal injury after use of a mini-cardiopulmonary bypass system. Ann Thorac Surg 2007;83:1760–66.
103. Gerritsen WB, van Boven WJ, Wesselink RM, et al. Significant reduction in blood loss in patients undergoing minimal extracorporeal circulation. Transfus Med 2006;16:329–34.
104. Remadi JP, Rakotoarivelo Z, Marticho P, Benamar A. Prospective randomized study comparing coronary artery bypass grafting with the new mini-extracorporeal circulation Jostra System or with

a standard cardiopulmonary bypass. Am Heart J 2006;151:198.
105. Beghi C, Nicolini F, Agostinelli A, et al. Mini-cardiopulmonary bypass system: results of a prospective randomized study. Ann Thorac Surg 2006;81:1396–400.
106. Beholz S, Zheng L, Kessler M, Rusche M, Konertz W. A new PRECiSe (priming reduced extracorporeal circulation setup) minimizes the need for blood transfusions: first clinical results in coronary artery bypass grafting. Heart Surg Forum 2005;8:E132–5.
107. Wiesenack C, Liebold A, Philipp A, et al. Four years' experience with a miniaturized extracorporeal circulation system and its influence on clinical outcome. Artif Organs 2004;28:1082–8.
108. van Boven WJ, Gerritsen WB, Waanders FG, Haas FJ, Aarts LP. Mini extracorporeal circuit for coronary artery bypass grafting: initial clinical and biochemical results: a comparison with conventional and off-pump coronary artery bypass grafts concerning global oxidative stress and alveolar function. Perfusion 2004;19:239–46.
109. Vaislic C, Bical O, Farge C, et al. Totally minimized extracorporeal circulation: an important benefit for coronary artery bypass grafting in Jehovah's witnesses. Heart Surg Forum 2003;6:307–10.
110. Folliguet TA, Villa E, Vandeneyden F, Laborde F. Coronary artery bypass graft with minimal extracorporeal circulation. Heart Surg Forum 2003;6: 297–301.

CHAPTER 33

Adjunctive Strategies to Impact Blood Transfusion in Cardiac Surgery

L. Ressler & Fraser Rubens
University of Ottawa Heart Institute, Ottawa, Ontario, Canada

Adjunctive strategies—introduction

Blood conservation in cardiac surgery encompasses a broad spectrum of technologies and strategies. Though few of these have undergone extensive clinical testing to the degree seen with antifibrinolytics, many, such as postoperative cell salvage, have made it into the mainstream in terms of incorporation into a broader accepted therapy for blood conservation.

In this chapter, we wish to recognize the potential for alternative ideas that have not previously been considered to impact transfusion. These concepts are not necessarily new. Many have been developed as tried and true procedures or patient management decisions, practiced by surgeons based on intuition with little support from clinical trials. Some, such as liberal reopening, have the potential to be expanded in the therapeutic algorithm as broader concepts to limit blood exposure. All have evolved to address surgical bleeding directly or indirectly, through steps primarily carried out on "our" side of the ether screen.

We are not publicly endorsing all of these strategies; however, our perception coupled with our clinical experience, suggests that now is the time to consider that these ideas are worthy of exploration and reconsideration. We anticipate that the readers may find these topics unconventional in terms of this field, but we believe that they are the ideas that provide "food for thought" for further clinical research.

Alternatives to Blood Transfusion in Transfusion Medicine, 2nd edition. Edited by A. Maniatis, P. Van der Linden, J.-F. Hardy.

A strategy of liberal reopening

As reviewed briefly in chapter 32, the physiologic insult of cardiac surgery coupled with the necessary anticoagulation and the relatively toxic effect of the blood-biomaterial interaction of cardiopulmonary bypass (CPB), results moderately frequently in postoperative bleeding. Excessive bleeding may be on the basis of a coagulopathy, or not infrequently, the surgeon may also miss surgical sites of bleeding at the time of closure of the median sternotomy wound, or small branches and vessels that were previously hemostatic due to spasm, may start to bleed shortly after the patient is returned to the ICU.

The impact of bleeding can be further complicated by the limited mediastinal space and the potential for cardiac compression with resulting hemodynamic compromise (cardiac tamponade). Pericardial effusions are relatively common after cardiac surgery, seen in up to 50–64% of cases, but luckily cardiac compromise is still relatively rare [1]. Regardless, surgical teams often must resort to reexploration of the wound (reopening) when excessive bleeding is detected or when there is evidence of tamponade and in most institutions, this requires a return to the operating room (OR) from the ICU. In virtually every case, during the time delay before reopening, the excessive bleeding often leads to a state of low output, accentuating the coagulopathy to which treating physicians respond by ordering more blood products. As discussed below, it is possible that a more rapid response to these crises with a more liberal, earlier reopening strategy may avoid this spiral and thus decrease the overall blood exposure.

The incidence of reopening after adult cardiac surgery generally ranges between 3 and 6% [2–4]. In a study by Choong et al., the most common indication for reexploration was persistent bleeding (82%) while the remaining cases underwent reexploration for tamponade [3]. The median duration from arrival in ICU to reexploration was 4.7 hours (IQR 2.9–9.7 hours) with the majority reexplored within 12 hours (82%) [3] (Figure 33.1). Patients can loose a great deal of blood before they ultimately get reopened with the median blood loss from chest tubes up to 1050 mL (IQR: 750–1575 mL, mean 1236 mL, range 100–10661 mL) [3]. If reopening occurs greater than 12 hours after ICU arrival, tamponade appears to be a more frequent indication for this intervention (44%) [3].

Patient factors associated with an increased risk for reopening include increased age [2–5], smaller body surface area or body mass index [3–5], and preoperative renal insufficiency [2]. Propensity-matched analysis also showed a relationship to preoperative unfractionated heparin (UFH) use ($p = 0.001$) [4], aspirin (ASA) use ($p = 0.004$) [3, 4], usage of the potent antiplatelet drug clopidogrel, and nonusage of antifibrinolytic agents (both $p < 0.035$) [3].

Operative factors shown to be associated with an increased risk of reopening have included nonelective cases [4], multiple distal anastomoses (greater than four) [4, 5] prolonged bypass times [2, 3, 5, 6], and the need for the use of an intra-aortic balloon pump (IABP) [5]. The type of procedure is also a factor as there is an increased risk with combined procedures, reoperations [6] and with procedures other than coronary artery bypass grafting (CABG) alone [2]. Unsworth-White et al. [7] followed 2221 patients; resternotomy for bleeding after CABG was seen in 2.3% but it was threefold more likely with valve cases (OR 3.4; 95% CI 2.1–5.4).

Trends suggest that the reopening rate is decreasing despite the increasing burden of age and comorbidity seen by most cardiac surgical teams. Work from the Northern New England Cardiovascular Disease Study Group (NNECVDSG) confirmed that the rate declined 46% from 3.6% to 2% of all cases from 1992 to 1994 as compared to the period 1995–1997 ($p < 0.001$) [8]. This is probably related to a myriad of processes of care and the increased popularity of use of antifibrinolytics. Interestingly, this decrease was seen despite the increased use of preoperative UFH and ASA [8].

Surgical causes (e.g., bleeding anastomoses, missed side branch) still appear to be the most common etiologic contributor to bleeding requiring reopening. In a clinical study by Unsworth-White et al., identifiable surgical causes of bleeding were found in 67% at reexploration, but concurrent coagulopathy was still common [7]. Similarly, in a clinical review of 82 patients who were reopened, 66% had surgical sites identified and 34% were coagulopathic [6]. Finally Charalambous et al. showed that of 240 patients reopened due to bleeding or tamponade, 55% had focal bleeding, 33% had diffuse bleeding and 11% had both [9].

The clinical relevance of reopening and tamponade

There is strong evidence that patients who require reopening for bleeding have worse outcomes than those who do not. Reopened patients have an increased inotrope need and an increased incidence of pulmonary/renal/abdominal complications, particularly if the bleeding has a medical cause (coagulopathy) as opposed to a surgical source [6]. Unsworth-White et al. used multiple forward stepwise logistic regression analysis to confirm that resternotomy for excess bleeding after cardiac surgery is a significant independent predictor of prolonged stay in the ICU ($p < 0.0001$), of the need for IABP ($p < 0.0001$) and of death ($p < 0.0001$) [7]. Dacey et al. also showed that mortality is threefold increased (9.5% versus 3.3%, $p < 0.001$) and the average length of stay is increased (14.5 days versus 8.6 days, $p < 0.001$) in patients requiring reopening [5]. Finally, Moulton et al. demonstrated that reoperation for bleeding was a strong independent predictor for operative mortality ($p < 0.005$), renal failure ($p = 0.0001$),

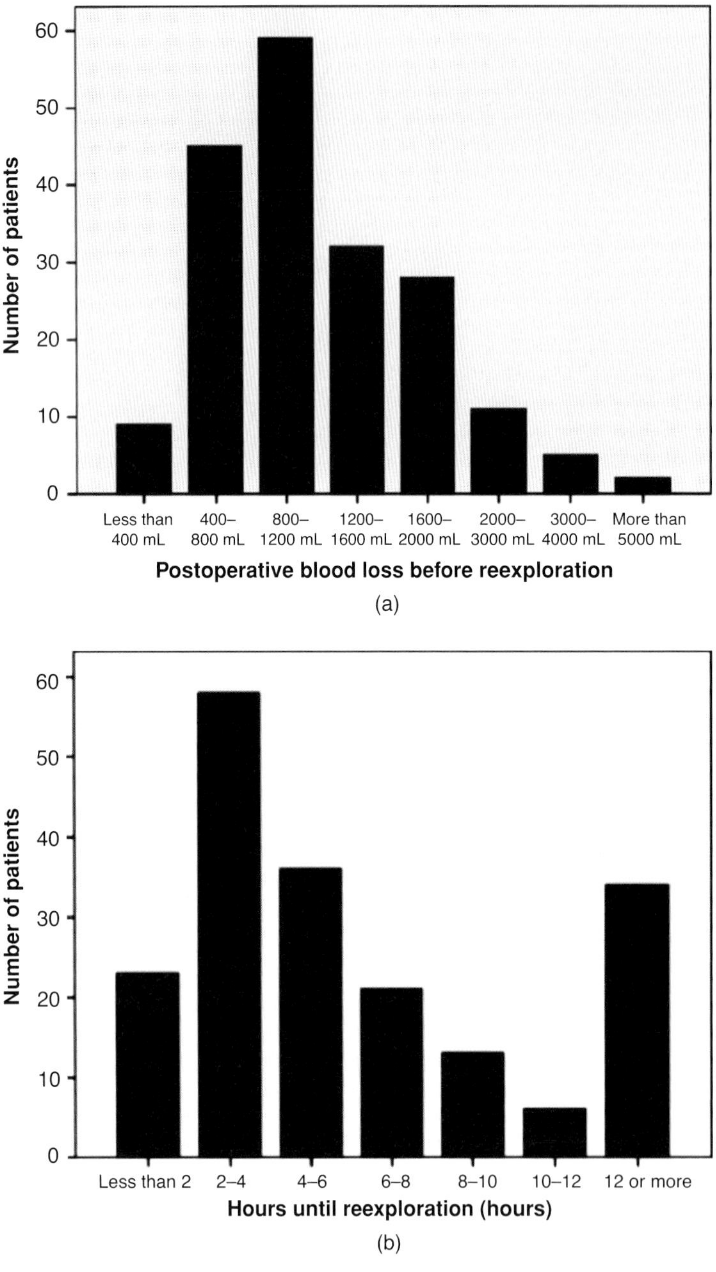

Figure 33.1 (a) Amount of bleeding in mL until reexploration for bleeding after coronary artery bypass surgery; (b) time in hours after coronary artery bypass surgery until reexploration. Data from Choong et al. [3], with permission from Elsevier.

prolonged mechanical ventilation ($p < 0.0001$), and atrial arrhythmias ($p = 0.006$) [2].

It is not clear that some of these complications could have been averted by earlier and more aggressive reopening to prevent the frequent massive transfusion and tamponade in bleeding patients; however, it appears that the amount of bleeding is proportional to the length of time the team waits prior to agreeing to reopen a patient [4]. Making a decision to *not* reopen due to procrastination is not

Table 33.1 Impact of late reopening on outcome [3].

	Reexplored <12 hours	Reexplored >12 hours	*p* value
Median total blood loss in liters (range)	2.1 (0.4–12.5)	2.6 (0.6–12.7)	0.22
Median ICU stay in days (range)	3 (0–97)	8.5 (2–37)	<0.001
IABP support (%)	22.3	44.1	0.01
Median RBC transfusion in units (range)	8 (1–59)	9.5 (3–32)	0.2
Hospital death (%)	7.0	29.4	<0.001

Abbreviations: ICU, intensive care unit; IABP, intra-aortic balloon pump; RBC, red blood cells.

a means to eliminate these problems and risks. In other words, just because there is an increased mortality with reopening, doesn't mean you can avoid the inevitable; longer delay may in fact lead to greater problems. Karthik et al. demonstrated that adverse outcomes were significantly higher when reopening was delayed greater than 12 hours after ICU arrival [4]. In this group, reopening was associated with increased inotrope use, increased need for prolonged mechanical ventilation, and prolonged hospital and ICU stay (all $p < 0.001$) as compared with a propensity-matched cohort not undergoing reopening [4]. In the delayed reopening group, there was a significantly increased rate of major complications (stroke, renal failure, and increased ICU stay) as compared to the small cohort who underwent reexploration in less than 12 hours (Table 33.1).

Reopening imposes a resource limitation in terms of OR time and staffing and some units have approached this problem by a critical analysis of the risk-benefit ratio of reopening without patient transfer immediately in the ICU. We recognize that there are many limitations to this approach in terms of the sterility of the environment such as lack of the negative pressure air flow; however, it is entirely possible that the delays imposed by waiting for transfer to a free operating theatre result in untoward hemodynamic compromise and increasing transfusion burden which by themselves likely increase the risk of infection to a greater degree than the theoretical lack of perfect sterility if reopening is done more rapidly in the ICU.

In fact, there does not appear to be strong evidence that reopening in the ICU is associated with an increased risk of infection. In a series reviewed by Charalambous et al. [9] of patients reopened in the ICU, there was a mortality rate of 6.7%, which varied little from the overall population and a 2.9% sternal wound infection rate, compatible to the rate seen in the group not undergoing reopening [9]. The authors concluded that returning to the operating theater delays reoperation thus carries high economic costs and imposes demands on OR times with frequent cancellations [9]. Similar findings were documented by Kaiser et al. [10] reporting on 49 cases reopened in ICU with no wound infections, and McKowen et al. [11] with 64 reexplorations in the ICU with a 3.1% incidence of infection. A study by Talamonti et al. [12] provides data supporting a more rapid reopening policy. In this retrospective review, patients who had undergone reopening were divided into those with and without subsequent sternal wound problems. The average time to reexploration in the group without problems was 7.6 hours, whereas it was 13.8 hours in those with wound problems. Thus delay in return was a significant risk factor for wound complications ($p < 0.001$) [12].

Conclusions—liberal reopening

It is possible that liberal early reopening may have a broader impact on patient outcome by minimizing overall bleeding and preventing the associated massive transfusions often seen as teams try to delay the inevitable. The indications for reopening must be flexible as we are faced with older, sicker patients, and potent antiplatelet agents. Currently there is no evidence that a strategy employing routine reopening in the ICU impacts wound infection rates. This unexpected finding may be due to

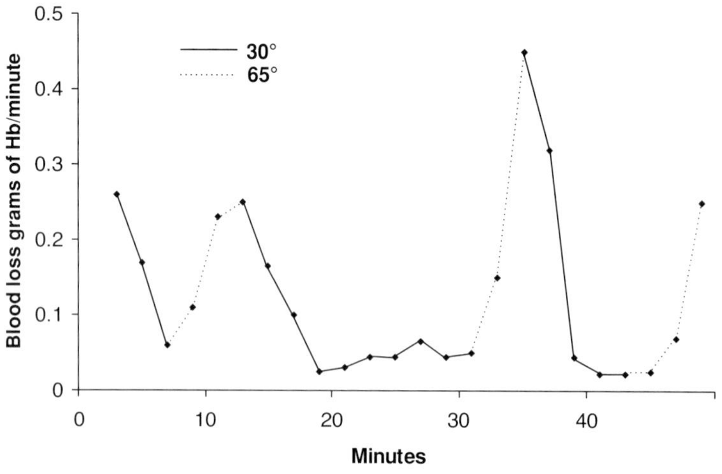

Figure 33.2 Amount of blood loss from experimental wound surface to which moist sponges at 30 and 65°C were alternately applied. Reproduced from Willman and Hanlon [19], with permission.

the minimization of transfusions before the coagulopathic spiral ensues. Unfortunately a culture has been created which discourages reopening as it is taken as a measure of quality without appropriately linking it to transfusion rates. We propose that further consideration of this controversial topic may indeed identify outcome measures that could test this hypothesis in the clinical setting. In fact, it is possible that when more clinical data is collected, it may become evident that early, liberal reopening to prevent transfusion may be a very important strategy to minimize patient complications.

Warm mediastinal irrigation

Hot water irrigation (HWI) for hemostasis has limited but accepted use in neurosurgery, and otolaryngology [13] but its historical roots derive from obstetrical surgery. The idea was first introduced by Milne-Murray at a meeting of the Edinburgh Obstetrical Society in 1886 [14]. The experiment that was presented involved a rabbit uterine vascular network. HWI caused vascular constriction which was sustained longer and ordinary tone was regained more slowly with no reactionary vascular congestion, as compared to cold irrigation which caused reactionary congestion associated with vessel dilation and increased hemorrhage. Based on these findings, HWI was subsequently successfully used to obtain hemostasis in postdelivery bleeding [15].

Potential mechanisms that have been proposed for the effect of HWI have included the activation of platelet aggregation, enhanced coagulation, and the induction of interstitial edema [16] with the latter causing perhaps external vascular compression. It has been known for many years that the ideal temperature for coagulation appears to be in the range of 36.5–40°C [17] (Figure 33.2). The ideal temperature of 40°C has been further supported based on histological analysis of the effect of HWI on nasal mucosa [18]. In this latter experiment, temperatures above this level had little additional benefit, and severe changes with epithelial necrosis were seen with temperatures greater than 52°C [18]. In a unique dog model, Willman et al. created split thickness skin graft wounds upon which gauze sponges soaked in saline at either 30°C or 65°C were applied for 6 minutes [19]. The sponges were rinsed to remove the blood, which was quantitated colorimetrically. As seen from Figure 33.3, bleeding reproducibly increased as soon as the higher temperature sponges were added to the wound. This supports that higher temperatures may cause more damage and increase bleeding, but it does not establish the optimum temperature in the range less than 52°C.

There is very little in the clinical literature on the use of HWI in any surgical subspecialty other than a single randomized clinical trial reported in the field of otolaryngology. In this study, Stangerup

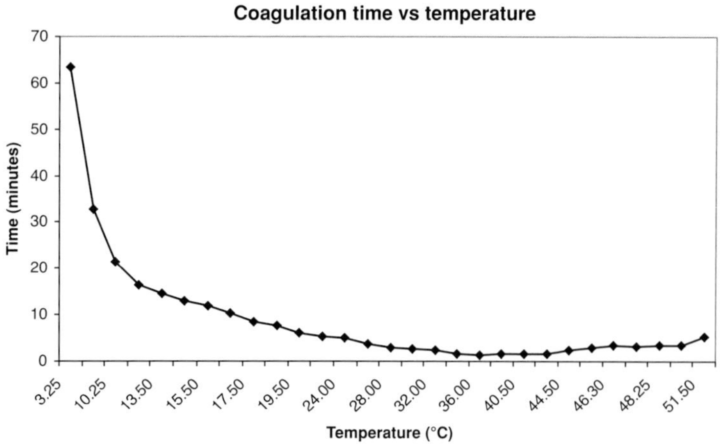

Figure 33.3 Coagulation times of human blood incubated in a controlled temperature bath. Data from Addis [17].

et al. [13] randomized 122 patients with posterior epistaxis to HWI or tamponade therapy with a foley balloon. Those treated with the HWI had decreased pain scores, more rapid cessation of bleeding and no evidence of mucosal necrosis clinically [13].

Conclusions: mediastinal warm irrigation

There are surgeons who routinely irrigate the surgical wound with copious amounts of warm saline solution. In the majority of cases, the primary goal is to wash out any contaminants and bacteria. In fact, this technique is widely used in the developing world as an alternative to antibiotic therapy. As an added benefit, there is evidence from other specialties and from animal models that this strategy may decrease overall bleeding. Therefore, we feel this procedure warrants further evaluation in our specialty as it is simple, cheap, and relatively easily tested in a clinical model.

Skeletonization of the internal thoracic artery

Other than the usual precautions involving steps to ensure hemostasis (accuracy of suturing, gentle handling of tissue, minimized tissue destruction, etc.) surgeons have been taught few technical skills that could influence bleeding in the mediastinum after CABG. Alternative means of tissue incision such as with the harmonic scalpel have received varied support, but there as yet has been little evidence that this technology may impact on transfusion [20]. On the other hand, options for the preparation of conduits used during bypass grafting should be considered as to their effect on postoperative bleeding. A critical step in the performance of coronary surgery is the harvest of the left internal thoracic artery (ITA) for its use for bypass of the left anterior descending artery. Traditionally this has been accomplished by the preparation with the electrocautery of the artery as a pedicle dissected from the chest wall with the accompanying fascia and the internal thoracic vein with a strip of tissue from 1 to 2 cm in width. This latter approach is fast and reproducible and most surgeons are comfortable with the distance provided between the artery and the dissection plane.

Recently, many groups of surgeons have promoted the use of skeletonization of the ITA as a means to minimize chest wall damage [21, 22]. This modified approach involves the isolated dissection of the artery with careful clipping of individual branches and preservation of chest wall structures including arterial collaterals, venous channels, and nerves. We have demonstrated that this approach results in preserved chest wall sensation and decreased chest wall pain, without compromise in conduit flow [23]. Skeletonization has been accepted by many groups due to its effect to minimize chest wall trauma, thus improving its acceptance in high-risk patient groups such as in the elderly [24, 25].

The minimized chest trauma associated with this technique appears to correlate with a decrease in blood loss as confirmed by Calafiori et al. [26] and Bonacchi et al. [27] and a decrease in transfusion requirements [26]. Sahar et al. [28] were also able to demonstrate that skeletonized bilateral ITA in the elderly was associated with less transfusion as compared to single ITA taken in a nonskeletonized fashion (1.9 ± 1.9 vs 4.3 ± 2.8 packed cells/patient, $p < 0.001$). Finally, Cartier et al. [29] have shown that the routine use of skeletonized ITA in off-pump surgery resulted in significantly decreased total blood loss as compared to a nonskeletonized cohort (325 ± 215 mL, vs 410 ± 230 mL) [29], however no difference in the incidence of reoperation for bleeding was observed between the groups (skeletonized 4.1% vs nonskeletonized 3.8%).

Skeletonization has not received universal acceptance in the cardiac surgery community for several reasons. It is technically demanding although we have shown that the procedure, with experience, can be completed successfully in almost the same time as with the nonskeletonized approach [23]. There are also concerns that the procedure may jeopardize the integral blood supply of the media and adventitia due to interruption of the vasa vasorum. However, there is little evidence to support this claim as previous research has confirmed that endoluminal nutrient support is more than adequate for arteries of this caliber [30]

Conclusions—skeletonization of the ITA

Skeletonization has proven to be a useful harvest technique for the ITA which is well-tolerated by patients, with data thus far supporting excellent short- and mid-term patency [20, 26]. Clinical observational studies have pointed to a benefit in terms of decreasing blood loss after bypass surgery. We believe the evidence is strong enough that the question of its value in decreasing transfusion exposure should be addressed in a large randomized controlled trial.

Mediastinal packing

Every cardiac surgeon has experienced cases of persistent bleeding related to fragile suture lines, diffuse coagulopathy, and the raw surfaces occasionally found after reoperative surgery. Invariably, these situations conclude long and laborious surgery where patience is weak and fatigue may render judgment more difficult. Not all surgeons are comfortable with the liberal use of powerful hemostatic adjuncts such as activated recombinant factor VII, particularly where unwanted thrombosis could jeopardize the principle target of surgery. Early in our training, therefore, we are taught techniques to pack with gauze to temporarily control bleeding while blood products are administered and heparin is reversed. As an extension of this approach in desperate situations of persistent bleeding, if the packing controls the bleeding and there is no cardiac compromise with the packs left in place, prolonged packing to achieve permanent hemostasis has been advised by some groups [31]

Packing of the chest with or without closure is utilized as a last-ditch resort in between 1.5 and 2.8% of cardiac cases [32]. Although the approach of delayed sternal closure may be used for severe myocardial edema, persistent bleeding was the cause listed for this management step in 32% of cases [32]. The cases are usually quite complex, such as after aortic dissection or endocarditis repair [31] but if used in coronary cases, graft compromise must be considered during the packing.

There are several alternative means by which packing can be accomplished. Berger et al. suggested the use of 4 × 24 inch sponges followed by complete closure of the chest [31] with removal of the packing 20–24 hours later. Bouboulis et al. used 30 × 30 cm and 10 × 10 cm 32 ply gauze (1 large, 3 small) with skin closure (leaving the sternum open) [33] with removal of the gauzes the next day (33 ± 19 hours). Interestingly, no difference has been seen in the incidence of late infection if the packs were removed in the ICU or the operating theatre [33]. Del Campo [34] recommended packing with a 2.5-cm gauze strip placed over the aorta in layers, brought through a left parasternal stab wound. The packing may be removed later once coagulation is corrected, without reopening the sternum. In an innovative step, as an alternative to gauze, Economopoulos et al. [35] used a pericardial fat pat dissected from the phrenic nerve, thus avoiding

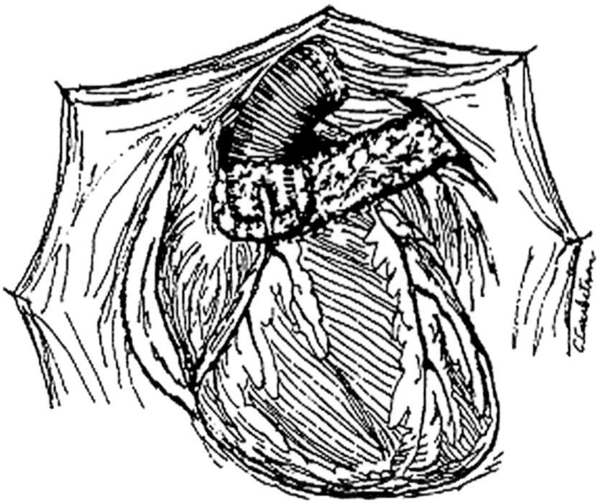

Figure 33.4 Pericardial fat pad utilized to pack around the aortic root. Data from Economopoulos et al. [35].

reopening to remove the pack as the "pack" is autologous. In this small series, all nine patients survived (Figure 33.4).

These techniques may be surprisingly successful in these desperate situations. In the largest series reported by Bouboulis et al., bleeding was controlled in 65/100 patients who were packed once and 29/100 more after reexploration and multiple packs (success 94%) but in 6 patients they were unsuccessful to control bleeding [33]. Despite the success in stopping the bleeding, this is a high-risk group with an overall mortality rate of 42%. Up to 24% had complications attributable to the packing technique and 16 patients out of these died [33]. In a series of 20 patients reported by Charalamous et al., packing for intractable bleeding with skin closure only was associated with an 85% survival rate [36]. Finally, Johnson et al. [37] reported on 13 patients who were packed after reexploration, reporting only 1 death and no infections.

Conclusions—mediastinal packing

Though infrequently collated in the literature, the overall successful experience of mediastinal gauze packing in situations of desperate bleeding that we have collected, supports that this technique should be formally taught and recognized in training programs. Further, we believe that this approach should not be quickly discarded as a feasible alternative to the use of activated recombinant factor VII.

Conclusions

We have introduced these ideas to stimulate discussion with regards to the impact of surgical decision-making on perioperative bleeding and its management. Some of these topics have not been considered in this context in the past, and most receive little attention in standard surgical textbooks, but rather are passed down through generations of surgeons without the benefit of scientific validation. The renewed recognition of the importance of transfusion as a contributor to patient morbidity should encourage us to reexamine these issues more closely with simple clinical trials. We hope this chapter will also encourage surgical teams to communicate other personally validated techniques to control bleeding and transfusion among the rest of our cardiovascular community.

References

1. Price S, Prout J, Jaggar SI, Gibson DG, Pepper JR. 'Tamponade' following cardiac surgery: terminology and echocardiography may both mislead. Eur J Cardiothorac Surg 2004;26:1156–60.
2. Moulton MJ, Creswell LL, Mackey ME, Cox JL, Rosenbloom M. Reexploration for bleeding is a risk factor for adverse outcomes after cardiac operations. J Thorac Cardiovasc Surg 1996;111:1037–46.
3. Choong CK, Gerrard C, Goldsmith KA, Dunningham H, Vuylsteke A. Delayed re-exploration for bleeding after coronary artery bypass surgery results in adverse outcomes. Eur J Cardiothorac Surg 2007;31:834–8.
4. Karthik S, Grayson AD, McCarron EE, Pullan DM, Desmond MJ. Reexploration for bleeding after coronary artery bypass surgery: risk factors, outcomes, and the effect of time delay. Ann Thorac Surg 2004;78:527–34.
5. Dacey LJ, Munoz JJ, Baribeau YR, et al. Reexploration for hemorrhage following coronary artery bypass grafting: incidence and risk factors. Northern New England Cardiovascular Disease Study Group. Arch Surg 1998;133:442–7.
6. Hall TS, Brevetti GR, Skoultchi AJ, et al. Reexploration for hemorrhage following open heart

surgery differentiation on the causes of bleeding and the impact on patient outcomes. Ann Thorac Cardiovasc Surg 2001;7:352–7.
7. Unsworth-White MJ, Herriot A, Valencia O, et al. Resternotomy for bleeding after cardiac operation: a marker for increased morbidity and mortality. Ann Thorac Surg 1995;59:664–7.
8. Munoz JJ, Birkmeyer NJ, Dacey LJ, et al. Trends in rates of reexploration for hemorrhage after coronary artery bypass surgery. Northern New England Cardiovascular Disease Study Group. Ann Thorac Surg 1999;68:1321–5.
9. Charalambous CP, Zipitis CS, Keenan DJ. Chest re-exploration in the intensive care unit after cardiac surgery: a safe alternative to returning to the operating theater. Ann Thorac Surg 2006;81:191–4.
10. Kaiser GC, Naunheim KS, Fiore AC, et al. Reoperation in the intensive care unit. Ann Thorac Surg 1990;49:903–7.
11. McKowen RL, Magovern GJ, Liebler GA, et al. Infectious complications and cost-effectiveness of open resuscitation in the surgical intensive care unit after cardiac surgery. Ann Thorac Surg 1985;40:388–92.
12. Talamonti MS, LoCicero J, III, Hoyne WP, Sanders JH, Michaelis LL. Early reexploration for excessive postoperative bleeding lowers wound complication rates in open heart surgery. Am Surg 1987;53:102–4.
13. Stangerup SE, Dommerby H, Siim C, Kemp L, Stage J. New modification of hot-water irrigation in the treatment of posterior epistaxis. Arch Otolaryngol Head Neck Surg 1999;125:686–90.
14. Vender JR, Miller J, Rekito A, McDonnell DE. Effect of hemostasis and electrosurgery on the development and evolution of brain tumor surgery in the late 19th and early 20th centuries. Neurosurg Focus 2005;18:e3.
15. Hansen TB. Hot water irrigation to obtain hemostasis. Bull Midwifes Copenh (Danish) 1890;3:8–10.
16. Kassam A, Snyderman CH, Carrau RL, Gardner P, Mintz A. Endoneurosurgical hemostasis techniques: lessons learned from 400 cases. Neurosurg Focus 2005;19:E7.
17. Addis T. The coagulation time of the blood in man. Q J Exp Physiol 1908;1:305–34.
18. Stangerup SE, Thomsen HK. Histological changes in the nasal mucosa after hot-water irrigation. An animal experimental study. Rhinology 1996;34:14–17.
19. Willman VL, Hanlon CR. The influence of temperature on surface bleeding, favourable effects of local hypothermia. Ann Surg 1956;143:660–63.
20. Higami T, Yamashita T, Nohara H, et al. Early results of coronary grafting using ultrasonically skeletonized internal thoracic arteries. Ann Thorac Surg 2001;71:1224–8.
21. Peterson MD, Borger MA, Rao V, Peniston CM, Feindel CM. Skeletonization of bilateral internal thoracic artery grafts lowers the risk of sternal infection in patients with diabetes. J Thorac Cardiovasc Surg 2003;126:1314–19.
22. De Paulis R, de Notaris S, Scaffa R, et al. The effect of bilateral internal thoracic artery harvesting on superficial and deep sternal infection: The role of skeletonization. J Thorac Cardiovasc Surg 2005;129:536–43.
23. Boodhwani M, Lam BK, Nathan HJ, et al. Skeletonized internal thoracic artery harvest reduces pain and dysesthesia and improves sternal perfusion after coronary artery bypass surgery: a randomized, double-blind, within-patient comparison. Circulation 2006;114:766–73.
24. Gurevitch J, Matsa M, Paz Y, et al. Effect of age on outcome of bilateral skeletonized internal thoracic artery grafting. Ann Thorac Surg 2001;71:549–54.
25. Kramer A, Mastsa M, Paz Y, et al. Bilateral skeletonized internal thoracic artery grafting in 303 patients seventy years and older. J Thorac Cardiovasc Surg 2000;120:290–97.
26. Calafiore AM, Vitolla G, Iaco AL, et al. Bilateral internal mammary artery grafting: midterm results of pedicled versus skeletonized conduits. Ann Thorac Surg 1999;67:1637–42.
27. Bonacchi M, Prifti E, Giunti G, et al. Respiratory dysfunction after coronary artery bypass grafting employing bilateral internal mammary arteries: the influence of intact pleura. Eur J Cardiothorac Surg 2001;19:827–33.
28. Sahar G, Meir A, Battler A, et al. Bilateral skeletonized internal mammary versus single-pedicled internal mammary grafting in the elderly. Isr Med Assoc J 2007;9:294–8.
29. Cartier R, Leacche M, Couture P. Changing pattern in beating heart operations: use of skeletonized internal thoracic artery. Ann Thorac Surg 2002;74:1548–52.
30. Goff SG, Wu HD, Sauvage LR, et al. Differences in reendothelialization after balloon catheter removal of endothelial cells, superficial endarterectomy, and deep endarterectomy. J Vasc Surg 1988;7:119–29.
31. Berger RL, Dunton RF, Leonardi HK, Karlson KJ. Pack and close approach to persistent postcardiopulmonary bypass bleeding. J Am Coll Surg 1994;178:353–6.

32. Mestres CA, Pomar JL, Acosta M, et al. Delayed sternal closure for life-threatening complications in cardiac operations: an update. Ann Thorac Surg 1991;51:773–6.
33. Bouboulis N, Rivas LF, Kuo J, et al. Packing the chest: a useful technique for intractable bleeding after open heart operation. Ann Thorac Surg 1994;57:856–60.
34. Del Campo C. Mediastinal packing for refractory non-surgical bleeding after open-heart surgery. Can J Surg 1985;28:55–6.
35. Economopoulos GC, Sfirakis PD, Zarkalis DA, Loukas LL. Pedicled pericardial fat pad: a useful hemostatic supplement. Ann Thorac Surg 1995;59:768–70.
36. Charalambous C, Zipitis CS, Keenan DJ. Outcome of primary chest packing and delayed sternal closure for intractable bleeding following heart surgery. Cardiovasc J S Afr 2002;13:231–4.
37. Johnson JA, Gundersen AE, Stickney ID, Cogbill TH. Selective approach to sternal closure after exploration for hemorrhage following coronary artery bypass. Ann Thorac Surg 1990;49:771–4.

SECTION 3
Anesthetic Techniques

CHAPTER 34

Anesthetic Techniques to Reduce Blood Loss

Dafydd Thomas
Intensive Therapy Unit, Morriston Hospital, Abertawe Bro Morgannwg University NHS Trust and Welsh Blood Service, Swansea, Wales, UK

Anesthetic techniques have an influence on perioperative blood loss, even if the main control of hemostasis belongs to the surgeon.

Essential factors that may influence blood loss in anesthetized patients include
1 Control of temperature;
2 Patient's positioning;
3 Anesthetic technique;
4 Induced hypotension which warrants special consideration (addressed in chapter 35).

Introduction

The anesthesiologist is regarded by many as someone who renders the patient unconscious to facilitate surgery and also tries to ensure that adequate pain relief is administered during the perioperative period. In addition the role extends to acting as a guardian of the unconscious or vulnerable patient. It incorporates a wide spectrum of duties ranging from the avoidance of undue and unguarded pressure on areas which may result in nerve damage damaged corneas or dislodged teeth to the longer term damage caused by unnecessary administration of drugs or blood components. This may lead to end-organ damage long after the successful surgery has been completed.

Alternatives to Blood Transfusion in Transfusion Medicine, 2nd edition. Edited by A. Maniatis, P. Van der Linden, J.-F. Hardy.

As our knowledge about the effect of allogeneic blood transfusion on recipient patients develops it has become apparent that not all patients need or indeed gain a net benefit from receiving blood components during the otherwise successful operative treatment. It is important that the use of allogeneic blood components is carefully evaluated on the physiological need of the patient and probably only administered when hemorrhage is life threatening or when withholding them would lead to a worse patient outcome. In the context of allogeneic blood transfusion there are a number of anesthetic interventions that can influence operative blood loss. It is unlikely that anesthetic techniques can eliminate the need for transfusion when there is massive blood loss but in other situations there may be a significant reduction in the amount of blood transfusion required or the techniques may help avoid transfusion altogether. The anesthetist can help limit the need for allogeneic transfusion by becoming involved in preoperative assessment as early as possible and by applying physiological and pharmacological understanding to the patient's perioperative care.

Preoperative assessment

Although there are chapters elsewhere in this textbook about various preoperative measures (Chapters 27–29), the anesthetist can by a number of small preoperative checks ensure that the patient's reserve to operative blood loss is maximized. The preoperative examination needs to occur far enough in advance so that the patient can be optimized for the anticipated physiological stress of surgery and anesthesia. It is important that preoperative hemoglobin values are as normal as can be achieved depending upon the underlying pathology. The goal is to ensure that patients present for elective surgery with a level of hemoglobin above 12 g/dL. This may be achieved with preoperative use of hemotinics such as oral or IV iron and in certain instances recombinant erythropoietin. Equal attention needs to be paid to concurrent drug therapy, e.g., acetyl salicylic acid, platelet inhibitors, and other anticoagulants such as coumarin therapy that may need to be stopped or substituted before surgery. In particular, patients presenting for orthopedic procedures may be taking nonsteroidal anti-inflammatory drugs which increase the risk of pre- and postoperative bleeding.

Application of physiological principles

Temperature control: maintenance of normothermia

All general anesthesia leads to an inability to control body temperature both because it prevents behavioral responses and it will impair autonomic thermoregulation. Anesthetized individuals become poiklothermic and loose heat to their environment. There is a three-phase response causing hypothermia, phase one occurring within 30 minutes and is mainly due to core peripheral heat distribution secondary to the induced vasodilation. The second phase is more gradual and is due to the decreased heat production due to a 20–40% reduction in basal metabolic rate. There is convective and radiation heat loss which is dependent on the difference between peripheral temperature and ambient temperature The loss is made worse by other environmental factors such as low humidity and the heat consumed when liquids evaporate from the body surface, such as wet drapes in contact with the patient's skin. The third phase is a plateau phase where heat loss is matched by metabolic heat production. At this temperature the patient is sufficiently cold to reach the lower threshold for vasoconstriction, which results in a restriction of further core to peripheral heat transfer.

The loss of heat if not minimized will lead to a drop in the patient's body temperature leading to hypothermia and less a efficient clotting ability, an increase in cardiac morbidity, and an increased chance of infection. Numerous studies have in fact shown how maintenance of normothermia in patients receiving general anesthesia for surgical operations can lead to a decrease in operative losses, a decrease in morbidity from cardiac events, and a decrease in the incidence of wound infection.

Patient heat loss can be minimized in a number of relatively simple ways:

1 The ambient temperature and humidity within the operating theater needs to be as high as possible although due consideration needs to be made to the comfort of the health care workers performing the surgery and anesthesia.

2 Humidification and perhaps warming of the dry inhaled gases. As the anesthetic cases are pressurized gases or volatile liquids they will be cold and dry. A simple heat and moisture filter, which can also have a bacterial filtration function, is routinely placed between the inspiratory and expiratory circuit and the patient to minimize heat loss from the patient and to warm and humidify inspired gases.

3 Warming under blankets can be used and warm air over blankets have also become commonplace to prevent or decrease the development of hypothermia in the patient.

4 All fluids administered need to be warmed during infusion. There are various devices that are able to adequately heat administered fluids even when the infusion rate is rapid and of large volume. The administration of 1 L of fluid at ambient room temperature can reduce core body temperature by −0.26°C (Table 34.1).

The routine use of a variety of warming techniques has become commonplace over the past decade as a result of a number of clinical reports highlighting the importance of such measures [1–5].

When considering all aspects of perioperative morbidity it is worth remembering that tolerance of anemia can also be affected by temperature. Consider the case of a patient who awakens from

Table 34.1 Prevention of perioperative temperature loss.

Maintain body heat preoperatively as this will prevent heat loss while waiting for anesthesia and aid venous cannulation	Preoperative forced air warmer
Active peripheral warming continued during anesthesia	Forced air warmer Radiant heat
Passive peripheral warming during anesthesia	Space blanket (less effective but cheaper and better than no attempt and conservation of heat at all)
Ensure all administered fluids and gases are warmed	Fluid warmers including level 1 type warmers for massive hemorrhage situations
	Heat and moisture airway filters Active humidification Cardioplulmonary bypass Amino acid infusion—thermogenesis

anesthesia feeling cold and who then starts to shiver. The increase in oxygen demand induced by shivering may alter the supply–demand balance of delivered oxygen. If the anesthetist has decided to allow permissive anemia in an attempt to reduce allogeneic transfusion then a shivering patient by increasing oxygen demand by 500% may compromise oxygen delivery and in particular myocardial oxygen demand resulting in myocardial ischemia. This adds another reason for the anesthetist to prevent hypothermia and therefore assist a safer perioperative course.

Prevention of excessive arterial and venous pressure at the operative site

One of the most basic physical principles learnt by the trainee anesthetist is the importance of pressure gradients. The understanding of gas and liquid flow through a tube is described by Poiseuille's Law for laminar flow through a cylinder.

$$\frac{\delta V}{\delta t} = \frac{[(P_a - P_b)\pi r^4]}{8\eta l}$$

where V is the volume of gas or liquid, P_a and P_b are the pressures at each end, l is the length of the tube, r is the radius, and η is the viscosity coefficient.

A relatively simplistic interpretation of this law when applied to a bleeding blood vessel means that the blood loss will be determined by the size of the hole in the blood vessel, the pressure difference between inside and the outside of the vessel, and the viscosity of the blood. If we accept this working principle then anything that the anesthetist does to minimize the pressure gradient between the inside the vessel and the atmospheric pressure outside the vessel in an open surgical wound will also minimize blood loss.

The aim therefore would be to try and decrease arterial blood pressure and venous pressure using a combination of pharmacological agents and a variety of anesthetic techniques.

Control of intrathoracic and abdominal pressure

Another major and common perioperative physiological disturbance that can occur during anesthesia and surgery is the alteration in normal thoracic and abdominal pressures. The use of mechanical ventilation and the use of positive end expiratory pressure (PEEP) can significantly reduce venous return and result in an increase in peripheral venous pressures [6].

Mechanical ventilation

This method of ventilation by definition is mechanical and not physiological. Also called positive pressure ventilation it increases intrathoracic pressure and removes the natural negative pressure caused by diaphragmatic movement which usually sucks air into the lungs. The change in airway pressure related to positive pressure ventilation leads to an increase in mean intrathoracic pressure which in turn results in a decrease in venous return of blood to the heart. The resultant obstruction to venous flow increases peripheral venous pressure and leads to an increase in the blood loss. It is possible to minimize this effect on peripheral venous pressure using the postural adjustments described below under patient positioning. The net effect of reversing the pressures within the thorax means that the positive pressure leads to a decrease in venous return, an increase in venous pressure and the potential for greater venous oozing and overall blood loss.

Venous return can be further inhibited by the application of PEEP further increasing thoracic pressure. While this can also decrease cardiac output the effect is not a desirable one in terms of a blood saving as the negative effect on cardiac function is brought about by a minor tamponade effect on heart.

A more positive effect, however, is the avoidance of sympathetic nervous system stimulation resulting from hypercapnea and hypoxia, which can result in increased bleeding. However providing hypercapnea and hypoxia are avoided by using high gas flows spontaneous ventilation has been shown by some investigators to decrease bleeding (Figure 34.1a and b).

A study by Modig on 38 patients undergoing a total hip replacement showed a significant reduction on bleeding when spontaneous ventilation was used compared to mechanical ventilation 1145 mL versus 1541 mL [7].

Abdominal laparoscopy

Likewise the increase in intra-abdominal pressure secondary to pneumoperitoneum, a prerequisite for laparoscopic techniques, may lead to decreased venous return and an increase in peripheral venous pressures. Carbon dioxide is used as the insufflation gas as it is very soluble and minimizes air embolism but will lead to hypercapnea, which in turn will lead to venous congestion. The mitigation against the excessive abdominal pressure and hypercapnea is a need for mechanical ventilation and muscle relaxation [8, 9].

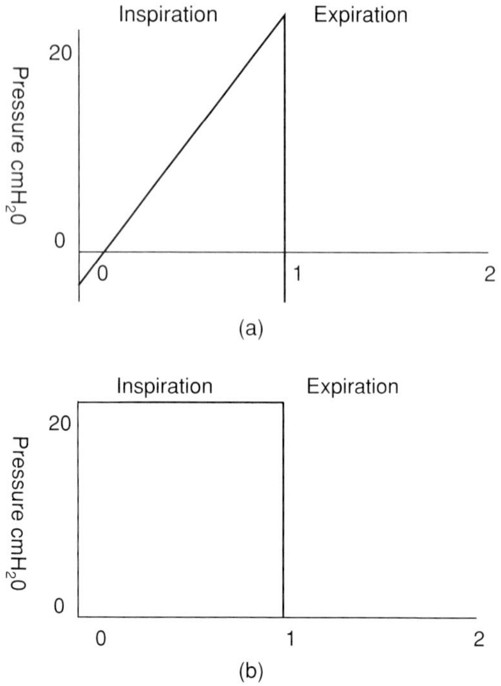

Figure 34.1 (a) Waveform produced by a volume-controlled ventilator. (b) Waveform produced by a pressure-generated ventilator.

Each intervention in itself may only result in a minor increase in blood loss but when taken as a whole may significantly alter the overall loss. The poor positioning of a patient may easily reverse any potential benefit that may occur as a result of anesthetic technique on blood loss. The use of position to alter both venous congestion and contribute to blood pressure control can transform the operative field, as with operations on the middle ear, making the surgery possible or quicker because of better vision for the surgical intervention.

Positioning

The correct positioning of the anesthetized patient or of a patient receiving regional anesthesia is dependent upon the attentive anesthetist. If a patient is unconscious as with general anesthesia or unaware of a part of their body because of regional or spinal anesthesia there is an inability to appreciate the normal afferent neural signals warning about abnormal or damaging pressure or position.

There are a number of nerves that need protection but in addition there are cardiovascular considerations. Excessive pressure for prolonged periods can lead to the development of localized pressure areas, venous occlusion with associated decrease in venous return and edema distal to the obstruction or even worse an arterial or arteriolar obstruction leading to hypoxic ischemic damage. In addition the decreased venous flow can lead to excessive venous pressure and resultant bleeding. The prone position leads to the greatest embarrassment of venous return as the abdominal compression leads to a significant obstruction of the venous system. It can be avoided by correct support to minimize pressure and allowing unrestricted abdominal movement. This is of particular importance during spinal surgery, which is usually performed in the prone position. The avoidance of pressure on the abdomen results in less vena caval pressure and less diversion of blood through collateral vertebral vessels (Baston's plexus) [10–12].

A second factor that can reduce venous pressure is the maintenance of paralysis and avoidance of coughing or straining, which may increase venous pressure. This is easily achieved with the monitoring of neuromuscular blockade while under general anesthesia. Third, the raising of the operative site above the level of the heart results in better venous return and reduces venous pooling at the surgical site. Caution is required to prevent air embolism with this latter technique [13, 14]. The surgeon and anesthetist need to take steps to minimize its occurrence and to monitor for and be able to treat such a complication, which can prove fatal.

The regional versus general anesthesia debate

There may be reasons apart from blood loss why a particular anesthetic technique is chosen over another, e.g., the use of regional anesthesia because of the poor respiratory reserve of someone with obstructive airways disease or the patient request to remain awake for the operative birth of a child. There is a generally held belief that regional anesthesia such as neuroaxial blockade, e.g., epidural or subarachnoid spinal anesthesia is associated with a reduced perioperative blood loss [15–19]. The evidence is conflicting and of course direct comparison between studies is not possible because of inherent variables between the patients and surgical techniques studied. In addition many of the studies lack proper randomization and suitable control groups and arterial blood pressure was not controlled for studies monitoring intraoperative blood loss. The use of regional techniques is persuasive when looking at the thrombo-embolic events and of course the other benefits of regional techniques such as less interference with the respiratory system and a better quality of postoperative pain relief without central sedation ensures continued popularity of this method of anesthesia.

In line with the basic principles outlined earlier epidural anesthesia has been associated with lower mean arterial pressures, right atrial pressures, mean pulmonary pressures, and mean peripheral venous pressures compared with patients undergoing general anesthetic techniques [8] and may therefore offer a theoretical advantage over general anesthesia. Sharrock showed that in 30 patients undergoing total hip arthroplasty under epidural anesthesia with similar mean arterial pressures differences in cardiac output induced by low dose epinephrine did not alter blood loss [20].

Hip replacement surgery

Two meta-analyses conducted by Pitner et al. and by Bradway JAP published in 1993 showed a benefit in terms of decreased blood loss in Hip replacement surgery (THR) when epidural anesthesia was used [21, 22]. A more recent meta-analysis in elective hip replacement patients showed that blood loss was reduced when using neuroaxial block when compared with general anesthesia and other operative outcomes were better for those patients who received neuroaxial block, confirming the findings of the two earlier meta-analyses [23]. All these analyses assessed studies which used either epidural or intrathecal techniques. Niemi showed a decrease in blood loss when general anesthesia was combined with epidural when compared with general anesthesia alone [24]. The reduction of blood loss with epidural anesthesia has even allowed total knee replacement to be undertaken without tourniquet or excessive blood loss [25]. Another recent publication considering a similar operative group of patients showed that spinal anesthesia resulted in a 12% decrease in operative time and a reduction in estimated intraoperative blood loss (25%), rate of operative blood loss (38%), and a 50% decrease in intraoperative transfusion requirements. Patients receiving spinal anesthesia had higher postoperative hemoglobins at day 1 and 2 and 20% lower transfusion requirements. [26]. This benefit does not seem to be apparent in operations for femoral neck fractures when epidural anesthesia is used [27], but when subarachnoid anesthesia is used in elderly patients for a similar surgical intervention blood loss was lower when compared with general anesthesia [28, 29].

Spinal procedures

Epidural block reduces intraoperative blood loss, even under normotensive conditions. It appears to be caused mainly by venous hypotension in the lumbar spine, created by sympathetic block with arteriolar vasodilation, venous pooling in lower limbs, and reactive vasoconstriction in the lumbar vertebra [14, 30]. The same decrease in blood loss does not seem to occur in operations on the cervical and thoracic spine.

Pelvic procedures

A study in patients undergoing abdominal prostatectomy showed that when compared with general anesthesia there was a reduction of between 30 and 40% in blood loss when a regional technique was used [31]. The etiology of this decreased blood loss is difficult to explain. The reduction in blood loss has been demonstrated even when there are similar blood pressures in the regional and general anesthesia groups [32] while other workers have found a synergistic effect on blood loss when GA and epidural techniques are used together resulting in lower diastolic and systolic blood pressures perioperatively [33]. Thorud et al. showed a 69% reduction on blood loss between epidural anesthesia versus neurolept technique during abdominal prostatectomies [34]. Abrahms also showed a reduction in blood loss when transurethral prostatectomy was performed under epidural or spinal anesthesia [35]. The majority of other studies confirm a decrease in blood loss with regional technique [36–39] although Nielsen et al. [40] previously failed to confirm this benefit and, in a later study, Wong did not find any benefit in using spinal anesthesia for radical retropubic prostatectomy [41]. Other pelvic operations for cystectomy and cesarean section seem to experience less blood loss when performed under epidural anesthesia [42–47].

Local anesthetic infiltration

As the name suggests there are few systemic effects when this type of anesthesia is used. The local anesthetic only affects the nerves which come into contact and there is minimal systemic effect. In addition the use of epinephrine will both prolong the action of the anesthetic and minimize blood loss by vasoconstriction within the surgical field. Patient selection is of great importance; however, an uncooperative or nervous patient can make surgical intervention difficult despite adequate analgesia and anesthesia. Local anesthetics have also been shown to exert and effect on hemostasis by inhibiting platelet aggregation and the effect was dose dependent. However there is no clinical relevance with regard to surgical blood loss as a result of this platelet inhibition.

Plexus blocks

These are more elaborate techniques where the deposit of local anesthetic is within a closed area or within a fascial plane allowing block of a plexus of nerves as the description suggests. An example is the deep cervical plexus block, which can be used very successfully to perform major vascular surgery such as carotid endarterectomy.

Again there is very little systemic effect from these types of block. The surgical field can be improved by altering posture despite a lack of systemic block as venous pressures can be altered by Trendelenburg or reverse Trendelenburg depending on which part of the body is being operated upon [48].

Hypotensive anesthesia

As with all anesthetic techniques employed to reduce blood loss, hypotensive anesthesia can aid the operative success by improving visibility in the surgical field. There are instances where this can have a major impact on the operative success such as eye, ear, and neurosurgery. In many other areas, however, caution needs to be exercised as hypotension while reducing vascular pressure and thereby reducing bleeding only lasts until the reversal of anesthesia. There is need to ensure that blood pressure is restored to normal values before surgical closure to ensure all bleeding points have been adequately dealt with. Another concern in dropping mean arterial pressure is the need to maintain adequate cerebral perfusion pressure. This is discussed further in the following chapter.

Conclusion

The anesthesiologist can play an integral role in many aspects of blood conservation. In addition to the techniques described above, by coordinating the many aspects of perioperative care, including preoperative optimization, operative blood salvage, and the withholding of allogeneic transfusion until there is physiological need, the anesthetist can help eliminate the need for allogeneic blood component transfusion in a large proportion of surgical patients.

References

1. Frank SM, Fleisher LA, Breslow MJ, et al. Perioperative maintenance of normothermia reduces the incidence of morbid cardiac events. JAMA 1997;277: 1127–34.
2. Schmied H, Kurz A, Sessler DI, Kozek S, Reiter A. Mild intraoperative hypothermia increases blood loss and allogeneic transfusion requirements during total hip arthroplasty. Lancet 1996;347:289–92.
3. Schmied H, Schifere A, Sessler DI, Meznik C. The effects of red cell scavenging, hemodilution and active warming on allogenic blood requirements in patients undergoing hip or knee arthroplasty. Anesth Analg 1998;86:387–91.
4. Winkler M, Akca O, Birkenberg B, et al. Aggressive warming reduces blood loss during hip arthroplasty. Anesth Analg 2000;91:978–84.
5. Rajagopalan S, Mascha E, Na J, Sessler DI. The effects of mild perioperative hypothermia on blood loss and transfusion requirement. Anesthesiology 2008; 108(1):71–7.
6. Prys-Roberts C. Effects of mechanical ventilation on the heart and pulmonary circulation. SNPM 1978;T.3:1919–26.
7. Bertrand D, Hannhart B, Laxenaire MC. Haemodynamic effects of inspiratory and expiratory resistances in anaesthetic breathing systems during induced hypotension. Eur J Anaesthesiol 1985;2(4):353–9.
8. Modig J. Regional anaesthesia and blood loss. Acta Anaesthesiol Scand Suppl 1998;89:44–8.
9. Whaba RW, Mazzama J. Ventilatory requirements during laparoscopic cholecystectomy. Can J Anaesth 1993;40:206–10.
10. Relton JE, Hall JE. Reduction of haemorrhage during spinal fusion combined with internal metallic fixation using a new scoliosis operating frame. Br J Bone Joint Surg 1967;49(2):327–32.
11. Lee TC, Yang LC, Chen HJ. Effect of patient position and hypotensive anaesthesia on inferior vena caval pressure. Spine 1998;23(8):941–7; discussion 947–8.
12. Bostman O, Hyrkas J, Hirvensalo E, et al. Blood loss, operating time and positioning of the patient in lumbar disc surgery. Spine 1990;15(5):360–63.
13. Park CK. The effect of patient positioning on intra-abdominal pressure and blood loss in spinal surgery. Anaesth Analg 2000;91(3):552–7.
14. Tate DE, Friedman RJ. Blood conservation in spinal surgery. Review of current techniques. Spine 1992;17:1450–56.
15. Richman JM, Rowlingson AJ, Maine DN, Courpas GE, Weller JF, Wu CL. Does neuraxial anesthesia reduce intraoperative blood loss? A meta-analysis. J Clin Anesth 2006;18(6):427–35.
16. Modig J Beneficial effects on intra-operative and post-operative blood loss in total hip replacement when performed under lumbar epidural anesthesia. An explanatory study. Acta Chir Scand 1989;550(Suppl.): 95–100; discussion 100–103.
17. Modig J, Karlstrom G. Intra- and post-operative blood loss in total hip replacement when performed under lumbar epidural versus general anaesthesia. Eur J Anaesthesiol 1987;4(5):345–55.
18. Dauphin A, Raymer KE, Stanton EB, Fuller HD. Comparison of general anesthesia with and without lumbar epidural for total hip arthroplasty: effects of

epidural block on hip arthroplasty. J Clin Anesth 1997;9(3):200–203.
19. Guay J. The effect of neuraxial blocks on surgical blood loss and blood transfusion requirements: a meta-analysis. J Clin Anesth 2006;18(2):124–8.
20. Sharrock NE, Mineo R, Go G. The effect of cardiac output on intraoperative blood loss during total hip arthroplasty. Reg Anaesth 1993;18(1):24–9.
21. Pitner RC, Mathie J. Is regional anaesthesia (RA) more effective than general anaesthesia(GA) in reducing intraoperative blood loss? A meta analysis. Anesthesiology 1993;79(Suppl. 3A):A1070.
22. Bradway JAP. A meta-analysis of regional vs. general anaesthesia in total hip arthroplasty. Anesthesiology 1993;(Suppl. 3A):A1064.
23. Mauerman WJ, Shilling AM, Zuo Z. A comparison of neuraxial block versus general anesthesia for elective total hip replacement: a meta-analysis. Anesth Analg 2006;103(4):1018–25.
24. Niemi TT, Pitkanen M, Syrjala M, Rosenberg PH. Comparison of hypotensive epidural anaesthesia and spinal anaesthesia on blood loss and coagulation during and after total hip arthroplasty. Acta Anaesthesiol Scand 2000;44(4):457–64.
25. Juelsgaard P, Larsen UT, Sorensen JV, Madsen F, Soballe K. Hypotensive epidural anesthesia in total knee replacement without tourniquet: reduced blood loss and transfusion. Reg Anesth Pain Med 2001;26(2):105–10.
26. Maurer SG, Chen AL, Hiebert R, et al. Comparison of outcomes of using spinal versus general anaesthesia in total hip arthroplasty. Am J Orthop 2007;36(7):E101–6.
27. Sorenson RM, Pace NL. Anesthetic techniques during surgical repair of femoral neck fractures. A meta-analysis. Anesthesiology 1992;77(6):1095–1104.
28. Covert CR, Fox GS. Anaesthesia for hip surgery in the elderly. Can J Anaesth 1989;36(3 Pt 1):311–19.
29. Davis FM, Laurenson VG. Spinal anaesthesia or general anaesthesia for emergency hip surgery in elderly patients. Anaesth Intensive Care 1981;9(4):352–8.
30. Kakiuchi M. Reduction of blood loss during spinal surgery by epidural blockade under normotensive general anesthesia. Spine 1997;22(8):889–94.
31. Madsen RE, Madsen PO. Influence of anesthesia form on blood loss in transurethral prostatectomy. Anesth Analg 1967;46(3):330–32.
32. Malhorta VS, Girardi R. Comparison of epidural anesthesia, general anesthesia and combined epidural general anesthesia for radical prostatectomy. Anesthesiology 1994;81(Suppl. 3A):A973.
33. O'Connor PJ, Hanson J, Finucane BT. Induced hypotension with epidural/general anesthesia reduces transfusion in radical prostate surgery. Can J Anaesth 2006;53(9):873–80.
34. Thorud T, Lund I, Holme I. The effect of anesthesia on intra-operative and post-operative bleeding during abdominal prostatectomies: a comparison of neurolept anesthesia, halothane anesthesia and epidural anesthesia. Acta Anaesthesiol Scand Suppl 1975;57:83–8.
35. Abrams PH, Shah PJ, Bryning K, et al. Blood loss during transurethral resection of the prostate. Anaesthesia 1992;37(1):71–3.
36. Shir Y, Raja SN, Frank SM, et al. Intraoperative blood loss during radical retropubic prostatectomy: epidural versus general anaesthesia. Urology 1995;45(6):993–9.
37. Albertsen PC. General versus spinal anesthesia in patients undergoing radical retropubic prostatectomy: results of a prospective, randomized study. J Urol 2005;174(3):931.
38. Dunet F, Pfister Ch, Deghmani M, Meunier Y, Demeilliers-Pfister G, Grise P. Clinical results of combined epidural and general anesthesia procedure in radical prostatectomy management. Can J Urol 2004;11(2):2200–204.
39. Salonia A, Crescenti A, Suardi N, et al. General versus spinal anesthesia in patients undergoing radical retropubic prostatectomy: results of a prospective, randomized study. Urology 2004;64(1):95–100.
40. Nielsen KK, Andersen K, Asbjorn J, et al. Blood loss in transurethral prostatectlomy;epidural versus general anaesthesia. Int Urol Nephrol 1987;19(3):287–92.
41. Wong RP, Carter HB, Wolfson A, Faustin C, Cohen SR, Wu CL. Use of spinal anesthesia does not reduce intraoperative blood loss. Urology 2007;70(3):523–6.
42. Donald DM. Blood Loss during major vaginal surgery. Bt J Anaesth 1968;40:233–9.
43. Ryan DW. Anaesthesia for cystectomy. A comparison of two anaesthetic techniques. Anaesthesia 1982;37(5):554–60.
44. Ladjevic N, Likic-Ladjevic I, Dzamic Z, Acimovic M, Dragicevic D, Durutovic O. Combined general and epidural anaesthesia versus general anaesthesia for radical cystectomy. Acta Chir Iugosl 2007;54(4):89–91.
45. Lertakyamanee J, Chinachoti T, Tritrakarn T, Muangkasem J, Somboonnanonda A, Kolatat T. Comparison of general and regional anesthesia for cesarean section: success rate, blood loss and satisfaction

from a randomized trial. J Med Assoc Thai 1999; 82(7):672–80.

46. Andrews WW, Ramin SM, Maberry MC, et al. Effect of type of anaesthesia on blood loss at elective repeat cesarean section. Am J Perinatol 1992:9(3):197–200.

47. Gilstrap LCIH, Hankins JC, Patterson DV. Effect of type of anaesthesia on blood loss at cesarian section. Obstet Gynaecol 1987;69:328–32.

48. Tetzlaff JE, Yoon HJ, Brems J. Interscalene brachial plexus block for shoulder surgery. Reg Anesth 1994;19(5):339–43.

CHAPTER 35

Controlled Hypotension Decreases Blood Transfusion Requirement: Fact or Fallacy?

Richard P. Dutton

University of Maryland School of Medicine; R Adams Cowley Shock Trauma Center, University of Maryland Medical System, Baltimore, MD, USA

Introduction

Controlled hypotension has long been advocated as a means of reducing blood loss during long elective surgeries. "Controlled" or "deliberate" hypotension refers to intraoperative maintenance at a systolic blood pressure (SBP) of 65–90 mmHg, or a mean arterial pressure (MAP) of 50–70, lower than normal but within the autoregulatory range for the brain and other organ systems. Controlled hypotension is used during head and neck, spine, and pelvic operations, but may be part of the anesthetic plan in other large elective surgeries. More recently, controlled hypotension has been advocated as a means of reducing blood loss during emergency surgery for trauma. This chapter will explain the techniques used for achieving and sustaining intraoperative hypotension, discuss the postulated physiology of this technique, and examine the scientific evidence that supports its use.

Techniques and physiology

Intraoperative blood pressure is governed by a number of factors (Figure 35.1). Intraoperative hypotension can be achieved through four distinct approaches. Each approach has particular technical and physiologic implications.

In the presence of ongoing hemorrhage, as with a trauma case or large elective surgery, the simplest means of achieving hypotension is to underresuscitate the patient, such that intravascular volume is reduced relative to intravascular capacity. Reduced filling of the right heart will lead to a reduction in cardiac output by way of Starling forces, accompanied by a state of systemic vasoconstriction driven by sympathetic activation and increased levels of circulating catecholamines [1]. Trauma patients presenting to the Emergency Department (ED) who are hypotensive and in hemorrhagic shock are profoundly vasoconstricted. When anesthetized there may be a profound drop in SBP, due both to the direct negative inotropic and vasodilatory effects of the anesthetic and to the indirect effect of reduced catecholamine outflow. In addition, animal studies have demonstrated increased sensitivity of the brain to both sodium thiopental and propofol in the setting of hemorrhagic shock, which may contribute to relative overdosing of these agents [2]. Blood pressure will be labile when hypotension is achieved by fluid restriction, with exaggerated swings both up and down in response to episodes of increased bleeding or to bolus fluid administration (Figure 35.2). Patients who are hypotensive due to fluid restriction are in shock by definition and are suffering from decreased peripheral perfusion. While vital organs will tolerate

Alternatives to Blood Transfusion in Transfusion Medicine, 2nd edition. Edited by A. Maniatis, P. Van der Linden, J.-F. Hardy.

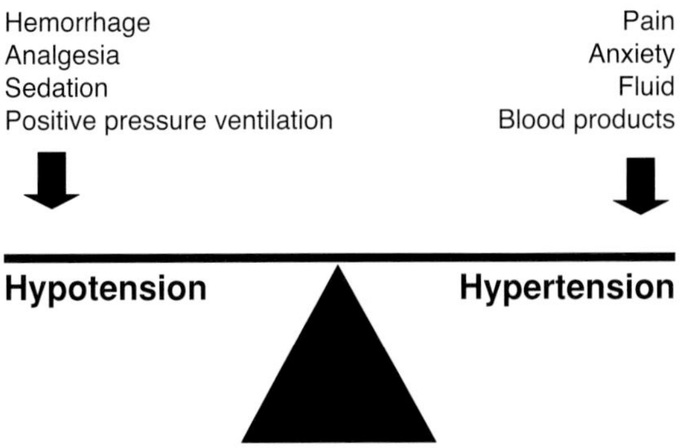

Figure 35.1 Factors influencing intraoperative blood pressure.

shock well for short periods, there exists the potential for inducing subsequent organ system failure as a consequence of hypoperfusion. This may be appropriate for short periods when management of uncontrolled hemorrhage is the overwhelming priority (see discussion of trauma cases below), but is not a rational approach for elective cases or when alternatives exist. In general, controlled hypotension in elective cases depends on simultaneous restoration and preservation of normal circulating fluid volume, and the largest potential pitfall of delayed hypotensive management is the failure to recognize and treat developing hypovolemia.

More commonly hypotension is induced and maintained with the addition of a systemic vasodilator to an otherwise stable anesthetic. Nitroglycerin and nitroprusside are the most commonly advocated agents, but prostaglandin E1, beta-receptor antagonists, calcium channel antagonists, angiotensin-converting enzyme inhibitors, and clonidine have all been used for this purpose [3]. The potent short-acting intravenous agents are typically administered by continuous infusion, offering flexibility in titration and more rapid resolution of hypotension at the end of the case. Induced hypotension with vasodilating medication follows induction of a stable anesthetic and fluid balance first, making subsequent determinations of anesthetic depth and fluid volume requirement easier: once a stable level of anesthesia and hypotension is achieved, any subsequent fall in SBP is likely to be the result of surgical blood loss or a change in stimulation level. Hypotension maintained in this way is characterized by dilation of peripheral vascular beds with increased blood flow (low pressure, high flow), which sustains peripheral tissue perfusion better than the low pressure, low flow state created by fluid restriction. Whether this condition can predispose to "steal" of perfusion from sensitive cardiac or cerebral vascular beds is unknown but has been postulated as a risk of this technique [4].

A third approach to controlled intraoperative hypotension, and the easiest for the anesthesiologist to achieve, is deliberate overdosing of conventional anesthetic agents. Increasing the administered concentration of isoflurane, for example, requires no additional equipment or supplies. This technique acts through the mechanisms of vasodilatation and negative inotropy common to most sedative/hypnotic medications. In the hands

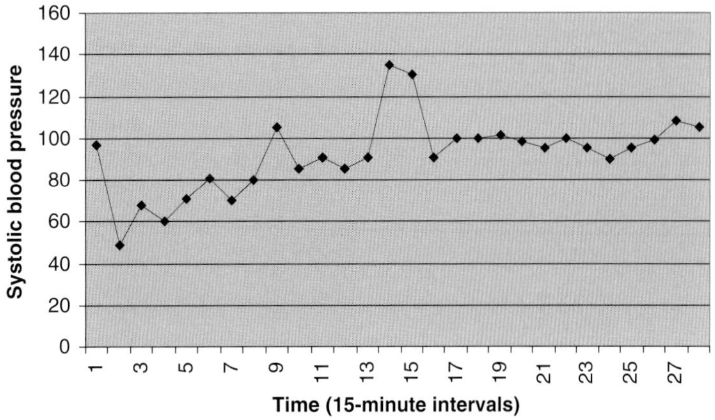

Figure 35.2 Deliberate hypotensive management of a trauma case. This patient was undergoing operative debridement and packing of a Grade V liver injury. Hypotension was achieved through deliberate restriction of fluids with a target systolic blood pressure of 80 mmHg. Note the typical oscillations of pressure caused by fluid boluses in the presence of ongoing hemorrhage, and the normalization of pressure once hemorrhage was operatively controlled, even without further fluid administration (about the 10th interval).

of an experienced anesthesia provider the resulting hypotension is easy to titrate. With the modern generation of ultra short-acting volatile and intravenous medications, hypotension is also easy to reverse when no longer indicated. As with the use of nonanesthetic vasodilators, the resulting hypotension is in the low-pressure, high-flow category, presenting a similar picture of preserved peripheral perfusion with the potential for central steal. This approach works better in younger, euvolemic patients, in whom the vasodilatory effects of the anesthetic can be used to advantage, and the negative inotropic effects tolerated. In older or more debilitated patients the cardiac depressant effects of high dose anesthetic agents may lead to a low-pressure, low-flow state that is not as beneficial as induction of hypotension with nitroglycerin or nitroprusside.

A final mechanism for achieving deliberate hypotension is the use of a central neuraxial block. Spinal or epidural anesthesia reliably produces hypotension through the mechanism of lower body sympatholysis and subsequent reduction in vascular tone. This technique is more difficult to titrate and harder to reverse when no longer desired, but central neuraxial blocks have demonstrated a proven benefit over general anesthesia in major hip and lower abdominal surgery [5], and reduced blood loss due to controlled hypotension may be one reason. Fluid loading to compensate for increased intravascular space runs the risk of fluid overload when the sympathectomy resolves, especially in older patients with limited cardiac and renal reserve. The physiology of controlled hypotension from regional anesthesia, while fitting into the same low-pressure, high-flow model already described, may be different from hypotension induced by systemic vasodilators because only a portion of the body is involved, with preserved vasoconstrictive mechanisms above the level of the block. Further, the venous dilation observed, with very low central pressure, may have its own direct effects on surgical site hemorrhage [6, 7]. Hypotension by way of a regional anesthetic is typically reserved for those patients who are receiving this sort of anesthetic for other reasons, or those who will benefit postoperatively from epidural analgesia.

Benefits of controlled hypotension

The principal benefit of controlled hypotension is reduction in intraoperative blood loss, which has been well documented in a number of different surgical procedures [3, 6–18]. Summary data from the orthopedic literature cites a 50% reduction in blood loss during total hip replacement with deliberate hypotension [8]. It should be remembered, however, that reduced blood loss may or may not translate to a tangible improvement in outcome for the patient.

Reduced blood loss is most beneficial when it results in a reduced transfusion requirement. The benefits of reducing transfused volume, or avoiding transfusion altogether, have been well enumerated elsewhere in this volume. Briefly, they include reduced immune suppression, reduced incidence of postoperative pulmonary complications (including transfusion associated lung injury), reduced risk of an allergic or febrile reaction, reduced risk of bacterial transmission, and reduced risk of infection with CMV, hepatitis, or HIV.

In many surgical cases reduced intraoperative blood loss does not equate with a reduction in transfusion, because the surgery is limited enough that transfusion is unlikely. Defining a benefit of deliberate hypotension in these cases is harder. It is impossible to demonstrate a difference in clinical outcome between a laparoscopic cholecystectomy patient who loses 100 mL and one who loses 200 mL, but the difference between losing 500 mL vs 1000 mL in a total hip replacement might be more apparent, even if neither patient is transfused. The patient with the greater blood loss is thought to be at greater risk for postoperative complications such as myocardial infarction, wound break down, or prolonged ileus [19], but studies to document this difference are hard to perform, and largely lacking in the literature. Reduction in blood loss per se thus becomes a benefit of deliberate intraoperative hypotension only when considering cases that will approach or cross the transfusion threshold.

A secondary benefit of reduced surgical bleeding is improved visualization of the surgical field, leading to more rapid and technically improved operations. This is a common subjective motivator for the use of controlled hypotension in surgeries such as cranial aneurysm clipping [20], endoscopic sinus surgery [21], microscopic ear or facial surgery [22, 23], and spine surgery in the prone position [8–10]. Many studies of controlled hypotension have documented reductions in surgical time in parallel with reductions in blood loss. Although difficult to prove, reduced surgical time should also reduce the incidence of wound or deep tissue infection. Hypotension during aneurysm surgery may also benefit the patient by reducing the risk of rupture during surgical dissection and temporary occlusion [21], although the clinical evidence supporting this approach is sparse and conflicting. Recent literature on this topic has focused on the risks of hypotension in patients with injured brain tissue and disrupted autoregulatory mechanisms, especially if exposure of the aneurysm will require significant retraction (and thus compression) of brain tissue [24, 25].

Risks of controlled hypotension

The principal risk of controlled hypotension is hypoperfusion and organ system injury. A MAP of 50 mmHg is usually taken as the lowest acceptable target for controlled hypotension, specifically because this is the lower limit of cerebral autoregulation in normal patients. Below this level cerebral perfusion becomes a direct function of blood flow, making tissue ischemia more probable. The autoregulatory threshold for other organs is similar, although the brain's dependence on aerobic metabolism makes it the organ at greatest risk in most patients. Cerebral effects of controlled hypotension have been studied using transcranial Doppler [26], demonstrating preserved blood flow at low pressures and near-infrared cerebral oximetry [27], and demonstrating reduced tissue oxygen tension. In neither study did any patient have a demonstrable neurologic defect, indicating that the changes in physiology observed were within the range of normal tolerance.

Mortality and morbidity following deliberate intraoperative hypotension is rare, and attributing negative outcomes to the technique is difficult because of numerous confounding factors such as the patient's underlying health and the organ-specific risks of the surgery itself. For example, very few patients emerge from anesthesia with a new central neurologic deficit, and the ones that do have almost all had brain or spinal surgery. On the contrary, subtle diffuse cognitive deficits following anesthesia are common [28], especially in older patients, and the impact of deliberate hypotension on this outcome has not been rigorously studied. Improved intraoperative monitoring, development of sophisticated and validated tests of cognition, and growing interest in postoperative cognitive deficits will likely shed more light on this risk over the coming decade.

The risks of controlled hypotension are strongly affected by the patient's premorbid condition. Chronic hypertension, especially when poorly controlled, leads to changes in the autoregulatory thresholds of the brain and other organ systems, making the patient effectively hypotensive at a much higher blood pressure. If normal end points are used to manage this patient, significant hypoperfusion may result. Similarly, many specific organ system pathologies can cause an increased sensitivity to hypoperfusion, including brain trauma, coronary artery disease, chronic liver disease, and renal insufficiency. The use of controlled hypotension is therefore contraindicated in patients with uncontrolled hypertension, end-organ pathology, or pregnancy [3].

The risk of myocardial hypoperfusion from deliberate hypotension is likely real, but very small. In theory, reduced blood flow across fixed coronary lesions creates an ischemic risk through the mechanism of steal [4], but in practice deliberate intraoperative hypotension is seldom associated with S-T segment changes on ECG, enzyme leak, or other evidence of myocardial injury, and studies have shown improvement in coronary perfusion [29]. This may be a feature of patient selection or it may be a function of the beneficial effects of afterload reduction and decreased metabolic demand under general anesthesia.

Renal dysfunction following controlled hypotension is unlikely. Glomerular filtration rate and urine production fall when blood pressure is low, a manifestation of renal cell "hibernation" in response to hypotension [30]. Renal cells do not become ischemic, however, unless hypotension is severe, prolonged, and accompanied by vasoconstriction. Urine output returns when blood pressure is allowed to normalize. Hepatic dysfunction is similarly unlikely, with blood flow in the liver preserved over wide variations in systemic pressure [31, 32].

Newly identified risks of controlled hypotension include focal ischemia of the spine or optic nerve. While controlled hypotension is highly effective at reducing blood loss during long spinal surgery cases, distraction of the spinal cord during manipulation, and hardware placement puts it at risk for ischemic injury [10, 33]. Neurophysiologic monitoring, including somato-sensory evoked potentials, motor-evoked potentials, and even the traditional wake-up test have become the standard of care for spinal surgery specifically because of their ability to indicate spinal ischemia [10], and the first response to an observed change in neurologic function is typically an effort to raise the blood pressure and increase perfusion.

Posterior ischemic optic neuropathy (PION) is the most common cause of blindness following anesthesia and is strongly associated with long spine cases in the prone position [34]. Once thought to be due to direct pressure on the eye, PION is now understood to be the result of intraoperative hypoperfusion. While length of surgery and increased intraoperative blood loss are cited as independent risk factors in the latest review of the American Society of Anesthesiologists (ASA) visual loss registry [35], and hypotension is not, it seems clear that hypoperfusion is at the root of this disease, and is likely the result of many factors including position, anemia, vasoconstriction, and hypotension. While still very rare, the devastating nature of this complication has moderated enthusiasm for controlled hypotension in major spine cases.

Controlled hypotension in elective surgery

Controlled hypotension has been shown to significantly reduce blood loss in clinical trials in total hip arthroplasty [5–8, 17], total knee arthroplasty (without a tourniquet) [16], spinal fusion [10], major orthognathic surgery [14, 15], and radical prostate surgery [18]. Based on this data, controlled hypotension has also been recommended as a technique for reducing blood loss in major craniofacial surgery, neurologic tumor resection, radical pelvic or abdominal surgery [11–13], and radical mastectomy, although these more uncommon conditions have not been studied prospectively. Deliberate hypotension is also an important consideration when the patient undergoing a large operation will not accept blood products (i.e., in Jehovah's Witness patients [9]) or is a difficult crossmatch due to multiple anti-RBC antibodies.

Deliberate hypotension to facilitate the surgical view of the operative field has been recommended in sinus surgery [21, 23], microsurgery of the ear [22], and intracranial aneurysm surgery [20]. The use of deliberate hypotension to improve surgical visibility in sinus surgery has been challenged [21], but this technique remains the standard in most practices. In aneurysm surgery, as was noted previously, the immediate benefits of hypotension to visualization, manipulation and control of the aneurysm must be carefully weighed against the potential for ischemia in retracted brain tissue [24, 25]. Prudent practice at present includes the use of continuous arterial pressure monitoring, neurophysiologic monitoring of affected brain segments, maintenance of normovolemia, and the capability on hand to immediately raise or lower the patient's blood pressure in response to changing surgical requirements [20]. Deliberate hypotension can then be employed selectively only at the time of aneurysm manipulation and only for as long as electrophysiologic monitoring indicates the continued adequacy of cerebral perfusion.

Studies comparing different techniques for controlled hypotension have largely failed to demonstrate any difference in overall blood loss between hypotension achieved with specific vasodilators, hypotension achieved with anesthetic agents, and hypotension due to epidural anesthesia. As noted previously, all three of these techniques result in a low-pressure, high-flow state that should preserve tissue perfusion as long as vascular volume is maintained. The choice of technique for controlled hypotension should therefore be made on the basis of other factors, such as the patient's benefit from epidural analgesia postoperatively, the patient's tolerance of anesthetic versus vasodilating medications, the logistics of the anesthetic delivered, and the experience of the provider. Because most of the benefits of controlled hypotension accrue from avoidance of transfusion, the likelihood that RBCs will be needed should always be a consideration. Deliberate hypotension should be reserved for cases with significant blood loss and the potential for transfusion or the specific surgical need for a bloodless field (i.e., microsurgery of the head and neck).

Controlled hypotension in resuscitation from hemorrhagic shock

Fluid administration is the cornerstone of resuscitation, and aggressive administration of fluid to the trauma patient has been strongly recommended in basic texts for at least five decades [36]. This therapy was supported by early studies of shock which demonstrated the intracellular migration of fluid in response to ischemia, producing an intravascular fluid deficit in excess of the actual volume of bleeding [37]. Further, the aggressive use of fluids has a strong visceral appeal to providers: by Starling's law an increase in intravascular volume will result in an immediate increase in cardiac output and blood pressure in most hemorrhaging patients, often making their blood pressure "normal" within a matter of minutes. This effect may even be exaggerated in young, previously healthy patients who are profoundly vasoconstricted as the result of blood loss.

It was not until the development of sophisticated mammalian models of *uncontrolled* hemorrhage in the late 1980s that this approach was challenged. It is now recognized that fluid administration to a patient with *active* hemorrhage is like pouring water into a bucket with a hole in the bottom; increasing SBP and venous pressure only results in more rapid hemorrhage. Both hypotension and regional vasoconstriction are essential functional components of the systemic response to bleeding. Returning blood pressure to normal is problematic because rebleeding is likely to occur when fragile early clots are washed away. Further damage occurs because most resuscitation in the field and ED is carried out with isotonic crystalloid solutions, which neither clot nor carry oxygen. Significant dilution of both RBC mass and clotting factors is likely.

Animal trials using a swine model of uncontrolled aortic hemorrhage have consistently demonstrated a reduction in rebleeding, improvement in tissue oxygen delivery, and improved survival when fluid resuscitation is targeted to a lower than normal blood pressure [38, 39]. This observation has been confirmed in an elegant rat model of hemorrhagic shock incorporating a variety of resuscitation strategies [40]. The absence of resuscitation leads to a high mortality, as does resuscitation targeted to normal vital signs. It is only in animals resuscitated to a lower than normal target pressure (MAP 50–60) that survival is improved. A consensus panel organized in 1993 to summarize this area of research concluded that deliberate hypotension was consistently beneficial in mammalian models of uncontrolled hemorrhagic shock, and urged the translation of this research to clinical practice [41].

The most important human trial of deliberate under-resuscitation was conducted in Houston in the early 1990s [42]. Hypotensive victims of penetrating torso trauma were randomized based on the day of the month to receive conventional intravenous fluid therapy or no fluid at all during prehospital and ED care. At the time of reaching the operating room (OR) there was a 2-L difference between groups in the amount of fluids received, but no difference in SBP (the effect of spontaneous hemostasis and auto-resuscitation, as seen in Figure 35.2, above). The fluid restricted group had significantly better survival. This landmark study was published in 1994, and subsequently criticized for its enrollment mechanism, its restriction to penetrating trauma victims, its "all or none" resuscitation strategy, and its failure to continue fluid restriction beyond the start of surgery (i.e., until the definitive control of ongoing hemorrhage) [43].

A similar study performed in Baltimore in the late 1990s corrected many of these faults [44]. This trial enrolled both blunt and penetrating trauma victims, used titration of fluids based on high or low blood pressure targets, and continued therapy until hemostasis had been achieved. This study did not show improved survival, due both to a smaller number of patients enrolled and to improved overall outcomes in trauma care, but the results suggested that deliberate hypotension was at least as safe as the traditional approach. Despite the inconclusive outcome of this study increasing experience with deliberate hypotension has led most large trauma centers to adopt this approach, and "hypotensive resuscitation" is now a common practice.

Two important caveats apply to the use of deliberate hypotension in resuscitation from traumatic shock. First is the underlying physiology. Unlike patients presenting for elective surgery, these patients are already hypotensive and often profoundly vasoconstricted when they arrive in the OR. Administration of anesthetic agents and conversion from spontaneous to positive pressure ventilation may produce profound hypotension and even loss of a palpable pulse. For this reason, deliberate hypotension is often achieved by significant underdosing of anesthesia and analgesia. This creates the potential for intraoperative recall and subsequent psychological complications. In addition, it makes these patients physiologically different from the animal models of uncontrolled hemorrhage described above, which are necessarily conducted under general anesthesia. To date there have been no clinical trials in trauma comparing vasoconstricted hypotension sustained through fluid restriction and the more physiologically sound approach of keeping the patient hypotensive through the use of anesthetics, while providing enough fluid to tolerate the vasodilatation that results. In theory it is blood pressure that is most important to ongoing hemorrhage, while tissue perfusion is the key to avoiding long-term sequelae from shock. Vasodilatation at a low pressure should produce the best overall outcomes. There is tantalizing laboratory data that supports this view [45], but as yet no confirmation in humans.

The second caveat to the use of deliberate hypotension in trauma patients concerns the composition of administered fluids. Most of the laboratory data cited, as well as the clinical trials performed to date, initiated resuscitation with isotonic crystalloid solutions. Dilution of coagulation factors and oxygen-carrying capacity is part of the pathophysiology of aggressive resuscitation, and certainly contributes to the poor outcomes observed. This problem can be mitigated, however, by the use of RBC and plasma as initial resuscitation fluids, and it is possible that the blood pressure achieved is less important when normal blood composition is preserved. Experienced traumatologists have long advocated the early use of uncrossmatched type-O RBC [46], while preliminary data from the US Army experience in Iraq suggests that early use of plasma is associated with improved outcomes in patients requiring massive transfusion [47]. Beyond even these concerns is the observation that lactated Ringers solution—the most commonly used isotonic crystalloid—may be proinflammatory in trauma patients, and may contribute directly to the development of organ system failure [48].

All in all, controlled hypotension during early resuscitation and hemostatic surgery for actively bleeding trauma patients is the recommended approach. Hypotension will facilitate early clot formation, may improve surgical visibility, and will likely reduce the overall transfusion requirement. This technique, however, should not be applied in a vacuum. Enough fluid should be administered to allow a deep level of anesthesia, and RBC and plasma should be administered early enough to preserve functional blood composition.

Conclusion

Controlled intraoperative hypotension is a valuable anesthetic technique that can reduce or eliminate transfusions in both major elective surgeries and emergency surgery for traumatic hemorrhage. Like most techniques, controlled hypotension carries both risks and benefits. Knowledge of the physiology of blood pressure control, and the manner in which anesthetic agents can influence the surgical procedure, is essential for the skilled anesthesiologist, and will allow the application of controlled hypotension in the patients and at the times that it is most likely to be beneficial.

References

1. Dutton RP. Current concepts in hemorrhagic shock. In: Weiss, Shamir (eds) *Anesthesiology Clinics of North America*, Vol. 25. Elsevier, Philadelphia, 2007, pp. 23–34.
2. Johnson KB, Egan TD, Kern SE, McJames SW, Cluff ML, Pace NL. Influence of hemorrhagic shock followed by crystalloid resuscitation on propofol: a pharmacokinetic and pharmacodynamic analysis. Anesthesiology 2004;101:647–59.
3. Shander A, Rijhwani T. Anesthesia techniques in blood conservation. In: Spiess BD, Spence RK, Shander A (eds) *Perioperative Transfusion Medicine (2e)*. Lippincott Williams & Wilkins, Philadelphia, 2006, pp. 435–50.
4. Hickey RF, Verrier ED, Baer RW, et al. A canine model of acute coronary artery stenosis: effects of deliberate hypotension. Anesthesiology 1983;59:226–36.
5. Mauermann WJ, Shilling AM, Zuo Z. A comparison of neuraxial block versus general anesthesia for elective total hip replacement: a meta-analysis. Anesth Analg 2006;103:1018–25.
6. Chin SP, Abou-Madi MN, Eurin B, et al. Blood loss in total hip replacement: extradural v. phenoperidine analgesia. Br J Anaesth 1982;54:491–5.
7. Rosberg B, Fredin H, Gustafson C. Anesthetic techniques and surgical blood loss in total hip arthroplasty. Acta Anaesthesiol Scand 1982;26:189–93.
8. Sollevi A. Hypotensive anesthesia and blood loss. Acta Anaesthesiol Scand Suppl 1988;89:39–43.
9. Brodsky JW, Dickson JH, Erwin WD, et al. Hypotensive anesthesia for scoliosis surgery in Jehovah's Witnesses. Spine 1991;16:304–6.
10. Grundy BL, Nash CL Jr, Brown RH. Deliberate hypotension for spinal fusion: prospective randomized study with evoked potential monitoring. Can Anaesth Soc J 1982;29:452–62.
11. Ahlering TE, Henderson JB, Skinner DG. Controlled hypotensive anesthesia to reduce blood loss in radical cystectomy for bladder cancer. J Urol 1983;129:953–4.
12. Powell JL, Mogelnicki SR, Franklin EW, et al. A deliberate hypotensive technique for decreasing blood loss during radical hysterectomy and pelvic lymphadenopathy. Am J Obstet Gynecol 1983;147:196–202.
13. Donald JR. The effect of anesthesia, hypotension, and epidural analgesia on blood loss in surgery for pelvic floor repair. Br J Anaesth 1969;41:155–66.
14. Dolman RM, Bentley KC, Head TW, English M. The effect of hypotensive anesthesia on blood loss and operative time during LeFort I osteotomies. J Oral Maxillofac Surg 2000;58:834–9.
15. Praveen K, Narayanan V, Muthusekhar MR, Baig MF. Hypotensive anaesthesia and blood loss in orthognathic surgery: a clinical study. Br J Oral Maxillofac Surg 2001;39:138–40.
16. Juelsgaard P, Larsen UT, Sorensen JV, Madsen F, Soballe K. Hypotensive epidural anesthesia in total knee replacement without tourniquet: reduced blood loss and transfusion. Reg Anesth Pain Med 2001;26:105–10.
17. Eroglu A, Uzunlar H, Erciyes N. Comparison of hypotensive epidural anesthesia and hypotensive total intravenous anesthesia on intraoperative blood loss during total hip replacement. J Clin Anesth 2005;17:420–25.
18. O'Connor PJ, Hanson J, Finucane BT. Induced hypotension with epidural/general anesthesia reduces transfusion in radical prostate surgery. Can J Anaesth 2006;53:873–80.
19. Sorensen LT, Hemmingsen U, Kallehave F, et al. Risk factors for tissue and wound complications in gastrointestinal surgery. Ann Surg 2005;241:654–8.
20. Drummond JC, Patel PM. Neurosurgical anesthesia. In: Miller RD (ed.) *Miller's Anesthesia*, 6th edn. Elsevier Churchill Livingstone, Philadelphia, 2005, pp. 2149.
21. Jacobi KE, Bohm BE, Rickauer AJ, Jacobi C, Hemmerling TM. Moderate controlled hypotension with sodium nitroprusside does not improve surgical conditions or decrease blood loss in endoscopic sinus surgery. J Clin Anesth 2000;12:202–7.
22. Scholtes JL. Deliberate hypotension for middle ear microsurgery. Acta Anaesthesiol Belg 1981;32:195–211.
23. Heerman J, Neues D. Intranasal microsurgery of all paranasal sinuses, the septum, and the lacrimal sac with hypotensive anesthesia. 25 years' experience. Ann Otol Rhinol Laryngol 1986;95:631–8.
24. Chang HS, Hongo K, Nakagawa H. Adverse effects of limited hypotensive anesthesia on the outcome of patients with subarachnoid hemorrhage. J Neurosurg 2000;92:271.
25. Foroohar M, Macdonald RL, Roth S, et al. Intraoperative variables and early outcome after aneurysm surgery. Surg Neurol 2000;54:304.
26. Fukusaki M, Kanaide M, Inadomi C, et al. Human middle cerebral artery flow velocity during controlled hypotension combined with

hemodilution-transcranial Doppler study. J Clin Anesth 2005;17:177–81.
27. Han SH, Bahk JH, Kim JH, et al. The effect of esmolol-induced controlled hypotension in combination with acute normovolemic hemodilution on cerebral oxygenation. Acta Anaesthesiol Scand 2006;50: 863–8.
28. Newman S, Stygall J, Hirani S, Shaefi S, Maze M. Postoperative cognitive dysfunction after noncardiac surgery: a systematic review. Anesthesiology 2007;106:572–90.
29. Mikhail MS, Thangathurai D, Thaker KB, Hutchinson SJ, Black DR, Chandraratna PA. Echocardiographic assessment of coronary blood flow velocity during controlled hypotensive anesthesia with nitroglycerin. J Cardiothorac Vasc Anesth 2000;14:565–70.
30. Lessard MR, Trepanier CA. Renal function and hemodynamics during prolonged isoflurane-induced hypotension in humans. Anesthesiology 1991;74:860–65.
31. Andel D, Andel H, Horauf K, et al. The influence of deliberate hypotension on splanchnic perfusion balance with use of either isoflurane or esmolol and nitroglycerin. Anesth Analg 2001;93:1116–20.
32. Pakulski C, Nowicki R, Kowalczyk P, et al. The influence of controlled hypotension on splanchnic mucosal perfusion using gastric tonometry in patients undergoing resection of meningioma. Med Sci Monit 2002;8:CR28–30.
33. Yeoman PM, Gibson MJ, Hutchinson A, et al. Influence of induced hypotension and spinal distraction on feline spinal somatosensory evoked potentials. Br J Anaesth 1989;63:315–20.
34. Ho VT, Newman NJ, Song S, Ksiazek S, Roth S. Ischemic optic neuropathy following spine surgery. J Neurosurg Anesthesiol 2005;17:38–44.
35. Lee LA, Roth S, Posner KL, et al. The American Society of Anesthesiologists Postoperative Visual Loss Registry: analysis of 93 spine surgery cases with postoperative visual loss. Anesthesiology 2006;105:652–9.
36. Committee on Trauma. *American College of Surgeons: Advanced Trauma Life Support Program for Doctors*. American College of Surgeons, Chicago, 1997.
37. Shires GT, Coln D, Carrico J, et al: Fluid therapy in hemorrhagic shock. Arch Surg 1964;88:688–93.
38. Riddez L, Johnson L, Hahn RG. Central and regional hemodynamics during fluid therapy after uncontrolled intra-abdominal bleeding. J Trauma 1998;44:1–7.
39. Stern A, Dronen SC, Birrer P, Wang X. Effect of blood pressure on haemorrhagic volume in a near-fatal haemorrhage model incorporating a vascular injury. Ann Emerg Med 1993;22:155–63.
40. Capone A, Safar P, Stezoski SW, Peitzman A, Tisherman S. Uncontrolled hemorrhagic shock outcome model in rats. Resuscitation 1995;29:143–52.
41. Shoemaker WC, Peitzman AB, Bellamy R, et al. Resuscitation from severe hemorrhage. Crit Care Med 1996;24:S12–23.
42. Bickell WH, Wall MJ, Pepe PE, et al. Immediate versus delayed resuscitation for hypotensive patients with penetrating torso injuries. N Engl J Med 1994;331:1105–9.
43. Dutton RP. Low pressure resuscitation from hemorrhagic shock. In: Dutton RP, Sharar S, Hurford W (eds) *International Anesthesia Clinics: Trauma*, Vol. 40. 2002, pp. 19–30.
44. Dutton RP, Mackenzie CF, Scalea TM. Hypotensive resuscitation during active hemorrhage: impact on in-hospital mortality. J Trauma 2002;52:1141–6.
45. Shaftan GW, Chiu C, Dennis C, Harris B. Fundamentals of physiologic control of arterial hemorrhage. Surgery 1965;58:851–6.
46. Dutton RP, Shih D, Edelman BB, Hess JR, Scalea TM. Safety of uncrossmatched Type-O Red cells for resuscitation from hemorrhagic shock. J Trauma 2005;59:1445–9.
47. Gonzalez EA, Moore FA, Holcomb JB, et al. Fresh frozen plasma should be given earlier to patients requiring massive transfusion. J Trauma 2007;62:112–9.
48. Alam HB, Rhee P. New developments in fluid resuscitation. Surg Clin North Am 2007;87:55–72.

CHAPTER 36

Acute Normovolemic Hemodilution

Javad Bidgoli & Philippe Van der Linden
Department of Anesthesiology,CHU Brugmann-HUDERF,Université Libre de Bruxelles, Brussels, Belgium

Increasing awareness of the potential adverse effects of allogeneic blood transfusion, but also the occurrence of intermittent blood shortages have prompted both physicians and patients to search alternatives to the use of donor blood. Acute normovolemic hemodilution (ANH) was introduced into clinical practice in the 1970s to reduce requirements for allogeneic blood products [1,2]. ANH entails the removal of blood from a patient either immediately before or shortly after the induction of anesthesia and its simultaneous replacement by an appropriate volume of crystalloids and/or colloids to maintain "normovolemia" [3, 4]. As a result, blood subsequently lost during surgery will contain proportionally less red blood cells (RBCs) per milliliter, thus reducing the loss of autologous erythrocytes. Potential benefits of ANH therefore include all the advantages associated with a reduction in allogeneic blood exposure, including a reduction of transfusion reactions from exposure to donor's blood antigens and a decreased exposure to blood-borne pathogens. When compared to other blood conservation techniques, ANH offers several inherent advantages: it is quite inexpensive and easily available, it improves tissue oxygenation because of decreased blood viscosity and it provides fresh autologous blood units for later transfusion after the achievement of surgical hemostasis. However, the real efficacy of ANH in reducing allogeneic blood transfusion remains controversial. This review aims to describe the physiology, limits and clinical use of ANH.

Alternatives to Blood Transfusion in Transfusion Medicine, 2nd edition. Edited by A. Maniatis, P. Van der Linden, J.-F. Hardy.

Physiological compensatory mechanisms

The acute reduction in RBCs concentration induced by hemodilution elicits intrinsic compensatory mechanisms, which allow the maintenance of adequate oxygenation at the tissue level [5, 6]. The development of these mechanisms is closely related to the improvement of whole blood fluidity achieved by hemodilution providing the maintenance of "normovolemic" conditions. The basic determinants of blood fluidity are the red cell concentration, the plasma viscosity, the cell-to-cell interactions and the prevailing shear rate (i.e., the mean linear flow velocity). The lower the shear rate, the more pronounced is the improvement in blood fluidity based on changes in hematocrit [3]. Elicited compensatory mechanisms mainly involve an increase in cardiac output and an increase in tissue oxygen extraction.

Increase in cardiac output

At the systemic level, improvement in blood fluidity results in an increase of venous return and a reduction of left ventricular afterload. Enhancement of shear rate with subsequent release of nitric oxide also contributes to systemic vasodilation [7], while hemodilution-induced stimulation of aortic chemoreceptors increase the sympathetic activity of the heart, resulting in improved myocardial performance [8]. All of these phenomena are responsible for the increase in cardiac output, mainly through a rise in stroke volume, but also to some extent through an increase in heart rate. Indeed, in awake subjects undergoing ANH, an increase in stroke volume and heart rate has been observed, whereas in anesthetized patients, the increase in cardiac output is essentially related to the rise in stroke volume, but also to some extent to an increase in heart rate [4, 9]. The physiologic response of cardiac output to ANH appears to be dependent on the presence of an intact autonomic nervous system. In animals deprived of their autonomic nervous system, the heart rate did not increase during isovolemic anemia and the increase in cardiac output was significantly lower than in intact animals [10]. Alpha-adrenergic tone to capacitance vessels also appears essential for an adequate cardiac output response to anemia [11]; it is possible that this enhanced venomotor tone results from hemodilution-induced stimulation of aortic chemoreceptors [12].

Increase in tissue oxygen extraction

The second compensatory mechanism aims at a better matching of oxygen delivery to oxygen demand at the tissue level. This mechanism, which allows for increased blood oxygen extraction entails physiologic alterations at both the systemic and microcirculatory level. At the systemic level, a better matching of oxygen delivery to tissue oxygen demand requires a redistribution of blood flow to areas of high metabolic demand from areas of low one. Several experimental studies demonstrated cerebral and coronary vasodilation during isovolemic hemodilution, blood flow in these areas increasing out of the proportion of the rise in cardiac output [13]. Vasoconstriction develops in the hepatic, renal, mesenteric, and splanchnic areas, with the results that blood flow to these organs contributes less to the overall increase in blood flow. This regional redistribution of blood flow during isovolemic hemodilution is partly due to alpha-adrenergic stimulation, but seems unaltered in the presence of beta-adrenergic blockade [14]. At the microcirculatory level, several physiologic alterations develop to provide a more efficient utilization of the remaining blood oxygen content. The most important effect is an increase in RBC velocity resulting from increased arteriolar pressure, which, alone, stimulates arterial vasomotion [15]. Increased flow velocity and enhanced vasomotion provide a better spatial and temporal distribution of RBCs within the capillary network. This will result in improved tissue oxygen extraction capabilities [16]. Lastly, a right shift of the oxygen dissociation curve related to a rise in the RBC 2–3 diphosphoglycerate level may reduce the affinity of hemoglobin for oxygen and therefore improve oxygen availability. This mechanism, however, takes some time to occur and has been demonstrated only in chronic anemia [17].

Effects of anesthesia

Anesthesia can alter the physiologic adjustments to isovolemic hemodilution at different levels (Table 36.1). Most anesthetic agents depress the cardiovascular and the autonomic nervous system in a dose-dependent manner. Therefore, the most striking effect of anesthesia would be a decreased cardiac output response to isovolemic hemodilution. The effects of anesthesia on the cardiac output response were assessed in patients undergoing major abdominal surgery in whom moderate intentional hemodilution (target hemoglobin of 8.0 g/dL) was part of the blood conservation program [9]. In the awake patients, intentional hemodilution was associated with a significant increase in the cardiac index, which was related to an increase in both the heart rate and the stoke index. This increase in cardiac index compensated for the decrease in

Table 36.1 Effects of anesthesia on the physiologic response to hemodilution.

1. Effects on the cardiac output response
   a. Alteration in cardiac loading conditions
   b. Negative inotropic effect
   c. Depressed autonomic nervous system activity
2. Effects on the O_2 extraction response
   a. Vasodilation
   b. Depressed sympathetic nervous system activity
3. Effects on gas exchange
   a. Decreased functional residual capacity
4. Effects on tissue oxygen demand
   a. Relief of pain, stress, anxiety
   b. Decreased muscular activity
   c. Decreased myocardial O_2 demand (negative chronotropic and inotropic effect)

hemoglobin concentration, so that oxygen delivery remained unaltered. However oxygen consumption increased, resulting in an increase in the oxygen extraction ratio. In the anesthetized patients, intentional hemodilution resulted in a significantly smaller increase in cardiac index, which was solely related to a raise in the stroke index. Therefore, oxygen delivery decreased, but oxygen consumption remained unchanged as the oxygen extraction ratio increased. The increase in oxygen consumption observed in awake patients has been attributed at least in part to an increased in myocardial oxygen demand associated with the increased heart rate. Similar observations have been reported in awake volunteers undergoing severe isovolemic hemodilution [18]. In the Ickx et al. study [9], when the awake patients were anesthetized, all the measured parameters returned to values similar to those obtained in patients undergoing hemodilution while anesthetized. Therefore, performing hemodilution before or after induction of anesthesia did not result in a significant different physiologic response at the time of surgery.

Limits of hemodilution

As described above, maintenance of tissue oxygenation during ANH results from an increase in cardiac output and oxygen extraction. Several experimental and clinical studies have demonstrated the involvement of both mechanisms even in the early stage of ANH [19]. The relative contribution of these mechanisms will depend on the ability of the organism to recruit them [20]. They allow the maintenance of tissue oxygen balance until the hemoglobin concentration falls to about 3 to 4 g/dL (hematocrit 10–12%). Below this "critical" value, oxygen delivery can no longer match tissue oxygen demand and cellular hypoxia will develop. Several experimental studies reported this "critical hemoglobin value [21–23]. Van Woerkens et al. [24] studied a Jehovah's Witness patient who died from extreme hemodilution, and they observed a critical hemoglobin concentration of 4 g/dL.

The efficacy of the mechanisms preserving tissue oxygen delivery when the oxygen carrying capacity of the blood is reduced depends primarily on the maintenance of an adequate circulating blood volume. Indeed, hypovolemia blunts the effects of decreased blood viscosity on venous return [25]. Although "normovolemic" conditions are difficult to define, replacement of the blood and fluid losses with at least a volume of substitute having the same expanding effect on the intravascular volume is required.

Tolerance to acute isovolemic hemodilution not only depends on the integrity of the compensatory mechanisms described above, but also on the level of tissue oxygen demand. For a given cardiac output and oxygen extraction response, any increase in tissue oxygen demand will require a higher hemoglobin concentration.

ANH and the cardiac patient

Maintenance of myocardial oxygen delivery during ANH depends essentially on the increase in the coronary blood flow as oxygen extraction is already nearly maximal at the level of the heart under resting conditions [13]. This is achieved by a reduction in coronary vascular resistance related to the decreased blood viscosity but also to specific coronary vasodilation. Heart rate and possibly myocardial contractility have been shown to increase during hemodilution [26, 27], which results in an augmentation of myocardial oxygen demand. When hematocrit is reduced to about 10%, myocardial oxygen consumption more than double, as it has been demonstrated in dogs [28]. In these conditions, coronary vasodilation is nearly maximal. Below such a hematocrit, coronary blood flow can no longer match the increased myocardial oxygen demand and ischemia develops, ultimately resulting in cardiac failure.

As myocardial O_2 supply essentially depends on an increased coronary blood flow, during ANH, the coronary reserve, i.e., the ratio between maximal and resting coronary blood flow is significantly reduced in these conditions [29]. This indicates the vulnerability of the heart during ANH, especially if higher work demands on the myocardium should coexist. Among healthy conscious subjects undergoing acute isovolemic reduction of hemoglobin to 5 g/dL, Leung et al. [30] observed that those who developed reversible ST-segment depression on the Holter ECG monitoring were also those who exhibited the higher maximal heart rate. This higher heart rate may have contributed to the development of an imbalance between myocardial supply and demand, resulting in ECG evidence of myocardial ischemia. In patients with coronary artery disease (CAD), coronary blood flow is limited by the atherosclerotic lesions. Experimental data in animals with extrinsically applied coronary stenosis have demonstrated a complete exhaustion of the coronary reserve. In these animals, cardiac failure developed at a significantly higher hematocrit than in controls [31]. The lowest tolerable hemoglobin concentration in CAD patients remains unknown and probably depends on several factors, including the severity of the disease [32]. Observational studies have shown an association between anemia, defined as a hematocrit <30%, and increased mortality in patients with cardiovascular disease [33, 34]. In these circumstances, however, there are no definitive data showing that blood transfusion either mitigates myocardial ischemia or improves survival [35–37]. There is increasing evidence that tolerance of CAD patients to isovolemic anemia closely depends on the level of myocardial oxygen demand. In anesthetized patients scheduled for CABG surgery, several studies demonstrated that moderate ANH (target hematocrit value 27–33%) is well tolerated [38–40], and might even have some cardioprotective effects when associated with a reduction of the myocardial metabolic demand [41].

However, any increase in myocardial oxygen demand in these conditions could be associated with the development of myocardial ischemia and cardiac dysfunction. Tonkovic et al. [42] assessed before surgery the hemodynamic response to moderate dose of dobutamine in hemodiluted CAD patients scheduled for off-pump surgery. Patients were hemodiluted to a target hemoglobin concentration of either 9.5–10.5/dL (moderate ANH) or 7.5–8.5 g/dL (severe ANH). Dobutamine infusion at a rate of 5 μg/kg/minute was associated with a significant increase in cardiac index in patients undergoing moderate ANH, but not in patients undergoing severe ANH. The dobutamine infusion was associated with an increase in heart rate and blood pressure in both groups, but resulted in the more severe hemodiluted patients in the development of myocardial oxygen supply–demand imbalance as evidenced by a decrease in stroke volume index and left ventricular stroke work index [43]. Recent clinical data confirm that tolerance of CAD patients to moderate anemia is closely related to the level of heart rate [44]. The anesthetic technique also may play a role. The early postoperative period is certainly critical in hemodiluted CAD patients, because they have to face with an increased tissue metabolic demand.

ANH and hemostasis

Hemodilution could affect hemostasis in different ways. First, it will dilute not only plasmatic factors, but also cellular coagulation factors, like platelets and of course RBCs. RBCs have been shown to interfere with hemostasis through a mechanical effect (they push away the platelets to the periphery of the vessels) but also through biological effects related to the release of intracellular adenosine diphosphate and to the generation of thrombin [45]. The clinical consequences (i.e., importance of perioperative bleeding) of these interactions between RBCs and hemostasis remain to be determined. Singbartl et al. suggested that, during advanced hemodilution, the decrease in coagulation factors and platelets may be more limiting than low hemoglobin values [46].

Hemodilution could also affect hemostasis through the direct effects of plasma substitution fluids on the platelets and the coagulation mechanisms [47]. These effects are more marked with dextrans than with gelatins and albumin. For hydroxyethyl starches, these effects appear closely related to the intrinsic properties of the different solutions, such as a high in vitro molecular weight and a high degree of hydroxyethyl substitution [48].

Despite the evidence that ANH may directly interfere with normal hemostasis, there is no evidence from the literature that ANH is associated with increased perioperative bleeding. In a first meta-analysis evaluating the efficacy of ANH in reducing perioperative allogeneic blood transfusion,

Bryson et al. [49] reported that ANH had a small and insignificant effect on the volume of blood lost in the intra- and postoperative period. In a second meta-analysis, Segal et al. [50] reported that the volume of intraoperative blood loss was similar in the ANH and the usual care groups, but total (intra- and postoperative) blood loss was significantly less in the ANH groups. The authors also noted that ANH was more effective in reducing perioperative blood loss in orthopedic and cardiac surgery than in other surgical specialties [50].

Practical aspects

Intentional hemodilution can be performed just before or shortly after the induction of anesthesia. Performing hemodilution after induction of anesthesia has gained wider acceptance, because it is more comfortable for the patient without increasing the period of anesthesia before the onset of surgery [3].

Calculating blood volume collection

Different formulas and nomograms have been developed to determine the volume of blood that should be withdrawn to reach the target hematocrit or hemoglobin concentration [51, 52]. The simplified formula proposed by Gross et al. [52] is one of the most often used (Table 36.2). Whatever the formula used isovolemia as a starting point is essential to adequate calculation for the allowable collected blood volume. Clinical experience indicates that it is not easy to achieve precisely the desired target hematocrit or hemoglobin level, by blinded adherence to the hemodilution nomogram. It has been therefore recommended to measure onsite hematocrit or hemoglobin concentration intermittently by means of a portable measuring system [53]. More recently, Meier et al. [54] have proposed a new mathematical model that seems to predict more accurately the exchangeable blood volume. This algorithm, which can be easily obtained from the authors, might therefore enhance patient safety.

Table 36.2 Technique of intentional hemodilution.

$$\text{ABV} = \text{EBV} \times \frac{\text{H0} - \text{HT}}{(\text{H0} + \text{HT})/2}$$

ABV: autologous blood to be collected
EBV: estimated blood volume
H0: initial hematocrit or hemoglobin concentration
HT: target hematorit or hemoglobin concentration
Substitution fluids:
- Crystalloids: ratio 3:1
- Colloids: ratio 1:1 (except gelatins: 1.5:1)

Blood is withdrawn from a venous or an arterial line, collected in labeled citrate phosphate dextrose (CPD) bags (450 mL/bag) stored at room temperature for up to 6 hours

Technique

Depending on the patient characteristics, up to 2–2.5 L of blood are withdrawn from a venous or an arterial line in standard collection bags containing anticoagulant, usually citrate–phosphate–dextrose (CPD). In cardiac surgery the technique has to be adapted taking into account the underlying cardiac disease that reduces the tolerance of the patient to severe hemodilution and the importance of the priming volume used in the cardiopulmonary bypass (CPB) [55, 56]. The bags containing the autologous blood are numbered sequentially, labeled and stored at room temperature in the operating theatre to preserve platelet function. Aseptic technique is of utmost importance during the procedure. The blood bags usually contain anticoagulant for 450–500 mL of blood. From time to time, collected units should be gently agitated to ensure adequate mixing. In case significantly less blood is collected into the bags, hemostasis of the patient may be altered during transfusion due to the high concentration of the anticoagulant in the stored unit [3]. On the other hand, collecting more than 450–500 mL per bag could result in massive blood clotting in the bag due to insufficient anticoagulant. Colloids and/or crystalloids can be used to maintain normovolemia, the volume to be administered depending on the physiochemical characteristics of the substitute that is used (Table 36.2). Normothermia must be maintained throughout the surgical procedure (with the possible exception of the CPB time in cardiac surgery), as it is crucial to insure adequate hemostasis.

Autologous blood will be transfused once the transfusion trigger (hematocrit or hemoglobin concentration) has been reached. Depending on the patient characteristics, the clinical situation and the ongoing blood loss and/or the likelihood of achieving surgical hemostasis, this trigger may vary somewhat between 20 and 30% hematocrit or 7 and 10 g/dL hemoglobin. Transfusion of the autologous blood will be performed in the inverse order of collection, the first unit collected, which is the richest in RBCs, platelets and coagulation factors, being transfused preferably at the end of the procedure, or when surgical bleeding has been controlled. For cardiac surgery patients, blood collected just before going on bypass contains heparin and will be ideally transfused during protamine administration. For safety reasons (i.e., bacterial contamination) any autologous blood unit kept at room temperature must be transfused within 6 hours from harvesting [4].

Monitoring

During intentional hemodilution, physiologic compensatory mechanisms play an essential role in maintaining tissue oxygenation [5]. Adequate monitoring of cardiorespiratory parameters is therefore of major importance in patients undergoing hemodilution [3, 57]. The extent of this monitoring will vary, depending on the patient's clinical status (preexisting disease, preoperative treatment, etc.), the type and the duration of the surgical procedure, and the degree of hemodilution (Table 36.3).

Table 36.3 Hemodynamic monitoring in the perioperative period.

1. Hemodilution to a hematocrit of 25%
   a. Continuous monitoring
      i. ECG monitor (lead II and V5)
      ii. Online ST-segment analysis
      iii. Invasive arterial pressure
      iv. Pulse oximetry
      v. Urine output
   b. Intermittent monitoring
      i. Central venous pressure
      ii. Arterial blood gas analysis
      iii. Hemoglobin or hematocrit measurements
2. Hemodilution to a hematocrit of 20%
   a. Additional monitoring
      i. Central venous blood gas analysis
      ii. Arterial lactate
   b. Facultative
      i. Non invasive cardiac output measurements
      ii. Pulmonary artery catheter
      iii. Continuous cardiac output measurement (pulmonary or arterial catheter)
      iv. Continuous mixed venous O_2 saturation (SvO_2) measurement
      v. Transesophageal echocardiography

Adapted from Kreimeier and Messmer [3] and Trouwborst et al. [57].

Efficacy

Theoretical aspects

The basic concept behind ANH is that patients undergoing such procedure will lose less erythrocytes per milliliter of lost blood during surgery and after transfusion of the collected autologous blood in the immediate postoperative period [3]. Consequently, ANH is most efficacious when a high blood volume can be collected before a surgical procedure associated significant blood loss [4]. Several authors have developed equations to calculate the efficacy of ANH as a function of surgical blood loss, initial hematocrit, target post-ANH hematocrit, and hematocrit used as the transfusion trigger [58–60]. Presuming a "usual" surgical patient without preoperative anemia, and a transfusion decision based exclusively on a trigger hemoglobin concentration of 6–7 g/dL, Weiskopf [61] calculated a minimal fractional blood loss of 50% to enable any saving of allogeneic RBCs with ANH. Expressed as a fraction of the patient's blood volume, 55–77% of total blood volume must be lost during surgery in order to achieve savings of about 180 mL of RBCs, which represents one standard blood unit. In this mathematical model, however, fractional blood loss is overestimated because blood loss subsumes both the volume of blood removed during ANH and the volume of blood lost during the surgical procedure. The calculation of fractional blood loss should

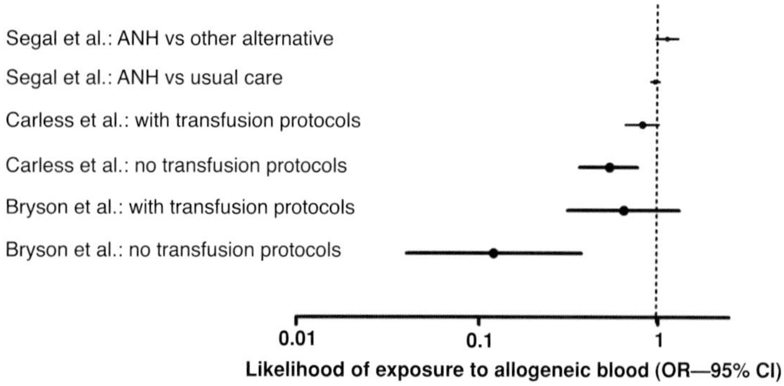

Figure 36.1 Difference in exposure to allogeneic blood reported in the three meta-analyses. For the Bryson et al. [49] and the Carless et al. [62] analyses, data are presented according to the presence or not of a protocol to guide allogeneic blood transfusion. For the report by Segal et al. [50], comparisons between ANH vs usual care and ANH vs another blood conservation method are presented. Data are presented as odd ratio (OR) with 95% confidence intervals (solid lines).

be exclusively based on intraoperative blood loss. In this case, the "effective" fractional blood loss will be found at about 25% [4]. The usefulness of the different published models in clinical practice is also limited by the fact that some of them do not take into account postoperative blood loss and/or the use of a higher hemoglobin concentration as postoperative transfusion trigger. Moreover, some authors assume that once the transfusion trigger has been reached, available autologous blood will be transfused continuously, on a milliliter-for-milliliter basis, which does not correct for the effective RBC mass substituted.

Results from the literature

Efficacy of ANH as a blood conservation technique remains controversial. Three meta-analyses have systematically reviewed the literature to determine whether ANH was effective in reducing the likelihood of patient's exposure to allogeneic blood in the perioperative period [49, 50, 62]. Most of the studies reviewed were performed in the setting of cardiac or orthopedic surgery. Efficacy of ANH was found to be relatively modest in terms of likelihood of exposure to allogeneic blood and units transfused. It closely depends on the use or not of protocols to guide transfusion practice (Figures 36.1 and 36.2). However, the authors of these three meta-analyses emphasized the fact that proper evaluation of the published results was hampered by the relative poor quality of the studies and the marked heterogeneity observed between trials, partly explained by study factors (patient populations, target hematocrit values, transfusion triggers, ANH technique, etc.). There was no obvious increase in adverse events with ANH, but the incidence of complications was poorly reported.

As reported in the different published mathematical models [58–61], the efficacy of ANH depends on the amount of blood collected, the hematocrit (or hemoglobin concentration) used as the transfusion trigger, and the volume of surgical blood loss. Two prospective randomized studies confirmed these observations. They have evaluated the efficacy of ANH in patients undergoing major hepatic resection [63, 64]. Most enrolled patients were ASA I or II. Mean or median volume of blood collected was about 2000 mL in both studies. The transfusion threshold was clearly defined in both studies, a hematocrit of 20% in the first one [63], and a hemoglobin of 7 g/dL during the procedure and 8 g/dL thereafter in the second one [64]. In the Matot et al. study [63], median estimated intraoperative blood loss was 800 mL (100–7500), and ANH reduced significantly the likelihood of exposure to allogeneic RBCs units. The authors observed that ANH was especially efficacious in patients having lost 71–90% of their calculated blood volume. In the study by Jarnagin et al. [64], median estimated blood loss was also 800 mL (100–4000), and ANH reduced the likelihood of exposure to allogeneic RBCs units only in patients with intraoperative blood loss equal or superior to 800 mL. Further confirmation of the different factors that influence the efficacy of ANH was brought by Spahn et al. study [65], in which a perfluorocarbon-based O_2 carrier was used to enhance ANH in patients undergoing major abdominal surgery. All these

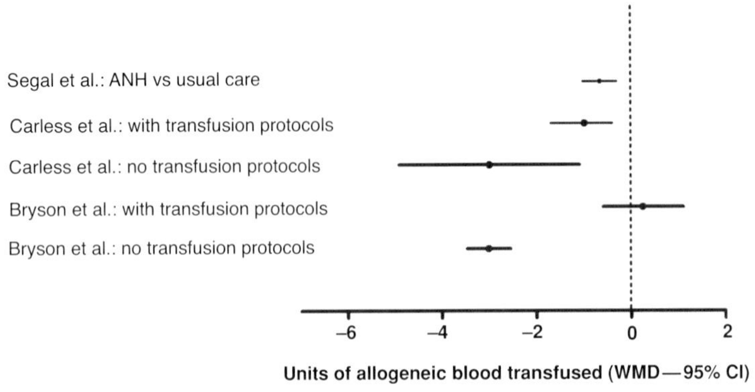

Figure 36.2 Difference in allogeneic blood units transfused. For the Bryson et al. [49] and the Carless et al. [62] analyses, data are presented according to the presence or absence of a protocol guiding blood transfusion. For the report by Segal et al. [50], comparison between ANH vs usual care is presented. There was insufficient data to compare ANH to another blood conservation method. Data are presented as weight mean differences (WMD) with 95% confidence intervals (solid lines).

observations, however, indicate that efficient ANH requires quite significant expertise in the field from the care given team.

Developing a blood conservation strategy

Acute normovolemic hemodilution should be considered as one of the components of an overall strategy aiming at reducing patient's exposure to allogeneic blood products, the so-called "blood conservation" approach. This approach implies that the developed strategy should focus on the individual patient, as opposed to a strategy linked to a surgical or a medical procedure [66]. As a rule, combining techniques decreases allogeneic blood exposure. However, the effects of merging different methods are not as predictable as it may seem at first glance. The efficacy of combining different techniques should also take into account the relative costs of these alternatives [67]. Last but not least, to be really effective, a blood conservation approach also requires the adoption of a standardized multidisciplinary blood transfusion policy [68]. Any clinician who decides to transfuse a patient at a higher transfusion trigger than the others will ruin the efforts of the whole team.

Developing a blood conservation strategy starts with the establishment of a reliable system of data collection, both at the surgical team and the hospital levels. The choice of the techniques being applied will primarily depend on the type of clinical situation one faces. Identifying patients' risks for transfusion should alter patient management perioperatively to decrease their transfusion rate and make more efficient use of blood resources [69]. Any addition to a set of existing blood conservation methods needs careful assessment to avoid useless or even counter-productive efforts. As a good example, Casati et al. [70] evaluated the effects of moderate ANH added to a comprehensive blood-sparing protocol in patients undergoing off-pump coronary surgery. They reported a significant reduction in the likelihood of allogeneic blood exposure and a decrease in the total number of RBCs units transfused in the group of patients undergoing ANH.

Because the interests of patients and clinicians may change over time, the developed blood conservation strategy must be continuously monitored and adapted to the need of specific surgical populations [66].

Conclusions

Acute normovolemic hemodilution entails the removal of blood from a patient shortly after the beginning of the surgical procedure, and its replacement with crystalloids or colloids to maintain the circulating blood volume. It is a relatively simple, cheap, and effective tool to avoid or reduce allogeneic blood transfusion. Factors that influence the efficacy of the technique have been clearly identified. This reduces the field of application of ANH to patients undergoing high bleeding risk surgery in whom a great volume of blood can be collected. Knowledge of the physiologic compensatory mechanisms that occur during normovolemic hemodilution and their limits are essential for the safe use of the technique. In addition, the anesthesiologist must be familiar with its practical aspects. Although ANH has a place in different types of surgery, it must be regarded as an integral part of a blood conservation strategy tailored to the individual patient's needs and adapted to specific surgical procedures.

References

1. Klövekorn WP, Laks H, Pilon RN, Anderson WP, Mac Callum JR, Moore FD. Effects of acute hemodilution in man. Eur Surg Res 1973;5:27–8.
2. Bauer H, Pichlmaier H, Ott E, Klövekorn WP, Sunder-Plasmann L, Messmer K. Autotransfusion durch akute, preoperative hemodilation. Eerste klinische Erfahrungen. Langenbecks Arch Chir 1974;185–9.
3. Kreimeier U, Messmer K. Perioperative hemodilution. Transfus Apher Sci 2002;27:59–72.
4. Jamnicki M, Kocian R, Van Der Linden P, Zaugg M, Spahn DR. Acute normovolemic hemodilution: physiology, limitations, and clinical use. J Cardiothorac Vasc Anesth 2003;17:747–54.
5. Van Der Linden P. The physiology of acute isovolaemic anaemia. Acta Anaesthesiol Belg 2002;53: 97–103.
6. Hébert PC, Van Der Linden P, Biro GP, Qun Hu L. Physiologic aspects of anemia. Crit Care Clin 2004;20: 187–212.
7. Doss DN, Estafanous FG, Ferrario CM, Brum JM, Murray PA. Mechanism of systemic vasodilation during normovolemic hemodilution. Anesth Analg 1995;81:30–34.
8. Chapler CK, Cain CM. The physiologic reserve in oxygen carrying capacity: studies in experimental hemodilution. Can J Physiol Pharmacol 1986;64: 7–12.
9. Ickx B, Rigolet M, Van Der Linden P. Cardiovascular and metabolic response to acute normovolemic anemia: effects of anesthesia. Anesthesiology 2000;93: 1011–16.
10. Glick G, Plauth WH, Braunwald EB. Role of the autonomic nervous system in the circulatory response to acutely induced anemia in unanesthetized dogs. J Clin Invest 1964;43:2112–24.
11. Chapler CK, Cain SM. Effects of alpha-adrenergic blockade during acute anemia. J Appl Physiol 1982;52:16–20.
12. Szlyk PC, King CE, Jennings B, Cain SM, Chapler CK. The role of the aortic chemoreceptors during acute anemia. Can J Physiol Pharmacol 1984;62:519–23.
13. Fan FC, Chen RYZ, Schuessler GB, Chien S. Effects of hematocrit variations on regional hemodynamics and oxygen transport in the dog. Am J Physiol 1980;238: H545–52.
14. Crystal GJ, Ruiz JR, Rooney MW, Salem MR. Regional hemodynamics and oxygen supply during isovolemic hemodilution in the absence and the presence of high-grade beta-adrenergic blockade. J Cardiothorac Vasc Anesth 1988;2:772–80.
15. Messmer K, Gutierrez G, Vincent JL. *Blood Rheology Factors and Capillary Blood Flow, Tissue Oxygen Utilization*. Springer-Verlag, Berlin, Heidelberg, New-York, 1991, pp. 103–13.
16. Van Der Linden P, Gilbart E, Paques P, Simon C, Vincent JL. Influence of hematocrit on tissue O_2 extraction capabilities during acute hemorrhage. Am J Physiol 1993;264:H1942–7.
17. Rodman T, Close HP, Purcell MK. The oxyhemoglobin dissociation curve in anemia. Ann Intern Med 1960;52:295–301.
18. Weiskopf RB, Viele MK, Feiner J, et al. Human cardiovascular and metabolic response to acute, severe isovolemic anemia. JAMA 1998;279:217–21.
19. Spahn DR, Leone BJ, Reves JG, Pasch T. Cardiovascular and coronary physiology of acute isovolemic hemodilution: a review of nonoxygen-carrying and oxygen-carrying solutions. Anesth Analg 1994;78: 1000–1021.
20. Lieberman JA, Weiskopf RB, Kelley SD, et al. Critical oxygen delivery in conscious humans is less than 7.3 ml O_2. kg^{-1}. min^{-1}. Aneshesiology 2000;92:407–13.
21. Wilkerson DK, Rosen AL, Sehgal LR, Gould SA, Sehgal HL, Moss GS. Limits of cardiac output compensation in anemic baboon. Surgery 1988;103:665–70.
22. Räsänen J. Supply-dependent oxygen consumption and mixed venous oxyhemoglobin saturation during isovolemic hemodilution in pigs. Chest 1992;101:1121–4.
23. Van Der Linden P, De Groote F, Mathieu N, et al. Critical haemoglobin concentration in anaesthetized dogs: comparison of two plasma substitutes. Br J Anaesth 1998;81:556–62.
24. van Woerkens ECSM, Trouwborst A, van Lanschot JJB. Profound hemodilution: what is the critical level of hemodilution at which oxygen delivery-dependent

oxygen consumption starts in an anesthetized human? Anesth Analg 1992;75:818–21.
25. Richardson TQ, Guyton AC. Effects of polycythemia and anemia on cardiac output and other circulatory factors. Am J Physiol 1959;197:1167–70.
26. Weiskopf RB, Feiner J, Hopf H, et al. Heart rate increases linearly in response to acute isovolemic anemia. Transfusion 2003;43:235–40.
27. Habler OP, Kleen MS, Podtschaske AH, et al. The effect of acute normovolemic hemodilution (ANH) on myocardial contractility in anesthetized dogs. Anesth Analg 1996;83:451–8.
28. Von Restorff W, Hfling B, Holtz J, Bassenge E. Effect of increased blood fluidity through hemodilution on general circulation at rest and during exercise in dogs. Pflugers Arch 1975;357:25–34.
29. Geha AS. Coronary and cardiovascular dynamics and oxygen availability during acute normovolemic anemia. Surgery 1976;80:47–53.
30. Leung JM, Weiskopf RB, Feiner J, et al. Electrographic ST-segment changes during acute, severe isovolemic hemodilution in humans. Anesthesiology 2000;93:1004–10.
31. Levy PS, Kim SJ, Eckel PK, et al. Limit to cardiac compensation during acute isovolemic hemodilution: influence of coronary stenosis. Am J Physiol 1993;265:H340–49.
32. Tircoveanu R, Van Der Linden P. Hemodilution and anemia in patients with cardiac disease: what is the safe limit? Curr Opin Anaesthesiol 2008;21:66–70.
33. Nelson AH, Fleisher LA, Rosenbaum SH. Relationship between postoperative anemia and cardiac morbidity in high-risk vascular patients in the intensive care unit. Crit Care Med 1993;21:860–66.
34. Hogue CW, Goodnough LT, Monk T. Perioperative myocardial ischemic episodes are related to hematocrit level in patients undergoing radical prostatectomy. Transfusion 1998;38:1070–77.
35. Wu WC, Rathore SS, Wang Y, Radford MJ, Krumholz HM. Blood transfusion in elderly patients with acute myocardial infarction. N Engl J Med 2001;345:1230–36.
36. Rao SV, Jollis JG, Harrington RA, et al. Relationship of blood transfusion and clinical outcomes in patients with acute coronary syndromes. JAMA 2004;292:1555–62.
37. Hébert PC, Yetisir E, Martin C, et al. Is a low transfusion threshold safe in critically ill patients with cardiovascular diseases? Crit Care Med 2001;29:227–34.
38. Spahn DR, Schmid ER, Seifert B, Pasch T. Hemodilution tolerance in patients with coronary disease who are receiving chronic B-adrenergic blocker therapy. Anesth Analg 1996;82:687–94.
39. Herregods L, Moerman A, Foubert L, et al. Limited intentional normovolemic hemodilution: ST-segment changes and use of homologous blood products in patients with left main coronary artery stenosis. J Cardiothorac Anesth 1997;11:18–23.
40. Licker M, Sierra J, Tassaux D, Diaper J. Continuous haemodynamic monitoring using transoesophageal Doppler during acute normovolaemic hemodilution in patients with coronary artery disease. Anaesthesia 2004;59:108–15.
41. Licker M, Ellenberger C, Sierra J, et al. Cardioprotective effects of acute normovolemic hemodilution in patients undergoing coronary artery bypass surgery. Chest 2005;128:838–47.
42. Tonkovic D, Husedzinovic I, Barisin S, et al. Hemodynamic response to moderate dobutamine dose in OPCAB surgery during acute normovolemic hemodilution. Can J Anaesth 2005;52:214–215.
43. Van Der Linden P, De Hert S. Normovolemic hemodilution and the heart. Can J Anaesth 2005;52:130–32.
44. Cromheecke S, Lorsomradee S, Van Der Linden PJ, De Hert SG. Moderate acute isovolemic hemodilution alters myocardial function in patients with coronary artery disease. Anesth Analg 2008;107:1145–52.
45. Ouakine-Orlando B, Samama CM, Samama CM, et al. *Hématocrite et hémostase, Hémorragies et thromboses périopratoires: approche pratique*. Masson, Paris, 2000, pp. 113–19.
46. Singbartl K, Innerhofer P, Radvan J, et al. Hemostasis and hemodilution: a quantitative mathematical guide for clinical practice. Anesth Analg 2003;96:929–35.
47. Van Der Linden P, Ickx BE. The effects of colloid solutions on hemostasis. Can J Anaesth 2006;53:S30–39.
48. Kozek-Langenecker SA. Effects of hydroxyethyl starch solutions on hemostasis. Anesthesiology 2005;103:654–60.
49. Bryson GL, Laupacis A, Wells GA. Does acute normovolemic hemodilution reduce perioperative allogeneic transfusion ? A meta-analysis. Anesth Analg 1998;86:9–15.
50. Segal JB, Blasco-Colmenares E, Norris EJ, Guallar E. Preoperative acute normovolemic hemodilution: a meta-analysis. Transfusion 2004;44:632–44.
51. Bourke DL, Smith TC. Estimating allowable hemodilution. Anesthesiology 1974;41:609–12.
52. Gross JB. Estimating allowable blood loss: corrected for dilution. Anesthesiology 1983;58:277–80.
53. Polasek J, Taeger K. Zur Anwendbarkeit eines transportablen Hämoglobinmeβsystems in operativen und

intensivmedizinischen Routinebetrieb. Anasth Intensivmed 1990;31:268–70.
54. Meier J, Kleen MS, Habler OP, Messmer K. New mathematical model for the correct prediction of the exchangeable blood volume during acute normovolemic hemodilution. Acta Anaesthesiol Scand 2003;47:37–45.
55. Van Der Linden P, Sakr P. Acute normovolemic hemodilution in cardiac surgery. Transfus Altern Transfus Med 2005;7:11–19.
56. Van Der Linden P, Dierick A. Blood conservation strategies in cardiac surgery. Vox Sang 2007;92: 103–12.
57. Trouwborst A, van Bommel J, Ince C, Henny P. Monitoring normovolaemic haemodilution. Br J Anaesth 1998;81:73–8.
58. Feldman JM, Roth JV, Bjoraker DG. Maximum blood savings by acute normovolemic hemodilution. Anesth Analg 1995;80:108–13.
59. Kick O, Daniel E. Mathematical considerations in the practice of acute normovolemic hemodilution. Transfusion 1997;37:141–3.
60. Weiskopf RB. Mathematical analysis of isovolemic hemodilution indicates that it can decrease the need for allogeneic blood transfusion. Transfusion 1995;35:37–41.
61. Weiskopf RB. Efficacy of acute normovolemic hemodilution assessed as a function of fraction of blood volume lost. Anesthesiology 2001;94: 439–46.
62. Carless P, Moxey A, O'Connell D, Henry D. Autologous transfusion techniques: a systematic review of their efficacy. Transfus Med 2004;14:123–44.
63. Matot I, Scheinin O, Jurim O, Eid A. Effectiveness of acute normovolemic hemodilution to minimize allogeneic blood transfusion in major liver resections. Anesthesiology 2002;97:794–800.
64. Jarnagin WR, Gonen M, Maithel SK, et al. A prospective randomized trial of acute normovolemic hemodilution compared to standard intraoperative management in patients undergoing major hepatic resection. Ann Surg 2008;248:360–69.
65. Spahn DR, Waschke KF, Standl T, et al. Use of perflubron emulsion to decrease allogeneic blood transfusion in high-blood-loss non-cardiac surgery: results of a European phase 3 study. Anesthesiology 2002;97:1338–49.
66. Baele P, Van Der Linden P. Developing a blood conservation strategy in the surgical setting. Acta Anaesthesiol Belg 2002;53:129–36.
67. Nuttall GA, Oliver WC, Jr, Ereth MH, et al. Comparison of blood conservation strategies in cardiac surgery patients at high risk for bleeding. Anesthesiology 2000;92:674–82.
68. Van Der Linden P, De Hert S, Daper A, et al. A standardized multidisciplinary approach reduces the use of allogeneic blood products in patients undergoing cardiac surgery. Can J Anaesth 2001;48:894–901.
69. Moskowitz DM, Klein JJ, Shander A, et al. Predictors of transfusion requirements for cardiac surgical procedures at a blood conservation center. Ann Thorac Surg 2004;77:626–34.
70. Casati V, Benussi S, Sandrelli L. Intraoperative moderate acute normovolemic hemodilution associated with a comprehensive blood-sparing protocol in off-pump surgery. Anesth Analg 2004;98:1217–23.

CHAPTER 37
Hyperoxic Hemodilution

Jens Meier[1], *Konrad Messmer*[2] *& Oliver Habler*[3]
[1]Department of Anesthesiology, Intensive Care Medicine and Pain Control, Johann Wolfgang Goethe-University, Frankfurt, Germany
[2]Institute for Surgical Research, Ludwig-Maximilians-University, Munich, Germany
[3]Clinic of Anesthesiology, Intensive Care Medicine, and Pain Control, Nord-West Hospital, Frankfurt, Germany

Introduction

Intraoperative surgical blood loss is initially replaced by infusion of red cell-free crystalloidal or colloidal solutions. Although the resulting hemodilution reduces the red cell mass and the hemoglobin (Hb) concentration [1], it is known for long that adequate tissue oxygenation does not depend on "normal" Hb concentrations [2–4]. As long as normovolemia is maintained tissue oxygenation is preserved by an increase of cardiac output (CO) and arterial oxygen extraction (O_2-ER) during acute dilutional anemia until a so-called "critical" hemoglobin concentration (Hb_{crit}) is reached [1].

In this situation, beside red blood cell transfusion, arterial oxygen content can be rapidly increased by ventilating the patient with pure oxygen (hyperoxic ventilation or HV), thus enhancing the amount of physically dissolved oxygen in plasma (hyperoxia). As a consequence the immediate transfusion of red blood cells can be avoided in this situation, and the resulting gain in time may at least enable the surgeon to achieve definite control of bleeding or to complete the surgical intervention before red blood cell transfusion becomes necessary. In the best case HV can delay or even avoid the transfusion of allogeneic blood this way. It can be assumed that this approach might reduce the overall amount of blood transfused. The technique of bridging acute blood losses by a combination of HV and acellular volume substitution is called "hyperoxic hemodilution," and has been introduced to the literature in 1998 (Figure 37.1) [5].

In experimental and clinical studies, HV has emerged as a simple, safe, and effective intervention to enlarge the margin of safety for hemodynamic compensation and tissue oxygenation in hemodiluted subjects experiencing major blood loss allowing the avoidance of immediate blood transfusion at a preset transfusion trigger. The hyperoxia-associated microcirculatory dysregulation and impaired tissue oxygenation that are known to take place in the presence of a physiologic Hb concentration are not encountered in hemodiluted subjects. "Hyperoxic hemodilution" may therefore be considered a cost-effective, safe, and efficient supplement to reduce allogeneic transfusion during surgical interventions associated with high blood losses.

Fluid replacement of surgical blood loss

The transfusion of allogeneic blood is expensive and—although safer than ever before—is still associated with potential complications (acute transfusion reaction due to "clerical error," transfusion related bacterial and viral infection, immunosuppression, transfusion associated lung injury or TRALI). To reduce both costs and immanent risks, allogeneic transfusion should be either completely avoided or at least minimized during surgical procedures. This can be achieved by (1) intraoperative transfusion of autologous blood

Alternatives to Blood Transfusion in Transfusion Medicine, 2nd edition. Edited by A. Maniatis, P. Van der Linden, J.-F. Hardy.

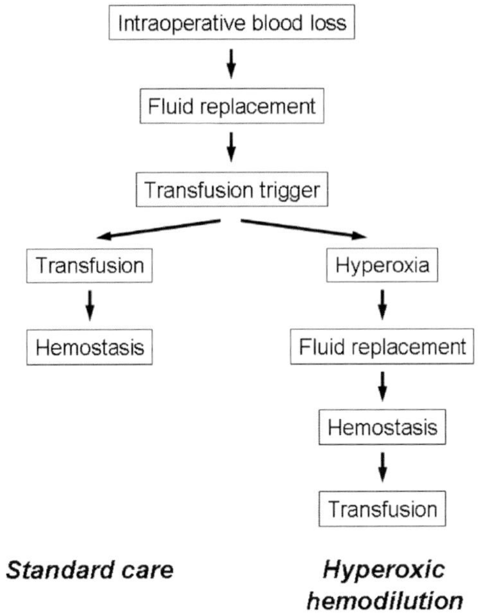

Figure 37.1 Flow chart of the blood sparing technique "hyperoxic hemodilution." Usually intraoperative blood losses are substituted with acellular solutions until a preset transfusion trigger is met. In this case arterial oxygen content can be increased either by the transfusion of blood (left side, "standard care"), or by the ventilation with pure oxygen (right side, "hyperoxic hemodilution"). This approach allows to delay blood transfusion until surgical hemostasis can be achieved.

collected preoperatively (autologous blood donation, acute normovolemic hemodilution) or intraoperatively (blood salvage); (2) reduction of the amount of blood loss (skillful surgical technique, deliberate hypotension, administration of antifibrinolytic drugs); and (3) acceptance of low intraoperative Hb concentrations.

Since it is known for a long time that survival does not depend on a "normal" Hb concentration [6] an intraoperative blood loss is initially replaced by erythrocyte-free crystalloidal or colloidal solutions (e.g., Ringer's lactate, dextran, hydroxyethyl starch, gelatine). As long as normovolemia is maintained the resulting dilutional anemia is compensated for without risk of tissue hypoxia by an increase of CO (through an increase of ventricular stroke volume) and enhanced O_2-ER [1, 2]. In the ideal case, a surgical blood loss can be "bridged" without allogeneic blood transfusion by intraoperative normovolemic hemodilution. However, once the Hb concentration has dropped to values recommended as the lower intraoperative limit (Hb 6 g/dL in healthy subjects or Hb 8–10 g/dL in patients with preexisting cardiovascular disease [7,8]) or so-called "transfusion-trigger" parameters (e.g., oxygen consumption, mixed-venous oxygen partial pressure, ST-segment-depression in ECG) indicate the exhaustion of the compensatory mechanisms for dilutional anemia usually transfusion of red blood cells is initiated to increase arterial oxygen content and to preserve a margin of safety for tissue oxygenation and organ function. When transfusion has to be started before definite surgical control of bleeding, the overall need for transfusion increases due to the partial loss of the red blood cells transfused.

As an alternative to the immediate transfusion of red blood cells, ventilation with pure oxygen (HV) can be performed to rapidly raise arterial oxygen content by increasing the amount of physically dissolved oxygen in plasma [5].

Effects of HV on arterial oxygen content and oxygen delivery

The quantity of oxygen (mLO_2) transported to all organs, the so-called oxygen delivery DO_2 can be calculated as:

$$DO_2 = CO \times CaO_2$$

where CO is the cardiac output in mL/min and CaO_2 is the arterial oxygen content.

The artertial oxygen content CaO_2 is defined as the sum of Hb bound oxygen and physically dissolved oxygen:

$$CaO_2 = \frac{SaO_2}{100} \times Hb \times 1.34 + 0.0031 \times paO_2$$

where SaO_2 is the arterial saturation of oxygen, Hb is the hemoglobin concentration in g/dL, and paO_2 is the arterial oxygen partial pressure. Since SaO_2 is a function of paO_2 the amount of oxygen transported to organs solely depends on three variables: CO, Hb, and paO_2.

As stated above, as an alternative to the immediate transfusion of red blood cells ventilation with pure oxygen (HV) can be employed to rapidly raise CaO_2 by increasing paO_2 and SaO_2. However, since during normoxic ventilation (FiO_2 0.21) nearly all erythrocytes are saturated with oxygen (i.e., $SaO_2 > 98\%$), increasing FiO_2 to 100% will usually mainly result in an increase of physically dissolved oxygen. As a consequence the total amount of oxygen additionally transported in this situation (ΔCaO_2) only slightly increases as compared to normoxic ventilation [5]. Furthermore, it has been demonstrated by a number of investigators for many different situations that HV fails to increase DO_2 despite a small but significant increase of CaO_2 [5, 9–11], a phenomenon clearly challenging the efficacy of HV to improve oxygen transport and, thereby, tissue oxygenation. The underlying mechanism seems to be a significant reduction of CO during HV, independent of the amount of oxygen transported to the organs [12]. This decline of CO induced by general vasoconstriction ("*hyperoxic vasoconstriction*") is believed not to be a compensatory mechanism owing to an increase of arterial oxygen content, but to be a typical, undesirable side effect of HV jeopardizing nutritive organ blood flow [12, 13].

Hyperoxic vasoconstriction

Molecular oxygen causes vasoconstriction. This effect of hyperoxia on large vessels as well as on microvessels (arterioles, venules) has been extensively demonstrated in vitro (isolated vessel segments [14]) and in vivo (intravital microscopy [15], laser doppler flowmetry [16], etc.). It seems to be locally mediated [17] by products of the arachidonic acid metabolic pathway (e.g., 20-hydroxyeicosa-tetraenoic acid, briefly 20-HETE [18]) and can be completely blocked by indomethacin [19] and cytochrome P-450 inhibitors [18]. It has been demonstrated by Lindbom and Arfors that this hyperoxic vasoconstriction reduces the density of perfused capillaries in proportion to the increase of the ambient pO_2 or partial pressure of oxygen [20]. As a consequence hyperoxia has been shown to increase systemic vascular resistance and to decrease CO and oxygen consumption in dogs with normal Hb concentration [21]. The simultaneously observed deterioration of tissue oxygenation has been interpreted as to reflect impaired local oxygen delivery due to hyperoxic vasoconstriction and abnormal spatial and temporal distribution of microvascular blood flow [20, 22, 23]. As a consequence hyperoxia at normal Hb concentrations is considered harmful concerning tissue integrity and function.

In experiments carried out in hemodiluted dogs (Hb 7 g/dL) hyperoxia completely reversed the hemodilution-induced increase of cardiac index (CI) and partially reversed the decrease of systemic vascular resistance (Figure 37.2) [24]. Nevertheless, the normal Gaussian distribution of single tissue pO_2 values measured by means of an oxygen sensitive multiwire surface electrode was preserved during hyperoxia (Figure 37.3). A higher number of hypoxic tissue pO_2 values (0–15 mmHg) was not detected and the shifting of the histograms to the right (increase of tpO_2 median) may even indicate improved tissue oxygenation. Moreover nonlinear analysis of blood flow distribution did not reveal any increase in heterogeneity of microcirculatory blood flow during hyperoxia in hemodiluted animals [25, 26]. Furthermore, in a more recent study, Cabrales et al. demonstrated that ventilation with pure oxygen at very low Hb levels (Hb 3.5 g/dL) did not result in a significant reduction of arteriolar diameter, arteriolar red blood cell velocity, or functional capillary density [27], changes of microvascular perfusion that have previously been observed by Tsai et al. during HV at normal Hb concentrations [22]. These findings demonstrate the pivotal role of the actual Hb concentration on the microcirculatory effects of hyperoxia. The increase of organ blood flow induced by hemodilution (i.e., normovolemic anemia) increases shear stress at the vessel wall which in turn induces the release of endothelium derived relaxing factor (i.e., nitric oxide or NO) and hence vasodilation [28, 29]. It can therefore be speculated that in dilutional anemia the microcirculatory dysregulation due to hyperoxia is counteracted by NO-release and might therefore play a minor role during HV.

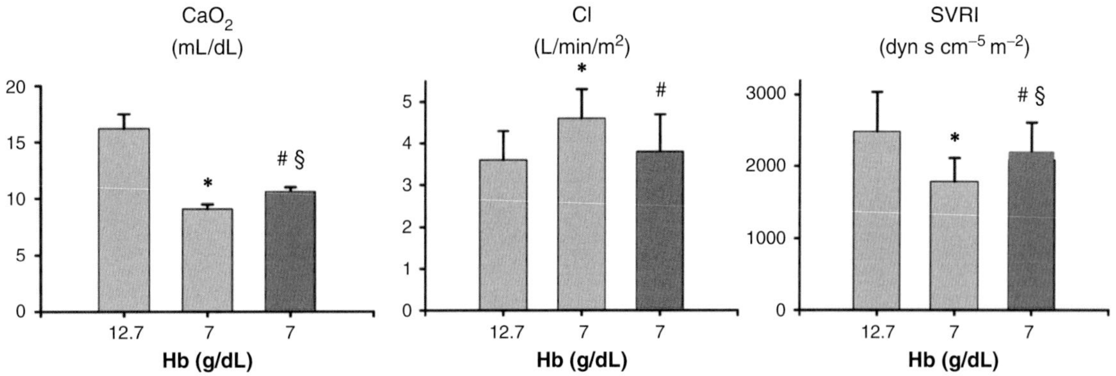

Figure 37.2 Changes in arterial oxygen content (CaO_2), cardiac index (CI), and systemic vascular resistance index (SVRI) upon normovolemic hemodilution on room-air ventilation (21% oxygen) to a Hb concentration of 7 g/dL and after subsequent onset of hyperoxic ventilation or HV (100% oxygen). Adapted from Habler et al. [24]. $^{*}p < 0.05$; "Hb 12.7 g/dL, room air" vs "Hb 7 g/dL, room air"; $^{\#}p < 0.05$; "Hb 7 g/dL, room air" vs "Hb 7 g/dL, HV"; $^{\S}p < 0.05$; "Hb 12.7 g/dL, room air" vs "Hb 7 g/dL, HV."

Oxygen toxicity

It has been known for long that ventilation with pure oxygen for hours or days results in deleterious effects on lung function in humans and, ultimately, in death from hyperoxic lung injury in laboratory animals [30,31]. The changes of pulmonary morphology during HV are very similar to changes induced by other kinds of acute lung injury (initial exudative phase defined by inflammation, atelectasis, and edema formation, which is followed by a fibroproliferative phase with irreversible loss of respiratory function) [32]. However, these effects are only important for prolonged phases of HV. It has been demonstrated by Davis et al. that HV for nearly 17 hours indeed lowers the structural or

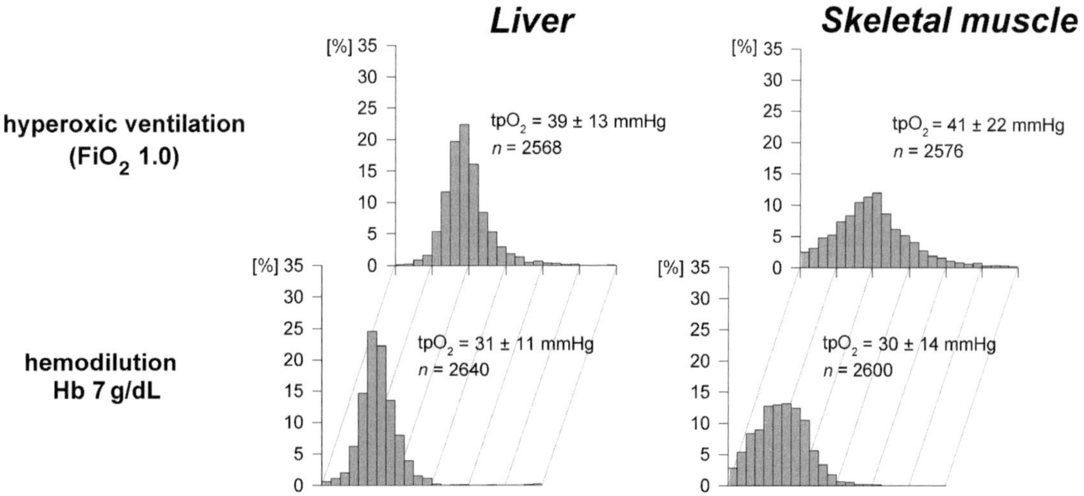

Figure 37.3 Frequency distribution of tissue pO_2 values measured on the surface of the liver and a skeletal muscle by use of an oxygen sensitive surface electrode (MDO electrode) in anesthetized dogs hemodiluted to Hb 7 g/dL under room-air ventilation (21% oxygen) and after onset of HV (100% oxygen). Adapted from Habler et al. [24]. $p < 0.05$; "Hb 7 g/dL, FiO_2 0.21" vs "Hb 7 g/dL, FiO_2 1.0."

functional barriers that normally prevent alveolar-capillary "leak" and induces processes that can culminate in fibrosis of the alveolar wall, but eventually does not result in a change of the total number or type of lung inflammatory and immune effector cells recovered by lavage [33]. Therefore, HV might be considered a safe short-term measure, but it has been demonstrated recently that HV induces significant endothelial activation by ROS signaling with subsequent expression of adhesion molecules [34] within 90 minutes. However, these early endothelial effects themselves do not constitute an injury because endothelial responses were fully reversible after 90 minutes of hyperoxia [34].

Hyperoxia as an alternative to red blood cell transfusion in surgical blood loss

Despite the relatively small effects of HV on arterial oxygen content and the absence of its effects on oxygen delivery, HV has proven an effective and simple measure to stabilize tissue oxygenation during moderate and extreme anemia. Furthermore, there is a noteworthy multitude of experimental and some clinical data supporting the hypothesis that HV might be an effective and safe method to bridge periods of acute anemia in order to delay blood transfusion despite its prima facie minor effect on oxygen transport.

Experimental data

Under the "protection" of hyperoxia, intraoperative hemodilution may be extended to Hb concentrations lower than those usually accepted as trigger for red blood cell transfusion as demonstrated in experimental and clinical studies [35, 36]. In dogs initially hemodiluted on room-air ventilation to Hb 7 g/dL, subsequent HV allowed for further hemodilution to the extreme value of Hb 3 g/dL without encountering significant changes in tissue oxygenation [24] and cardiac performance [37]. Moreover, in pigs ventilated with room air and diluted until the occurrence of manifest tissue hypoxia (Hb 2.6 g/dL), subsequent ventilation with pure oxygen was not only able to effectively reverse tissue hypoxia [11], but allowed to extend the dilution to Hb 1.2 g/dL, i.e., almost complete blood exchange before the signs of tissue hypoxia reoccurred [10]. Beyond that it has been demonstrated that HV lowers the individual Hb_{crit} as compared to normoxic ventilation (FiO_2 0.21: Hb_{crit} = 2.4 g/dL vs FiO_2 0.6: Hb_{crit} = 1.5 g/dL, $p < 0.05$) [38]. Furthermore, in the presence of hemodilution-induced tissue hypoxia, effective tissue utilization of physically dissolved plasma-oxygen has been demonstrated by a significantly higher survival rate of pigs ventilated with pure oxygen as compared to pigs remaining under room-air ventilation [39]. Therefore, it can be speculated that HV ensures tissue oxygenation during extreme anemia despite its negative effects at the microcirculatory level at physiological Hb concentrations. However, some organs benefit more than others from HV during moderate and extreme anemia. Especially intestinal, hepatic, and renal blood flow are less suspicious for a distinct decrease of nutritive organ blood flow during ventilation with pure oxygen [40].

Recently it has been demonstrated that HV also ensures survival during hypovolemic anemia, and as a consequence it can be stated that HV also might be an effective therapeutic option during shock [9]. However, once more it has to be pointed out, that these positive effects are drastically diminished if HV is initiated and maintained at normal Hb levels. This has been demonstrated in a model of severe methemoglobinemia, where HV during normocytemic tissue hypoxia (i.e., reduction of oxygen transporting red cell mass without changing rheological properties of blood) failed to improve oxygen transport and tissue oxygenation noticeably, and as a consequence, resulted only in a negligible increase of survival time [41].

At normal Hb concentrations hyperoxic vasoconstriction might not only endanger tissue oxygenation at the microcirculatory level, but might have the ability to improve macrohemodynamics, since extreme anemia not only threatens myocardial oxygen supply by a decline of arterial oxygen content, but also by a decline of mean aortic pressure and thus coronary perfusion pressure. It can therefore be speculated that the stabilization of MAP and CPP by HV-induced vasoconstriction may increase tolerance to extreme anemia and thus improve outcome. This view is substantiated by a recent study, where it has been demonstrated that application of norepinephrine during extreme anemia improves oxygen transport, tissue oxygenation, and survival via stabilization of MAP and CPP [42,43]. Summing up, it appears that HV might be advantageous during moderate and extreme anemia at the macrocirculatory level, whereas its potentially negative effects on the microcirculation are negligible at low Hb levels.

Clinical data

So far only a few studies exist investigating the effects of HV on oxygen transport, tissue oxygenation, and transfusion needs in the perioperative period; however, there are some clinical investigations describing advantageous effects accompanying perioperative hyperoxia like the reduction of postoperative nausea and vomiting [44] as well as a reduced incidence of perioperative wound infections [45,46].

Weiskopf et al. investigated the effects of HV on cognitive function and memory during profound anemia (Hb 5.7 $\pm$ 0.3 g/dL) in awake, healthy volunteers [47]. The findings of the authors support the hypothesis that increasing paO_2 to 350 mmHg or greater by breathing oxygen reverses all of the negative effects of acute anemia. This can be confirmed as significant improvement of cerebral tissue oxygenation by HV during profound anemia.

In a recent clinical study, Suttner et al. demonstrated that HV is similar to the transfusion of allogeneic blood in improving several parameters of oxygen transport but is clearly superior in improving tissue oxygenation in volume-resuscitated patients with a Hb concentration in the range from 7.5 g/dL to 8.5 g/dL [48]. It can therefore be stated that HV is an effective method to ameliorate tissue oxygenation in the perioperative period in anemic patients; however, the influence of HV on transfusion needs was not analyzed in this study. The same authors investigated the effects of HV on skeletal muscle tissue oxygenation during sodium nitroprusside-induced hypotension [49]. The observed improvement of local tissue oxygenation in this study seems to be most likely due to an increase in convective oxygen transport and the attenuation of hyperoxemia-induced arteriolar vasoconstriction by sodium nitroprusside. This finding supports the hypothesis that HV is void of negative effects on the microcirculation, if hyperoxic vasoconstriction is diminished by peripheral vasodilation.

The only clinical study investigating the effects of HV on the possibility to delay blood transfusions at a preset transfusion trigger was performed by Spahn et al. in patients experiencing major intraoperative bleeding during orthopedic surgery. In the patients the indication for red cell transfusion (based on the appearance of physiologic trigger parameters) could be reversed in two-thirds of the patients by the simple switch from ventilation with 40% oxygen to ventilation with pure oxygen [36]. This maneuver enabled continuation of acellular volume substitution and thereby intraoperative hemodilution, and as a consequence the definite need for red blood cell transfusion could be postponed for 27–60 minutes (median 30 minutes) [36]. This gain in time at least enables the surgeon to achieve definite control of bleeding or to complete the surgical intervention before red blood cell transfusion becomes necessary. The augmentation of blood oxygen transport capacity to reduce inspiratory oxygen fraction to values allowing extubation of the patient may then be achieved by exclusive transfusion of autologous red blood cells collected in the perioperative period.

However, up to now no controlled clinical trial exists that clearly demonstrates a reduction of transfusion needs by a blood sparing protocol based on HV. Admittedly it has to be pointed out that there is good evidence that the onset of HV ensures sufficient oxygen transport and tissue oxygenation during extreme anemia and many other pathological conditions, and as a consequence should always be considered as a first line measure whenever a transfusion trigger is reached and blood is not available immediately.

Conclusion

Achievement of the goal to reduce the overall amount of blood transfused during the perioperative period requires a multimodal approach. One cornerstone of this concept is to delay the transfusion of allogeneic blood as long as possible in order to avoid unnecessary premature blood transfusion. However, this requires acceptance of rather low Hb levels. It has been demonstrated that in this situation ventilation with pure oxygen ensures tissue oxygenation and survival, and can therefore be used to bridge intraoperative periods of acute, significant anemia without the transfusion of red blood cells. The deliberate acceptance of distinct intraoperative anemia in combination with hyperoxia with the aim to avoid unnecessary premature blood transfusion has been introduced to the literature as "hyperoxic hemodilution," a procedure where a preset transfusion trigger can be undercut, and impending tissue hypoxia can be avoided by the ventilation with pure oxygen. Further studies are required to demonstrate the efficacy of this method to reduce the perioperative transfusion needs.

References

1. Habler OP, Messmer KF. The physiology of oxygen transport. Transfus Sci 1997;18:425–35.
2. Messmer K, Sunder-Plassmann L, Klövekorn W, Hopler K. Circulatory significance of hemodilution: rheological changes and limitations. Adv Microcirc 1972;4: 1–77.
3. Spahn DR, Leone BJ, Reves JG, Pasch T. Cardiovascular and coronary physiology of acute isovolemic hemodilution: a review of nonoxygen-carrying and oxygen-carrying solutions. Anesth Analg 1994;78: 1000–1021.
4. Zollinger A, Hager P, Singer T, Friedl HP, Pasch T, Spahn DR. Extreme hemodilution due to massive blood loss in tumor surgery. Anesthesiology 1997;87:985–7.
5. Habler O, Messmer K. Hyperoxaemia in extreme haemodilution. Br J Anaesth 1998;81 Suppl. 1: 79–82.
6. Kronecker H. Kritisches und Experimentelles über lebensrettende Infusionen von Kochsalzlösungen bei Hunden. Correspondenzblatt für schweizer Ärzte 1886;16:447–55.
7. College of American Pathologists. Practice parameter for the use of red blood cell transfusions. Arch Pathol Lab Med 1998;122:130–38.
8. American Society of Anesthesiologists. Practice guidelines for blood component therapy. Anesthesiology 1996;84:732–47.
9. Meier J, Kemming GI, Kisch-Wedel H, Blum J, Pape A, Habler OP. Hyperoxic ventilation reduces six-hour mortality after partial fluid resuscitation from hemorrhagic shock. Shock 2004;22:240–47.
10. Meier J, Kemming G, Meisner F, Pape A, Habler O. Hyperoxic ventilation enables hemodilution beyond the critical myocardial hemoglobin concentration. Eur J Med Res 2005;10:462–8.
11. Kemming GI, Meisner FG, Kleen M, et al. Hyperoxic ventilation at the critical haematocrit. Resuscitation 2003;56:289–97.
12. Baron JF, Vicaut E, Hou X, Duvelleroy M. Independent role of arterial O_2 tension in local control of coronary blood flow. Am J Physiol 1990;258: H1388–94.
13. Habler O, Kleen M, Kemming G, Zwissler B. Hyperoxia in extreme hemodilution. Eur Surg Res 2002;34:181–7.
14. Carrier OJ, Walker JR, Guyton AC. Role of oxygen in autoregulation of blood flow in isolated vessels. Am J Physiol 1964;206:951–4.
15. Duling BR. Oxygen sensitivity of vascular smooth muscle. II. In vivo studies. Am J Physiol 1974;227: 42–9.
16. Pakola SJ, Grunwald JE. Effects of oxygen and carbon dioxide on human retinal circulation. Invest Ophthalmol Vis Sci 1993;34:2866–70.
17. Bachofen M, Gage A, Bachofen H. Vascular response to changes in blood oxygen tension under various blood flow rates. Am J Physiol 1971;220:1786–92.
18. Harder DR, Narayanan J, Birks EK, et al. Identification of a putative microvascular oxygen sensor. Circ Res 1996;79:54–61.
19. Messina EJ, Sun D, Koller A, Wolin MS, Kaley G. Increases in oxygen tension evoke arteriolar constriction by inhibiting endothelial prostaglandin synthesis. Microvasc Res 1994;48:151–60.
20. Lindbom L, Arfors KE. Mechanisms and site of control for variation in the number of perfused capillaries in skeletal muscle. Int J Microcirc Clin Exp 1985;4: 19–30.
21. Lodato RF. Decreased O_2 consumption and cardiac output during normobaric hyperoxia in conscious dogs. J Appl Physiol 1989;67:1551–9.
22. Tsai AG, Cabrales P, Winslow RM, Intaglietta M. Microvascular oxygen distribution in awake hamster window chamber model during hyperoxia. Am J Physiol Heart Circ Physiol 2003;285:H1537–45.
23. Thorborg P, Malmqvist LA, Lund N. Surface oxygen pressure distributions in rabbit skeletal muscle: dependence on arterial pO_2. Microcirc Endothelium Lymphatics 1988;4:169–92.

24. Habler OP, Kleen MS, Hutter JW, et al. Effects of hyperoxic ventilation on hemodilution-induced changes in anesthetized dogs. Transfusion 1998;38:135–44.
25. Kleen M, Habler O, Hutter J, et al. Normovolaemic haemodilution and hyperoxia have no effect on fractal dimension of regional myocardial perfusion in dogs. Acta Physiol Scand 1998;162:439–46.
26. Kleen M, Habler O, Hutter J, et al. Hemodilution and hyperoxia locally change distribution of regional pulmonary perfusion in dogs. Am J Physiol 1998;274:H520–28.
27. Cabrales P, Tsai AG, Frangos JA, Briceño JC, Intaglietta M. Oxygen delivery and consumption in the microcirculation after extreme hemodilution with perfluorocarbons. Am J Physiol Heart Circ Physiol 2004;287:H320–30.
28. Doss DN, Estafanous FG, Ferrario CM, Brum JM, Murray PA. Mechanism of systemic vasodilation during normovolemic hemodilution. Anesth Analg 1995;81:30–34.
29. de Wit C, Schäfer C, von Bismarck P, Bolz SS, Pohl U. Elevation of plasma viscosity induces sustained no-mediated dilation in the hamster cremaster microcirculation in vivo. Pflugers Arch 1997;434:354–61.
30. Caldwell PR, Lee WLJ, Schildkraut HS, Archibald ER. Changes in lung volume, diffusing capacity, and blood gases in men breathing oxygen. J Appl Physiol 1966;21: 1477–83.
31. Crapo JD, Barry BE, Foscue HA, Shelburne J. Structural and biochemical changes in rat lungs occurring during exposures to lethal and adaptive doses of oxygen. Am Rev Respir Dis 1980;122:123–43.
32. Crapo JD. Morphologic changes in pulmonary oxygen toxicity. Annu Rev Physiol 1986;48:721–31.
33. Davis WB, Rennard SI, Bitterman PB, et al. Pulmonary oxygen toxicity. Early reversible changes in human alveolar structures induced by hyperoxia. N Engl J Med 1983;309:878–83.
34. Brueckl C, Kaestle S, Kerem A, et al. Hyperoxia-induced reactive oxygen species formation in pulmonary capillary endothelial cells in situ. Am J Respir Cell Mol Biol 2006;34:453–63.
35. Habler OP, Kleen MS, Hutter JW, et al. Hemodilution and intravenous perflubron emulsion as an alternative to blood transfusion: effects on tissue oxygenation during profound hemodilution in anesthetized dogs. Transfusion 1998;38:145–55.
36. Spahn DR, van Brempt R, Theilmeier G, et al. Perflubron emulsion delays blood transfusions in orthopedic surgery. European perflubron emulsion study group. Anesthesiology 1999;91:1195–208.
37. Habler O, Kleen M, Hutter J, et al. IV perflubron emulsion versus autologous transfusion in severe normovolemic anemia: effects on left ventricular perfusion and function. Res Exp Med 1998;197:301–18.
38. Pape A, Meier J, Kertscho H, et al. Hyperoxic ventilation increases the tolerance of acute normovolemic anemia in anesthetized pigs. Crit Care Med 2006;34: 1475–82.
39. Meier J, Kemming GI, Kisch-Wedel H, Wölkhammer S, Habler OP. Hyperoxic ventilation reduces 6-hour mortality at the critical hemoglobin concentration. Anesthesiology 2004;100: 70–76.
40. Meier J, Pape A, Kleen M, Hutter J, Kemming G, Habler O. Regional blood flow during hyperoxic haemodilution. Clin Physiol Funct Imaging 2005;25:158–65.
41. Meier J, Pape A, Lauscher P, Zwissler B, Habler O. Hyperoxia in lethal methemoglobinemia: effects on oxygen transport, tissue oxygenation, and survival in pigs. Crit Care Med 2005;33:1582–8.
42. Meier J, Pape A, Loniewska D, et al. Norepinephrine increases tolerance to acute anemia. Crit Care Med 2007;35:1484–92.
43. Walsh TS, Saleh E. Anemic heart: best kept under pressure? Crit Care Med 2007;35:1615–17.
44. Greif R, Laciny S, Rapf B, Hickle RS, Sessler DI. Supplemental oxygen reduces the incidence of postoperative nausea and vomiting. Anesthesiology 1999;91:1246–52.
45. Greif R, Akça O, Horn EP, Kurz A, Sessler DI. Supplemental perioperative oxygen to reduce the incidence of surgical-wound infection. Outcomes research group. N Engl J Med 2000;342:161–7.
46. Belda FJ, Aguilera L, García de la Asunción J, et al. Supplemental perioperative oxygen and the risk of surgical wound infection: a randomized controlled trial. JAMA 2005;294:2035–42.
47. Weiskopf RB, Feiner J, Hopf HW, et al. Oxygen reverses deficits of cognitive function and memory and increased heart rate induced by acute severe isovolemic anemia. Anesthesiology 2002;96:871–7.
48. Suttner S, Piper SN, Kumle B, et al. The influence of allogeneic red blood cell transfusion compared with 100% oxygen ventilation on systemic oxygen transport and skeletal muscle oxygen tension after cardiac surgery. Anesth Analg 2004;99:2–11.
49. Suttner SW, Lang K, Boldt J, Kumle B, Maleck WH, Piper SN. The influence of hyperoxic ventilation during sodium nitroprusside-induced hypotension on skeletal muscle tissue oxygen tension. Anesthesiology 2002;96:1103–8.

CHAPTER 38

Intraoperative and Postoperative Cell Salvage

Ernil Hansen[1] *& Hans Gombotz*[2]

[1]Department of Anesthesiology, Regensburg University Medical Center, Regensburg, Germany

[2]Department of Anesthesiology and Intensive Care, General Hospital Linz, Linz, Austria

Cell salvage is defined as the reinfusion of wound blood salvaged during or after surgery. As a method of autologous transfusion it plays an important role in the context of perioperative blood saving strategies, having assumed standard of care status for many surgical procedures [1–12]. While the use of normovolemic hemodilution and predonation of autologous blood has diminished in recent years, the impact of cell salvage is consolidated and even still increasing.

The principle of cell salvage is to continuously collect intra- or postoperatively shed blood from the surgical field into a dedicated reservoir. It is then processed by cell separation and washing with saline, and concentrated before retransfusion or reinfused unwashed after filtration. In contrast to both allogeneic or autologous banked blood, these fresh, unstored red blood cells (RBC) have full functional capacities like oxygen delivery to tissues and unchanged survival rate, indicating that cell salvage has no significant detrimental effects on erythrocytes [13]. In addition, as autologous, unstored cells they do neither cause allosensitization nor immunomodulation.

Blood salvage is probably the most effective part of a multimodal blood saving strategy including a restrictive transfusion trigger, predonation of autologous blood, intra- and postoperative cell salvage, and other adjuvant drug therapies. These blood conservation methods can be combined according to the surgical procedure, the patients' individual needs and the skills of the responsible physicians [4, 14].

Alternatives to Blood Transfusion in Transfusion Medicine, 2nd edition. Edited by A. Maniatis, P. Van der Linden, J.-F. Hardy.

Retransfusion of unwashed wound blood

Simple devices for the retransfusion of unwashed, filtered whole blood are on the market [15–18]. However, these devices have primarily been designed for the salvage of slowly oozing blood rather than rapid hemorrhage [18]. With the development of new generations of safe, fully automated, and easy-to-use cell separators, the importance of simple autotransfusion of unwashed blood has largely shifted from the intraoperative toward the postoperative phase [4, 19, 20]. Main fields of application are knee and hip replacement surgery [5, 7, 8, 11, 20, 21], and pericardial drainage following heart surgery [5, 7, 12, 22].

Using these devices shed blood is usually collected without adding an anticoagulant and filtered through a microaggregate filter to remove tissue debris and other unwanted materials. Collection time must be limited to 6 hours to prevent bacterial growth [23].

Arguments against retransfusion of unwashed wound blood

Retransfusion of whole wound blood was at the very beginning of transfusion medicine. Nowadays however, there are many concerns about the transfusion of unwashed blood [24]:

1 The risks of allogeneic transfusion that once stimulated all the transfusion alternatives have been decreased significantly. Large scientific and financial efforts have been made to cope with even small risks of allogeneic transfusion like prion transmission, but the same high standards need to be applied to autologous transfusion. From our growing knowledge about contamination in wound blood and its pathophysiological consequences, it is evident that autologous blood transfusion may not necessarily be superior when compared to allogeneic transfusions in all circumstances [25]. Wound blood contains products and mediators of humoral and cellular activation as well as cell lysis. The transfusion of such bioactive contaminants raises concern and does not meet the high standards of modern transfusion medicine, as, for instance, in some countries the allowed extend of hemolysis in blood products is regulated.

2 Quality management (QM) and quality assurance as recommended for intra- and postoperative autotransfusion [23, 26] cannot be applied to unwashed shed blood, as no valid parameters for quality control are available. In addition, the quality of this product can hardly be improved: Neither anticoagulation [27] nor the use of heparin-coated lines [28], nor the use of leukocyte depletion filters [29, 30], which may even aggravate cell activation and mediator release, shows any improvement. During bleeding and collection the blood contacts damaged tissue and artificial surfaces, while humoral and cellular blood components of coagulation, inflammation, and immune response are activated or damaged (Table 38.1). After retransfusion these cells and mediators express their normal local pathophysiological function systemically. Most of these mediators act in cascade systems, so once generated they tend to induce and amplify further reactions resulting in even more activation products [31]. These bioactive substances are elevated 10- to 10,000-fold in the shed blood [32], and after retransfusion levels, exceed the concentrations induced by surgery [24, 31]. Some have been identified as the main mediators of coagulopathy, disseminated intravascular coagulation (DIC), adult respiratory distress syndrome, systemic inflammatory response, and multiorgan failure. The individual load of a specific wound blood with multiple bioactive contaminants is unknown. In addition, the capacity of an individual patient to cope with that burden is not predictable. The usual recommendation to limit the amount of wound blood to be retransfused to small volumes, namely < 500 mL or 1000 mL for risk reduction has no sound evidence base. [5, 11, 33–36]. No dose-relationship to severity and rate of side effects has been observed. In addition, with increasing age and morbidity patients will show limitations in their compensatory capabilities more frequently.

3 Severe complications have been reported after retransfusion of unwashed shed blood. A number of case reports demonstrate organ dysfunction or even organ failure. The clinical side effects can aggravate coagulation [37], airway [38], and pulmonary, renal, cardiac, circulatory, and central nervous functions [39–41]. Also lethal complications have been documented [17, 42–44]. The observation of increased interferon and natural killer cell precursors in patients after retransfusion of unwashed wound blood [45] has been taken as evidence for general immunostimulation. But this rather reflects the experimental finding that after addition of a mixture of all kinds of potent mediators all kind of effects are to be expected including immunostimulatory effects, depending on the test system used to look at immune functions. A clinical study in more than 4000 orthopedic patients at least showed the highest overall wound infection rate after postoperative retransfusion of unwashed blood in comparison to cell salvage and predonation of autologous blood [8]. Also, in cardiac patients postoperative retransfusion of unwashed shed blood was associated with increased sternal or systemic infections [46, 47].

4 Due to the low hematocrit in wound blood, the blood saving effect can be considered small or even absent. Little blood saving has been demonstrated in a recent meta-analysis for the retransfusion of mediastinal drainage blood in cardiac surgery [5], and in several studies on postoperative autotransfusion in orthopedic surgery [48, 49], respectively. The causes found were the low hematocrit of the

Table 38.1 Bioactive contaminants demonstrated in unwashed wound blood.

Coagulation activation	
Thrombin generation:	TATIII↑, F_1/F_2SP↑, ATIII↓
Fibrin generation:	FG↓, FGDP↑, FM↑
Activation/loss of factors:	FXIIa↑, FXIIIa↑, PTT↓, FVc↓, FXIII↓
Platelet activation/degradation	
Serotonin↑, histamine↑, PAI-1↑, PDEGF↑, βTG↑, TxA_2↑, TxB_2↑↑, PF4↑	
Fibrinolysis activation	
FDP↑, AP↓, PAP↑, PG↓, D-dimers↑, tPA↑	
Leucocyte activation/degradation	
IL1↑, IL4↑, IL6↑↑, IL8↑, IL10↑, TNF, sTNFR↑, IL-1Ra↑, leukotrienes↑, elastase↑, EPX↑, MPX↑, PGE_2, ECP↑, PGI_2↑	
Complement activation	
C′I↓, C′3↓, C′5↓, C′3a↑, C′5a↑, terminal C′-complex (sC′5a-9)↑	
Hemolysis/cytolysis	
fHb↑, LDH↑, CK↑, CK-MB↑, K^+↑, lipids, microaggregates	
Inflammation activation	
free radicals, endothlins, NO, phospholipaseA_2, kallikrein	

Levels 10- to 100-fold decreased or increased.

AP, antiplasmin; βTG, β-thromoglobulin; C′3a, activated complement factor 3; CK, creatinine kinase; ECP, eosinophilic cationic protein; EXP, eosinophilic protein X; FDP, fibrin degradation products; FG, fibrinogen; FGDP, fibrinogen degradation products; fHb, free plasma hemoglobin; FM, fibrin monomers; FSP, fibrin split products; FXIII, coagulation factor XIII; FXIIa, activated coagulation factor XII; IL, interleukin; MPX, myeloperoxidase; PAI, plasminogen activator inhibitor; PAP, plasmin–antiplasmin complex; PF4, platelet factor 4; PG, plasminogen; PGE_2, prostaglandin E_2; PTT, prothrombin time; sC′5a-9, terminal complement complex; sTNFR, soluble receptor for tumor necrosis factor; TAT, thrombin–antithrombin.

drained blood, the small or restricted volumes collected (representing only a small proportion of the total blood loss), and an increase in blood loss [32, 38, 50, 51]. Therefore this method cannot be assumed cost-effective, especially as these systems create the same costs also in cases without retransfusion [52].

Although several clinical studies demonstrate equivalent safety and efficacy for systems without cell washing [11, 15–17, 21, 22], caution is warranted because

- Patient numbers are generally too small for risk evaluation especially when compared to other transfusion risks
- Side effects are not consequently reported (for example the common observation of fever or infection signs was not attributed to the retransfusion of drained blood)
- Also inconsistencies, like the report of saving 2 units of blood after retransfusion of 300 mL of shed blood of low hematocrit [5].

Nevertheless, there may still be an indication for these simple devices in developing countries. However, it has to be taken into consideration, that retransfusion of unwashed wound blood, of this mixture of cellular debris, enzymes, and potent cytokines released by cell activation or lysis, and humoral factors like fibrin split products, D-dimers, activated complement [19, 19, 33, 34, 38, 41], and of many more (see Table 38.1), may trigger severe hemostatic disturbances like DIC [41, 44] or systemic inflammatory reactions [30, 53]. Retransfusion of this "activated cytolytic soup" is not an appropriate part of modern transfusion medicine [24, 54].

Cell separation and washing

All the detrimental side effects can be avoided by using cell separation and washing. This procedure does not only highly improve the quality of the blood to be retransfused but also enables the implementation of QM and assurance [19, 21, 34, 41, 55–57]. Under standard conditions almost all of these mediators are removed by the cell salvage procedure. As only RBCs are saved and retransfused, simultaneous volume and plasma replacement has to be provided, especially after processing large quantities of shed blood [3].

Methods

Several devices are available for processing wound blood by cell separation and cell washing. They all are based on the principle of centrifugation, where RBCs are separated from plasma and other fluids, including the wash solution, continuously or intermittently [58–61].

Elimination of soluble contaminants

The elimination of the soluble contaminants is achieved in two steps:

1 With the increasing sediment of RBCs filling the centrifuge bowl most of the hemolytic plasma is discarded

2 The remaining supernatant is diluted by the wash solution rinsing the RBCs.

Therefore, the elimination of contaminants is insufficiently reflected by the decreased concentrations of the substances (not changing during cell separation), but is better defined as the reduction of their total amounts [elimination rate = (volume of product supernatant × concentration of marker, e.g., protein, in product supernatant)/(volume of shed blood supernatant × concentration of marker in shed blood supernatant) × 100%]. Usually an elimination of 95–99% is achieved, equivalent to a reduction of all soluble contaminants to 1/20–1/100. Thereby heparin, procoagulants, cytokines, enzymes, and other potentially harmful substances are removed together with the plasma [49, 59, 60]. In the case of heparin this relates to less than 5 IU retransfused with every unit of processed autologous blood. However, it is important to know that washout is never complete, but sufficient to avoid any clinical side effects [62]. In addition, the volume load for the patient is reduced by concentrating the RBCs through the elimination of wound secretions, irrigation fluids, and anticoagulant solution.

Elimination of larger particles

Larger particles and cell aggregates are removed by the microaggregate filter in the collection reservoir. Separation of the remaining particles is dependent on their density and size, according to the sedimentation equation. Leukocytes are removed with the buffy coat to varying degrees [60]. Despite their activation in the wound, at the artificial surfaces and at the filter of the reservoir, their retransfusion is obviously without any clinical consequences [63, 64]. Thus, additional leukodepletion is unnecessary and might even stimulate cytokine release from the activated white blood cells [65]. Only under experimental conditions with artificially low bowl filling and excessive wash volumes, can significant leukocyte and platelet activation be observed in the centrifugation bowl. This can lead to the so-called "cell salvage syndrome" [66, 67]. The elimination of platelets together with the plasma and the buffy coat is variable und usually misinterpreted by standard measurements in cell counters due to size shift and membrane vesicles generated from lysed cells [68]. In addition, most of them are dysfunctional and do not cause any clinical side effects.

Practical recommendations

For the initial collection of wound blood only a sterile reservoir, a double-lumen suction catheter, and a solution for anticoagulation are necessary. The washing device may be set up once sufficient wound blood has accumulated. Using this "standby-collection" procedure time and expenses can be saved. Only for expected massive bleeding, e.g., in vascular surgery or polytrauma patients the complete cell salvage system should be ready from the beginning of surgery. Anticoagulation of the shed blood is usually achieved with heparin (30,000 IU in 1000 mL saline). Citrate (0.24%) or acid citrate dextrose might be used as well, especially in patients with HIT II [23]. After "priming" the collection system with 100–200 mL of anticoagulant solution [8], the flow is adjusted to an anticoagulant/blood ratio of 1:5–1:7. Shed blood is aspirated from the surgical field, anticoagulated at the suction tip, and stored in a plastic (cardiotomy) reservoir equipped with a microaggregate filter (40–150 μm). A limitation of suction to −150 or −200 mmHg (= −0.3 mbar) is recommended [23] to prevent hemolysis. Actually, these recommendations are based on older studies using outdated banked blood [69]. However, studies using freshly donated or fresh wound blood showed only a minimal hemolysis rate (< 0.4%) without limitation of negative suction pressure (−0.6 mbar) [70]. Thus faster control of the bleeding can be obtained.

After setup of the washing disposal, the anticoagulated and filtered wound blood is pumped into a rotating separation chamber in the centrifuge. Then the RBC sediment to the wall of the centrifuge bowl, while the hemolytic plasma is discarded to the waste bag. The RBC sediment is rinsed with wash solution (saline), and then the washed, packed RBCs are suspended in saline (Hct 50–70%) and pumped into a transfusion bag [71].

Using a Latham bowl (e.g., Cell Saver, Electa) the washing procedure is a *discontinuous* process consisting of a filling, washing, and emptying phase (Figure 38.1). Centrifugation bowls of different sizes are available (125–225 mL for adults and 55–70 mL for children). Whenever the amount or type of surgical debris requires more extensive washing, processing cycles can be repeated manually. On the contrary, washing can be skipped in emergency cases. After completion of each cycle, the bowl can be refilled as many times as required [4, 58–61]. Modern sensor technology monitoring input and output blood Hct as well as washout (Electa) allows quality control and optimization of programs according to different requirements.

The OrthoPAT system, a small autotransfusion device designed for automatic postoperative processing of drainage blood, has a centrifugation chamber which is a flexible disk (Figure 38.2). The blood and wash solution is moved by extension and contraction of a silicone membrane instead of a roller pump [72]. The discontinuous process uses wash volumes limited by the maximal chamber volume of 100 mL and results in a product with a hematocrit of 70%. Although this system is specially constructed for postoperative autotransfusion in orthopedics and heart surgery (cardioPAT), all available cell salvage machines can also be used for this purpose after connection of the drains to the reservoir used during surgery.

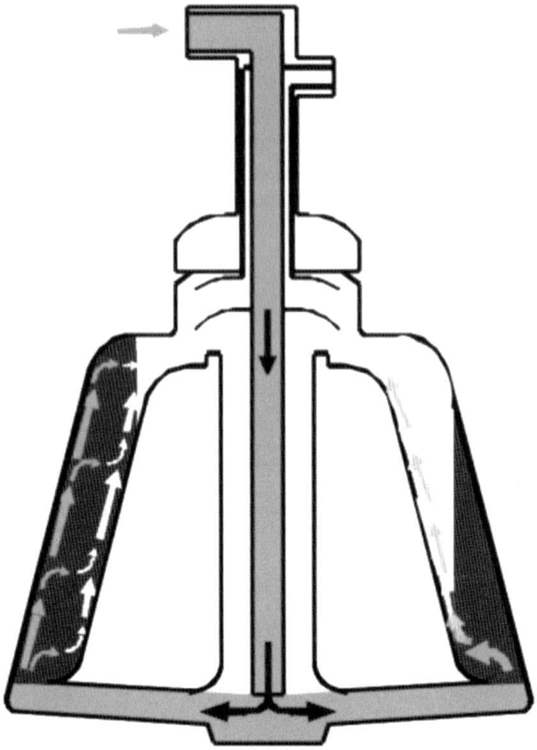

Figure 38.1 Principle of the Latham bowl (Cell Saver, Electa). Left side showing wash solution flowing through the RBC sediment, right side showing wash solution bypassing the RBC sediment in a partially filled bowl.

In contrast to these discontinuous systems operating in batches or units the CATS (Continuous AutoTransfusion System) allows *continuous* blood processing [71–74]. The separation chamber represents a blood channel in the shape of a double spiral, where separation and washing steps are performed simultaneously (Figure 38.3). Once the system is filled (approx. 30 mL RBC), all additional blood pumped into the loop leads to an overflow of washed RBC (hematocrit 60–70%) from the continuously rotating separation chamber [71–74].

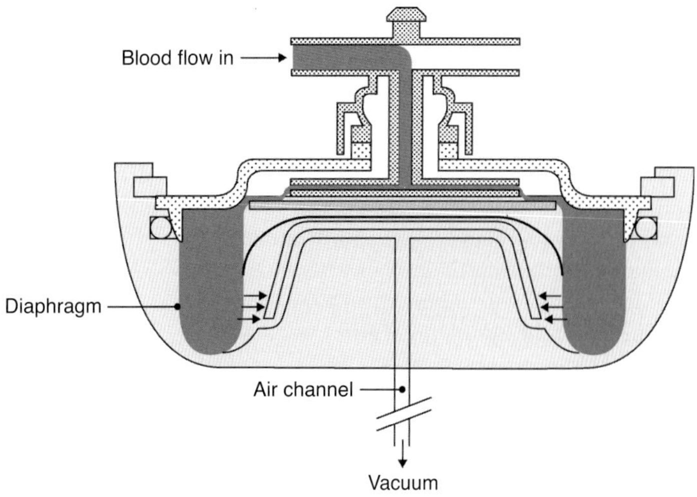

Figure 38.2 Principle of the dynamic disc (OrthoPAT). Blood flow into the centrifugation chamber by vacuum-driven expansion of a silicone membrane.

Cost-effectiveness

In contrast to increasing costs for laboratory tests (e.g., cross match) as well as for allogeneic blood, cost efficacy of cell salvage is easily achieved with proper indication and standby-collection. Former calculations of cost-effectiveness that recommended only application of cell salvage in procedures with anticipated or collected blood loss of $\geq$ 1000 mL [3,75,76] did not account for the sharp rise in the cost of allogeneic blood and the enormous additional costs that arise from its ineffective use and serious adverse effects [77–79]. Besides, such volumes of the collected blood, e.g., 1000 mL, are not reliable measures for the effectiveness of cell salvage, since the hemoglobin content of wound blood shows high variation.

Adverse effects

In general processed blood should be retransfused without delay. To avoid transfusion errors an ABO-bedside test should be performed for identity control, whenever the transfusion bag is disconnected

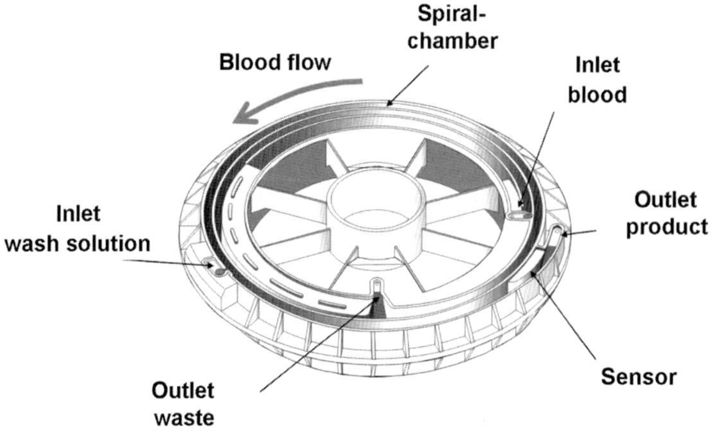

Figure 38.3 Principle of the continuous autotransfusion system (CATS).

or distanced from the patient. Air embolism is avoided by air detectors incorporated in the devices. In case of pressure transfusion any air in the transfusion bag has to be removed by transferring the processed blood to another transfusion bag. The recommendation to limit the collection time to 6 hours is based on the observation of increasing bacterial growth in drained blood after that time, and applies only partially to intraoperative blood salvage with a reservoir emptied and blood processed several times during the procedure. In 20–80% of cases skin- and air-borne bacteria can be detected in salvaged and processed blood in low numbers without any clinical consequences [80–82].

Dilutional coagulopathy is not a side effect of blood salvage, but a side effect of blood loss and its exclusive substitution with washed RBCs. Thus, extensive loss of plasma and platelets may require substitution of appropriate allogeneic components in addition to the autologous RBC saved and processed [19, 55]. Incomplete filling of Latham-bowls should be avoided, since this may lead to insufficient plasma washout [83].

Indications and contraindications

Intra- and postoperative cell salvage must be part of a total blood conservation program and should be considered—if there is no contraindication—for all surgical procedures with major blood loss [3, 84, 85]. Unfortunately, estimates of surgical blood loss by preoperatively available data are very difficult to obtain and unreliable, even for planned and uncomplicated surgery [86, 87]. Therefore, the anesthesiologist's individual experience and knowledge of institutional circumstances (based on retrospective analyses), the type of procedure, and the patient's red cell reserve, body mass and gender are the most helpful parameters in predicting intraoperative blood loss [87]. An answer to this dilemma is the use of standby-collection, where anticoagulated shed blood is collected into an inexpensive reservoir. Only if the amount of blood is large enough to justify the use of cell salvage, should it be processed [4]. This less expensive and simple strategy allows use of intraoperative autotransfusion in cases of unexpected blood loss, thereby expanding application of cell salvage.

Cardiac surgery

One of the major indications for cell salvage is cardiac surgery. According to recent guidelines of the Society of Thoracic Surgeons and the Society of Cardiovascular Anesthesiologists there is a level A evidence for the use of red cell salvage in cardiac operations using cardiopulmonary bypass (CPB) [12], whereas preoperative platelet- or plasmapheresis is not recommended. Besides the reduction of blood loss and transfusion requirements [88, 89], several reports document the safety of cell salvage. Neither adverse CNS effects [53] nor increased infectious complications occur and there is an overall reduced complication rate [90] and reduced systemic inflammation. Salvage from the pump during CPB may cause adverse side effects. Low volumes of blood processed to remove contaminants from prolonged uncontrolled cardiotomy suction with excessive aspiration of air and lipids may impair cerebral microcirculation [91]. On the contrary, excessive blood volumes washed may cause loss of plasma and coagulation factors [92]. There exists only level C evidence, for the use of salvaged pump blood shortly after completion of cardiopulmonary bypass as a means of blood conservation. Postoperatively retransfusion of shed mediastinal blood is considered reasonable (level B evidence) when cell washing is used. Direct retransfusion of shed mediastinal blood from postoperative chest tube drainage is not recommended and may cause adverse side effects [12]. Also in off-pump cardiac surgery is cell salvage recommended [93].

Orthopedics

Cell salvage has been shown to work efficiently in major orthopedic surgery [5, 8, 11, 14, 21, 87], namely in studies using washed and processed shed blood [6]. In a meta-analysis cell washing was associated with greater blood-sparing effect than retransfusion of unwashed cells [7, 19]. Therefore, even in procedures with low intraoperative blood loss like primary knee or hip replacement postoperatively drained and collected blood should be washed [24]. Higher blood loss and, as a consequence, a higher benefit of cell salvage is documented in revision hip surgery, spondylodesis, or scoliosis surgery [94]. The impact of orthopedic fat found in processed blood is unclear, as a fat embolism has never been demonstrated after retransfusion. If a lipid layer is observed in the transfusion bag, it should simply not be transfused.

Vascular surgery

Several studies have shown a reduction of rate and the amount of allogeneic transfusions by using cell salvage in abdominal aortic aneurysm repair [10, 17, 18, 33, 95]. This was not the case in one study with liberal transfusion trigger [96]. In addition, a reduced risk of infectious complications and SIRS was observed compared to allogeneic transfusion [95]. In smaller vascular surgery like aortofemoral bypass operations [10] there is no sufficient evidence for a clear advantage of cell salvage [95].

Polytrauma

Nowadays cell salvage is an essential part of modern emergency medicine [97]. In acute emergency cases of severely traumatized patients with intense hemorrhage, the use of intraoperative autotransfusion enables optimal repair, and may literally be life-saving due to its fast availability and due to a possibly limited supply of allogeneic blood. Thus supplemental autologous RBC supply provided by the comparably simple cell salvage procedure may be extremely helpful. For these reasons, it is recommended that a cell saving device should be available in emergency rooms or emergency operating units. Also, the attending staff should be well-trained and competent in its use [4]. The same applies to other procedures in general surgery with high blood loss, like liver transplantation [98].

Pediatric surgery

While cell salvage is established for adolescents and older children, as in scoliosis surgery [94], new technical developments—as for example a small Latham-bowl (BT55, Sorin), a CATS (Fresenius) or a smaller device with a dynamic disc designed for postoperative autotransfusion (OrthoPAT, Haemonetics) give hope for application of blood salvage even in smaller children and infants. According to a recent study all three devices allowed processing of small volumes with comparable results under clinically relevant conditions [99]. However, these systems are limited at a body weight of about 10 kg, where a loss of 30–40% of the estimated total blood volume has to be tolerated by the infant before enough autologous blood for a relevant transfusion (10% of its blood volume) is available. Similar limitations have been observed in clinical application in infants with craniosynostosis [100]. This may not be the absolute limit in the future, since none of these devices have actually been optimized for this indication.

Cancer surgery

The demand for blood and blood products in cancer surgery is high and continuously increasing. In general about 30% of all banked blood is used in tumor surgery [101], and in hospitals routinely using cell salvage in tumor surgery this amounts to 50–60% of the cell saver applications [102–104]. Transfusion related immunomodulation induced by both the allogeneic barrier and by storage lesions of banked blood with subsequent increased risk of postoperative infections and tumor recurrence [105] is especially relevant to these patients. Thus, intraoperative cell salvage seems favorable. However it is considered contraindicated, as malignant tumor cells contaminating the wound blood from the operative field would get access to the circulation with its subsequent potential of generating metastases after retransfusion [1, 23, 106]. Clinical studies that have not found adverse effects on tumor recurrence or survival rate [106, 107] are unable for statistical reasons to demonstrate or to exclude the risk of tumor cell dissemination after retransfusion of salvaged wound blood [108]. Instead, demonstration of viable, proliferating, invasive, and tumorigenic tumor cells in the shed blood in high incidence (>90%) and with high cell counts (up to 10^7 cells) underlines the contraindication for retransfusion of untreated shed blood of cancer patients [109, 110].

To overcome this contraindication a method is required to effectively eliminate the contaminating cancer cells. Several authors have claimed elimination of tumor cells by leukocyte depletion filters [111–114], but in these studies the basic principles of leukocyte depletion filter testing have not been appreciated, i.e., characterization by reduction rate (calculated from cell numbers before and after (!) filtration, improvement of detection sensitivity of the test system, declaration of the achieved detection sensitivity. Actually, when tested with native tumor cells instead of cell lines and with sensitive detection techniques, leukocyte depletion filters show only limited capacity to reduce the number of tumor cells in blood [9, 115]. Residual tumor cells after filtration, as have been demonstrated [116–118], are not acceptable, since the capability of single cells to cause metastasis has been shown [119].

On the contrary, because of the well-known radiosensitivity of tumor cells at least a 12-log reduction in proliferating cells is to be expected from a 50 Gy gamma irradiation. The effectiveness of such wound blood irradiation has been tested and confirmed by eradication of any cell proliferation or DNA metabolism [120, 121]. Radiation failure, well known in radiotherapy of cancer, is excluded because with well oxygenated cell suspension and with unfractionated irradiation dose radioresistant cells in hypoxic areas or chances for DNA repair are lacking. The safety of blood irradiation with regard to RBC quality has been tested and was demonstrated by minimal hemolysis, minimal potassium release, normal levels of 2,3 DPG and ATP, and by an unimpaired 24-hour survival rate [122]. Thus, blood irradiation with 50 Gy can be regarded as safe by eliminating the risk of tumor cell dissemination without impairing RBC quality. It represents the only method described to guarantee elimination of tumor cells and to overcome the contraindication of blood salvage in tumor surgery.

Meanwhile, more than 1000 cancer patients have been successfully treated with this combination of two well-established methods: intraoperative blood salvage and blood irradiation. Effective reduction in allogeneic blood transfusions and saving of blood resources have been documented [103, 104, 121, 123]. The method proved feasible as irradiation facilities are usually available at tumor centers. In addition, for Jehovah's Witness patients the method described may be the only way to receive more extensive oncologic surgery at all [124]. Preliminary data of a study on surgery of spinal metastasis suggest improved outcome of the patients with cell salvage [123].

Bacterial contamination

Contamination of the surgical field by bacteria is a major clinical concern, since neither cell washing, nor filtration, nor antibiotics can sufficiently remove bacteria from the processed blood (only 1–2 log reduction) [106, 125, 126]. Therefore, the use of cell salvage in all kinds of septic surgery as well as urologic surgery in contact with urine (if bacterial infection cannot be excluded), enoral or endonasal procedures in contact with mucosa, and blunt abdominal injuries is unsafe and not recommended, except as an ultimate life-saving procedure [1, 2, 23]. Bacterial contamination of the surgical field should not be confused with the frequent detection of air- or skin-borne bacteria in small numbers in salvaged wound blood, which has no clinical impact [80–82, 127]. In contrast, a high incidence of bacteremia with high numbers of highly pathogenic germs and clinical signs of postoperative infection (fever, shivering) have been reported after cell salvage in transurethral procedures, maxillofacial surgery, or penetrating abdominal trauma [128, 129]. Some reports show that most patients who had received contaminated wound blood from abdominal trauma as part of resuscitation in life-threatening hemorrhage survived, probably due to concomitant administration of antibiotics [130, 131], but with modern blood banking allogeneic blood would seem the better choice and these indications should be rare. According to modern transfusion medicine, intentional induction of bacteremia should not be part of medical therapy, and cell salvage from a site with expected or known bacterial contamination is strictly contraindicated [23].

Obstetrics

Under normal circumstances blood loss is low and blood transfusion is a rare event in obstetrics.

Although cell salvage has been considered contraindicated because of the risk of amniotic fluid embolism, induction of DIC, and transmission of fetal cells, recently the general use of cell saving has been proposed [132]. Safe applications have been reported [133] in a number of patients too small for risk evaluation, but one fatal case as well [134]. Experimental data show insufficient removal (1–2 log reduction) of fetal squamous cells, or insufficient removal of tissue factor [135–137] by cell washing and leukocyte depletion filters. Thus, cell salvage should be limited only to life-threatening obstetric hemorrhage [138].

Quality management

Medical societies and hospital administrations call for QM of medical treatment, especially in transfusion medicine including blood salvage. Most of all, a system of QM is necessary to guarantee the high quality of this autologous blood and the benefits of autologous transfusion, and to support further improvement. Since QM should not just describe all available methods [36], but rather is a matter of decisions and commitments, it should be definite, clear, and written down in a QM-handbook. Such QM of blood salvage has been proposed [26] and established, and first experiences have been reported [83, 139]. Structure quality of blood salvage can be improved by defining responsibilities, documenting procedures and (hospital-specific) indications and contraindications. Process quality should be supported by a clear description of the techniques used, by the definition of parameters and procedures for quality assurance, and by a profound understanding of the methods of blood salvage [70, 99]. For respective evaluations of autotransfusion devices, disposals, programs, and process variables, testing with freshly donated blood with defined hemolysis is recommended [83] instead of using outdated banked blood. Data on the effects of various process variables on product quality support improvements in performance and reactions to specific clinical challenges [140].

Quality controls

Quality controls should test

• Product quality by measuring volume and hematocrit of the washed RBC, with a threshold value of hematocrit >50% (once per each application)

• Process quality by determining of RBC recovery and plasma elimination, with a threshold value of RBC recovery >80% and of protein elimination >90% (quarterly for each autotransfusion device in use) [26].

Clear actions should be defined if these criteria are not met.

RBC recovery is calculated from the produced amount of RBC divided by the amount of RBC taken from the reservoir. Similarly, for determination of *plasma elimination* the total amount and not only the concentration of a soluble substance in the supernatant should be compared before and after processing. Although several parameters can be used to determine plasma elimination rate, total protein concentration is preferable. In contrast to free plasma hemoglobin its correct determination is simple and fast in routine laboratories. Microbiological testing is unnecessary since it has neither consequence nor clinical relevance.

Advantages of blood salvage

Blood salvage using processing of the wound blood carries many advantages including high and fast availability, high cost efficacy, high effectiveness, reduction of transfusion risks, high quality of the salvaged blood, and possibly an improvement in outcome [123].

Efficacy

Cell savers are available in most hospitals performing major surgical procedures. In Germany, for example, there are 160,000 procedures of intraoperative cell salvage per year. With a mean rate of 80% leading to retransfusion and a mean of 2.9 units processed per procedure this corresponds to about 371,000 units of autologous blood per year, equivalent to 9% of all transfusions (a rate never reached by predonation). These devices are set up for use within a few minutes. Cell salvage is also accepted by Jehovah's Witnesses and makes control of blood loss and the surgery available to these patients. Within a few minutes washed RBC are produced out of the collected wound blood and thus available for retransfusion. In emergency cases this may represent the fastest source of compatible hemotherapy.

In the light of increasing costs of banked blood and with proper indication and standby-collection cell salvage is cost-effective. Cost efficacy is usually already reached with 1 unit of processed blood, and increases with every further unit prepared. It becomes even greater if performed by the anaesthesiologist or the nurse with no additional staff necessary Cost efficacy is further increased, if the better function and viability of fresh autologous RBC are taken into account instead of just comparing hemoglobin content.

Cell salvage is highly efficient in blood saving by retransfusion 50–60% of the RBC lost, and is accompanied by an equivalent reduction in allogeneic transfusions. This supports blood supply in cases of high blood loss and saves blood resources for patients with rare blood groups or irregular antibodies.

Quality

High safety and an extremely low rate of side effects are reported for cell salvage using processing, even though elimination of contaminants from cell lysis and activation in wound blood can never be complete (95–99%). This autologous blood is neither immunogenic, nor antigenic and without transfusion reactions or alloimmunization. In contrast to banked allogeneic or predonated autologous blood it is not immunosuppressive. The allogeneic barrier and storage lesions may lead to an increased postoperative infection rate and tumor recurrence. There is no risk of overtransfusion as it is blood-loss-dependent. A major advantage is that the indication for fresh autologous blood transfusion is more liberal, and thus the known disadvantages of anemia, a major determinant for bad outcome, can be avoided. In addition, with a lower risk of undertransfusion efficacy of chemotherapy and radiotherapy in cancer patients is not impaired.

Fresh, unstored, unrefrigerated, washed RBC are of excellent quality, having normal morphology and membrane characteristics, normal function of oxygen transport and release (2,3 DPG, p50), normal viability (ATP, 24 hours survival), but no load of potassium or free hemoglobin. This strikingly contrasts with banked allogeneic or autologous blood, where function is recovered within hours to days only, where in addition, at the end of the allowed storage time 25–30% of RBCs are lost and hemolyzed 1 day after transfusion and also microcirculation is impaired.

Outcome

The impact of cell salvage on outcome is rather unclear, but retrospective data in surgery of spinal metastasis suggest a highly significantly improved outcome (survival) of tumor patients [123]. Both anemia and allogeneic transfusions are associated with worse outcome. So, for instance, in cardiac patients during cardiopulmonary bypass, anemia and hemodilution lead to increased mortality, perioperative stroke, myocardial infarction, low-output failure, and renal or multiorgan failure. Allogeneic transfusions do not reverse this risk, but may even increase it further [12]. Thus, both aspects of cell salvage, namely reduction of blood loss and autologous transfusion, should be beneficial. Actually, only few outcome studies are available and most are of low quality [7]. Therefore, well-performed large-scale prospective studies are needed. In orthopedic surgery with intermediate blood loss and with multifactorial outcome parameters like hospital stay, mobilization, or postoperative infections a study like this has to involve hundreds of patients. The higher the blood loss and transfusion rates, and with hard outcome parameters like survival time in cancer patients a smaller group size is sufficient. In contrast to the studies on colorectal cancer surgery with low transfusion rates and with predonated blood carrying storage lesions, that failed to show a difference between autologous and allogeneic transfusion [141, 142], chances to see a difference between allogeneic and autologous blood transfusion therefore are much higher with cell salvage. If the better outcome of cancer patients observed after intraoperative autotransfusion [123] could be confirmed in prospective studies, this method would become state-of-the-art treatment.

References

1. Dzik WH, Sherburne B. Intraoperative blood salvage: medical controversies. Transfus Med Rev 1990;4:208–35.
2. Tawes RL. Intraoperative autotransfusion: advantages, disadvantages, and contraindications. Semin Vasc Surg 1994;7:95–7.
3. Tawes RL. Clinical applications of autotransfusion. Semin Vasc Surg 1994;7:89–90.
4. Gombotz H, Kulier A. Reduction in the use of donated blood in surgical medicine. Anaesthesist 1995;44:191–218.
5. Huet C, Salmi LR, Fergusson D, et al. A meta-analysis of the effectiveness of cell salvage to minimize perioperative allogeneic blood transfusion in cardiac and orthopedic surgery. Anesth Analg 1999;89:861–9.
6. Rubens FD, Boodhwani M, Lavalee G, Mesena T. Perioperative red blood cell salvage. Can J Anaesth 2003;50(Suppl. 6):S31–40.
7. Careless P, Moxey A, O'Conell D, Henry D. Autologous transfusion techniques: a systematic review of their efficacy. Transfus Med 2004;14:123–44.
8. Rosencher N, Kerkkamp HEM, Macheras G, et al. Orthopedic surgery transfusion hemoglobin European overview (OSTHEO) study: blood management in elective knee and hip arthroplasty in Europe. Transfusion 2003;43:459–69.
9. Hansen E. Cell salvage in the presence of malignancy. Transfus Altern Transfus Med 2003;5:472–7.
10. Alvarez GG, Fergusson DA, Neilipovitz DT, Hebert PC. Cell salvage does not minimize perioperative allogeneic blood transfusion in abdominal vascular surgery: a systematic review. Can J Anesth 2004;51:425–31.
11. Munoz M, Campos A, Munoz E, et al. Red cell salvage in orthopedic surgery. Transfus Altern Transfus Med 2006;8:41–51.
12. Society of Thoracic Surgeons Blood Conservation Guideline Task Force, Ferraris VA, Ferraris SP, et al. Perioperative blood transfusion and blood conservation in cardiac surgery: the society of thoracic surgeons and the society of cardiovascular anesthesiologists clinical practice guideline. Ann Thorac Surg 2007;83(Suppl. 5):S27–86.
13. Kent P, Ashley S, Thorley PJ, et al. 24-hour survival of autotransfused red cells in elective aortic surgery: a comparison of two intraoperative autotransfusion systems. Br J Surg 1991;78:1473–5.
14. Huo MH, Paly WL, Keggi KJ. Effect of preoperative autologous blood donation and intraoperative and postoperative blood recovery on homologous blood transfusion requirement in cementless total hip replacement operation. J Am Coll Surg 1995;180:561–7.
15. Duchateau J, Nevelsteen A, Suy R, et al. Autotransfusion, during aorto-iliac surgery. Eur J Vasc Surg 1990;4:349–54.
16. Bartels C, Claeys L, Ktenidis K, et al. Intraoperative whole blood autotransfusion, during venous thrombectomy. J Cardiovasc Surg 1994;35: 109–14.
17. Ouriel K, Shortell CK, Green RM, DeWeese JA. Intraoperative autotransfusion in aortic surgery. J Vasc Surg 1993;18:16–22.
18. Kalra M, Beech MJ, al-Khaffaf H, Charlesworth D. Autotransfusion in aortic surgery: the Haemocell System 350 cell saver. Br J Surg 1993;80:32–5.
19. Tawes RL, Sydorak GR, DuVall TB. Postoperative salvage: a technological advance in the "washed" versus "unwashed" blood controversy. Semin Vasc Surg 1994;7:98–103.
20. Blaylock RC, Carlson KS, Morgan JM, et al. In vitro analysis of shed blood from patients undergoing total knee replacement surgery. Am J Clin Pathol 1994;101:365–9.
21. Shenolikar A, Wareham K, Newington D, et al. Cell salvage autotransfusion in total knee replacement surgery. Transfus Med 1997;7:277–80.
22. Cross MH. Autotransfusion in cardiac surgery. Perfusion 2001;16:391–400.
23. AABB. *Guidelines for Blood Recovery and Reinfusion in Surgery and Trauma*. American Association of Blood Banks, Bethesda, 1997.
24. Hansen E, Pawlik M. Reasons against the retransfusion of unwashed wound blood. Transfusion 2004;44(Suppl. 2):45–53.
25. Laffey JG, Boylan JF, Cheng DC. The systemic inflammatory response to cardiac surgery: implications for the anesthesiologist. Anesthesiology 2002;97:215–52.
26. Hansen E, Altmeppen J. Proposal for internal quality management in intra- and postoperative blood salvage. Infus Ther Transfus Med 2002;29:147–50.

27. Handel M, Winkler J, Hornlein RF, et al. Influence of acid-citrate-dextrose anticoagulation on blood quality in retransfusion systems after total knee arthroplasty. Arch Orthop Trauma 2002;122:269–73.
28. Kvarnström A, Schmidt A, Tylman M, et al. Complement split products and proinflammatory cytokines in intraoperatively salvaged unwashed blood during hip replacement: comparison between heparin-coated and non-heparin-coated autotransfusion systems. Vox Sang 2008;95:33–8.
29. Cross MH. Cell salvage and leukodepletion. Perfusion 2001;16(Suppl.):61–6.
30. Dalen T, Bentsson A, Engstrom KG. Inflammatory mediators in autotransfusion drain blood after knee arthroplasty, with and without leucocyte reduction. Vox Sang 2003;85:31–9.
31. Duchow J, Ames M, Hess T, Seyfert U. Activation of plasma coagulation by retransfusion of unwashed drainage blood after hip joint arthroplasty. J Arthroplasty 2001;16:844–9.
32. Krohn CD, Reikeras O, Brosstad F. Fibrinolytic activity and postoperative salvaged untreated blood for autologous transfusion in major orthopaedic surgery. Eur J Surg 2001;167:168–72.
33. Long GW, Glover JL, Bendick PJ, et al. Cell washing versus immediate reinfusion of intraoperatively shed blood during abdominal aortic aneurysm repair. Am J Surg 1993;166:97–102.
34. Bartels C, Bechtel JV, Winkler C, Horsch S. Intraoperative autotransfusion, in aortic surgery: comparison of whole blood autotransfusion, versus cell separation. J Vasc Surg 1996;24:102–8.
35. Yomtovian R. Autologous transfusion complications. In: Popovsky MA (ed.) *Transfusion Reactions*. American Association of Blood Banks, Bethesda, 1996, pp. 237–80.
36. AABB. *Guidance for Standards for Perioperative Autologous Blood Collection and Administration*. American Association of Blood Banks, Bethesda, 2002.
37. De Haan J, Schonberger J, Haan J, et al. Tissue type plasminogen activator and fibrin monomers synergistically cause platelet dysfunction during retransfusion of shed blood after cardiopulmonary bypass. J Thorac Cardiovasc Surg 1993;106:1017–23.
38. Woda R, Jetzlaff JE. Upper airway oedema following autologous blood transfusion from wound drainage system. Can J Anaesth 1992;39:290–92.
39. Kitano T, et al. Unwashed shed blood infusion causes deterioration in right ventricular function after coronary artery surgery. Anaesth Intensive Care 2000;28:642–5.
40. Stump DA, Rogers AT, Hammon JW, et al. Cerebral emboli and cognitive outcome after cardiac surgery. J Cardiothorac Vasc Anesth 1996;10: 113–19.
41. Vertrees RA, Conti VR, Lick SD, et al. Adverse effects of postoperative infusion of shed mediastinal blood. Ann Thorac Surg 1996;62:717–23.
42. Duncan SE, Edwards WH, Dale WA. Caution regarding autotransfusion. Surgery 1974;76:1024–30.
43. Azzopardi N, Yabri M. A fatal reaction following scavenged autologous blood transfusion. Anaesth Intensive Care 1993;21:335–6.
44. Milne A, Drummond GB, Paterson DA, et al. Disseminated intravascular coagulation after aneurysma repair, intraoperative salvage autotransfusion, and aprotinin. Lancet 1994;344:470–71.
45. Gharehbaghian A, Haque KMG, Truman C, et al. Effect of autologous salvaged blood on postoperative natural killer cell precursor frequency. Lancet 2004;363:1025–30.
46. Dial S, Nguyen D, Menzies D. Autotransfusion of shed mediastinal blood: a risk factor for mediastinitis after cardiac surgery? Results of a cluster investigation. Chest 2003;124:1847–51.
47. Body SC, Birmingham J, Parks R, et al. Safety and efficacy of shed mediastinal blood transfusion after cardiac surgery: a multicenter observational study. J Cardiothorac Vasc Anesth 1999;13:410–16.
48. Mauerhan DR, Nussman D, Mokris JG, Beaver WB. Effect of postoperative reinfusion systems on hemoglobin levels in primary total hip and total knee arthroplasties. A prospective randomized study. J Arthroplasty 1993;8:523–7.
49. Grimaldi NA, Sicuranza M, Eck JC. Perioperative autotransfusion systems in TKA are not necessary. Orthopedics 2006;29:1027–9.
50. Schirmer U, Hemmer W, Lindner KH, et al. Shed mediastinal blood in 500 elective cardiac surgery patients: is there enough for retransfusion routinely? J Cardiovasc Surg 1997;38:45–50.
51. Martin J, Robitaille D, Perrault LP, et al. Reinfusion of mediastinal blood after heart surgery. J Thorac Cardiovasc Surg 2000;120:499–504.
52. Rizzi L, Bertracchi P, Ghezzi LM, et al. Postoperative blood salvage in hip and knee arthroplasty: a prospective study on cost effectiveness in 161 patients. Acta Orthop Scand 1998;69:31–4.
53. Svenmarker S, Engstrom KG. The inflammatory response to recycled pericardial suction blood and the influence of cell-saving. Scand Cardiovasc J 2003;37:158–64.

54. Waters JH, Dyga RM. Postoperative blood salvage: outside the controlled world oft he blood bank. Transfusion 2007;47:362–5.
55. Trubel W, Gunen E, Wuppinger G, et al. Recovery of intraoperatively shed blood in aortoiliac surgery: comparison of cell washing with simple filtration. Thorac Cardiovasc Surg 1995;43:165–70.
56. Perttila J, Leino L, Poyhonen M, Salo M. Leucocyte content in blood processed by autotransfusion devices during open-heart surgery. Acta Anaesthesiol Scand 1995;39:445–8.
57. Jewell AE, Akowuah EF, Suvarna SK, et al. A prospective randomised comparison of cardiotomy suction and cell saver for recycling shed blood during cardiac surgery. Eur J Cardiothorac Surg 2003;23:633–6.
58. Williamson KR, Taswell HF. Intraoperative blood salvage: a review. Transfusion 1991;31:662–75.
59. Burman JF, Westlake AS, Davidson SJ, et al. Study of five cell salvage machines in coronary artery surgery. Transfus Med 2002;12:173–9.
60. Serrick CJ, Scholz M, Melo A, et al. Quality of red blood cells using autotransfusion devices: a comparative analysis. J Extra Corpor Technol 2003;35:28–34.
61. Reeder G. Autotransfusion theory of operation: a review of the physics and hematology. Transfusion 2004;44(Suppl.):S35–9.
62. Amand T, Pincemail J, Blaffart F, et al. Levels of inflammatory markers in the blood processed by autotransfusion devices during cardiac surgery associated with cardiopulmonary bypass circuit. Perfusion 2002;17:117–23.
63. Innerhofer P, Wiedermann FJ, Tiefenthaler W, et al. Are leukocytes in salvaged washed autologous blood harmful for the recipient? The results of a pilot study. Anesth Analg 2001;93:566–72.
64. Nohé B, Ries R, Ploppa A, et al. Effects of intraoperative blood salvage on leukocyte recruitment to the endothelium. Anesthesiology 2005;102:300–307.
65. Ilmakunnas M, Pesonen EJ, Ahonen J, et al. Activation of neutrophils and monocytes by a leukocyte-depleting filter used throughout cardiopulmonary bypass. J Thorac Cardiovasc Surg 2005;129:851–9.
66. Bull BS, Bull MH. The salvaged blood syndrome: a sequel to mechanochemical activation of platelets and leukocytes? Blood Cells 1990;16:5–20.
67. Tawes RL, Jr, Duvall TB. Is the "salvaged-cell syndrome" myth or reality? Am J Surg 1996;172:172–4.
68. Lorentz A, Waibel H, Becker P, et al. Routine automated laboratory methods are inadequate to determine the number of platelets in blood salvaged and processed for autotransfusion. Infus Ther Transfus Med 2000;27:33–6.
69. Gregoretti S. Suction-induced hemolysis at various vacuum pressures: implications for intraoperative blood salvage. Transfusion 1996;36:57–60.
70. Hansen E, Kling J, Roth G. The myth of suction pressure limitation in blood salvage. Anästh Intensivmed 2006;47(Suppl.):118–22.
71. Dai B, Wang L, Djaiani G, Mazer CD. Continuous and discontinuous cell-washing autotransfusion systems. J Cardiothorac Vasc Anesth 2004;18:210–17.
72. Geiger P, Platow K, Bartl A, et al. New developments in autologous transfusion systems. Anaesthesia 1998;53(Suppl. 2):32–5.
73. Florio G, Valbonesi M, Lercari G, et al. The Fresenius continuous autotransfusion, system (CATS): preliminary studies and application. Int J Artif Organs 1996;19:431–4.
74. Bengtsson A, Avall A, Tylman M, et al. Effects on complement activation of a new continuous autotransfusion, system. Transfus Med 1997;7:107–13.
75. Solomon MD, Rutledge ML, Kane LE, Yawn DH. Cost comparison of intraoperative autologous versus homologous transfusion. Transfusion 1988;28:379–82.
76. Goodnough LT, Monk TG, Sicard G, et al. Intraoperative salvage in patients undergoing elective abdominal aortic aneurysm repair: an analysis of cost and benefit. J Vasc Surg 1996;24:213–18.
77. Goodnough LT, Brecher ME, Kanter MH, Aubuchon JP. Transfusion, medicine. First of two parts—blood transfusion. N Engl J Med 1999;340:438–47.
78. Waters JR, Meier HH, Waters JH. An economic analysis of costs associated with development of a cell salvage program. Anesth Analg 2007;104:869–75.
79. Shander A, Hofmann A, Gombotz H, et al. Estimating the costs of blood: past, present, and future directions. Best Pract Res Clin Anaesthesiol 2007;21(2): 271–89.
80. Ezzedine H, Baele P, Robert A. Bacteriologic quality of intraoperative autotransfusion. Surgery 1991;109:259–64.
81. Bland LA, Villarino ME, Arduino MJ, et al. Bacteriologic and endotoxin analysis of salvaged blood used in autologous transfusions during cardiac operations. J Thorac Cardiovasc Surg 1992;103: 582–8.
82. Sugai Y, Sugai K, Fuse A. Current status of bacterial contamination of autologous blood for transfusion. Transfus Apher Sci 2001;24:255–9.

83. Hansen E, Bechmann V, Altmeppen J, et al. Quality management in blood salvage: implementation of quality assurance and variables affecting product quality. Transfus Med Hemother 2004;31: 221–7.
84. Hayes SL, Torella F, McCollum CN. Cell salvage—state of the art and cost-effectiveness. Transfus Altern Transfus Med 2003;5:446–52.
85. Waters JH. Indications and contraindications of cell salvage. Transfusion 2004;44(Suppl. 12):40–44.
86. Nuttall GA, Santrach PJ, Oliver WC, et al. The predictors of red cell transfusions in total hip arthroplasties. Transfusion 1996;36:144–9.
87. Lisander B, Ivarsson I, Jacobsson SA. Intraoperative autotransfusion is associated with modest reduction of allogeneic transfusion in prosthetic hip surgery. Acta Anaesthesiol Scand 1998;42:707–12.
88. Hall RI, Schweiger IM, Finlayson DC. The benefit of the Hemonetics cell saver apparatus during cardiac surgery. Can J Anaesth 1990;37:618–23.
89. Laub GW, Dharan M, Riebman JB, et al. The impact of intraoperative autotransfusion, on cardiac surgery. A prospective randomized double-blind study. Chest 1993;104:686–9.
90. Deleuze P, Intrator L, Liou A, et al. Complement activation and use of a cell saver in cardiopulmonary bypass. ASAIO Trans 1990;36:179–81.
91. Brooker RF, Brown WR, Moody DM, et al. Cardiotomy suction: a major source of brain lipid emboli during cardiopulmonary bypass. Ann Thorac Surg 1998;65:1651–5.
92. Despotis GJ, Filos KS, Zoys TN, et al. Factors associated with excessive postoperative blood loss and hemostatic transfusion requirements: a multivariate analysis in cardiac surgical patients. Anesth Analg 1996;82:13–21.
93. Niranjan G, Asimakopoulos G, Karagounis A, et al. Effects of cell saver autologous blood transfusion on blood loss and homologous blood transfusion requirements in patients undergoing cardiac surgery on- versus off-cardiopulmonary bypass: a randomised trial. Eur J Cardiothorac Surg 2006;30:271–7.
94. Verma RR, Williamson JB, Dashti H, et al. Homologous blood transfusion is not required in surgery for adolescent idiopathic scoliosis. J Bone Joint Surg 2006;88:1187–91.
95. Mercer KG, Spark JI, Berridge DC, et al. Randomized clinical trial of intraoperative autotransfusion in surgery for abdominal aortic aneurysm. Br J Surg 2004;91:1443–8.
96. Clagett GP, Valentine RJ, Jackson MR, et al. A randomized trial of intraoperative autotransfusion during aortic surgery. J Vasc Surg 1999;29:22–30.
97. Cavallieri S, Riou B, Roche S, et al. Intraoperative autologous transfusion in emergency surgery for spine trauma. J Trauma 1994;36:639–43.
98. Phillips SD, Maguire D, Deshpande R, et al. A prospective study investigating the cost effectiveness of intraoperative blood salvage during liver transplantation. Transplantation 2006;81:536–40.
99. Hansen E, Kling J, Roth G. Processing small volumes in blood salvage: characterization of ELECTA, CATS and OrthoPAT. Anästh Intensivmed 2006;47(Suppl.):123–30.
100. Dahmani S Dahmani S, Orliaguet G, et al. Perioperative blood salvage during surgical correction of craniosynostosis in infants. Br J Anaesth 2000;85:550–55.
101. Friedman BA, Burns TL, Schork MA. A study of blood utilisation by diagnosis, month of transfusion, and geographic region of the United States. Transfusion 1979;19:511–25.
102. Hansen E, Altmeppen J, Taeger K. Practicability and safety of intra-operative autotransfusion with irradiated blood. Anaesthesia 1998;53(Suppl. 2):42–3.
103. Valbonesi M, Bruni R, Lercari G, et al. Autoapheresis and intraoperative blood salvage in oncologic surgery. Transfus Sci 1999;21:129–39.
104. Hansen E, Bechmann V, Altmeppen J. Intraoperative blood salvage in cancer surgery: safe and effective? Transfus Apher Sci 2002;27:153–7.
105. Nielsen HJ. Detrimental effects of perioperative blood transfusion. Br J Surg 1995;82:528–37.
106. Park KI, Kojima O, Tomoyoshi T. Assessment of the availability of intraoperative autotransfusion in urological operations. J Urol 1997;157:1777–80.
107. Zulim RA, Rocco M, Goodnight JE, et al. Intraoperative autotransfusion, in hepatic resection for malignancy. Is it safe? Arch Surg 1993;128:206–11.
108. Hansen E, Altmeppen J, Taeger K. Autologous haemotherapy in malignant diseases. In: Kretschmer G, Blauhut B (eds) *Blood, Blood Products and Blood Saving Techniques. Vol. 11: Clinical Anaesthesiology*, Baillière Tindall, London, 1997, pp. 335–50.
109. Hansen E, Wolff N, Knuechel R, et al. Tumor cells in blood shed from the surgical field. Arch Surg 1995;130:387–93.
110. Cheng DLW, Savannah GA, Liu BCS, et al. Intraoperative autotransfusion during radical prostatectomy: detection and significance of micrometastasis using reverse transcription polymerase

chain reaction. Proc Am Urol Assoc 1995;153: 655.

111. Miller GV, Ramsden CW, Primrose JN. Autologous transfusion: an alternative to transfusion with banked blood during surgery for cancer. Br J Surg 1991;78:713–15.
112. Torre GC, Ferrari M, Favre A, et al. A new technique for intraoperative blood recovery in the cancer patient. Eur J Surg Oncol 1994;20:565–70.
113. Kongsgaard UE, Wang MY, Kvalheim G. Leucocyte depletion filter removes cancer cells in human blood. Acta Anaesthesiol Scand 1996;40:118–20.
114. Catling S, Williams S, Freites O, et al. Use of a leucocyte filter to remove tumour cells from intra-operative cell salvage blood. Anaesthesia 2008;63:1332–8.
115. Hansen E, Altmeppen J, Hansen K, Taeger K. Leucocyte depletion filters do not eliminate cancer cells contaminating blood. Transfusion 1999;39:S239.
116. Jones CC, Stammers AH, Fristoe LW, et al. Removal of hepatocarcinoma cells from blood via cell washing and filtration techniques. J Extra Corpor Technol 1999;31:169–76.
117. Liang TB, Li DL, Liang L, et al. Intraoperative blood salvage during liver transplantation in patients with hepatocellular carcinoma: efficiency of leukocyte depletion filters in the removal of tumor cells. Transplantation 2008;85:863–9.
118. Hansen E. Failed evidence of tumour cell removal from salvaged blood after leukocyte depletion. Transfus Med 2006;16:213–14.
119. Fidler IJ, Talmadge JE. Evidence that intravenously derived murine pulmonary metastases can originate from the expansion of a single tumor cell. Cancer Res 1986;46:5167–71.
120. Hansen E, Knuechel R, Altmeppen J, Taeger K. Blood irradiation for intraoperative autotransfusion in cancer surgery: demonstration of efficient elimination of contaminating tumor cells. Transfusion 1999;39:608–14.
121. Hansen E, Bechmann V, Altmeppen J. Intraoperative blood salvage in oncologic surgery—answers to current questions. Infus Ther Transfus Med 2002;29:138–41.
122. Hansen E, Altmeppen J, Marienhagen J, Taeger K. Quality of blood salvaged and irradiated during cancer surgery. Transfusion 1999;39(Suppl.):S256.
123. Hansen E, Pawlik M, Altmeppen J, Bechmann V. Advantages of intraoperative blood salvage with blood irradiation in cancer surgery. Transfus Med Hemother 2004;31:286–92.
124. Hansen E. Intraoperative blood salvage in tumor surgery in a Jehovah's witness. Transfus Alternat Transfus Med 2002;4(Suppl.):60.
125. Boudreaux JP, Bornside GH, Cohn I. Emergency autotransfusion: partial cleansing of bacteria-laden blood by cell washing. J Trauma 1983;23:31–5.
126. Waters J, Tuohy MJ, Hobson DF, Procop G. Bacterial reduction by cell salvage washing and leukocyte depletion filtration. Anesthesiology 2003;99:652–5.
127. Feltracco P, Michieletto E, Barbieri S, et al. Microbiologic contamination of intraoperative blood salvaged during liver transplantation. Transplant Proc 2008;39:1889–91.
128. Ozmen V, McSwain NE, Nichols RL, et al. Autotransfusion, of potentially culture-positive blood (CPB) in abdominal trauma: preliminary data from a prospective study. J Trauma 1992;32:36–9.
129. Rohling RG, Zimmermann AP, Breymann C. Transfusion of washed and centrifuged shed RBCs during maxillofacial surgery affects cytokine concentrations. Transfusion 2000;40:1352–6.
130. Thomas MJG. Infected and malignant fields are an absolute contraindication to intraoperative cell salvage: fact or fiction? Transfus Med 1999;9:269–78.
131. Bowley DM, Barker P, Boffard KD. Intraoperative blood salvage in penetrating abdominal trauma: a randomised, controlled trial. World J Surg 2006;30:1074–80.
132. Thomas D. Facilities for blood salvage (cell saver technique) must be available in every obstetric theatre. Int J Obstet Anesth 2005;14:48–52.
133. Potter PS, Waters JH, Burger GA, Mravovic B. Application of cell-salvage during Cesarean section. Anesthesiology 1999;90:619–21.
134. Oei SG, Wingen CBM, Kerkkamp HEM. Cell salvage: how safe in obstetrics? Int J Obstet Anesth 2000;9:143.
135. Bernstein HH, Rosenblatt MA, Gettes M, Lockwood C. The ability of the haemonetics 4 cell saver system to remove tissue factor from blood contaminated with amniotic fluid. Anesth Analg 1997;85: 831–3.
136. Catling SJ, Williams S, Fielding AM. Cell salvage in obstetrics: an evaluation of the ability of cell salvage combined with leucocyte depletion filtration to remove amniotic fluid from operative blood loss at caesarean section. Int J Obstet Anesth 1999;8: 79–84.
137. Waters JH, Biscotti C, Potter PS, Phillipson E. Amniotic fluid removal during cell salvage in the cesarean section patient. Anesthesiology 2000;92:1519–22.

138. Gombotz H. Blood salvage in obstetric hemorrhage. Con Transfus Altern Transfus Med 2007;9(Suppl. 1):14–15.
139. Hansen E. Quality management in intraoperative blood salvage. Transfus Alternat Transfus Med 2002;4(Suppl.):59–60.
140. Reents W, Babin-Ebell J, Misoph MR, et al. Influence of different autotransfusion devices on the quality of salvaged blood. Ann Thorac Surg 1999;68:58–62.
141. Busch OR, Hop WC, Hoynck van Papendrecht MA, et al. Blood transfusions and prognosis in colorectal cancer. N Engl J Med 1993;328:1372–6.
142. Heiss MM, Mempel W, Delanoff C, et al. Blood transfusion-modulated tumor recurrence: first results of a randomized study of autologous versus allogeneic blood transfusion in colorectal cancer surgery. J Clin Oncol 1994;12:1859–67.

SECTION 4
Special Settings

CHAPTER 39

Anemia and Red Blood Transfusion in Critical Care

Tim Walsh
Anaesthetics, Critical Care and Pain Medicine, New Edinburgh Royal Infirmary, Edinburgh, Scotland, UK

Introduction

Anemia occurs frequently during critical illness. Recent studies have increased our understanding of the causes of anemia and how well it is tolerated by critically ill patients. Red blood cell (RBC) transfusion remains the standard treatment of anemia, but new methods of treatment using erythropoiesis-stimulating agents have also been recently evaluated.

Definition of anemia

Anemia is a hemoglobin concentration in blood that is below the expected value, when age, gender, pregnancy, and certain environmental factors, such as altitude, are taken into account. It results in a reduction in red cell mass and a decrease in the oxygen-carrying capacity of the blood. The World Health Organization (WHO) defines anemia as a hemoglobin <13 g/dL (hematocrit <39%) for adult males and <12 g/dL (hematocrit <36%) for adult nonpregnant females. The WHO has further classified anemia as mild (9.5–10.9 g/dL), moderate (8.0–9.4 g/dL), severe (6.5–7.9 g/dL), and life-threatening (<6.5 g/dL).

Alternatives to Blood Transfusion in Transfusion Medicine, 2nd edition. Edited by A. Maniatis, P. Van der Linden, J.-F. Hardy.

Prevalence of anemia during critical illness

The prevalence of anemia among critically ill patients is influenced by factors that include patient case mix, illness severity, preexisting comorbidity, and the blood transfusion practice employed. The Transfusion Requirements In Critical Care (TRICC) study (described later) has resulted in a more consistent use of restrictive triggers [1]. Typical median pretransfusion hemoglobin values in recent studies have been 7.8–8.5 g/dL [2–6].

Anemia at ICU admission

Several large studies have documented the prevalence of anemia at ICU admission. A cohort study of 3534 patients admitted to 146 western European ICUs with varying case-mix (the ABC study) found that the mean hemoglobin concentration at ICU admission was 11.3 g/dL [5]. Sixty-three percent of patients had a hemoglobin concentration <12 g/dL at ICU admission and 29% of patients had an admission hemoglobin concentration <10 g/dL. In this study, 13% of patients had a recent history of anemia. Fifty percent of patients admitted to ICUs with a hemoglobin concentration <10 g/dL had no history of either acute bleeding or other documented causes of anemia. Anemia was more frequent and more severe in older patients. A similarly designed study evaluated 4892 admissions to ICUs in the United States (the CRIT study) [2]. This study found a similar mean hemoglobin concentration at ICU admission (11.0 g/dL), and almost two-thirds of patients had a hemoglobin concentration

Table 39.1 Estimates of the prevalence of anemia at admission to intensive care.

Variable	Estimate of value or prevalence
Mean hemoglobin concentration at ICU admission	10.5–11.3 g/dL
Proportion of patients with	
Hemoglobin concentration <12 g/dL	60–70%
Hemoglobin concentration <9 g/dL	20–30%
Prevalence of preexisting anemia at ICU admission	13%

<12 g/dL at ICU admission. As in the ABC study, 13% of patients had anemia as a comorbidity on admission. A cohort study of 1023 sequential admissions to 10 Scottish ICUs found that the median hemoglobin concentration at ICU admission was 10.5 g/dL [7]. At ICU admission, 25% of patients had a hemoglobin concentration <9 g/dL. Based on these studies, 20–30% of patients have moderate to severe anemia (hemoglobin concentration <9 g/dL) at ICU admission, but only 10–15% have documented preexisting anemia (Table 39.1).

Anemia during ICU stay

The evolution of anemia among nontransfused nonbleeding critically ill patients is difficult to study both ethically and in practice. Nguyen and colleagues found that among nonbleeding ICU patients who did not receive RBC transfusions, hemoglobin concentrations decreased by a mean 0.52 g/dL/day [8]. On average, hemoglobin concentrations decreased by 0.66 g/dL/day for the first 3 days and by 0.12 g/dL/day thereafter. This early rapid decrease in hemoglobin values was also found in a prospective observational single center cohort study of patients receiving >24 hours of intensive care [9]. Several studies show that the period of most rapid decrease in hemoglobin concentration is the first 3–4 days in the ICU, following which a plateau is reached, which is strongly influenced by the RBC transfusion practice used. Typically 40–50% of all ICU patients receive RBC transfusions, depending on the individual case mix of populations and the transfusion trigger used (Table 39.2)

Epidemiological studies indicate that the mean hemoglobin concentration of ICU populations, irrespective of admission hemoglobin concentration, converges toward 9.5–10 g/dL over the first 4–5 days in the ICU when transfusion triggers of 8–9 g/dL are used. This phenomenon is strongly influenced by transfusion practice, particularly for longer term ICU patients who have an incidence of moderate–severe anemia of 70–80%. A consequence is a high prevalence of anemia at ICU discharge. A study of 766 ICU survivors found that >80% of patients were anemic at ICU discharge, and 25% had a hemoglobin of <9 g/dL.

These data show that the "hit" of critical illness frequently results in acute anemia, which is present at ICU admission or develops within the first 24–48 hours. Once present, anemia persists in most patients until ICU discharge unless modified by blood transfusion practice.

Anemia after ICU discharge

During the period between ICU and hospital discharge and in the period after discharge home, many patients suffer fatigue, breathlessness, and other morbidity frequently associated with anemia. A single center study found that 77.4% of all ICU survivors were anemic when discharged home from hospital and 32.5% had a hemoglobin concentration <10.0 g/dL [10]. Fifty percent of patients who spent >7 days in ICU had a hemoglobin concentration <10 g/dL when discharged home. Cohort studies indicate that only 11–13% of patients are transfused after ICU discharge, typically at hemoglobin values of 8–9 g/dL or less [2, 5]. These data suggest that anemia persists after ICU discharge, and many patients remain anemic when discharged from hospital. The importance of anemia to functional recovery is unknown.

Table 39.2 Hemoglobin transfusion triggers and transfusion rates in intensive care for recent large epidemiological studies of anemia and/or blood transfusion in intensive care units.

Study (reference)	Study acronym	Study size	Case mix	Mean (SD) population APACHE II score	Transfusion trigger	Proportion of admissions transfused (%)
Vincent et al. [5]	ABC study	3534	Mixed multicenter ICUs	14.8 (7.9)	Mean 8.4 (SD 1.3)	37
Rao et al. [4]	None	1247	Mixed multicenter general ICUs	Transfused patients 19.0 (8.8) Non-transfused patients 16.3 (9.3)	"Hemorrhage" 8.5 (IQR: 7.8–9.3) "Low hemoglobin" 8.5 (IQR: 7.8–8.9)	53
Corwin et al. [2]	CRIT study	4892	Mixed multicenter ICUs	19.7 (8.2)	Mean 8.6 (SD1.7)	44
French et al. [3]	None	1808	Mixed general ICU	Not given	Mean 8.2 (range: 4.4–18.7)	19.8
Walsh et al. [6]	ATICS study	1023	Mixed adult general ICUs (excluding cardiac)	19.8 (7.7)	Median 7.8 (IQR: 7.3–8.5)	39.5

Etiology of anemia during critical illness

The etiology of anemia during critical illness is multifactorial in most patients. Contributing factors are considered below and listed in Table 39.3.

Hemodilution

Critically ill patients frequently develop intravascular hypovolemia requiring fluid resuscitation. Current practice is to administer crystalloid or colloid solutions during resuscitation and withhold red cell transfusion unless patients have severe hemorrhage. Relatively modest hemodilution can cause anemia without decreasing red cell mass. Hemodilution contributes to the rapid decrease in hemoglobin described during early ICU treatment.

Table 39.3 Causes of anemia during critical illness.

- Preexisting chronic anemia
  - Acquired anemia
    - Hemodilution
    - Blood loss
      - Blood sampling
      - Hemorrhage
    - Reduced red cell survival
    - Reduced red cell production
      - Abnormal iron metabolism
      - Nutritional deficiencies
      - Inappropriate erythropoietin production
    - Abnormal red cell production

Blood loss

Blood loss is a significant cause of anemia in intensive care patients. Potential sources of blood loss are diagnostic blood sampling and hemorrhage from body sites.

Blood sampling

Early studies found that, on average, a critically ill patient lost 1–2 units of blood through blood sampling during their hospital stay [11, 12], or up to 30% of the total blood transfused in the ICU [13, 14]. More recent data indicate that 30–40 mL per 24 hours are removed in blood samples [5], with more blood sampled in sicker patients and those receiving renal replacement therapy [5, 15, 16].

Hemorrhage

There are many potential sources of bleeding in critically ill patients. The contribution from gastrointestinal bleeding is probably overstated with modern resuscitation and management [17, 18], but may be relevant in high-risk patients including those receiving mechanical ventilation, or with coagulopathy and renal failure [19]. Recent ICU-based transfusion studies suggest that between 20 and 55% of all transfusion events are associated with bleeding [3–6], and about 20% of ICU patients experience at least one episode of significant bleeding during ICU stay [6].

Reduced red cell survival

It is likely that critical illness, and sepsis in particular, reduces red cell lifespan but direct evidence for this is lacking. Experimental data show that inflammatory mediators, such as TNF-α and IL-1, can decrease erythrocyte survival time in other settings [20], and oxidative stress has been shown to induce premature apoptosis among red cells [21].

Reduced red cell production

Anemic critically ill patients have inappropriately low reticulocyte counts compared with the healthy response to anemia [16, 22, 23]. Bone marrow suppression appears to be associated with the presence or persistence of an inflammatory state. Several mechanisms may be involved, many of which are implicated in the anemia of chronic disease. Corwin coined the term "acute anemia of chronic disease" to describe the abnormal erythropoiesis that occurs during critical illness [24]. This term is useful because there appear to be many similarities between erythropoiesis during acute and chronic inflammatory conditions, including cancer. A number of factors, which normally regulate or limit red cell production, could contribute to reduced red cell production during critical illness. Typical biochemical parameters for anemic patients during critical illness are shown in Table 39.4.

Iron metabolism

Acute inflammation decreases the iron available for erythropoiesis. The interpretation of iron indices in inflammatory states is difficult because serum ferritin is increased and serum transferrin is decreased as part of the acute phase response [25]. ICU patients typically have a low serum iron, total iron binding capacity, and serum iron/total iron binding capacity ratio, but the serum ferritin concentration is normal or more usually elevated [16, 23, 26]. During inflammation, iron is transferred into macrophages, where it is incorporated into ferritin, reducing serum iron but increasing storage iron [27]. This is associated with low transferrin saturation reflecting reduced available iron for erythropoeisis [20, 28]. Circulating soluble transferrin receptor concentrations (sTFR) are normal in anemic critically ill patients [23, 29]. These shed receptors are increased in iron deficiency and during active erythropoeisis further supporting a lack of absolute

Table 39.4 Biochemical characteristics of anemia in critically ill patients.

	Change	Comment
Serum iron	↓	Similar to anemia of chronic disease
Total iron binding capacity	↓	
Serum iron/total iron binding capacity ratio	↓	
Ferritin	↑	"Positive" acute phase protein
Transferrin	↓	"Negative" acute phase protein
Transferrin saturation	↓	
Soluble transferring receptor concentration	N	Increase thought to indicate iron deficiency or new erythropoeisis
Percent hypochromic red cells	N/↑	Indicative of functional iron deficiency
Vitamin B12 and folate	N	
Erythropoietin concentration	N/slight increase	Inappropriately low for degree of anemia May be transiently increased in acute renal failure

iron deficiency in most cases. No large studies have examined the effect of iron therapy alone on anemia during critical illness, but in one small study, daily intravenous iron disaccharide therapy alone for 14 days did not increase reticulocyte counts or have any beneficial effect compared to the control group [23]. Based on these data, there is little to support routine iron supplementation as part of intensive care treatment, unless erythropoietin is being used (see later).

Functional iron deficiency is a term used to describe the inability to incorporate iron into hemoglobin for normal red cell production, often despite adequate body stores of iron [30]. It is associated with reduced reticulocyte hemoglobin concentration (CHR) and increased percent hypochromic red cells in peripheral blood both of which have been demonstrated in the critically ill [31, 32].

B12 and folate metabolism

There are few studies evaluating the prevalence of vitamin B12 or folate deficiency in intensive care patients either on admission or during prolonged illness. Rodriguez and colleagues found evidence of deficiency in only 2% of ICU patients [26]. The relation between these and other nutritional deficiencies and anemia are unknown. Based on available evidence, these vitamins do not limit red cell production in most anemic critically ill patients.

Inappropriately low circulating erythropoietin concentrations

The normal response to anemia is to increase erythropoietin release from the kidneys. Appropriate values for circulating erythropoietin concentration have been established in otherwise healthy patients with various degrees of anemia [33]. Using these data as reference for a healthy response to anemia, many studies consistently show that critically ill patients have inappropriately low erythropoietin concentrations for their degree of anemia [16, 23, 34–36]. The blunted erythropoietin response during critical illness probably results from inhibition of the erythropoietin gene by inflammatory cytokines (Figure 39.1) [24, 37].

Abnormal RBC maturation

Inflammatory cytokines such as tumor necrosis factor α, interleukin-1, and interleukin-6 have been shown to directly inhibit red cell formation [20, 38, 39]. Elevated concentrations of these cytokines are frequently present in the circulation of critically ill patients, particularly those with inflammation and/or sepsis. In addition, other circulating factors such as interferon γ have been shown to induce apoptosis of erythroid precursors in experimental studies and could be important during critical illness. These factors, together with a relative deficiency of circulating erythropoietin and decreased

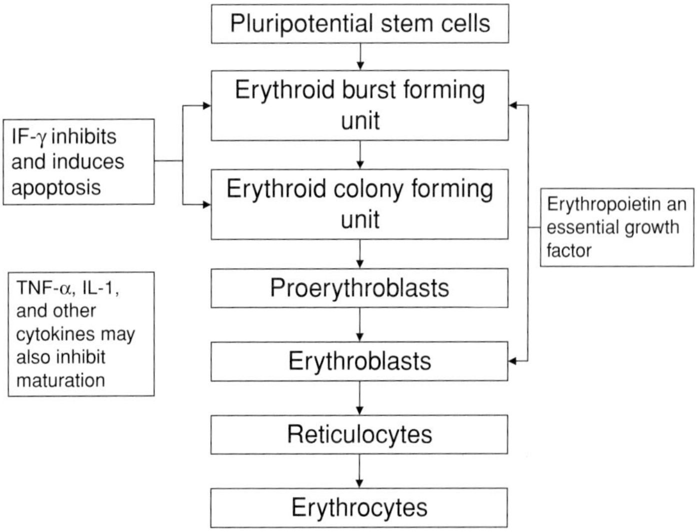

Figure 39.1 Schematic diagram showing stages in red blood cell maturation from pluripotential stem cells and the sites of action of potential inhibitors during critical illness.

iron availability may explain the poor erythroid response that occurs in response to anemia (Figure 39.1). Reticulocyte counts are usually not increased in anemic critically ill patients unless stimulated by pharmacological doses of erythropoietin, which also suggests a bone marrow hyporeactivity [23, 26].

Summary of factors contributing to anemia during critical illness

Blood loss contributes to anemia but is rarely the only explanation for anemia. During resuscitation with colloid and crystalloid solutions hemodilution contributes to a decreased hemoglobin concentration, but potentially without altering red cell mass. A major factor resulting in the development and persistence of anemia is reduced new RBC production. This appears to result from a combination of inappropriately low circulating erythropoietin and a hyporeactive bone marrow.

Management of anemia

Reduction of red cell loss

Simple interventions to decrease sampling volumes are likely to decrease the prevalence of anemia and transfusion requirements, especially for sicker and longer term ICU patients [12, 40].

RBC transfusion

The established method for managing anemia in the ICU is allogeneic red cell transfusion. The key question in deciding how to use red cell transfusion in the ICU is identifying the *most appropriate transfusion trigger* and the *target hemoglobin range* for each patient. Several concepts are useful in deciding when to treat anemia using allogeneic red cell transfusion.

Critical hemoglobin concentration

The "critical hemoglobin concentration" is usually defined as the hemoglobin below which oxygen consumption (VO_2) is supply-dependent assuming normovolemia is maintained [41, 42]. This is unlikely to be a fixed value, but varies between organs and is dependent on the metabolic activity of the tissue and oxygen extraction capabilities. Studies in dogs, pigs, and baboons [43, 44] have demonstrated this critical Hb concentration in animal models to be around 4 g/dL.

A classic series of studies of acute normovolemic hemodilution in healthy volunteers and surgical patients suggest that the critical hemoglobin concentration in humans is <5 g/dL [45–47]. At these levels, there was no evidence of anaerobic metabolism based on lactate concentrations and whole body oxygen consumption. These studies are supported by case reports from Jehovah's Witness patients [48]. It is unclear how applicable these data are to critically ill patients, in whom cellular oxygen demand may be high, alterations to microcirculatory flow occur, and comorbidity is common [49].

Acceptable hemoglobin concentration during critical illness

An acceptable hemoglobin concentration is the degree of anemia that is the best balance between the risks of red cell transfusion and the risks of low hemoglobin concentration. There are three broad groups of evidence concerning the acceptable hemoglobin concentration for critically ill patients. The first is the TRICC trial [1], the second is cohort studies that have examined transfusion practice in critically ill groups of patients, and the third is pathophysiological studies that examined the effect of transfusions on indices of tissue hypoxia in critically ill patients.

The TRICC trial

This study showed that a restrictive transfusion strategy is at least as effective as and possibly superior to a liberal transfusion strategy in critically ill patients and provides compelling evidence that a hemoglobin concentration in the 7–9 g/dL range, using a trigger of 7 g/dL, is well tolerated by most critically ill patients and has no overall adverse effect on mortality [1]. Among patients aged <55 years and among the subgroup with admission APACHE II score <20, there was a statistically significantly better 30 days mortality among patients in the restrictive group. The study was not powered for subgroup analyses, but when these were carried out, there was no statistically or clinically important difference in ventilation times

[50] or in mortality for patients with cardiovascular disease [51]. The survival curves were reversed for the sub group of patients classified as having ischemic heart disease at study entry, although the severity and relation to the primary ICU diagnosis were unclear and the subgroup was small. This finding suggests uncertainty regarding the safety of restrictive transfusion triggers for patients with ischemic heart disease. Outcomes were also similar for the 203 patients admitted with trauma and a small cohort with brain injury [52]. Data from the TRICC trial indicate possible harm from RBC transfusions (or a benefit from anemia) during critical illness. Possible contributing factors include transfused leucocytes (the TRICC trial was carried out before universal leucodepletion), an adverse effect related to red cell storage (RBC storage age was typically >15 days), or an effect related to blood rheology. The difference in red cell exposure was 33% (100% liberal group vs 67% restrictive group) and mean difference in red cell use was 2.8 units (5.3 RBCs/patient vs 2.5 RBCs/patient). These data suggest that relatively small differences in RBC exposure could impact significantly on patient outcome. The mechanism for the difference in outcomes observed is unclear. There was an excess of cardiac complications in the liberal group and these patients also developed greater organ failures. Although increased infection is often associated with blood transfusions, infectious complications were similar between the groups.

The TRICC trial strongly supports the use of restrictive transfusion triggers and target hemoglobin of 7–9 g/dL in younger less severely ill patients. The trial findings are less certain for older sicker patients, especially those with cardiac comorbidity, but still support a restrictive use of blood transfusions in ICU patients.

Cohort studies examining the association between blood transfusions and outcomes during critical illness

There are many cohort trials investigating the association between patients' outcomes including mortality, infections, and hospital stay, and blood transfusions [53]. These observational studies are all potentially affected by confounding by other variables. Despite this, there is a strong signal associating adverse outcomes with receiving blood transfusions in most studies. Several studies have used propensity matching to evaluate the contribution of blood transfusions to outcome, although this is difficult for complex patient populations such as the critically ill. Early propensity matched studies found greater mortality in transfused versus nontransfused patients [2, 5], but this was not confirmed in a more recent study [54]. The introduction of leucodepletion could explain this difference over time. Systematic review and meta-analysis of leucodepletion trials show inconsistent effects on infections and mortality in critically ill and high-risk surgical populations [55, 56]. The largest study, undertaken around the introduction of universal leucodepletion to the Canadian blood service, showed a small (1%) reduction in mortality [57].

Overall, cohort studies strongly support the avoidance of blood transfusions in the critically ill whenever possible, and further support the TRICC trial findings.

Effect of blood transfusions on indices of tissue hypoxia during critical illness

When blood transfusions are administered to increase hemoglobin concentration in the absence of bleeding, the terms used in published studies to describe the indication include "diminished/reduced physiological reserve," "altered tissue perfusion," "tissue hypoxia," and "coronary disease" [5, 9]. These indicate a clinical concern that the patient either has or is at risk for tissue hypoxia or organ specific ischemia. These indications usually account for 40–80% of transfusion episodes in the ICU [2–5, 9].

Many studies have assessed the effect of blood transfusions on indices of tissue hypoxia during critical illness. These have used measures of ischemia at a "whole body" level such as VO_2, plasma or whole blood lactate concentration, mixed venous oxygen saturation (SvO_2), or mixed venous oxygen partial pressure (PvO_2). Regional indices include gastric tonometry derived indices (pHi and "PCO_2 gap"). The methodological quality, the baseline hemoglobin concentration, and the red cell product used varied widely between these studies. Despite this the majority of studies fail to demonstrate a clinically important improvement in measures of oxygenation, despite increasing calculated oxygen delivery [41, 58]. Even transfusion with very fresh red cells (storage age ≤5 days) did not improve clinical indices of tissue hypoxia in euvolemic critically ill patients [59]. These data show that although clinicians frequently transfuse because they are concerned about inadequate oxygen delivery to tissues, this does not usually result in measurable improvements using currently available indices of tissue hypoxia. These data also support the TRICC study findings that hemoglobin of 7–9 g/dL is safe for most critically ill patients.

Possible exceptions to the restrictive strategy used in the TRICC trial

The patient with chronic ischemic heart disease

The only published subgroup analysis for the TRICC trial in which the survival lines were reversed in favor of a liberal strategy, but with nonsignificant outcome difference, was for patients with ischemic heart disease at study entry [51]. The evidence for the safest transfusion trigger for patients with ischemic heart disease is inadequate and of particular concern to many clinicians [60]. This subject has been recently reviewed in detail [61]. Retrospective cohort studies have found associations between anemia and excess mortality among patients with nonacute coronary disease compared with patients without coronary disease at hemoglobin concentrations <9–10 g/dL [62, 63]. However, in the TRICC trial the numbers of adverse cardiac events was actually fewer in the restrictive group [1]. Specifically, the number of myocardial infarctions was smaller among the patients managed with restrictive transfusion triggers, who were more anemic during their critical illness.

Most experts agree that critically ill patients with chronic ischemic heart disease can be managed with a transfusion trigger of 7–8 g/dL, and a target hemoglobin of 7–9 g/dL, unless there is evidence of myocardial ischemia.

The patient with an acute coronary syndrome

The evidence for patients with acute coronary syndromes in the ICU is reviewed in Chapter 20.

Early severe sepsis

Goal directed therapy during early severe sepsis improved mortality in a single center randomized trial [64]. The intervention algorithm used central venous oxygen saturation <70% as a trigger for interventions to increase global oxygen delivery. Part of this algorithm was blood transfusion to maintain a hematocrit ≥30% (hemoglobin ≥10g/dL), but it is unclear how important this component was to improving mortality. The patients in the goal directed therapy group received significantly more blood transfusions and had a higher hemoglobin concentration. Several large multicenter studies are currently ongoing to evaluate the benefits of early goal-directed sepsis therapy. Until further studies are done, higher target hemoglobin concentrations of 9–10 g/dL (hematocrit 30%) should be considered for patients during the early phase of severe sepsis, but only if the central venous oxygen saturation is <70%. Current evidence only supports this higher target during the first 6 hours of resuscitation. After this, current evidence supports the restrictive approach used in the TRICC trial.

The patient with traumatic brain injury

There are clear associations between hypoxia, hypotension, inadequate resuscitation, and adverse outcomes from traumatic brain injury (TBI). The relationship between anemia during neurointensive care, following initial stabilization, and adverse outcomes is unclear. Expert opinion frequently suggests higher hemoglobin concentrations for these patients with the rationale of reducing cerebral ischemia. A subgroup analysis of the TRICC trial in 67 patients with TBI found no difference in 30-day mortality, but did not compare longer term neurological outcomes [52]. Several small studies found associations between blood transfusion and improvement in direct measures of cerebral oxygenation, but it was unclear whether these related to improved cerebral perfusion or were directly attributable to improvement in hemoglobin concentration [65, 66].

The current evidence base regarding safe hemoglobin concentration for patients with TBI (or other acute neurological injuries) is unclear.

Erythropoietin therapy

The inappropriate endogenous erythropoietin response to anemia found in critically ill patients makes exogenous administration a potential treatment. Studies have shown that exogenous erythropoietin concentration can increase reticulocyte counts in critically ill patients [23]. The optimum dose of erythropoietin, including the frequency of dosing, is unclear. Supplemental iron therapy is important, but the optimum dose and method of administration are also uncertain. Three large industry sponsored randomized placebo-controlled trials have evaluated the clinical effectiveness of erythropoietin in critically ill patients [22, 67, 68]. These are summarized in Table 39.5. These trials indicate that rHuEPO can increase hemoglobin compared to placebo treatment, but the effect on RBC use is small. Higher overall doses of rHuEPO with more frequent dosing were more effective that once weekly regimens. Inadequate iron supplementation, especially using the enteral route, may decrease the effectiveness of rHuEPO. A feature of these trials was the relatively low transfusion rate in the control group (50–60%) and the use of transfusion triggers significantly >7 g/dL. The most recent trial, in which transfusion practice was most restrictive, found no blood sparing effect. The clinical effectiveness of rHuEPO in patients at higher risk of transfusion is uncertain, particularly if more restrictive transfusion triggers are used. In the EPO-3 trial an increase in thrombotic events was found in rHuEPO treated patients, which is consistent with findings in other patient groups in whom concerns regarding the risk-benefit profile of rHuEPO have been raised. A decrease in mortality among trauma patients was also observed

Table 39.5 Summary of the three largest (industry sponsored) trials of erythropoietin in critical care.

Trial	Patients numbers	Erythropoietin regimen in intervention group	Outcome
EPO-1 study [67]	160	300 units/kg subcutaneously day 3 for 5 days, then alternate days for minimum 2 weeks or ICU discharge	Lower mean red cell use in rHuEPO group (2.1 vs 3.8 units per patient)
			Higher HCT in rHuEPO group at end of trial (35.1 vs 31.6) Lower transfusion exposure during study in rHuEPO group (45% vs 55%)
EPO-2 study [22]	1302 (medical, surgical, and trauma patients)	40,000 rHuEPO weekly from day 3 for 3 doses (fourth dose for patients in ICU on day 21)	10% reduction in transfusion exposure (60.4% vs 50.5%)
			19% reduction in red cell use per ICU day (0.6 red cell units per admission) No difference in mortality or reported adverse events (mortality rates 14–15%)
EPO-3 study [68]	1460 (stratified as trauma; non-trauma surgical; medical)	40 000 rHuEPO weekly up to 3 doses	No difference in red cell use overall or in subgroups
			Lower mortality in trauma patients receiving rHuEPO (3.5% vs 6.7%) Increase in thrombotic events in rHuEPO group

raising the possibility of nonerythrogenesis related benefits. A meta-analysis of all trials of rHuEPO in critically ill patients found that no overall effect on mortality. rHuEPO was associated with a decreased chance of receiving any blood transfusions (OR 0.73 (95% CI: 0.64–0.84)) and a mean decrease in RBC use of 0.41 units (0.10–0.74). It was noted that many of these studies were carried out before the widespread use of restrictive transfusion triggers, which would tend to decrease the treatment effect [69].

Two health economic evaluations of rHuEPO in the critically ill have been published, which come to opposite conclusions. Central to economic evaluation is the balance between the value of avoiding transfusion and the possible risks of receiving erythropoietin, neither of which are fully understood. In order to assess this balance high quality data concerning the attributable risks of both blood transfusions and erythropoietin therapy are needed in critically ill patients. Other than viral infection and transfusion errors, most data concerning transfusion risks, such as pneumonia or other infection, were generated from cohort studies of patients receiving nonleucodepleted blood and could be misleading. MacLaren and Sullivan [70] concluded that rHuEPO was cost effective against accepted parameters, but only if assumptions that allogeneic blood transfusions cause bacterial infections (common events in this population) were true. In contrast, Shermock and colleagues mainly considered viral infection, transfusion errors, and Transfusion Associated Lung Injury (rare events in this population) and found no evidence of cost effectiveness [71].

Conclusions and recommendations

Recommendations for the management of anemia during critical illness based on available evidence are summarized in Box 39.1. Further trials are required to define optimum use of blood during critical illness. Priority research questions include the management of elderly patients and those with chronic ischemic heart disease, the management of anemic patients with acute coronary syndromes, and the importance of the age of RBCs. The optimum management of anemia during recovery from critical illness requires investigation, because restrictive transfusion practice during ICU care results in a high prevalence of anemia following ICU discharge.

Summary

- Anemia is prevalent in critically ill patients
- The onset of anemia is rapid during the first 2–3 days of critical illness
- 40–50% of all critically ill patients receive RBC transfusions during ICU care
- Anemia persists into the post-ICU recovery period
- The etiology of the anemia of critical illness is multifactorial, and includes hemodilution, blood sampling, hemorrhage, and reduced RBC production
- Critically ill patients tolerate anemia levels of 7–9 g/dL without adversely effecting mortality and cardiorespiratory complications
- Younger (age <55 years) and less severely ill (APACHE II <20) patients benefit for transfusion avoidance using transfusion triggers of 7 g/dL
- There is less certainty regarding older patients and those with ischemic heart disease. In these cases decisions should be based on clinical judgment, but a target hemoglobin range of 7–9 g/dL is still appropriate in most cases
- Erythropoietin does not result in major reductions in RBC use, but the optimum dose and patient group, and a full understanding of the risk-benefit profile in the critically ill, are still uncertain. At present, erythropoietin is not licensed for use in critically ill patients as a blood-sparing agent

References

1. Hebert PC, Wells G, Blajchman MA, et al. A multicenter, randomized, controlled clinical trial of transfusion requirements in critical care. Transfusion Requirements in Critical Care Investigators, Canadian Critical Care Trials Group. N Engl J Med 1999;340(6):409–17.
2. Corwin HL, Gettinger A, Pearl RG, et al. The CRIT Study: anemia and blood transfusion in the critically ill–current clinical practice in the United States. Crit Care Med 2004;32(1):39–52.

3. French CJ, Bellomo R, Finfer SR, Lipman J, Chapman M, Boyce NW. Appropriateness of red blood cell transfusion in Australasian intensive care practice. Med J Aust 2002;177(10):548–51.
4. Rao MP, Boralessa H, Morgan C, et al. Blood component use in critically ill patients. Anaesthesia 2002;57(6):530–34.
5. Vincent JL, Baron JF, Reinhart K, et al. Anemia and blood transfusion in critically ill patients. JAMA 2002;288(12):1499–507.
6. Walsh TS, Garrioch M, Maciver C, et al. Red cell requirements for intensive care units adhering to evidence-based transfusion guidelines. Transfusion 2004;44(10):1405–11.
7. Walsh TS, Lee RJ, Maciver C, et al. Anaemia during and at discharge from intensive care: the impact of restrictive blood transfusion practice. Intensive Care Med 2006;32:100–109.
8. Nguyen BV, Bota DP, Melot C, Vincent JL. Time course of hemoglobin concentrations in nonbleeding intensive care unit patients. Crit Care Med 2003;31(2):406–10.
9. Chohan SS, McArdle F, McClelland DB, Mackenzie SJ, Walsh TS. Red cell transfusion practice following the transfusion requirements in critical care (TRICC) study: prospective observational cohort study in a large UK intensive care unit. Vox Sang 2003;84(3):211–18.
10. Walsh TS, Saleh EE, Lee RJ, McClelland DB. The prevalence and characteristics of anaemia at discharge home after intensive care. Intensive Care Med 2006;32(8):1206–13.
11. Henry ML, Garner WL, Fabri PJ. Iatrogenic anemia. Am J Surg 1986;151(3):362–3.
12. Smoller BR, Kruskall MS, Horowitz GL. Reducing adult phlebotomy blood loss with the use of pediatric-sized blood collection tubes. Am J Clin Pathol 1989;91(6):701–3.
13. Andrews NC. Anemia of inflammation: the cytokine-hepcidin link. J Clin Invest 2004;113(9):1251–3.
14. Eckardt KU. Anemia in critical illness. Wien Klin Wochenschr 2001;113(3–4):84–9.
15. Andrews T, Waterman H, Hillier V. Blood gas analysis: a study of blood loss in intensive care. J Adv Nurs 1999;30(4):851–7.
16. von Ahsen N, Muller C, Serke S, Frei U, Eckardt KU. Important role of nondiagnostic blood loss and blunted erythropoietic response in the anemia of medical intensive care patients. Crit Care Med 1999;27(12):2630–39.
17. Cook DJ, Griffith LE, Walter SD, et al. The attributable mortality and length of intensive care unit stay of clinically important gastrointestinal bleeding in critically ill patients. Crit Care 2001;5(6):368–75.
18. Pimentel M, Roberts DE, Bernstein CN, Hoppensack M, Duerksen DR. Clinically significant gastrointestinal bleeding in critically ill patients in an era of prophylaxis. Am J Gastroenterol 2000;95(10):2801–6.
19. Cook D, Heyland D, Griffith L, Cook R, Marshall J, Pagliarello J. Risk factors for clinically important upper gastrointestinal bleeding in patients requiring mechanical ventilation. Canadian Critical Care Trials Group. Crit Care Med 1999;27(12):2812–17.
20. Scharte M, Fink MP. Red blood cell physiology in critical illness. Crit Care Med 2003;31(Suppl. 12):S651–7.
21. Lang KS, Duranton C, Poehlmann H, et al. Cation channels trigger apoptotic death of erythrocytes. Cell Death Differ 2003;10(2):249–56.
22. Corwin HL, Gettinger A, Pearl RG, et al. Efficacy of recombinant human erythropoietin in critically ill patients: a randomized controlled trial. JAMA 2002;288(22): 2827–35.
23. van Iperen CE, Gaillard CA, Kraaijenhagen RJ, Braam BG, Marx JJ, van de WA. Response of erythropoiesis and iron metabolism to recombinant human erythropoietin in intensive care unit patients. Crit Care Med 2000;28(8):2773–8.
24. Corwin HL, Krantz SB. Anemia of the critically ill: "acute" anemia of chronic disease. Crit Care Med 2000;28(8):3098–9.
25. Biesma DH, van de WA, Beguin Y, Kraaijenhagen RJ, Marx JJ. Post-operative erythropoiesis is limited by the inflammatory effect of surgery on iron metabolism. Eur J Clin Invest 1995;25(6):383–9.
26. Rodriguez RM, Corwin HL, Gettinger A, Corwin MJ, Gubler D, Pearl RG. Nutritional deficiencies and blunted erythropoietin response as causes of the anemia of critical illness. J Crit Care 2001;16(1):36–41.
27. Weiss G, Goodnough LT. Anemia of chronic disease. N Engl J Med 2005;352(10):1011–23.
28. Hobisch-Hagen P, Wiedermann F, Mayr A, et al. Blunted erythropoietic response to anemia in multiply traumatized patients. Crit Care Med 2001;29(4):743–7.
29. Hutchinson C, Walsh TS, Black J, Ross JA. Soluble transferrin receptor assay as a marker of anaemia in critically ill patients. Br J Anaesth 2003;90(4):544P.
30. Goodnough LT, Skikne B, Brugnara C. Erythropoietin, iron, and erythropoiesis. Blood 2000;96(3):823–33.

31. Bellamy MC, Gedney JA. Unrecognised iron deficiency in critical illness. Lancet 1998;352(9144):1903.
32. Patteril MV, Davey-Quinn AP, Gedney JA, Murdoch SD, Bellamy MC. Functional iron deficiency, infection and systemic inflammatory response syndrome in critical illness. Anaesth Intensive Care 2001;29(5):473–8.
33. Beguin Y, Clemons GK, Pootrakul P, Fillet G. Quantitative assessment of erythropoiesis and functional classification of anemia based on measurements of serum transferrin receptor and erythropoietin. Blood 1993;81(4):1067–76.
34. Elliot JM, Virankabutra T, Jones S, et al. Erythropoietin mimics the acute phase response in critical illness. Crit Care 2003;7(3):R35–40.
35. Krafte-Jacobs B, Levetown ML, Bray GL, Ruttimann UE, Pollack MM. Erythropoietin response to critical illness. Crit Care Med 1994;22(5):821–6.
36. Rogiers P, Zhang H, Leeman M, et al. Erythropoietin response is blunted in critically ill patients. Intensive Care Med 1997;23(2):159–62.
37. Jelkmann W, Pagel H, Wolff M, Fandrey J. Monokines inhibiting erythropoietin production in human hepatoma cultures and in isolated perfused rat kidneys. Life Sci 1992;50(4):301–8.
38. Danielson B. R-HuEPO hyporesponsiveness–who and why? Nephrol Dial Transplant 1995; (Suppl. 10) 2:69–73.
39. Jongen-Lavrencic M, Peeters HR, Rozemuller H, et al. IL-6-induced anaemia in rats: possible pathogenetic implications for anemia observed in chronic inflammations. Clin Exp Immunol 1996;103(2):328–34.
40. O'Hare D, Chilvers RJ. Arterial blood sampling practices in intensive care units in England and Wales. Anaesthesia 2001;56(6):568–71.
41. McLellan SA, McClelland DB, Walsh TS. Anaemia and red blood cell transfusion in the critically ill patient. Blood Rev 2003;17(4):195–208.
42. Spahn DR, Casutt M. Eliminating blood transfusions: new aspects and perspectives. Anesthesiology 2000;93(1):242–55.
43. Rasanen J. Supply-dependent oxygen consumption and mixed venous oxyhemoglobin saturation during isovolemic hemodilution in pigs. Chest 1992;101(4):1121–4.
44. Van Der LP, Schmartz D, De Groote F, et al. Critical haemoglobin concentration in anaesthetized dogs: comparison of two plasma substitutes. Br J Anaesth 1998;81(4):556–62.
45. Leung JM, Weiskopf RB, Feiner J, et al. Electrocardiographic ST-segment changes during acute, severe isovolemic hemodilution in humans. Anesthesiology 2000;93(4):1004–10.
46. Weiskopf RB, Kramer JH, Viele M, et al. Acute severe isovolemic anemia impairs cognitive function and memory in humans. Anesthesiology 2000;92(6):1646–52.
47. Weiskopf RB, Viele MK, Feiner J, et al. Human cardiovascular and metabolic response to acute, severe isovolemic anemia. JAMA 1998;279(3):217–21.
48. Brimacombe J, Skippen P, Talbutt P. Acute anaemia to a haemoglobin of 14 g.l-1 with survival. Anaesth Intensive Care 1991;19(4):581–3.
49. Hebert PCM. The anemic patient in the intensive care unit: how much does the heart tolerate? Curr Opin Crit Care 2000;6(5):372–80.
50. Hebert PC, Blajchman MA, Cook DJ, et al. Do blood transfusions improve outcomes related to mechanical ventilation? Chest 2001;119(6):1850–57.
51. Hebert PC, Yetisir E, Martin C, et al. Is a low transfusion threshold safe in critically ill patients with cardiovascular diseases? Crit Care Med 2001;29(2):227–34.
52. McIntyre L, Hebert PC, Wells G, et al. Is a restrictive transfusion strategy safe for resuscitated and critically ill trauma patients? J Trauma 2004;57(3):563–8.
53. Marik PE, Corwin HL. Efficacy of red blood cell transfusion in the critically ill: a systematic review of the literature. Crit Care Med 2008;36(9):2667–74.
54. Vincent JL, Sakr Y, Sprung C, Harboe S, Damas P. Sepsis Occurence Acutely Ill Patie. Are blood transfusions associated with greater mortality rates? Anesthesiology 2008;108(1):31–9.
55. Vamvakas EC. WBC-containing allogeneic blood transfusion and mortality: a meta-analysis of randomized controlled trials. Transfusion 2003;43(7):963–73.
56. Vamvakas EC. White-blood-cell-containing allogeneic blood transfusion and postoperative infection or mortality: an updated meta-analysis. Vox Sang 2007;92(3):224–32.
57. Hebert PC, Fergusson D, Blajchman MA, et al. Clinical outcomes following institution of the Canadian universal leukoreduction program for red blood cell transfusions. JAMA 2003;289(15):1941–9.
58. Ho J, Sibbald WJ, Chin-Yee IH. Effects of storage on efficacy of red cell transfusion: when is it not safe? Crit Care Med 2003;31(12 Suppl.):S687–97.
59. Walsh TS, McArdle F, McLellan SA, et al. Does the storage time of transfused red blood cells influence regional or global indexes of tissue oxygenation in anemic critically ill patients? Crit Care Med 2004;32(2):364–71.

60. Walsh TS, McClelland DB, Lee RJ, et al. Prevalence of ischaemic heart disease at admission to intensive care and its influence on red cell transfusion thresholds: multicentre Scottish Study. Br J Anaesth 2005;94(4): 445–52.
61. Walsh TS, McClelland DB. When should we transfuse critically ill and perioperative patients with known coronary artery disease? Br J Anaesth 2003;90(6):719–22.
62. Carson JL, Duff A, Poses RM, et al. Effect of anaemia and cardiovascular disease on surgical mortality and morbidity. Lancet 1996;348(9034):1055–60.
63. Hebert PC, Wells G, Tweeddale M, et al. Does transfusion practice affect mortality in critically ill patients? Transfusion Requirements in Critical Care (TRICC) Investigators and the Canadian Critical Care Trials Group. Am J Respir Crit Care Med 1997;155(5):1618–23.
64. Rivers E, Nguyen B, Havstad S, et al. Early goal-directed therapy in the treatment of severe sepsis and septic shock. N Engl J Med 2001;345(19): 1368–77.
65. Leal-Noval SR, Rincon-Ferrari MD, et al. Transfusion of erythrocyte concentrates produces a variable increment on cerebral oxygenation in patients with severe traumatic brain injury – a preliminary study. Intensive Care Med 2006;32(11):1733–40.
66. Smith MJ, Stiefel MF, Magge S, et al. Packed red blood cell transfusdon increases local cerebral oxygenation. Crit Care Med 2005;33(5):1104–8.
67. Corwin HL, Gettinger A, Rodriguez RM, et al. Efficacy of recombinant human erythropoietin in the critically ill patient: a randomized, double-blind, placebo-controlled trial. Crit Care Med 1999;27(11):2346–50.
68. Corwin HL, Gettinger A, Fabian TC, et al. Efficacy and safety of epoetin alfa in critically ill patients. N Engl J Med 2007;357(10):965–76.
69. Zarychanski R, Turgeon AF, McIntyre L, Fergusson DA. Erythropoietin-receptor agonists in critically ill patients: a meta-analysis of randomized controlled trials. Can Med Assoc J 2007;177(7):725–34.
70. MacLaren R, Sullivan PW. Cost-effectiveness of recombinant human erythropoietin for reducing red blood cells transfusions in critically ill patients. Value Health 2005;8(2):105–16.
71. Shermock KM, Horn E, Lipsett PA, Pronovost PJ, Dorman T. Number needed to treat and cost of recombinant human erythropoietin to avoid one transfusion-related adverse event in critically ill patients. Crit Care Med 2005;33(3):497–503.

CHAPTER 40

Red Blood Cell Transfusions and Alternatives to Treat the Anemia of Prematurity

Ronald G. Strauss
University of Iowa College of Medicine, DeGowin Blood Center, University of Iowa Hospitals, Iowa City, IA, USA

Introduction

Several aspects of erythropoiesis that occur during the third trimester of gestation in term neonates (e.g., placental iron transport from the mother and high rates of erythropoiesis) are abbreviated in extremely preterm neonates. In addition, premature birth often is complicated by serious medical problems that are accompanied by phlebotomy, blood losses for laboratory testing, bleeding, and/or hemolysis which, in the setting of immature hematopoiesis, mandate red blood cell (RBC) transfusions. Extremely preterm neonates—particularly, those with birth weight <1.0 kg—nearly always receive allogeneic RBC transfusions [1]. Transfusion practices for neonates are controversial, vary from center to center, and often are based, largely, on logical assumptions. Although well-designed controlled clinical trials are being reported, they are not always mutually supportive and questions remain [2, 3]. Because firm indications for neonatal RBC transfusions do not exist, it is important to consider the underlying pathophysiology of anemia during infancy, the goals of transfusion and alternative therapies, and all aspects of the benefit to risk ratio, when making therapeutic decisions—particularly, whether or not and when to transfuse RBCs.

Although alternatives to allogeneic RBC transfusions exist for preterm infants (e.g., recombinant human erythropoietin [rHuEPO] and the transfusion of "autologous" placental blood), they are controversial because of unproven or incomplete efficacy and potential toxicities that are incompletely defined [1,4]. Accordingly, allogeneic RBC transfusions remain as the foundation of treatment for the anemia of prematurity. The mechanisms responsible for the anemia of prematurity and the possible therapeutic approaches will be critically analyzed in this chapter.

Pathophysiology of the anemia of prematurity

All infants experience a decline in circulating RBCs during the first weeks of life. This decline results both from physiological factors and, in sick preterm infants, from phlebotomy blood losses for laboratory testing. In healthy term infants, the nadir hemoglobin value rarely falls below 10 g/dL at an age of 10–12 weeks. This decline is more rapid (i.e., nadir at 4–6 weeks of age) and the blood hemoglobin concentration falls to lower levels in infants born prematurely—to approximately 8 g/dL in infants with birth weights of 1.0–1.5 kg and to approximately 7 g/dL in infants with birth weights <1 kg [1]. Because this postnatal drop in hemoglobin level in term infants is well tolerated and requires no therapy, it is commonly

Alternatives to Blood Transfusion in Transfusion Medicine, 2nd edition. Edited by A. Maniatis, P. Van der Linden, J.-F. Hardy.

referred to as the "physiological anemia of infancy." However, because the pronounced decline in hemoglobin concentration that occurs in many extremely preterm infants is associated with abnormal clinical signs and need for allogeneic RBC transfusions, the "anemia of prematurity" is not accepted as a normal, benign event [5].

Physiological factors play a role in the pathogenesis of the anemia of prematurity. Growth is extremely rapid during the first months of life, and RBC production by neonatal marrow must increase commensurately. It is widely accepted that the circulating life span of neonatal RBCs in the bloodstream is shorter than that of adult RBCs. However, this may be an artifact, in part, because studies of transfused autologous RBCs labeled with biotin or radioactive chromium may underestimate RBC survival in the infant's bloodstream for technical reasons [6]. In healthy adults—where body size is stable so that blood and RBC volumes are constant (i.e., not increasing with growing body size and commensurate increase in erythropoiesis), when no transfusions are given, and when large volumes of blood are not being taken for laboratory studies—the gradual disappearance of transfused labeled RBCs, caused by dilution with RBCs produced by the bone marrow, accurately reflects RBC survival in the bloodstream. In contrast, one or more of these confounding factors (i.e., growth, RBC transfusions, phlebotomy) exists in infants—particularly, sick preterms—to introduce error into the calculations performed when determining RBC survival, on the basis of disappearance of labeled RBCs.

A key reason that the hemoglobin nadir is lower in preterm than in term infants is the former group's diminished plasma erythropoietin (EPO) level in response to anemia [7]. Although anemia provokes EPO production in premature infants, the plasma levels achieved in anemic infants, at any given hematocrit (HCT), are lower than those observed in comparably anemic older persons [8]. Erythroid progenitor cells of preterm infants are quite responsive to EPO in vitro—a finding suggesting that inadequate production EPO is the major cause of physiological anemia, not marrow unresponsiveness [9].

The mechanisms responsible for the diminished EPO output by preterm neonates are only partially defined and, likely, are multiple. One mechanism is that the primary site of EPO production in preterm infants is in the liver, rather than kidney [10]. This dependency on hepatic EPO is important because the liver is less sensitive to anemia and tissue hypoxia—hence, a relatively sluggish EPO response to the falling HCT. The timing of the switch from liver to kidney is set at conception and is not accelerated by preterm birth. Viewed from a teleological perspective, decreased hepatic production of EPO under in utero conditions of tissue hypoxia may be an advantage for the fetus. If this were not the case, normal levels of fetal hypoxia in utero could trigger high levels of EPO and produce erythrocytosis and consequent hyperviscosity. Following birth, however, diminished EPO responsiveness to tissue hypoxia is disadvantageous and leads to anemia because it impairs compensation for low HCT levels caused by rapid growth, RBC losses due to phlebotomy, clinical bleeding, hemolysis, etc.

Diminished EPO production cannot entirely explain low plasma EPO levels in preterm infants because extraordinarily high plasma levels of EPO have been reported in some fetuses and infants [11,12]. Moreover, macrophages from human cord blood produce normal quantities of EPO messenger RNA and protein [13]. Thus, additional mechanisms contribute to diminished EPO plasma levels. For example, plasma levels of EPO are influenced by metabolism (clearance) as well as by production. Data in human infants [14] have demonstrated low plasma EPO levels due to increased plasma clearance, increased volume of distribution, more rapid fractional elimination, and shorter mean plasma residence times than comparative values in adults. Thus, accelerated catabolism accentuates the problem of diminished EPO production, so that the low plasma EPO levels are a combined effect of decreased synthesis plus increased metabolism.

Phlebotomy blood losses play a key role in the anemia of prematurity, particularly in the first few weeks. The modern practice of neonatology requires critically ill neonates to be monitored closely with serial laboratory studies such as blood gases, electrolytes, blood counts, and cultures. Small preterm infants are the most critically ill, require the most frequent blood sampling, and suffer the greatest proportional loss of RBCs because their circulating RBC volumes are smallest. In the past, the mean volume of blood removed for sampling has been reported to range from 0.8 to 3.1 mL/kg per day during the first few weeks of life for preterm infants requiring intensive care [15]. Promising "in-line" devices that withdraw blood, measure multiple analytes, and then reinfuse the sampled blood have been reported [16, 17]. They have decreased the need for RBC transfusions. However, until these devices are proven more extensively to be effective and safe, replacement of blood losses due to phlebotomy will remain a critical factor responsible for RBC transfusions given to critically ill neonates, particularly transfusions given during the first 4 weeks of life.

Table 40.1 Allogeneic RBC transfusions for the anemia of prematurity.

Maintain infant blood HCT per clinical status
>40% (35–45%*) for severe cardiopulmonary disease
>30% for moderate cardiopulmonary disease
>30% for major surgery
>25% (20–25%*) for symptomatic anemia
> 20% (not at all*) for asymptomatic anemia

*Reflects practices that vary among neonatologists.

RBC transfusions for the anemia of prematurity

Guidelines for transfusing RBCs to preterm neonates are controversial, and practices vary [1, 18–20]. This lack of a consistent approach stems from limited knowledge of the cellular and molecular biology of erythropoiesis during the perinatal period, an incomplete understanding of infant responses to anemia, and lack of definitive transfusion practice guidelines based on well-designed clinical trials. Generally, RBC transfusions are given to maintain a level of blood hemoglobin or HCT believed to be optimal for each neonate's clinical condition. Guidelines for RBC transfusions, judged to be reasonable by most neonatologists to treat the anemia of prematurity, are listed by Table 40.1. These guidelines are very general, and it is important that terms such as "severe" and "symptomatic" be defined to fit local transfusion practices/policies.

An important controversy that is still unresolved is the wisdom or lack, thereof of prescribing RBC transfusions to neonates using restrictive guidelines (i.e., low pretransfusion HCT values) versus liberal guidelines (i.e., conventional, relatively-high pretransfusion HCT values). Two randomized, controlled trials have been published and, although many of their results agree, they disagree in one extremely important way—specifically, whether preterm infants are at increased risk of brain injury when given RBC transfusions per restrictive guidelines [2, 3]. In both trials, preterm infants were randomly allocated to receive all small-volume RBC transfusions per either restrictive or liberal guidelines—with guidelines based on a combination of the pretransfusion HCT or hemoglobin level, age of the neonate, and clinical condition at the time each transfusion was given. Both studies found that neonates in the restrictive transfusions group received fewer RBC transfusions, without an increase in mortality or in morbidity based on several clinical outcomes. However, one critical discrepancy was present. Bell et al. [2] found increases in apnea, intraventricular bleeding, and brain leukomalacia in infants transfused per restrictive guidelines, whereas, Kirpalani et al. [3] found no differences between infants in the restrictive versus liberal groups. Moreover, rates of serious outcomes were fairly high in both groups of the Kirpalani study, perhaps, due to the extreme prematurity of the infants [3]. However, because neonates in the liberal RBC transfusion group of Bell et al. [2] likely had substantially higher blood HCT/hemoglobin levels than neonates in either of the groups of Kirpalani et al. [3], it is reasonable to speculate that the higher blood HCT levels, in some way, protected liberally transfused infants. Until more information is available, it seems wise to transfuse preterm neonates using conventional, relatively liberal guidelines (i.e., do not place infants at possible risks of undertransfusion).

Most RBC transfusions given to preterm neonates are small in volume (10–15 mL/kg) and are repeated frequently to maintain a HCT level deemed appropriate for each infant's clinical condition at the time of transfusion (Table 40.1). In neonates with severe respiratory disease, such as those requiring high volumes of oxygen with ventilator support, it is customary to maintain the HCT above 40% (hemoglobin concentration above 13 g/dL)—particularly when blood is being drawn frequently for testing. Some believe the HCT should be kept even higher [2]. This practice is based on the belief that transfused donor RBCs, containing adult hemoglobin, will provide optimal oxygen delivery throughout the period of diminished pulmonary function. Consistent with this rationale for ensuring optimal oxygen delivery in neonates with pulmonary failure, it seems logical to maintain the HCT above 40% in infants with congenital heart disease that is severe enough to cause either cyanosis or congestive heart failure.

Definitive studies are not available to establish the optimal HCT for neonates facing major surgery. However, it seems reasonable to maintain the HCT >30% because of limited ability of the neonate's heart, lungs, and vasculature to compensate for anemia. Additional factors include the inferior offloading of oxygen to tissues by the infant's own RBCs due to the diminished interaction between fetal hemoglobin and 2,3-DPG plus the developmental impairment of neonatal pulmonary, renal, hepatic, and neurological function. Because this transfusion guideline is simply a recommendation—not a firm indication—it should be applied with flexibility to individual infants facing surgical procedures of varying complexity (i.e., minor surgery may be judged not to require an HCT >30%).

The clinical indications for RBC transfusions in preterm infants who are not critically ill but, nonetheless, develop moderate anemia (HCT <24% or blood hemoglobin level <8 g/dL) are extremely variable. In general, infants who are clinically stable with modest anemia do not require RBC transfusions, unless they exhibit significant clinical problems that are ascribed to the presence of anemia or are predicted to be corrected by donor RBCs. As an example of such a clinical problem (reviewed in references 20, 21), proponents of RBC transfusions to treat disturbances of cardiopulmonary rhythms believe that a low blood level of RBCs contributes to tachypnea, dyspnea, apnea, and tachycardia, or bradycardia because of decreased oxygen delivery to the respiratory center of the brain. Transfusions of RBCs might decrease the number of apneic spells by improving oxygen delivery to the central nervous system. However, results of clinical studies have been contradictory [2, 20, 21].

Another controversial clinical indication for RBC transfusions is to maintain a reasonable HCT level as treatment for unexplained growth failure. Some neonatologists consider poor weight gain to be an indication for RBC transfusion, particularly if the HCT is <25% and if other signs of distress are evident (e.g., tachycardia, respiratory difficulty, weak suck, and cry, diminished activity). In this setting, growth failure has been ascribed to the increase in metabolic expenditure required to support the work of labored breathing. In the past, a HCT below 30% was of concern and often led to transfusion. However, results of clinical studies have not supported this practice [20, 21], and no apparent rationale exists to justify maintaining any predetermined HCT level by prophylactic, small-volume RBC transfusions in stable, growing infants who seem to be otherwise healthy.

In practice, the decision of whether or not to transfuse RBCs is based on the desire to maintain the HCT concentration at a level judged to be most beneficial for the infant's clinical condition. Investigators who believe this "clinical" approach is too imprecise have suggested the use of "physiological" criteria such as red cell mass [22], available oxygen [23], mixed venous oxygen saturation, and measurements of oxygen delivery and utilization [24] to develop guidelines for transfusion decisions. In one study of 10 human infants with severe (oxygen-dependent) bronchopulmonary dysplasia, improvement of physiological end points was shown (increased systemic oxygen transport and decreased oxygen use) as a consequence of small-volume RBC transfusions [24]. However, these promising but technically demanding methods are, at present, difficult to apply in the day-to-day practice of neonatology. The application, in infants, of data obtained from studies of animals and adult humans that correlate tissue oxygenation with the clinical effects of anemia and the need for RBC transfusions is confounded by the differences between infants and adults in hemoglobin oxygen affinity, ability to increase cardiac output, and regional patterns of blood flow. Another physiological factor, considered in transfusion decisions, is use of the circulating RBC volume/mass rather than the blood HCT or hemoglobin level. Although circulating RBC/mass is a potentially useful index of the blood's oxygen-carrying capacity, it cannot be predicted accurately from blood HCT or hemoglobin concentration levels; hence, it must be measured directly [25, 26]. Unfortunately, circulating RBC volume/mass measurements and other "physiologically" criteria for RBC transfusions are not widely available for clinical use.

Alternatives to neonatal RBC transfusions

Recognition of low plasma EPO levels and adequate erythropoietic activity in preterm infants provides a rational basis to consider rHuEPO as treatment for the anemia of prematurity. Because the inadequate quantity of EPO is the major cause of anemia, not a subnormal response of erythroid progenitors to EPO, it is logical to assume that rHuEPO will correct EPO deficiency and will effectively treat the anemia of prematurity. Unfortunately, rHuEPO has not been widely accepted in clinical neonatology practice because its efficacy is incomplete. On one hand, clonogenic erythroid progenitors from neonates respond well to rHuEPO in vitro and rHuEPO and iron effectively stimulate erythropoiesis in vivo as evidenced by increased blood reticulocyte and RBC counts in recipient infants (i.e., efficacy successful at the marrow level). On the other hand, when the primary goal of rHuEPO therapy is to eliminate RBC transfusions, rHuEPO often fails (i.e., efficacy at the clinical level has not been consistently successful) [4, 27].

By the end of 1999, over 20 controlled clinical trials assessing the efficacy of rHuEPO to eliminate RBC transfusions in the anemia of prematurity were published with inconsistent results. To investigate the extent and reasons for the inconsistencies, a meta-analysis was conducted of the controlled clinical studies published between 1990 and 1999 [27]. To be included, a reported study had to prospectively enroll a treatment group of preterm infants under 4 months of age treated with rHuEPO and a concurrent control group not given rHuEPO. Twenty-one reports were eligible for inclusion in the meta-analysis. However, because the experimental design and conduct of the studies was extremely variable, only four reports were judged to fulfill all of the highly desired characteristics of being effectively blinded, having high quality experimental design (i.e., randomized, placebo-controlled, all dropouts well-explained, etc.), using conservative RBC transfusion practices (rather than liberal transfusions which suppress endogenous erythropoiesis), and enrolling a majority of very preterm infants with birth weight <1.0 kg.

Two major conclusions emerged from the meta-analysis [27]. First, the controlled trials of rHuEPO to treat the anemia of prematurity differed from one another in multiple ways and, consequently, produced markedly variable results that could not be adequately explained. Hence, it was judged premature to make firm recommendations regarding use of rHuEPO in clinical practice to treat the anemia of prematurity. Second, when the four studies with highly desired characteristics were analyzed separately, rHuEPO was found to be efficacious in significantly reducing RBC transfusion needs. However, the magnitude of the effect of rHuEPO on reducing the total RBC transfusions given to infants throughout their initial hospitalization was, in fact, relatively modest and of questionable clinical importance. For example, in one trail, significantly fewer RBC transfusions were given during the study period to rHuEPO-treated infants than to placebo-treated controls (mean of 1.1 transfusions per infant vs 1.6, respectively), but rHuEPO exerted only a modest effect on overall RBC transfusion needs during the entire hospitalization (mean of 4.4 transfusions per infant for rHuEPO-treated infants vs 5.3 for placebo-treated infants) [27]. Although the meta-analysis was unable to recommend how to use rHuEPO in clinical practices, it was apparent that, 1) relatively large or stable preterm infants, shown to respond best to rHuEPO plus iron at the marrow level, are given relatively few RBC transfusions with today's conservative transfusion practices and, accordingly, have little need for rHuEPO when the goal is to avoid RBC transfusions; and 2) extremely small preterm infants, who are critically ill and unstable, have not consistently responded to rHuEPO plus iron when the outcome measure is to reduce need for RBC transfusions.

Because meta-analysis has not given firm guidelines for the use of rHuEPO, neonatologists must determine if more recent publications will facilitate evidence-based decision making for this issue. Several reports published after 2000 have provided useful information. Donato et al. [28] randomized 114 neonates with birth weight <1.25 kg to receive either rHuEPO or placebo during the first 2 weeks of life, followed by a 6 week treatment period during which all infants were given rHuEPO, iron, and folic acid. During the first 3 weeks of life, rHuEPO increased reticulocytes and HCT values, but there was no difference in RBC transfusions. However, at the end of all treatment (8 weeks), a subgroup of infants with birth weight <0.8 kg and phlebotomy losses >30 mL/kg, given rHuEPO shortly after birth, received fewer total RBC transfusions than infants initially given placebo (3.4 ± 1.1 vs 5.4 ± 3.7, $p < 0.05$). Similarly, Yeo et al. [29] found a modest advantage for a subgroup of very low birth weight infants given rHuEPO. Infants with birth weight 0.8–0.99 kg were given fewer RBC transfusions with rHuEPO than control infants not given rHuEPO (2.1 ± 1.9 vs 3.5 ± 1.6, $p < 0.04$). A randomized, blinded trial by Meyer et al. [30] found an advantage for very low birth weight infants given rHuEPO. Neonates with birth weight <1.7 kg plus criteria that predicted a likely need for RBC transfusions were randomized either to receive rHuEPO beginning shortly after birth or to experience a sham treatment to simulate placebo injections. Iron was given to all infants, but at a much lower dose (unfortunately) to control infants not given rHuEPO than to infants given rHuEPO, thus creating two variables/differences (rHuEPO and iron dose, rather than just rHuEPO) being assessed in treated versus control infants. There was no overall difference in RBC transfusions, but in a subset of infants with birth weight <1.0 kg, RBC transfusions given late (i.e., after 30 days of age) were reduced by rHuEPO versus controls (0.5 ± 0.7 vs 1.6 ± 1.1, $p = 0.01$).

Two reports defined rHuEPO "success" as maintaining an HCT of ≥30% without need for any RBC transfusions. Maier et al. [31] randomized 219 neonates with birth weights 0.5–0.99 kg to receive either early rHuEPO (from the first week of life for 9 weeks), late rHuEPO (from the fourth week of life for 6 weeks), or no rHuEPO. "Success" was modest (13% with early rHuEPO, 11% with late rHuEPO, 4% with no rHuEPO). Only early rHuEPO infants were significantly superior to no rHuEPO ($p = 0.026$). Avent et al. [32] randomized 93 neonates with birth weight 0.9–1.5 kg to receive either low dose rHuEPO (250 units/kg) high dose rHuEPO (400 units/kg), or no rHuEPO. Treatment began within 7 days of life and continued until discharge (median 32 days and maximum 74 days). "Success" was met by 75% of low dose rHuEPO infants, 71% of high dose rHuEPO, and 40% of no rHuEPO infants ($p < 0.001$). Interestingly, the number of RBC transfusions given to all infants treated with rHuEPO versus those with no rHuEPO was not significantly different. The authors concluded that rHuEPO does not significantly decrease RBC transfusions in infants, birth weight 0.9–1.5 kg, when phlebotomy losses are small and RBC transfusions are given per stringent transfusion guidelines.

The observation by Avent et al. [32] that the benefits of rHuEPO in reducing the number of RBC transfusions given can be equalled by stringent/conservative transfusion guidelines has been made by others. Franz and Pohlandt [33] assessed both the number of RBC transfusions given and RBC transfusion guidelines in four prospective, randomized trials of rHuEPO given to preterm neonates. To be selected for analysis, the clinical trials had to include ventilated infants (i.e., sick infants likely to receive RBC transfusions). The authors found that, when restrictive transfusion guidelines were followed, the number of RBC transfusions and the volume of RBCs transfused were similarly low in infants either given or not given rHuEPO [33]. Similarly, Amin and Alzahrani [34] found no difference in the number of RBC transfusions, whether or not rHuEPO was given to preterm infants with birth weight ≤1.0 kg, when

RBC transfusions were given per strict transfusion guidelines.

Another alternative to allogeneic RBC transfusions is use of placental blood as a source of autologous RBCs [35, 36]. Although collection, storage, and transfusion of placental blood postdelivery deserves careful consideration, at least three obstacles must be overcome before autologous transfusions of stored placental RBCs can be adopted for clinical use. One concern is that a sufficient quantity of RBCs will not be obtained consistently from placentas of preterm infants to avoid later allogeneic transfusions. The second issue is the sterility of placental blood. Since bacterial contamination of placental blood is a distinct possibility [35], extensive testing will be needed to ensure absolute safety. Finally, acceptable quality of stored placental blood must be maintained [36]. Because of these concerns collection and storage of placental blood has not been encouraged [37]. Instead, interest has been renewed in delayed clamping of the umbilical cord immediately postdelivery to expand neonatal blood volume and RBC volume/mass to, possibly, improve circulatory hemodynamics and increase tissue perfusion/oxygenation [26, 38, 39].

Acknowledgment

Supported in part by NIH Program Project Grant: P01 HL46925.

Note added in proof: After preparation of this manuscript, a paper was published which critically analyzed the controversy surrounding the transfusion of preterm neonates per liberal versus restricted guidelines (Strauss RG: 2008 Emily Cooley Lecture: Lessons learned from pediatric transfusion medicine clinical trials . . . a little child shall lead them. Transfusion 2009;49:1996–2004).

References

1. Strauss RG. Managing the anemia of prematurity: red blood cell transfusions versus recombinant erythropoietin. Transfus Med Rev 2001;15:213–23.
2. Bell EF, Strauss RG, Widness JA, et al. Randomized trial of liberal versus restrictive guidelines for red blood cell transfusions in preterm infants. Pediatrics 2005;115:1685–91.
3. Kirpalani H, Whyte RK, Andersen C, et al. The Premature Infants in Need of Transfusion (PINT) study: a randomized, controlled trial of a restrictive (low) versus liberal (high) transfusion threshold for extremely low birth weight infants. J Pediatr 2006;149:301–7.
4. Strauss RG. RBC transfusion and/or recombinant EPO therapy of the anemia of prematurity. ISBT Sci Ser 2006;1:11–14.
5. Wardrop CA, Holland BM, Veale KE, Jones JG, Gray OP. Nonphysiological anaemia of prematurity. Arch Dis Child 1978;53:855–60.
6. Strauss RG, Mock DM, Widness JA, Johnson K, Cress G, Schmidt RL. Post-transfusion 24-hour recovery and subsequent survival of allogeneic red blood cells in the bloodstream of newborn infants. Transfusion 2004;44:871–6.
7. Stockman JA, III, Graeber JE, Clark DA, McClellan K, Garcia JF, Kavey RE. Anemia of prematurity: determinants of the erythropoietin response. J Pediatr 1984;105:786–92.
8. Brown MS, Garcia JF, Phibbs RH, Dallman PR. Decreased response of plasma immunoreactive erythropoietin to "available oxygen" in anemia of prematurity. J Pediatr 1984;105:793–8.
9. Rhondeau SM, Christensen RD, Ross MP, Rothstein G, Simmons MA. Responsiveness to recombinant human erythropoietin of marrow erythroid progenitors from infants with the "anemia of prematurity". J Pediatr 1988;112:935–40.
10. Dame C, Fahnenstich H, Freitag P, et al. Erythropoietin mRNA expression in human fetal and neonatal tissue. Blood 1998;92:3218–25.
11. Snijders RJ, Abbas A, Melby O, Ireland RM, Nicolaides KH. Fetal plasma erythropoietin concentration in severe growth retardation. Am J Obstet Gynecol 1993;168:615–19.
12. Widness JA, Susa JB, Garcia JF, et al. Increased erythropoiesis and elevated erythropoietin in infants born to diabetic mothers and in hyperinsulinemic rhesus fetuses. J Clin Invest 1981;67:637–42.
13. Ohls RK, Li Y, Trautman MS, Christensen RD. Erythropoietin production by macrophages from preterm infants: implications regarding the cause of the anemia in prematurity. Pediatr Res 1994;35:169–70.
14. Widness JA, Veng-Pedersen P, Peters C, Pereira LM, Schmidt RL, Lowe LS. Erythropoietin pharmacokinetics in premature infants: developmental, nonlinearity, and treatment effects. J Appl Physiol 1996;80: 140–48.

15. Obladen M, Sachsenweger M, Stahnke M. Blood sampling in very low birth weight infants receiving different levels of intensive care. Eur J Pediatr 1988;147:399–404.
16. Widness JA, Madan A, Grindeanu LA, Zimmerman MB, Wong DK, Stevenson DK. Reduction in red blood cell transfusions among preterm infants: results of a randomized trial with an in-line blood gas and chemistry monitor. Pediatrics 2005;115:1299–306.
17. Madan A, Kumar R, Adams MM, Benitz WE, Geaghan SM, Widness JA. Reduction in red blood cell transfusions using a bedside analyzer in extremely low birth weight infants. J Perinatol 205;25: 2–25.
18. Ringer SA, Richardson DK, Sacher RA, Keszler M, Churchill WH. Variations in transfusion practice in neonatal intensive care. Pediatrics 1998;101:194–200.
19. Bednarek FJ, Weisberger S, Richardson DK, Frantz ID, III, Shah B, Rubin LP, for the SNAP II Study Group. Variations in blood transfusions among newborn intensive care units. J Pediatr 1998;133:601–7.
20. Ramasethu J, Luban NL. Red blood cell transfusions in the newborn. Semin Neonatol 1999;4:5–16.
21. Strauss RG. Red blood cell transfusion practices in the neonate. Clin Perinatol 1995;22:641–55.
22. Phillips HM, Holland BM, Abdel-Moiz A, et al. Determination of red-cell mass in assessment and management of anaemia in babies needing blood transfusion. Lancet 1986;1:882–4.
23. Jones JG, Holland BM, Veale KE, Wardrop CA. "Available oxygen," a realistic expression of the ability of the blood to supply oxygen to tissues. Scand J Haematol 1979;22:77–82.
24. Alverson DC, Isken VH, Cohen RS. Effect of booster blood transfusions on oxygen utilization in infants with bronchopulmonary dysplasia. J Pediatr 1988;113:722–6.
25. Strauss RG, Mock DM, Widness JA, Johnson K, Cress G, Schmidt RL. Post-transfusion 24-hour recovery and subsequent survival of allogeneic red blood cells in the bloodstream of newborn infants. Transfusion 2004;44:871–6.
26. Strauss RG, Mock DM, Johnson K, et al. Circulating red blood cell (RBC) volume, measured using biotinylated RBCs, is superior to the hematocrit to document the hematologic effects of delayed versus immediate umbilical cord clamping in preterm neonates. Transfusion 2003;43:1168–72.
27. Vamvakas EC, Strauss RG. Meta-analysis of controlled clinical trials studying the efficacy of recombinant human erythropoietin in reducing blood transfusions in the anemia of prematurity. Transfusion 2001;41:406–15.
28. Donato H, Vain N, Rendo P, et al. Effect of early versus late administration of human recombinant erythropoietin on transfusion requirements in premature infants: results of a randomized, placebo-controlled, multicenter trial. Pediatrics 2000;105:1066–72.
29. Yeo CL, Choo S, Ho LY. Effect of recombinant human erythropoietin on transfusion needs in preterm infants. J Paediatr Child Health 2001;37:352–8.
30. Meyer MP Sharma E, Carsons M. Recombinant erythropoietin and blood transfusion in selected preterm infants. Arch Dis Child Fetal Neonatal Ed 2003;88:F41–5.
31. Maier RE, Obladen M, Müller-Hansen I, et al. on behalf of the European Multicenter Erythrpoietin Beta Study Group. Early treatment with erythropoietin b ameliorates anemia and reduces transfusion requirements in infants with birth weights below 1000 g. J Pediatr 2002;141:8–15.
32. Avent M, Cory BJ, Galpin J, et al. A comparison of high versus low dose recombinant human erythropoietin versus blood transfusion in the management of anemia of prematurity in a developing country. J Trop Pediatr 2002;48:227–33.
33. Franz AR, Pohlandt F. Red blood cell transfusions in very and extremely low birthweight infants under restrictive transfusion guidelines: is exogenous erythropoietin necessary? Arch Dis Child Fetal Neonatal Ed 2001;84:F96–100.
34. Amin AA, Alzahrani DM. Efficacy of erythropoietin in premature infants. Saudi Med J 2002;23:287–90.
35. Anderson A, Fangman J, Wager G, Uden D. Retrieval of placental blood from the umbilical vein to determine volume, sterility, and presence of clot formation. Am J Dis Child 1992;146:36–9.
36. Bifano EM, Dracker RA, Lorah K, Palit A. Collection and 28-day storage of human placental blood. Pediatr Res 1994;36:90–94.
37. Strauss RG. Autologous transfusions for neonates using placental blood. A cautionary note. Am J Dis Chil 1992;146:21–2.
38. Kinmond S, Aitchison TC, Holand BM, Jones JG, Turner TL, Wardrop CA. Umbilical cord clamping and preterm infants: a randomized trial. Br Med J 1993;306:172–5.
39. Mercer JS, Vohr BR, McGrath MM, Padbury JF, Wallach M, Oh W. Delayed cord clamping in very preterm infants reduces the incidence of intraventricular hemorrhage and late-onset sepsis: a randomized, controlled trial. Pediatrics 2006;117:1235–42.

CHAPTER 41

Transfusion Alternatives in Orthopedic Surgery

Manuel Muñoz[1], *José Antonio García-Erce*[2] *& Jorge Cuenca*[3]
[1]Transfusion Medicine, School of Medicine, University of Málaga, Málaga, Spain
[2]Department of Hematology, University Hospital Miguel Servet, Zaragoza, Spain
[3]Department of Orthopedic Surgery, University Hospital Miguel Servet, Zaragoza, Spain

Introduction

Preoperative anemia may be present in up to 75% of surgical patients, depending on the underlying pathology for which they require surgery [1]. Iron deficiency (ID) and chronic inflammation, with or without ID, are the most common causes of preoperative anemia, although deficiencies of iron, folic acid, and/or vitamin B12 without anemia are also frequent, especially among elder population [2]. In this regard, in a recent series of 345 patients undergoing major elective orthopedic surgery, the prevalence of preoperative anemia was 18% because of hematinic deficiency (30%), chronic inflammation with or without ID (40%), and mixed or unknown cause (30%). Interestingly, ID was present in 18% of nonanemic patients, vitamin B12 deficiency in 21%, and folate deficiency in 7% [3]. These deficiencies might blunt the response to erythropoiesis-stimulating agents or delay the recovery from postoperative anemia.

In addition, 30% of patients in this series had a Hb level <13 g/dL [3], and it is well known that a low preoperative hemoglobin level is one of the major predictive factors for perioperative blood transfusion in orthopedic surgery with moderate to high perioperative blood loss [4, 5]. A European study including almost 4000 patients showed an inverse relationship between preoperative Hb values and the probability of receiving allogeneic blood transfusion (ABT) (e.g., 10–18% for Hb 150 g/L, 20–30% for Hb 130 g/L, 50–60% for Hb 100 g/L; 70–75% for Hb 80 g/L) [6]. Similarly, 30–70% of patients undergoing hip fracture repair received ABT perioperatively [7, 8], and the logistic regression analysis identified preoperative Hb value as an independent predictor of the need for ABT [8]. The limited physiologic reserve and the higher prevalence of unrecognized cardiovascular disease may still render the elderly population vulnerable to milder degrees of anemia when undergoing the stress of surgery. In this regard, Wu et al. [9] analyzed a retrospective cohort of 310,311 veterans aged 65 years or older who underwent major noncardiac surgery and found that the adjusted risk of 30-day postoperative mortality and cardiac morbidity begins to rise when preoperative hematocrit levels decrease to less than 39%.

On the other hand, major orthopedic procedures are associated with a significant perioperative blood loss. As a consequence, up to 90% of these patients develop postoperative anemia, which may be aggravated by inflammation-induced blunted erythropoiesis, especially through decreased iron availability (i.e., hepcidin-dependent downregulation of intestinal absorption and impaired mobilization from body stores) [10]. Correction of severe postoperative anemia often required ABT.

However, overall concerns about adverse effects of ABT (e.g., increased risk of postoperative

Alternatives to Blood Transfusion in Transfusion Medicine, 2nd edition. Edited by A. Maniatis, P. Van der Linden, J.-F. Hardy.

Table 41.1 Some blood conservation strategies in orthopedic surgery, with evidence-based grades of recommendation in regard to their blood-saving effect.

Strategy	Level of evidence	Grade of recommendation*
Restrictive transfusion protocol	I	B
Correction of anemia		
Iron	III	D
Recombinant Erythropoietin	I	A
Reduction of blood loss		
Antifibrinolytic agents	I	Not available†
Fibrin sealants	II	C
Avoid postoperative drain	I	B
Usage of autologous blood		
Preoperative donation	I	B
Perioperative cell salvage	I	B
Acute hemodilution	I	Not recommended

*Grade of recommendation: A, supported by at least 2 studies of level 1 (RTCs with large sample populations, clear objectives, and low or a very low risk of bias, or well-conducted meta-analyses or systematic reviews); B, supported by 1 study of level I; C, supported by studies of level II (RTCs with small sample populations, clear objectives, and moderate risk of bias); D, supported by studies of level III (Observational studies with contemporary controls); E, supported by studies of level IV (Observational studies with historical controls), or V (Non-analytic studies, e.g., case reports, case series, expert's opinion).

†Further evaluation of safety is required before recommending the use of antifibrinolytics in orthopedic surgery.

infection, fluid overload, transfusion-related acute lung injury) have prompted the review of transfusion practice and the search for alternatives to allogeneic transfusion (AAT), such as preoperative autologous blood donation, hemodilution, perioperative cell salvage, recombinant erythropoietin (rHuEPO), or administration of antifibrinolitics [11].

The main objective of this chapter is to provide updated evidence-based recommendations on the use of AAT in orthopedic surgical patients that enable physicians to improve the patient's clinical management (Table 41.1). The grade of recommendation was categorized from A (highest) to E (lowest) according to Delphi's methodology used in the Spanish Consensus Statement on Alternatives to Allogeneic Blood Transfusion [12].

Review of transfusion practice

As stated above, ABT is used as part of perioperative anemia treatment, but there is a large intercenter variability in the percentage of patients who receive ABT when undergoing a particular orthopedic surgical procedure. Very recently, in the Austrian benchmark study, Gombotz et al. [13] found a considerable variability in ABT rates, as 16–85% of patients undergoing primary total hip replacement (THR) and 12–87% of patients undergoing primary total knee replacement (TKR) received transfusions. They also found a considerable variability in blood loss (25–60% of total RBC mass for THR, 24–47% for TKR) that mainly reflects differences in surgical techniques, rather than patients' characteristics [13]. In the Orthopedic Surgery Transfusion Hemoglobin European Overview (OSTHEO) study a significant variability in transfusion triggers for TKR and THR patients was also observed [6]. In order to reduce variability in transfusion practice and ABT-related risks, scientific societies have developed evidence-based guidelines and recommendations on the indications of ABT. Although the final objective of these guidelines is a more rational and restrictive approach to its use, many clinicians are uncomfortable with low transfusion thresholds and as a result we are still overusing blood transfusing after elective and nonelective orthopedic surgery.

On the other hand, the randomized controlled trials conducted so far have offered contradictory results regarding the safety of restrictive transfusion triggers [14–16]. While two of them reported that a restrictive transfusion protocol resulted in the transfusion of appreciably fewer units of RBC, with no differences between groups regarding postoperative morbidity or mortality [14, 15], the third one found that a restrictive transfusion threshold (Hb <8 g/dL) may results in higher incidence of postoperative cardiovascular complications (10% vs 2%, $p = 0.05$) and 30-day mortality (8% vs 0%, $p = 0.02$) when compared with a liberal transfusion threshold (Hb <10 g/dL) [16]. The Transfusion Trigger Trial for Functional Outcome in Cardiovascular Patients Undergoing Surgical Hip Fracture Repair (FOCUS), which has been planned to be a 2600-patient, multicenter clinical trial, will most probably address the question of whether patients with cardiovascular disease or cardiovascular risk factors undergoing surgical repair of hip fracture benefit from a higher or lower transfusion trigger [17]. Meanwhile, the transfusion trigger used in these studies (Hb <8 g/dL) is likely to be representative of mainstream practice [18] and seems appropriate for older surgical patients with no risk factors for ischemia. In addition, attention must be paid to signs and symptoms of anemia, because they are variable depending on the patient's age, body temperature, medications, rate of volume loss, and comorbidities. Thus, the Hb transfusion trigger might be lowered for younger patients (7 g/dL) and should be increased (9 g/dL) for patients with organ dysfunction. Therefore, *the use of restrictive transfusion criteria should be the first measure to implement in a blood conservation program (Grade of recommendation B)*, although it is not the only strategy to reduce both the frequency and volume of ABT.

Stimulation of erythropoiesis

Orthopedic surgical patients at risk of receiving perioperative ABT should be identified on the basis of patient's RBC mass (reflected by hemoglobin concentration on the day before surgery), the lowest hemoglobin concentration that the patient can tolerate (transfusion trigger), and the expected blood loss (e.g., using Mercuriali's algorithm) [19]. Therefore, whenever clinically feasible, patients undergoing elective surgery with a high risk of developing severe postoperative anemia should have Hb level [20] and iron status (serum iron, ferritin, and transferrin saturation index) tested preferably 30 days before the scheduled surgical procedure. For patients older than 60 years, vitamin B12 and folic acid should also be measured [2]. Any deficiency should be corrected prior to surgery, and unexplained anemia should always be considered as secondary to some other process and, therefore, elective surgery should be deferred until an appropriate diagnosis has been made [20].

Iron

Preoperative oral iron reduces transfusion requirements in patients scheduled for knee arthroplasty [21, 22] (Grade of recommendation D). Similarly, perioperative administration of IV iron, with or without single doses of rHuEPO, plus the implementation of a restrictive transfusion protocol, in patients undergoing surgery for knee replacement or hip fracture repair resulted in a reduction of both the requirements for ABT and the postoperative morbidity (postoperative infection rate) [23, 27] (Grade of recommendation D).

Regarding postoperative anemia, the administration of oral iron after orthopedic surgery does not appear to be worthwhile [28,29] (Level of evidence II). However, iron sucrose has also been shown to be more effective in restoring postoperative Hb levels after spinal surgery in children (3 mg/kg/day) with respect to an historical control receiving oral iron [30], and postoperative iron sucrose reduced the requirements for ABT in hip arthroplasty [31], whereas others have found no effect [32] (Grade of recommendation E). In addition, perioperative IV iron administration may hasten the recovery from postoperative anemia and preserves iron stores in TKR patients, especially in patients with preoperative ferritin <100 ng/mL [33].

Safety

Although no serious life-threatening adverse events or increment in postoperative infection rate have been reported in the different studies reviewed above, the numbers of patients included in these studies are not large enough to draw definitive conclusions regarding the safety of IV iron agents. However, according to data from the United States Food and Drug Administration, the total number of reported adverse drugs events (ADEs) related to parenteral iron use was 1141 among approximately 30 million doses administered (approximately 38 ADEs per million), with 11 deaths (7 iron dextran, 3 iron gluconate, and 1 iron sucrose) [34]. In addition, several studies suggested that previously observed associations between iron administration and higher infection and mortality rates may have been due to confounding variables [35, 36]. Nevertheless, the administration of IV iron should be avoided in patients with pretreatment ferritin values >500 ng/mL or with ongoing bacteremia.

Recombinant human erythropoietin (rHuEPO)

In orthopedic surgical patients, rHuEPO is indicated before surgery to increase the procurement of autologous blood as well as in the perioperative period to increase Hb levels according to three main recommendations: 1) rHuEPO should only be given to patients scheduled for elective surgery where moderate–high blood loss is expected when their Hb is >10 g/dL and <13 g/dL; 2) the therapeutic goal is the increase of Hb level of at least 1 g/dL; and 3) rHuEPO should be discontinued when a Hb level of 15 g/dL is attained. The magnitude of this response is not depending on patient's age or gender, but on the administered rHuEPO dose and the availability of essential nutrients, such as iron (the use of IV iron may allow for a reduction of total rHuEPO dose), folate, or vitamin B_{12}.

In a meta-analysis of three randomized trials, including 684 patients with moderate anemia and scheduled for elective knee or hip arthroplasty, preoperative rHuEPO administration significantly reduced ABT rate (RR = 0.36, 95% CI 0.28–0.62) [37]. More recently, 2 prospective randomized controlled trials (896 patients) and a case-control study (770 patients) found a similar reduction in ABT rate (AOR = 0.63; 95% CI 0.21–0.49) [38–40]. The presence of inflammation does not seem to be a limiting factor, as patients with and without rheumatoid arthritis benefit equally from preoperative rHuEPO treatment [41] (Grade of recommendation A). In addition, perioperative rHuEPO treatment is also an alternative to PABD for patients deferred from the PABD program. However, the minimal effective rHuEPO dosage to reduce ABT rate in surgical patients is largely unknown, especially when administered together with IV iron [25, 38, 42].

Safety

Perioperative administration of rHuEPO to surgical patients is thought to have few adverse side effects (e.g., exaggerated increase in hematocrit, thrombocytosis, aggravation of hypertensive states, or thromboembolic complications), because it is a short-term treatment and its use is contraindicated for patients with comorbidities which may predispose to adverse side effects (e.g., uncontrolled arterial hypertension, previous acute myocardial infarction or stroke, unstable angina, severe carotid stenosis). However, the FDA alerted that the preliminary results of a 681 patient, multicenter, randomized, open-label study of rHuEPO (4 × 40,000 IU) compared to the standard of care orthopedic surgery showed that frequency of deep venous thrombosis in patients treated with rHuEPO was more than twice that of patients who received usual blood conservation care (4.7% vs 2.1%, respectively) (FDA Alert [11/16/2006, updated 2/16/2007 and 3/9/2007]). In addition, the latest findings on the negative impact of rHuEPO in survival in patients with cancer and kidney disease (http://www.emea.europa.eu/pdfs/human/press/pus/49618807en.pdf) have cast doubts regarding the recommendation of this drug as a first line treatment for anemia. This should be taken into account, carefully balancing risks and benefits, when prescribing and calculating the dosage of rHuEPO for orthopedic patients with any of these comorbidities.

Reduction of blood loss

There is a number of well known general perioperative strategies to reduce blood loss during major orthopedic procedures, including identification and correction of inherited or acquired coagulation abnormalities, patient's position to avoid blood pooling, choice of anesthesia and surgical technique, maintenance of normothermia, or deliberate hypotension [43]. In this section, we will focus on the utility of using antifibrinolytic drugs (aprotinin; tranexamic acid, TXA; epsilon-amino caproic acid, EACA), and fibrin glues, as well as in the possible advantage of avoiding postoperative drainage in the orthopedic surgical patient.

Antifibrinolytic agents

In major orthopedic surgery, the results of a recent meta-analysis including 43 clinical studies (23 with aprotinin, 20 with TXA, and 4 with EACA; 4 trials studied 2 different antifibrinolytics compared with placebo) suggests that the total perioperative blood loss was significantly reduced with the use of aprotinin and TXA resulting in a reduction of the proportion of patients requiring ABT (OR: 0.43, 95% CI 0.28–0.64, for aprotinin; OR: 0.17, 95% CI 0.11–0.24, for TXA) (Level of evidence I). In contrast, EACA did not lead to any significant difference in total blood loss or ABT requirements (OR: 0.71, 95%CI 0.29–1.73) (Level of evidence I) [44].

Safety

There remains a concern that these agents may promote a hypercoagulable state in settings of surgery at high risk of venous thromboembolism, such as orthopedic surgery. In addition, major concerns for aprotinin therapy also relate to hypersensitivity reaction and renal insufficiency, as well as its off-label use in orthopedic surgery. Although no increased risk of thromboembolism was found in this meta-analysis, unfortunately data were too limited for any conclusion regarding safety [44]. In this regard, a recent retrospective analysis found that, with respect to a control group ($n = 209$), routine administration of TXA during total knee arthroplasty to patients without history of thromboembolic disease ($n = 199$) was associated with a 67% reduction in RBC transfusions and, in those transfused, with a reduction in the number of units administered, but not with an increase in thromboembolic complications (2.9% vs 1.5%, respectively) [45].

In contrast, aprotinin has been recently withdrawn from the market due to the increased rate of postoperative severe renal dysfunction, cardiovascular and cerebrovascular thrombotic events, and death observed in cardiac surgical patients receiving this drug when compared to those observed with TXA or EACA. Under a limited use agreement, access to aprotinin is restricted to investigational use of the drug according to the procedures described in a special treatment protocol (FDA Safety Alert for Human Medical Products 2008).

Therefore, despite their efficacy in reducing ABT exposure, further evaluation of safety is required before recommending the use of antifibrinolytics in orthopedic surgery.

Fibrin sealants and glues

Fibrin sealants mimic the final phase of the coagulation pathway through the activation of fibrinogen by thrombin, which leads to the formation of a semirigid clot. Initially "home-made" in the operating room, fibrin glue preparations are now commercially available. Recognition of their potential as hemostatic agents has seen their use expanded across a range of surgical settings, although few randomized controlled trials have been published. In addition, they have been used as an adjunct to wound healing, tissue adhesion, and drug delivery [46].

In orthopedic surgery, two clinical trials including 111 patients undergoing TKR have demonstrated the benefits of fibrin sealants in reducing total blood loss, ABT rate (53% vs 26%, for control and fibrin glue, respectively) and ABT volume (0.9 U/patient vs 0.4 U/patient, respectively) [47,48]. In contrast, in a clinical trial including 69 patients undergoing THR, the use of autologous fibrin glue was not associated with a significant reduction in blood loss or ABT requirements [49]. Therefore, large, methodologically rigorous, randomized controlled trials of fibrin sealants are needed before issuing a definitive recommendation on their use (Level of evidence II).

Safety

Transmission of infection by fibrin sealant preparations has long been a source of concern and debate. However, there are no cases of serious viral transmission after the reported use of commercial fibrin sealant, although the theoretical possibility of nvCJD transmission when using bovine thrombin must be borne in mind. On the other hand, bovine thrombin can be immunogenic, and patients often develop antibodies to plasma proteins in bovine thrombin preparations. Commercial fibrin sealant use in patients who have previously been exposed to aprotinin should be done with caution [46]. Autologous fibrin products lack these side effects.

Postoperative drainage

The use of closed-suction drainage systems after total joint replacement is a common practice. The theoretical advantage for the use of drains is a reduction in the occurrence of wound hematomas and infection. The pooled results of a meta-analysis of randomized trials that compared patients managed with closed-suction drainage systems and those managed without a drain following elective hip and knee arthroplasty (18 studies, 3495 patients) indicated that a drained wound was associated with a significantly greater need for ABT (RR: 1.43; 95% CI 1.19–1.72) (Level of evidence I). In addition, there were no significant differences between the groups regarding the occurrence of wound infection (RR: 0.73; 95% CI 0.47–1.14), wound hematoma (RR: 1.73; 95% CI 0.74–4.07), reoperations for wound complications (RR: 0.52; 95% CI 0.13–1.99), limb-swelling, venous thrombosis, or hospital stay [50]. In addition, in hip surgery patients, no statistically significant differences were detected between the low vacuum and high vacuum systems with regards to blood loss, blood transfusion, and postoperative adverse events [51]. More recent studies indicated that closed suction drainage increases the transfusion requirements after elective hip ($n = 552$) and femoral fractures ($n = 200$) [52, 53], whereas drain clamping with intra-articular injection of saline with adrenaline is more effective than postoperative autologous blood transfusion after knee arthroplasty ($n = 212$) [54]. However, further randomized trials with use of larger numbers of patients with full reporting of outcomes are indicated before the absence of any benefit of drains, particularly for the outcome of wound infection, can be proven.

Usage of autologous blood

Preoperative autologous blood donation (PABD)

PABD consists of obtaining and storing patient's own blood previously to surgery in order to administrate it if necessary afterwards. This is the only autotransfusion modality under regulation in Europe, can be performed as standard blood donation or erythropheresis, and can be used safely in children and elderly populations.

In a meta-analysis of 3 randomized trials (169 patients), PABD significantly reduced ABT rate (RR = 0.16, 95% CI 0.07–0.36) [55]. This reduction in ABT rate was also observed in 18 observational controlled studies (19,239 patients) (RR = 0.29; 95% CI 0.25–0.34) [55]. Similar results were reported by the OSTHEO study (3996 patients) [6] (Grade of recommendation B)

In addition, a meta-analysis of 11 randomized trials (825 patients) showed that the administration of rHuEPO as adjuvant of PABD significantly reduced the exposure to ABT in orthopedic surgery patients (OR = 0.42, 95% CI 0.28–0.62) (Grade of recommendation B) [37]. A prospective randomized trial found PABD with rHuEPO to be more effective in reducing ABT rate than any of these alternatives alone [56]. The administration of rHuEPO to children and adolescents undergoing scoliosis surgery improved the effectiveness of PABD [57]. The effectiveness of different rHuEPO doses (50 IU/kg, 25 IU/kg, or placebo) in facilitating PABD and reducing ABT rate in children undergoing spinal surgery was evaluated in a double-blind, placebo-controlled, randomized trial. Only those patients receiving 50 IU/kg donated the requested PABD units and avoided ABT [58].

The efficacy of PABD in avoiding ABT exposure is lower when a transfusion protocol is implemented (RR = 0.49; 95% CI 0.37–0.63) than when it is not (RR = 0.15; 95% CI 0.06–0.37) [55]. Moreover, to avoid PABD disadvantages (overcollection, overtransfusion, breakthrough transfusion, outdating, wasting, etc.) it should only be performed in patients undergoing an elective surgical procedure in which the estimated risk of transfusion is higher than 20–30% [11], as well as in patients with antibodies against public RBC antigens, for whom it is difficult to get compatible donor blood.

Safety

PABD is not associated with an increase in either the morbidity or mortality rates or the length of hospital stay, but it must be taken into account that the risk of side effects during PADB is higher than during conventional blood donation, and that PABD increases the risk of exposure to any kind of transfusion [55]. However, PABD is contraindicated in patients with positive results for human immunodeficiency virus (HIV), hepatitis B virus (HBV), or hepatitis C virus (HCV), active bacterial infection, uncontrolled arterial hypertension, autoimmune disease, severe aortic stenosis, unstable angina, disseminated malignancy, severe occlusive cerebrovascular disease, or history of epilepsy or seizures. PABD should be avoided during the first and third trimester of pregnancy, and in patients with Hb <11 g/dL. As for children, the volume of each donation must be lower than 13% of their theoretical circulating blood volume, unless simultaneous volume replacement is performed.

Perioperative red cell salvage (PRCS)

PRCS is defined as the collection of patient's blood in surgical procedures in which blood loss is significant. Intraoperative cell salvage (ICS) should be indicated for patients undergoing surgical procedures with an estimated blood loss >1500 mL in which the recovery of 1.2–2 packed red cell units may be anticipated. Postoperative cell salvage (PCS) must be restricted to elective orthopedic procedures with an anticipated postoperative blood loss between 750–1500 mL, allowing for the recovery of at least the equivalent of one unit of packed red cells.

In a meta-analysis of 11 randomized trials (900 patients), PCS with unwashed filtered blood significantly reduced ABT rate (RR = 0.33, 95% CI 0.25–0.43) [55]. Similarly, the results of 8 randomized trials (655 patients) using ICS and/or PCS with washed blood showed a significant reduction in ABT rate (RR = 0.42, 95% CI 0.33–0.53) [55, 59] (Grade of recommendation B). In four observational studies in patients undergoing TKR (1746 patients, >100 patients per study arm, 2004–2007) postoperative salvage and return of unwashed filtered shed blood significantly decreased the requirements for ABT with respect to controls (13% vs 43%, respectively; RR = 0.30, 95% CI 0.29–0.38) [60, 61]. In addition, a prospective randomized study showed that for knee replacement surgery, PCS with filtered blood is as efficacious in reducing ABT as the preoperative donation of one autologous blood unit [62], whereas others found no benefit from the use PCS [63, 64]. Finally, it is worth noting that PRCS contribution to ABT reduction was decreased when a transfusion protocol was adopted [55].

Safety

The results of two meta-analyses of randomized trials and observational studies indicate that PCRS (ICS/PCS) is not associated with an increase in either the morbidity or mortality rates or the length of hospital stay, although isolated cases of serious adverse effects have been reported [55, 65].

Acute normovolemic hemodilution (ANH)

ANH consists of the extraction and anticoagulation of a predicted blood volume from the patient and its simultaneous exchange for a cell free crystalloid and/or colloid solution to maintain normovolemia [66]. A meta-analysis of randomized trials on the use of ANH in orthopedic surgery showed no significant reduction in ABT rate (RR = 0.77, 95% CI 0.51–1.04) [55]. The results of 7 observational controlled studies in different types of surgery (2 cardiac, 2 hepatic, 2 urologic, and 1 orthopedic), the use of ANH reduced by 55% the probability of receiving ABT (RR = 0.45, 95% CI 0.29–0.70), with a reduction in ABT volume of 2.8 units per patient (IC 95% 1.7–4.0) [55]. However, ANH contribution to ABT reduction is virtually eliminated when associated to a transfusion protocol (RR = 0.81, 95% CI 0.65–1.00) [55,67]. Therefore, ANH should only be used in combination with other blood sparing measures, for selected patients undergoing surgery, and at institutions where the logistics of blood removal and replacement can be undertaken without detracting from patient care [11, 66] (Level of evidence I).

Safety

Although in three meta-analysis ANH was not associated to either an increased rate of morbidity (myocardial infraction, myocardial ischemia, alteration of left ventricular function, deep venous thrombosis, stroke, hypotension, or transfusion reaction), postoperative infection or mortality or to prolonged length of hospital stay, the analyzed studies had low evidence level and did no allow to discriminate the effects of ANH from confounder factors [55,67]. A meta-analysis showed ANH to reduce the rate of postoperative thrombosis (RR = 0.44, 95% CI 0.21–0.93) suggesting a possible beneficial rheological effect of ANH. However, the author disclosed that the available data were insufficient to draw a definitive conclusion [55].

Summary

Several major orthopedic surgical procedures including hip and knee arthroplasty, hip fracture repair, and spinal fusion may result in significant blood loss and the need for ABT. However, overall concerns about adverse effects of ABT have prompted the review of transfusion practice (i.e., the promotion of restrictive transfusion protocols) and the search for transfusion alternatives, to decrease or avoid the use of ABT. These strategies include the following: general considerations (e.g., bleeding tendency or relevant drug therapy), correction of perioperative anemia, pharmacologic and nonpharmacologic measures to reduce blood loss, preoperative autologous donation, and perioperative blood salvage. We reviewed the efficacy and safety of these strategies and, where appropriate, gave evidence-based recommendation on their use in orthopedic surgery (Table 41.1). It is worth noting that some of the recommendations given in this chapter are not supported by a high level of evidence, and this must be borne in mind when making decisions regarding their application to a particular patient. Finally, although many of these techniques are effective alone, the goal of performing major orthopedic surgical procedures without the use of ABT and without placing the patient at risk for anemia-related complications may be better accomplished by combining several of these techniques into a defined algorithm, as the one proposed by Wong et al. [68].

References

1. Shander A, Knight K, Thurer R, Adamson J, Spence R. Prevalence and outcomes of anemia in surgery: a systematic review of the literature. Am J Med 2004;116:58S–69S.
2. Guralnik JM, Eisenstaedt RS, Ferrucci L, Klein HG, Woodman RC. The prevalence of anemia in persons aged 65 and older in the United States: evidence for a high rate of unexplained anemia. Blood 2004;104:2263–8.
3. Muñoz M, García-erce JA, Cuenca J, Bisbe E. Pharmacological management of perioperative anaemia: our experience with intravenous iron in orthopaedic surgery. ISBT Sci Ser 2007;2:257–63.
4. García-Erce JA, Solano VM, Cuenca J, Ortega P. La hemoglobina preoperatoria como único factor predictor de las necesidades transfusionales en la artroplastia de rodilla. Rev Esp Anestesiol Reanim 2002;49:254–60.
5. Salido JA, Marín LA, Gómez LA, Zorrilla P, Martínez C. Preoperative hemoglobin levels and the need for transfusion after prosthetic hip and knee surgery: analysis of predictive factors. J Bone Joint Surg Am 2002;84-A:216–20.
6. Rosencher N, Kerkkamp HE, Macheras G, et al. Orthopedic Surgery Transfusion Hemoglobin European Overview (OSTHEO) study: blood management in elective knee and hip arthroplasty in Europe. Transfusion 2003;43:459–69. Level III.
7. Poses RM, Berlin JA, Noveck H, et al. How you look determines what you find: severity of illness and

variation in blood transfusion for hip fracture. Am J Med 1998;105:198–206.
8. García-Erce JA, Cuenca J, Solano VM. Factores predictivos de la necesidad de transfusión en la fractura subcapital de cadera en pacientes mayores de 65 años. Med Clin (Barc) 2003;120:161–6.
9. Wu WC, Schifftner TL, Henderson WG, et al. Preoperative hematocrit levels and postoperative outcomes in older patients undergoing noncardica surgery. JAMA 2007;297:2481–8.
10. Van Iperen CE, Kraaijenhagen RJ, Biesma DH, Beguin Y, Marx JJM, Van de Wiel A. Iron metabolism and erythropoiesis after surgery. Br J Surg 1998;85:41–5.
11. Scottish Intercollegiate Guidelines Network. Perioperative blood transfusion for elective surgery. A national clinical guideline. www.sign.ac.uk, 2001 (Updated March 2009; accessed February 2010).
12. Leal R, Muñoz M, Páramo JA, García-Erce JA, for the Spanish Expert Panel on Alternatives to Allogeneic Blood Transfusion: Spanish consensus statement on alternatives to allogeneic blood transfusions: the Seville's document. TATM 2006;8:178–202.
13. Gombotz H, Rehak PH, Shander A, Hofmann A. Blood use in elective surgery: the Austrian benchmark study. Transfusion 2007;47:1468–80.
14. Carson JL, Terrin ML, Barton FB, et al. A pilot randomized trial comparing symptomatic vs. haemoglobin-level-driven red blood cell transfusions following hip fracture. Transfusion 1998;38:522–9. Level II.
15. Grover M, Talwalkar S, Casbard A, et al. Silent myocardial ischaemia and haemoglobin concentration: a randomized controlled trial of transfusion strategy in lower limb arthroplasty. Vox Sang 2006;90:105–12. Level II.
16. Foss NB, Kristensen MT, Jensen PS, Palm H, Krasheninnikoff M, Kehlet H. The effects of liberal versus restrictive transfusion thresholds on ambulation after hip fracture surgery. Transfusion 2009;49:227–34. Level II.
17. Carson JL, Terrin ML, Magaziner J, Chaitman BR, Apple FS, Heck DA, Sanders D, FOCUS Investigators. Transfusion trigger trial for functional outcomes in cardiovascular patients undergoing surgical hip fracture repair (FOCUS). Transfusion 2006;46:2192–206.
18. Carson JL, Hill S, Carless P, Hébert P, Henry D. Transfusion triggers: a systematic review of the literature. Transfus Med Rev 2002;16:187–99.
19. Mercuriali F, Inghilleri M. Proposal of an algorithm to help the choice of the best transfusion strategy. Curr Med Res Opin 1996;13:465–78.
20. Beris P, Muñoz M, García-Erce JA, Thomas D, Maniatis A, Van der Linden P. Peri-operative anaemia management: consensus statement on the role of intravenous iron. Br J Anaesth 2008;100:599–604.
21. Andrews CM, Lane DW, Bradley JG. Iron pre-load for major joint replacement. Transfus Med 1997;7:281–6. Level II.
22. Cuenca J, García-Erce JA, Martínez F, Cardona R, Pérez-Serrano L, Muñoz M. Preoperative haematinics and transfusion protocol reduce the need for transfusion after total knee replacement. Int J Surg 2007;5:89–94. Level IV.
23. Cuenca J, García-Erce JA, Muñoz M, Izuel M, Martínez AA, Herrera A. Patients with pertrochanteric hip fracture may benefit from preoperative intravenous iron therapy: a pilot study. Transfusion 2004;44:1447–52. Level IV.
24. Cuenca J, García-Erce JA, Martínez AA, Solano VM, Molina J, Muñoz M. Role of parenteral iron in the management of anaemia in the elderly patient undergoing displaced subcapital hip fracture repair: preliminary data. Arch Orthop Trauma Surg 2005;125:342–7. Level IV.
25. García-Erce JA, Cuenca J, Muñoz M, et al. Perioperative stimulation of erythropoiesis with intravenous iron and erythropoietin reduces transfusion requirements in patients with hip fracture. A prospective observational study. Vox Sang 2005;88:235–43. Level III.
26. Cuenca J, Garcia-Erce JA, Martinez F, Pérez-Serrano L, Herrera A, Muñoz M. Perioperative intravenous iron, with or without erythropoietin, plus restrictive transfusion protocol reduce the need for allogeneic blood after knee replacement surgery. Transfusion 2006;46:1112–9. Level III.
27. García-Erce JA, Cuenca J, Haman-Alcober S, Martínez AA, Herrera A, Muñoz M. Efficacy of preoperative recombinant human erythropoietin administration for reducing transfusion requirements in patients undergoing surgery for hip fracture repair. An observational cohort study. Vox Sang 2009;97:260–7. Level III.
28. Sutton PM, Cresswell T, Livesey JP, Speed K, Bagga T. Treatment of anaemia after joint replacement. J Bone Joint Surg (Br) 2004;86-B:31–3. Level II.
29. Mundy GM, Birtwistle SJ, Power RA. The effect of iron supplementation on the level of haemoglobin after lower limb arthroplasty. J Bone Joint Surg (Br) 2005;87-B:213–7. Level II.
30. Bernière J, Dehullu JP, Gall O, Murat I. Intravenous iron in the treatment of postoperative anemia in

surgery of the spine in infants and adolescents. Rev Chir Orthop 1998;84:319–22. Level IV.

31. Muñoz M, Naveira E, Seara J, Palmer JH, Cuenca J, García-Erce JA. Role of parenteralron on tranfusion requirements after total hip replacement. A pilot study. Transfus Med 2006;16:137–42.
32. Karkouti K, McCluskey SA, Ghannam M, Salpeter MJ, Quirt I, Yau TM. Intravenous iron and recombinant erythropoietin for the treatment of postoperative anemia. Can J Anesth 2006;53:11–19. Level III.
33. García-Erce JA, Cuenca J, Martínez F, Cardona R, Pérez-Serrano L, Muñoz M. Perioperative intravenous iron may transfusion requirements and hasten the recovery from postoperative anaemia after knee replacement surgery. Transf Med 2006;16:335–41.
34. Chertow GM, Mason PD, Vaaga-Nilsen O, Ahlmén J. Update on adverse drug events associated with parenteral iron. Nephrol Dial Transplant 2006;21:378–82.
35. Feldman HI, Joffe M, Robinson B, et al. Administration of parenteral iron and mortality among hemodialysis patients. J Am Soc Nephrol 2004;15:1623–32. Level III.
36. Hoen B, Paul-Dauphin A, Hestin D, Kessler M: EPIBACDIAL: a multicenter prospective studiy of risk factors for bacteremia in chronic hemodyalysis patients. J Am Soc Nephrol 1998;9:869–76.
37. Laupacis A, Fergusson D. Erythropoietin to minimize perioperative blood transfusion: a systematic review of randomized trials. Transfus Med. 1998;8:309–17. Level I.
38. Feagan BG, Wong CJ, Kirkley A, et al. Erythropoietin with iron supplementation to prevent allogeneic blood transfusion in total hip joint arthroplasty. Ann Intern Med. 2000;133:845–54. Level I.
39. Weber EWG, Slappendel R, Hémon Y, et al. Effects of epoetin alfa on blood transfusions and postoperative recovery in orthopaedic surgery: the European Epoetin Alfa Surgery Trial (EEST). Eur J Anaesthesiol. 2005;22:249–57. Level I.
40. Karkouti K, McCluskey SA, Evans L, Mahomed N, Ghannam M, Davey R. Erythropoietin is an effective clinical modality for reducing RBC transfusion in joint surgery. Can J Anesth. 2005;52:363–8. Level III.
41. Slappendel R, Weber EW, Hemon YJ, et al. Patients with and without rheumatoid arthritis benefit equally from preoperative epoetin-alpha treatment. Acta Orthop 2006;77:677–83. Level II.
42. Rosencher N, Poisson D, Albi A, Aperce M, Barré J, Samana CM. Two injections of erythropoietin correct moderate anemia in most patients awaiting orthopedic surgery. Can J Anesth 2005;52:160–65. Level II.
43. Habler O. Indications for perioperative blood transfusion in orthopedic surgery [Review]. TATM 2006;8:17–28.
44. Zufferey P, Merquiol F, Laporte S, et al. Do antifibrinolytics reduce allogeneic blood transfusion in orthopedic surgery? Anesthesiology 2006;105:1034–46. Level I.
45. Lozano M, Basora M, Peidro L, et al. Effectiveness and safety of tranexamic acid administration during total knee arthroplasty. Vox Sang 2008;95; 39–44. Level IV.
46. MacGillivray TE. Fibrin sealants and glues [Review]. J Card Surg 2003;18:480–85.
47. Levy O, Martinowitz U, Oran A, Tauber C, Horoszowski H. The use of fibrin tissue adhesive to reduce blood loss and the need for blood transfusion after total knee arthroplasty. A prospective, randomized, multicenter study. J Bone Joint Surg Am 1999;81A:1580–88. Level II.
48. Wang GJ, Hungerford DS, Savory CG, et al. Use of fibrin sealant to reduce bloody drainage and hemoglobin loss after total knee arthroplasty: a brief note on a randomized prospective trial. J Bone Joint Surg Am 2001;83A:1503–5. Level II.
49. Lassen MR, Solgaard S, Kjersgaard AG, et al. A pilot study of the effects of Vivostat patient-derived fibrin sealant in reducing blood loss in primary hip arthroplasty. Clin Appl Thromb Hemost 2006;12:352–7. Level II.
50. Parker MJ, Roberts CP, Hay D. Closed suction drain for hip and knee arthroplasty. A meta-analysis. J Bone Joint Surg Am 2004; 86-A: 1146–52. Level I.
51. Muñoz M, Thomas D. To drain or not to drain after hip replacement surgery? TATM 2008;10:163–5.
52. Walmsley PJ, Kelly MB, Hill RM, Brenkel I. A prospective, randomized, controlled trial of the use of drains in total hip arthroplasty. J Bone Joint Surg Br 2005;87-B:1379–401. Level I.
53. Tjeenk RM, Vrancken Peeters MP, van den Ende E, Kastelein GW, Breslau PJ. Wound drainage versus non-drainage for proximal femoral fractures. A prospective randomized study. Injury 2005;36:100–104. Level II.
54. Tsumara N, Yoshiya S, Chin T, et al. A prospective comparison of clamping drain or post-operative salvage of blood in reducing blood loss after total knee arthroplasty. J Bone Joint Surg Br 2006;88-B:49–53. Level II.

55. Carless P, Moxey A, O'Connell D, Henry D. Autologous transfusion techniques: a systematic review of their efficacy. Transf Med 2004;14:123–44. Level I.
56. Bezwada HP, Nazarian DG, Henry DH, Booth RE. Preoperative use of recombinant human erythropoietin before total joint arthroplasty. J Bone Joint Surg Am 2003;85A:1795–800. Level II.
57. García-Erce JA, Solano VM, Sáez M, Muñoz M. Recombinant human erythropoietin facilitates autologous blood donation in children undergoing corrective spinal surgery. Transfusion 2004;44:1447–52. Level III.
58. Lee JH, Lee SH, Han J. Minimal effective dosage of recombinant human erythropoietin in spinal surgery. Clin Orthop 2003;412:71–6. Level II.
59. Huet C, Salmi LR, Fergusson D, Koopman-van Gements AW, Rubens F, Laupacis A. A meta-analysis of the effectiveness of cell salvage to minimize perioperative allogeneic blood transfusion in cardiac and orthopaedic surgery. International Study of Perioperative Transfusion (ISPOT) Investigators. Anesth Analg 1999;89:861–9. Level I.
60. Muñoz M, Ariza D, Garcerán MJ, Gómez A, Campos A. Benefits of postoperative shed blood reinfusion in patients undergoing unilateral total knee replacement. Arch Orthop Trauma Surg. 2005;125: 385–9. Level IV.
61. Muñoz M, Kühlmorgen B, Ariza D, Haro E, Marroquí A, Ramírez G. Which patients are more likely to benefit of postoperative shed blood reinfusion after unilateral total knee replacement? Vox Sang 2007;92:136–41. Level III.
62. Woolson ST, Wall WW. Autologous blood transfusion after total knee arthroplasty. A randomized, prospective study comparing predonated and postoperative salvage blood. J Arthroplasty 2003;18:243–9. Level II.
63. Mauerhan DR, Nussman D, Mokris JG, Beaver WB. Effect of postoperative reinfusion systems on hemoglobin levels in primary total hip and total knee arthroplasties. A prospective randomized study. J Arthroplasty 1993;8:523–7. Level III.
64. Glynn A, McCarthy T, McCarroll M, Murray P. A prospective audit of blood usage post primary total knee arthroplasty. Acta Orthop Belg 2006;72:24–8. Level III.
65. Hansen E, Pawlik M. Reasons against the retransfusion of unwashed wound blood [Review]. Transfusion 2004;44(1 Suppl.): 45S–53S.
66. Shander A, Rijhwani TS. Acute normovolemic hemodilution [Review]. Transfusion 2004; 44(12 Suppl.): S26–S34.
67. Segal JB, Blasco-Colmenares E, Norris EJ, Guallar E. Preoperative acute normovolemic hemodilution: a meta-analysis. Transfusion 2004;44:632–44. Level I.
68. Wong CJ, Vandervoort MK, Vandervoort SL, et al. A cluster-randomized controlled trial of a blood conservation algorithm in patients undergoing total hip joint arthroplasty. Transfusion 2007;47:832–41. Level I.

CHAPTER 42
Transfusion Alternatives in Obstetrics

Christian Breymann
Obsterics, Gynecology and Feto Maternal Medicine, Feto Maternal Haematology Research Group, Obstetric Research, University Hospital Zurich, Zurich, Switzerland

Introduction

Safe and effective treatment of anemia avoiding blood transfusion is one of the major challenges in most medical and surgical fields.

It is well known that both chronic and acute anemia have an important impact on the patients morbidity and mortality outcome, therefore it is clear that if ever possible any anemia should be treated as soon as it has been diagnosed.

In this review, an important alternative to heterologous blood or oral iron only will be presented, namely the parenteral iron sucrose complex (Venofer®), which has become the mainstay of today's parenteral iron therapy in various fields because of its safety profile and effectivity. Vast and increasing experience has been published lately in the fields such as obstetrics, nephrology, inflammatory bowel disease, cardiac disease, surgery, and others and it is the aim of this review to summarize data and implications for the use of iron sucrose as an alternative to blood transfusion in obstetrics.

Anemia—general aspects

Anemia, simply called "lack of blood," is a consequence of reduced red cell production which leads to reduced hemoglobin concentration. The hemoglobin level is then too low for age and gender and depends on defined cutoffs in various populations or conditions (e.g., pregnancy with related cutoffs during gestational age). Anemia results in a decrease of oxygen transport capacity in the blood, the risk of tissue hypoxia increases with the severity of anemia. The body's principal compensatory mechanism involves circulatory and ventilatory adaptations and the initiation of compensatory erythrocyte synthesis after the release of erythropoietin.

Clinically, the most important consequences are disturbances in oxygen-dependent metabolic processes and organ functions. Typical signs in chronic anemia include pallor of the skin, reduced physical and mental performance, fatigue, and listlessness, dyspnoea at rest, tachycardia, and cardiac symptoms. Acute, severe, and uncontrolled anemia results in circulatory collapse, metabolic lactacidosis, and finally organ failure, and shock with high mortality risk.

The common forms of anemia can be divided into at least three main groups: (1) anemia secondary to blood loss (acute and chronic) which secondarily leads to iron deficient erythropoiesis and hypochromic and microcytic erythrocytes (in chronic bleeding); (2) anemia resulting from reduced or ineffective erythropoiesis (e.g., iron deficiency anemia, infection, renal disorders, erythropoietin deficiency, B12, and folic acid deficiency and others); and (3) anemia due to excessive erythrocyte breakdown and hemolysis (e.g., hemoglobinopathies, congenital erythrocyte membrane defects, drug induced hemolysis, and others). It is clear that adequate therapy requires adequate understanding of the underlying cause of anemia, i.e., using correct differential diagnosis by clinical assessment and laboratory evaluations

Alternatives to Blood Transfusion in Transfusion Medicine, 2nd edition. Edited by A. Maniatis, P. Van der Linden, J.-F. Hardy.

for which the author refers to respective textbooks and guidelines.

Clinical features of the most common forms of anemia of pregnancy and the postpartum period

Anemia due to blood loss

During pregnancy

Anemia as a result of blood loss can occur during pregnancy, but is more common postpartum. Typical reasons for hemorrhage during pregnancy include placenta previa or gastrointestinal bleeding due to an inflammatory intestinal disorder (Crohn's disease, ulcerative colitis).

Blood losses during pregnancy can result in severe anemia, leading to a higher rate of prematurity and maternal symptoms [1]. In addition, the peripartum blood reserves are reduced, increasing the risk of postpartum anemia, and thus of blood transfusions for the mother [2].

During the puerperium

According to WHO criteria, postpartum anemia is defined as a hemoglobin level of less than 10.0 g/dL. In spite of preventative measures, particularly the treatment of anemia during pregnancy, postpartum anemia also has a high prevalence in Switzerland: 10–15% for moderate anemia (8.5–9.9 g/dL) and 1–2% for severe anemia (<8.5 g/dL).

Hemoglobin values fall below this level following blood loss of approximately 500 mL or more, provided that the prepartum hemoglobin levels are normal (>11.0 g/dL). In general, blood losses of up to 30% of the total blood volume (approximately 15 mL/kg of body weight) are readily compensated. It has been shown, that postpartum anemia prolongs hospital stay [3]. Blood losses of 1000 mL or more lead to greatly elevated maternal morbidity and mortality. Postpartum anemia is one of the most important causes of maternal mortality, particularly in developing countries. Where medical care is good, maternal deaths due to hemorrhage are rare, provided that uterotonic agents are administered promptly, together with volume substitution (infusions), surgical intervention, and the ready availability of blood for transfusion. Table 42.1 summarizes main causes of postpartum anemia and possible interventions and preventive actions.

Main causes of postpartum anemia

Atonic bleedings at birth

This is a consequence of protracted, uncontrollable bleeding due to so-called atony (failure of the uterus to contract after delivery). Blood losses of between 1000 and 3000 mL are possible and can be limited by the prompt use of uterotonic agents (prostaglandins, oxytocin, misoprostol). Severe, uncontrollable cases require surgical intervention (suturing the uterus to arrest the hemorrhage, including use of the B-Lynch technique, hysterectomy, etc.). Virtually all women with atonic hemorrhage have severe postpartum anemia (Hb < 8.5 g/dL). In this context it should be pointed out that there are still wide variations in policies of management of the third stage of labor and the immediate management of postpartum hemorrhage in Europe [2, 4, 5].

Coagulopathies

Coagulopathies associated with pre-eclampsia, HELLP syndrome (hemolysis, elevated liver enzymes, and low platelet count syndrome), or DIC (disseminated intravascular coagulation) lead to high blood losses, especially when treatment is delayed (late delivery, no coagulation factors, or plasma administered). In emergency cases, there is often no time for prompt substitution with coagulation factors; where this is the case, caesarean sections in particular are associated with high blood losses. Other typical situations include hemorrhage due to placenta previa or placenta accreta/increta (an abnormally adherent placenta), or premature separation of the placenta. Ninety percent of patients with placenta accreta or increta have blood losses of >2000 mL, increasing the risk of receiving donor blood transfusions [6].

Table 42.1 Main causes and risk factors for PPH and blood transfusion and possible preventive interventions.

Cause	Possible intervention
Placental abnormality (e.g., placenta previa)	Surgical at birth, anemia therapy
Multiparity	Anemia therapy (if present)
History of PPH	Anemia therapy (if present)
Prolonged 3D stage of labor	Uterotonics, operative delivery
Pre-eclampsia	Delivery at proper gestational age
Anemia at 24–29 WOG	Anemia therapy
Anemia before birth	Anemia therapy
Coagulation disorders	Coagulation factors, platelets, etc.
Type of anesthesia	Prefer spinal/epidural
Instrumental vaginal delivery	Surgical (if tissue lacerations)

Birth injuries

Injuries during labor and delivery can also lead to high blood losses. These include tears in the perineum, vagina, and cervix.

Iron deficiency as the major cause of preexisting anemia

Maternal risks

It is known that iron deficiency influences a whole series of body functions, such as physical and mental performance, enzymatic functions (e.g., those of the respiratory chain), thermoregulation, muscular functions, the immune response, and neurological functions. Only a few of these potential effects have been specifically investigated in iron-deficiency anemia.

In general, iron-deficiency anemia leads to numerous symptoms such as fatigue, a reduction in physical performance and fitness for work, increased cardiovascular stress (tachycardia, fall in blood pressure), reduced thermoregulation, and an increased predisposition to infections.

In the gravida, the tolerance for peripartum blood loss is greatly reduced [1, 2, 4].

Maternal mortality increases depending on the severity of the iron-deficiency anemia. Causes include an increased rate of cardiovascular failure, a high risk of hemorrhagic shock, higher rates of infection during the puerperium and impaired wound healing.

Maternal morbidity may also be associated with additional factors such as socioeconomic status, the level of medical care, nutritional status, etc.

A general problem in interpreting the available studies is that maternal and fetal outcome have been investigated in relation to the severity of the anemia, but not in relation to the duration or initial onset of the anemia, or indeed the severity, duration, or onset of iron deficiency.

Taking these limitations into account, several authors have postulated an association between maternal mortality and the degree of anemia; however, there are no prospective studies investigating this and it is not clear what level of hemoglobin is critical with respect to maternal mortality. It appears to lay at levels of less than 8–9 g/dL, but the association between moderate anemia and maternal morbidity is not clear. To date, there have been no studies investigating the association between iron-deficiency anemia before pregnancy and the course of pregnancy, and there are also no prospective studies on large populations demonstrating the effect of early intervention and treatment of anemia on maternal, fetal, and neonatal outcome [7].

Fetal risks

Maternal hemoglobin levels below 9.0 g/dL increase the risk of premature births (PMB), intrauterine growth retardation (IUGR), and intrauterine fetal death (IUFD).

The association between maternal hemoglobin and birthweight follows a U-shaped curve.

Hemoglobin levels of more than 11.0 g/dL and less than 9.0 g/dL are associated with a 2–3 times greater risk of a light-for-dates neonate. Hemoglobin levels of more than 12.0 g/dL at the end of the second trimester are associated with an increased risk of pre-eclampsia and intrauterine growth retardation, probably due to a lack of plasma volume expansion.

The "ideal" hemoglobin range with respect to the prevention of prematurity and IUGR babies appears to lie between 9.5 and 11.5 g/dL.

There is increasing evidence of an association between the timing and duration of iron deficiency and anemia, and of pathological feto-placental changes. The risk of a premature birth is increased if there is iron deficiency during early pregnancy. However, it is not clear whether this is primarily the result of a lack of oxygen supply, or more the consequence of iron not being released or utilized. Various studies have investigated the effect of the iron stores themselves on infant outcome. It was shown that ferritin levels correlate more closely with intrauterine growth retardation than do hemoglobin levels, and that even high ferritin levels, possibly as a result of infections, correlate with a high rate of intrauterine growth retardation. Ferritin levels that are too low, indicating depleted iron stores, appear to have a symmetrical association with growth retardation; with excessively high ferritin levels, this effect is asymmetrical [1, 8–11]

Treatment of iron-deficiency anemia in pregnancy

From the preceding chapters, it is clear that iron-deficiency states and anemia should be treated. Even in milder forms of anemia, it is often impossible to predict the course of the condition, or whether the situation is likely to worsen, and maternal and fetal risks increase as anemia becomes more severe.

Factors to be taken into account when deciding on the treatment approach to use include the time remaining until delivery, the severity of the anemia, additional risks (e.g., premature labor), maternal comorbidity and the patient's own wishes (e.g., refusal to receive donor blood to treat severe anemia). Thus, for example, a Jehovah's Witness with severe anemia 2 weeks before term needs different treatment than a woman with moderate anemia and no additional risk factors during the second trimester.

At present, the main treatment options for anemia include oral iron, parenteral iron, the stimulation of hemopoiesis with growth factors (e.g., recombinant human erythropoietin), and the administration of heterologous blood.

Iron for therapy of anemia

It is clear that iron therapy is the first choice for anemias, which are linked to iron deficient conditions. The iron therapy can be performed either as oral iron therapy or parenteral iron therapy.

Depending on the severity of anemia or other factors such as limited time for therapy (e.g., before surgery) also allogeneic blood is often used to rise hemoglobin values quickly, however there is increasing evidence and awareness that the use of allogeneic blood should be restricted as far as possible due to its inevitable risks and patients concerns.

The role of oral iron

Iron salts, especially iron sulphate, remain the mainstay for iron therapy in many conditions. Although the bioavailability of Fe (II) (ferrous) salts is generally acceptable, many patients suffer from side effects, resulting in poor compliance. Metal ions tend to induce an emetic effect, which can be ameliorated by chelation. An additional potential hazard with relatively high doses of Fe (II) salts is the generation of damaging hydroxyl radicals in the presence of vitamin C and oxygen.

The bioavailability of Fe (III) salts is lower compared with Fe (II) compounds and ferric (III) salts are not widely used, but new formulas are coming up such as iron polymaltose with equal bioavailability and better tolerance [4].

For oral iron, an increase in the hemoglobin concentration of at least 20 g/L after 3 weeks of treatment is considered an adequate response to therapy. Three to five days after start of therapy, reticolocytosis begins, and this reaches a peak after 8–10 days and then declines. The hemoglobin

Table 42.2 Recent studies with intravenous iron sucrose during pregnancy and postpartum for the treatment of anemia.

Reference	Period	Total dose (mg)	Effectiveness (Hb increase)
Breymann et al.	PP	800	2.1–3.5 (14 days)
Gravier	PP	400–600	3.8 (14 days)
Broche	PP	200–600	1.9 (7 days)
Bhandall	PP	400	2.6 (5 days)
Breymann et al.	PR	~800–1600	2.0 (25 days)
Bayoumeu	PR		1.6 (30 days)

PP, postpartum; PR, pregnancy.

increase should start after the reticulocyte peak. The response has to be evaluated with regard to confounding factors, such as poor compliance, malabsorption of iron, continuing blood loss and infection, and inflammatory or malignant disease. In various settings, parenteral iron therapy will be more effective than oral iron therapy (Table 42.2).

Focus on parenteral iron sucrose complex (Venofer®)

Iron sucrose as alternative to allogeneic blood transfusion

Severe anemia in surgery, obstetrics, and various medical fields can necessitate the use of blood transfusions, plasma products, and volume expanders. It is important to have strict criteria for or against the administration of blood replacement products and to be aware of the potentials and possible risks of these substances [2, 12].

The administration of donor blood is indicated if it is proven that the product has been safely manufactured and tested, and if the use can avert a life-threatening situation for the patient.

Furthermore, there needs to be a sufficiently high likelihood that patient's mortality and morbidity cannot be averted through the use of equivalent alternatives (e.g., hematinics and volume replacement alone). There is increasing accordance in the scientific community that the indiscriminate use of blood products must be avoided at all times. While blood products can be life-saving, they also involve a variety of inherent risks and complications. In many cases, blood transfusion is not necessary as it is often possible to avert bleeding situations that necessitate transfusion by anticipating problems and taking preventive action. Circumstances in which blood transfusions are given include, among others, immediately before surgery to raise hemoglobin or postsurgery to speed up recovery. Alternative methods, such as volume expanders and over all the prompt treatment and prevention of anemia, are safer, cheaper, and in most cases, equally effective. In respect to anemia therapy, there is increasing evidence that intravenous iron sucrose is a first line option for both prevention and therapy of various types of anemia and it is obvious that effective treatment of anemia leads to a reduction of the use of allogeneic blood.

Anemia in pregnancy and the postpartum period

Iron deficiency anemia is one the most common problems in pregnancy. Traditional treatment, i.e., oral iron therapy, or blood transfusion, both involve significant drawbacks. High doses of oral iron frequently cause side effects and noncompliance is common. As far as blood transfusions are concerned, because of the risk associated with allogeneic blood products, especially in this young and otherwise healthy population, transfusions are used only in the most severe cases and particularly in life-threatening situations.

Therefore, intravenous iron alone or in association with rHuEPO has been considered as an alternative in the management of iron deficiency in this setting [13–24].

Since the early 1990s, iron saccharate (Venofer®) has been the only parenteral iron product used during pregnancy and the puerperium at the Zurich University Hospital Obstetrics Clinic. Data on the safety of the iron saccharate complex were first collected in a multicenter study in 1998. The side effect rate following the administration of 2000 ampoules, with a maximum single dose of 200 mg i.v., was found to be less than 0.5% [4].

In accordance with Obstetrics Clinic guidelines, an incremental treatment plan is used in anemia. Prerequisites for the use of parenteral iron include extensive diagnostic investigations and fulfillment of the following inclusion criteria (Table 42.2).

The first hemoglobin test is normally carried out during the first trimester, with oral iron prescribed in the first instance only if the value is less than 10.0 g/dL. If the hemoglobin level on oral iron falls below 10.0 g/dL within 2–4 weeks, or if the Hb level on the first test is already less than 10.0 g/dL, we use the iron saccharate complex as the treatment of first choice.

Practical use of the iron saccharate complex at Zurich Clinic of Obstetrics

The substance is administered through a venous butterfly cannula, once correct positioning in the vein has been tested with NaCl. Iron saccharate can be administered undiluted as a bolus or diluted (e.g., to 100–200 mL with NaCl) as a short infusion. Administration of a test dose (1 mL) is required in different countries. The subsequent bolus injection is given over 5–10 minutes, the short infusion over approximately 20 minutes. The maximum single dose is 200 mg. We generally give two doses a week to achieve a target Hb value of 11.0 g/dL. The treatment can be given on an outpatient basis without any problems; in our experience, a long period of monitoring is not usually necessary following administration [25].

Between 1992 and 2005, over 500 pregnant women with anemia were treated at the Zurich Obstetrics Clinic. Tab. gives an overview of hematological data during treatment. The mean treatment duration was 25 (8–29) days, with a mean total dose of 1000 mg (400–1600 mg) Venofer®, corresponding to five doses of 200 mg. There are several studies on, and clinical experience with, the use of iron saccharate during pregnancy and postpartum. Overall, a high level of efficacy and safety was demonstrated in all studies [13, 16, 19, 26–28].

Postpartum

The treatment of *postpartum anemia* depends on the severity of the anemia and/or additional maternal risk factors or comorbidity. A young, healthy woman can compensate for heavy blood losses far better than a puerperal with a heart defect, who can decompensate even following less severe losses.

In addition, blood losses need to be viewed in relation to the body mass and the estimated total blood volume. Another consideration is that significant errors can be made particularly when estimating blood loss, since the blood loss is often underestimated, something that can readily be verified by comparing prepartum and postpartum hemoglobin levels.

In addition to volume replacement, treatment options include the administration of oral iron, parenteral iron, and heterologous (donor) blood. Another option to be considered is the administration of recombinant erythropoietin [17, 20, 22, 29–32].

Oral iron should be prescribed at hemoglobin levels of over 9.5 g/dL; 80–100 mg/day is sufficient in such cases. The iron supplementation should be continued for a period of several months, to provide iron not just for hemoglobin normalization, but also to normalize the iron stores. In one study, we were able to show that puerperal with iron deficiency but no anemia can replenish their iron stores through iron supplementation alone.

Thus, puerperal who have iron deficiency and anemia are particularly likely to have a high iron requirement. We therefore continue giving iron for at least 6 months. In most cases, giving oral iron is not enough when treating severe anemia, since the endogenous iron stores are usually depleted and not enough iron is provided to ensure sufficient erythropoiesis. As mentioned earlier, reasons for this include limited absorption, poor compliance at high doses due to adverse effects, and low plasma levels, which lead to functional iron deficiency. In addition, an inflammatory reaction can occur particularly following surgically assisted deliveries and caesarean section, leading to iron sequestration, so that the administered iron is not available for hemopoiesis.

One alternative is the parenteral administration of iron sucrose. The high plasma iron concentrations that occur shortly after i.v. administration bypass, the limited release of iron from the reticuloendothelial system and inhibited absorption through the intestinal mucosa, thus delivering sufficient quantities of iron for erythropoiesis. As in pregnancy, we follow an incremental treatment plan, using parenteral iron saccharate at hemogbobin levels of less than 9.5 g/dL.

More recently Broche et al. retrospectively analyzed data from 4292 patients who gave birth in their institution between April 2001 and March 2003. All patients who presented with postpartum anemia (Hb < 8 g/dL) within 48 hours of delivery ($n = 217$, i.e., 5% of all parturients), were included in the study. Two groups were distinguished on the basis of availability of i.v. iron sucrose (Venofer®) in the institution at the time of delivery. The analysis comprised clinical and laboratory outcomes.

Between April 2001 and March 2002, 103 patients received either blood transfusions ($n = 15$ [14.6%]) or oral iron ($n = 88$), while between April 2002 and March 2003, 114 patients received blood transfusion ($n = 5$ [4.4%]), oral iron ($n = 66$), or intravenous iron sucrose ($n = 43$). The mean total amount of Venofer® dose was 359 mg (range, 200–600). The mean increase in Hb concentration over 7 days in patients who received iron sucrose was significantly higher compared to those who received oral iron exclusively. The authors concluded that since the availability of i.v. iron sucrose (Venofer®) in their institution, the number of transfused patients has been divided by three; the increase in Hb concentrations has been significantly higher with iron sucrose than with oral iron in patients with postpartum anemia. Iron sucrose was well tolerated in this study. Recently Bhandal et al. have shown in a randomized study that a total dose of 400 mg intravenous iron sucrose was superior to oral iron treatment beginning from day 5 until 14 postpartum [14] (Table 42.2).

Stimulation of erythropoiesis with recombinant erythropoietin (rhEPO)

The growth factor recombinant human erythropoietin (rhEPO), a glycoprotein (molecular weight 30,400 Da), is identical to endogenous erythropoietin and acts as a selective growth and survival factor for erythroid cells. It has been used clinically since 1986, primarily in patients with renal anemia who have endogenous erythropoietin deficiency. Other indications have been added during recent years, including anemia in premature neonates, following autologous blood donation, in oncological patients, in HIV patients and for the perioperative treatment of anemia, e.g., in Jehovah's Witnesses [17, 20, 22, 29–32].

Since then, increasing experience has also been gained in the field of obstetrics, in the form of randomized studies of the treatment of postpartum anemia, primarily in the form of case reports in patients with renal failure and in Jehovah's Witnesses, and also in the treatment of severe iron-deficiency anemia during pregnancy. The results of the studies and observations are highly promising. The administration of recombinant erythropoietin reduces the time taken for the hemoglobin concentration to normalize, provided that enough iron is administered. The most effective way of achieving this is with parenteral iron. If the concomitant availability of iron is insufficient, the patient develops so-called functional iron deficiency, which prevents the synthesis of adequate amounts of hemoglobin.

According to available results, the combination of rhEPO and parenteral iron is superior to iron treatment alone with regard to bringing about an increase in the hemoglobin concentration, and can be considered as an option when treating severe anemia or if the patient refuses donor blood. The effect of rhEPO is dose-dependent; according to our own experience, single intravenous doses of 150–300 U/kg are sufficient, though a repeat dose may be needed in some cases. At our clinic, we try to ensure an optimum cost-benefit ratio by aiming to treat anemia during pregnancy and the puerperium according to an incremental plan, according to which we treat anemia either with iron alone or in combination with rhEPO, depending on severity. This plan can be individually tailored to the patient, taking into account any additional risks.

Thus, for example, if treating a Jehovah's Witness patient with placenta previa, we would use recombinant erythropoietin even in moderate anemia.

In addition to modern anesthetic and surgical techniques, our incremental anemia treatment plan has an important role in the prevention of anemia requiring transfusion following high peripartum blood losses. Thus, less than 1% of our obstetric patients now require donor blood transfusions.

> At this point, it should be stressed that, to date, rhEPO has only been used in pregnancy and postpartum within the context of study protocols as off label use.

Donor blood transfusions

Severe anemia during pregnancy and in the postpartum period can necessitate the use of blood transfusions, plasma products, and volume expanders.

It is important to have strict criteria for or against the administration of blood replacement products, and to be aware of the potentials and risks of these substances.

The administration of donor blood and/or plasma products is indicated if it is proven that the products in question have been safely manufactured and tested, and if their use can avert a life-threatening situation for the patient. Furthermore, there needs to be a sufficiently high likelihood that maternal death and morbidity cannot be averted through the use of equivalent alternatives (e.g., through volume replacement alone). Also, it has been shown recently, that transfusion of RBC has no impact on length of hospital stay in moderately anemic patients [2, 3].

The nonselective and indiscriminate administration of blood products must be avoided at all times. According to the literature, the rate of donor blood transfusions at specialist treatment centers is 1–2% (relative to the number of births). At the Zurich University Hospital's Obstetrics Clinic, the current rate is 0.5–1%.

Obstetric clinics and specialists should be prepared for emergency blood transfusions. The availability of refrigerated blood (especially blood group 0 Rhesus negative) and plasma products (e.g., fresh frozen plasma) is essential.

Risks of blood donor transfusion

While blood transfusions can be life-saving, they also involve a variety of inherent risks and complications. In many cases, blood transfusions are not necessary, as it is often possible to avert obstetric situations that necessitate transfusions by anticipating problems and taking preventative action [2, 3, 12].

Circumstances in which blood transfusions are given include, among others, immediately before surgery to raise hemoglobin, or postpartum to speed up recovery. Alternative methods, such as volume expanders and the prompt treatment and prevention of anemia, are safer, cheaper and, in most cases, equally effective.

Prescribing donor blood

Donor blood should be prescribed according to national criteria (or hospital-specific in-house criteria based on national guidelines). In addition, the patient's wishes and her individual situation must be taken into account.

The following points need to be considered:

- Expected benefit/risk for the patient's individual situation;
- The use of alternatives;
- Procedure to minimize any further blood loss;
- Specific clinical and/or laboratory test-related indications;
- The risk of a possible infection (differs according to country); and
- Facilities for monitoring and intervention if transfusion-related complications occur.

Other obstetric measures

The most important principle in deciding for or against a blood transfusion or the use of blood products is that they represent only one of many options in the management of the patient.

The primary principle in managing an acute, severe hemorrhage is the replacement of fluids (volume replacement) to maintain organ perfusion. Other measures include keeping to a minimum, the number of blood samples taken for testing, and use of the best surgical and anesthesiological techniques to minimize blood loss.

Maintaining fluid balance

Once stable conditions are achieved, i.e., following the replacement of high fluid losses and the cessation of the hemorrhage, the patient can be switched to fluid maintenance with crystalloids (dextrose/electrolyte mixture). These replace fluid losses through the skin, lungs, feces, and urine. In general, volume expanders of this sort are needed for up to about 48 hours in obstetric cases; the amounts given vary according to the initial hemoglobin level, fever, any additional intake of fluids by mouth, etc. Human plasma (e.g., FFP) should not be used for volume replacement.

Summary of the key principles for the use of blood transfusions in obstetrics

- Any anemia (including mild forms) should be treated promptly to avoid the need for later donor blood transfusions;
- In general, blood losses should be minimized;
- The hemoglobin level (hematocrit) alone can never be the sole criterion for a donor blood transfusion. Key factors include clinical findings, the hemorrhage situation, and the probability of averting significant morbidity or even death. In our experience, the critical hemoglobin level, provided that the circulation is stable, is approximately 6.0 g/dL (hematocrit approximately 18–20%);
- In case of acute blood loss, start giving oxygen and volume expanders immediately;
- Blood transfusions represent only one of many options;
- The decision to give a blood transfusion should be made according to the relevant guidelines;
- Transfusion risks should be weighed up when making the decision;
- The patient's wishes must be taken into account if at all possible;
- Trained staff should carry out and monitor the transfusion;
- The indications for, and circumstances of, a blood transfusion must be recorded, as must any complication; and
- In modern obstetrics, blood transfusions should be the exception rather than the rule.

Conclusion

Regarding the fact that prepartum hemoglobin is a strong predictor for the need of blood transfusion, it is a very clear conclusion that everything should be done to normalize low hemoglobin values during pregnancy and prior to delivery. In other terms, the better the peripartum hemoglobin, the lesser the chance to receive blood.

While there is no alternative to blood transfusion during acute and life threatening events, there are many options as alternatives to blood transfusion under cardiovascular stable conditions such as volume replacement and use of various pharmaceutical agents such as uterotonics, coagulation factors, and red cell stimulating agents, and heamatinics, especially parenteral iron preparations. The same is true for the postpartum period, where a women with severe anemia can be treated efficiently avoiding blood transfusion at the same time, also here especially by using effective and safe iron preparations. In a recent publication by Silverman et al., it was estimated that up to 32% of allogeneic blood was given inappropriately in the peripartum period because it was not given according to transfusion guidelines.

The same authors state that up to 11% of the women with transfusion could have avoided transfusion if they had aggressive iron treatment before birth.

Concerning the use of iron sucrose in obstetrics there is increasing evidence that iron sucrose is safe for the mother and the fetus using the recommended dosages and therapy regimens.

Iron sucrose is effective in pregnancy and postpartum in patients who do not respond to oral iron, who are non compliant to oral iron and in combination with rhEPO. In both periods, according to the present data, the expected Hb-increase and time for therapy are predictable in responding patients therefore it is questionable whether it is reasonable to wait for an oral iron response anyway in moderate to severe anemia. Indications for the use of iron sucrose complex are: preexisting (moderate–severe) anemia, no effect of oral iron, side effects of oral iron, refusing blood transfusion (e.g., Jehovah's Witness), limited time until delivery, coexisting risks (e.g., bowel disease, renal disease), pre- and postoperative period, and postpartum anemia.

Future fields of research are the evaluation of patient's satisfaction and quality of life, impact on costs and hospital stay, impact on blood transfusion frequency and mortality rate, and finally impact on other factors such as breast feeding behavior and neonatal outcome such as birth weight, prematurity and neonatal iron stores.

References

1. Scholl T, Reilly T. Anemia, iron and pregnancy outcome. J Nutr 2000;130:443–7.
2. Ekorema A. Blood transfusion in obstetrics and gynaecology. BJOG 1997;104:278–84.
3. Palo R, Ahonen J, Salo H, Salmenpera M, Krusius T, Mäki T. Transfusion of red blood cells: no impact on length of hospital stay in moderately anaemic patients. Acta Anaesthesiol Scand 2007;51:565–9.
4. Breymann C, Huch R. *Anaemia in Pregnancy and the Puerperium*, 2nd edn. Uni-Med Science, Bremen, 2006.
5. Winter C, Macfarlaine A, Tharaux CD, et al. Variations in policies for management of third stage of labour and in the immediate management of postpartum haemorrhage. BJOG 2007;114:845–54.
6. Force HaTT. Investigation and clinical management of haemorrhagic disorders in pregnancy. J Clin Pathol 1994;47:100–108.
7. Allen LH. Pregnancy and iron deficiency: unresolved issues. Nutr Rev 1997;55(4):91–101.
8. Hercberg S, Galan P, Preziosi P. Consequences of iron deficiency in pregnant women: current issues. Clin Drug Invest 2000;19(suppl 1):1–7.
9. Kaltreider F, Kohl S. Epidemiology of preterm delivery. Clin Obstet Gynecol 1980;23:17.
10. Siega-Riz A, Adair L, Hobel C. Maternal hematological changes during pregnancy and the effect of iron status on preterm delivery in a west Los Angeles population. Am J Perinatol 1989;15(9):515–22.
11. Sifakis S, Pharmakides G. Anemia in pregnancy. In: *Hematological Problems in Pregnancy*. Science NYAo, New York, 1999, pp. 125–36.
12. Silverman J, Barrett J, LCallum J. The Appropriateness of red Cell Transfusions in the peripartum patient. Obstet Gynecol 2004;104(5):1000–1004.
13. Al R, Unlubilgin E, Kandemir O, Yalvac S, Cakir L, Haberal A. Intravenous versus oral iron for treatment of anaemia in pregnancy. Obstet Gynecol 2005;106(6):1335–40.
14. Bhandal N, Russell R. Intravenous versus oral iron therapy for postpartum anaemia. BJOG 2006;113(11):1248–52.
15. Breymann C. Iron deficiency and anaemia in pregnancy: modern aspects of diagnosis and therapy. Blood Cells Mol Dis 2002;29:506–16.
16. Breymann C. The use of iron sucrose complex for anemia in pregnancy and the postpartum period. Semi Hematol 2006;43(4 Suppl. 6):S 28–31.
17. Breymann C, Zimmermann R, Huch R, Huch A. Use of rhEPO in combination with parenteral iron for the treatment of postpartum anemia. Eur J Clin Invest 1996;23:123–6.
18. Broche D, Gay C, Branger SA, Grangeasse L, Terzibachian J. Acute postpartum anaemia. Clinical practice and interest of intravenous iron. Gynecol Obstet Fertil 2004;32:613–19.
19. Dede A, Uygur D, Yilmaz B, Mungan T, Ugur M. Intravenous iron sucrose complex vs oral ferrous iron sulfate for postpartum iron deficiency anemia. Int J Gynaecol Obstet 2004;90:238–9.
20. Dodd J, Dare M, Middleton P. Treatment for women with postpartum iron deficiency anaemia (Cochrane Systematic Review). In: *The Cochrane Pregnancy and Childbirth Database Library*. Oxford, 2004.
21. Gravier A. Avoiding postpartum transfusions: the utility of intravenous iron supplementation (translation). J Gynecol Obstet Biol Reprod 1999;28: 77–8.
22. Huch R, Huch A. Erythropoietin in obstetrics. In: Spivak JL (ed) *Hematol Oncol Clin North Am*. W.B. Saunders Comp, Philadelphia, London, Sydney, 1994, pp. 1021–40.
23. Koenig H, Levine E, Resnick D, Meyer W. Use of rhEPO in a Jehovah's Witness. J Clin Anesth 1993; 5:244–7.
24. Krafft A, Breymann C, Huch R, Huch A. Intravenous iron sucrose in two pregnant women with inflammatory bowel disease and severe iron deficiency anemia. Acta Obstet Gynecol Scand 2000;79:720–22.
25. Hoigné R, Breymann C, Künzi U, Brunner F. Parenteral iron therapy: problems and possible solutions. Schweiz Med Wochenschr 1998;128:528–35.
26. Carretti N, Rosa PM. Intravenous iron therapy in pregnancy anemia: haematological response in relation to gestationale age. Gynecol Obstet Invest 1999;47:217–22.
27. Chamate E. Treatment of iron deficiency anemia in pregnancy and the immediate puerperium and other ferropenic conditions with saccharated iron administered intravenously in fractionated doses. In: *XIVth*

International Congress of Haematology. Sao Paolo, Brasil, 1972.
28. Danielson BG, Geisser P, Schneider W. *Iron Therapy with Special Emphasis on Intravenous Administration*. Vifor (International) Inc., St. Gallen, 1996.
29. Breymann C, Major A, Richter C, Huch R, Huch A. Recombinant human erythropoietin and parenteral iron in the treatment of pregnancy anemia: a pilot study. J Perinat Med 1995;23:89–98.
30. Breymann C, Richter R, Hüttner C, Huch R, Huch A. Effectiveness of rhEPO and iron sucrose vs iron therapy only, in patients with postpartum anaemia and blunted erythropoiesis. Eur J Clin Invest 2000; 30(2):154–61.
31. Zimmermann R, Breymann C, Huch R, Huch A. Subcutaneous and intravenous rhEPO are both effective as a single shot therapy in postpartum anaemia. Clin Invest 1994;72:S25–30.
32. Zimmermann R, Breymann C, Richter C, Huch R, Huch A. rhEPO treatment of postpartum anaemia. J Perinat Med 1995;23:111–16.

PART 8
Legal and Ethical Issues in Transfusion Medicine

CHAPTER 43

Ethical Aspects of Informed Consent: American Models

Ronald E. Domen
Department of Pathology, Division of Clinical Pathology, Penn State College of Medicine, Milton S. Hershey Medical Center, Hershey, Pennsylvania, USA

Historical background of informed consent

Ethical reflection on the physician–patient relationship has been a part of medicine since ancient times. The Code of Hammurabi (1727 BC) and the Hippocratic Oath (421 BC), for example, sought to define proper conduct for physicians toward their patients, and to protect patients from harm and injustice [1]. In the United States, the first Code of Medical Ethics came from the American Medical Association (AMA) in 1847 and over the ensuing years it became widely accepted [2]. Despite the growth and acceptance of the AMA's code, as well as ethical codes from other medical organizations that subsequently were developed, the high ideals of patient autonomy and informed consent remained elusive concepts until well into the twentieth century [2]. The concept that patients should be "participants" in medical decision-making, and that physicians should view patients as "partners," ran counter to the prevailing attitude of paternalism by physicians. Fragments of a growing concern for the issues of patient autonomy, of obtaining patient consent before performing medical treatment, and of truthfulness in the physician–patient relationship are scattered about in various medical writings in the early part of the twentieth century, but prior to the 1950s the issue of consent, or patient-centered healthcare was not given serious consideration by the medical profession.

The legal requirement for physicians to obtain the consent of their patients prior to surgery dates back to at least as early as the 1767 British case of *Slater v. Baker & Stapleton* [3]. The physician in this case had embarked on an orthopedic procedure without first obtaining the patient's consent. The judge concluded that obtaining a patient's consent was the usual practice of physicians, as well as a professional duty, and that the physician should have first obtained the patient's consent before the medical intervention [3].

A number of legal precedents throughout the twentieth century were instrumental in helping to establish support for the informed consent process in the United States. The 1914 case of *Schloendorff v. Society of New York Hospital* was one of the first and most influential cases in the early history of informed consent [4]. Mary Schloendorff consented to undergo a pelvic examination under anesthesia but stipulated that no surgery was to be performed. Despite her expressed wishes, the surgeon proceeded to remove a tumor. The patient suffered complications and sued. Justice Cardozo wrote in 1914 that "Every human being of adult years and sound mind has a right to determine what shall be done with his own body; and a surgeon who performs an operation without his patient's consent, commits an assault, for which he is liable in damages. This is true except in cases of emergency where the patient is unconscious and

Alternatives to Blood Transfusion in Transfusion Medicine, 2nd edition. Edited by A. Maniatis, P. Van der Linden, J.-F. Hardy.

where it is necessary to operate before consent can be obtained [4]."

The 1957 case of *Salgo v. Leland Stanford, Jr. University Board of Trustees* added the term "informed" to consent [5]. Mr. Salgo suffered injury following a medical intervention and he argued that he was not properly informed of the potential risks. The *Salgo* court highlighted the duty to disclose risks and alternatives as part of the process of obtaining consent for medical interventions and that a "full disclosure of facts [is] necessary to an informed consent [5]."

Additional court decisions related to informed consent followed in the 1960s and 1970s but three landmark decisions in 1972 are generally recognized as being significant to underpinning the concepts of the informed consent process. *Canterbury v. Spence, Cobbs v. Grant,* and *Wilkinson v. Vesey* all upheld the duty of physicians to disclose risks and alternatives to patients, a patient's right of self-decision and the exercise of choice, and the obligation to inform the patient in language and terms that the patient can understand [6–8].

To this day, legal cases continue to define and uphold the informed consent process to include non-invasive medical therapies, the duty of the physician to inform the patient of medically reasonable alternative treatments, and the physician's ethical and professional responsibility to provide relevant information that will allow the patient to make an informed decision.

The ethical basis for informed consent

As noted above, legal precedent has heavily impacted the development and promotion of informed consent. However, the ethical justification for informed consent is also well established and recognized. The Nuremberg Code, formulated in 1947, articulated the concept of informed consent as it applied to research subjects and was one of the first documents to provide an ethical basis for the protection of human subjects. The Nuremberg Code states that, "The voluntary consent of the human subject is absolutely essential [9]." It further stipulates that it is the "personal duty and responsibility" of knowledgeable individuals to obtain the subjects' consent, and to ensure that they understand and comprehend what is being presented to them [9]. The World Medical Association's Declaration of Helsinki (1964) and The Belmont Report (1979) also uphold the ethical principle of informed consent [10, 11]. Several important, fundamental principles of bioethics have applicability to the specific issue of informed consent [12–14]. For example,

- Autonomy (respect for persons): respect for individual decision-making, privacy, freedom of will, and self-determination; as well as the protection of those with diminished autonomy. Respect for persons through the process of informed consent.
- Beneficence: action(s) intended to benefit others; promoting the welfare of the patient, blood donor, or research subject; minimizing harm; acts of kindness, altruism, etc., that go beyond strict obligation.
- Confidentiality and Privacy: protection from unwanted intrusions into one's personal, physical, or psychological space; the right to be free from unwanted bodily contact.
- Justice: fair, equitable, and appropriate treatment that is due, owed, or deserved.

Autonomy is often considered to be the most important ethical principle that supports the obligation and duty for the informed consent process but, in this context, many bioethicists caution against placing too much weight on one moral principle and would prefer to place equal value on all of the applicable ethical principles [14]. In addition to the recognized principles of autonomy, beneficence, confidentiality, and justice, other areas of medical ethics also support the need for informed consent. Virtue ethics, for example, would argue that the virtues of integrity, fidelity, justice, compassion, etc., should become a part of the medical character and are fundamental to the *virtuous* practice of medicine [15]. The virtuous person—the person of integrity—would be a person who not only recognizes and accepts respect for autonomy but who interprets its application (e.g., informed consent) in the most morally sensitive way, and who can be trusted to respect the subtleties of the moral claim to autonomy. According to virtue ethics, the ethics of character and virtue—of personal responsibility and conscience—remain the final determinants to safeguard patients, blood donors, and research subjects [15]. Thus, obtaining valid informed consent is a moral obligation and duty that is firmly grounded in bioethics.

In the bioethics literature, as well as in most legal definitions, the informed consent process usually contains the following major elements or concepts [15, 16].

- Disclosure: sharing of material information by the healthcare professional.
- Comprehension: ability to understand information by the patient, blood donor, or research subject.
- Voluntariness: freedom in making decisions by the patient, blood donor, or research subject.
- Competence: ability of the individual to understand and make decisions.
- Consent: decision and authorization.

Some ethicists would add specific treatment plans or "recommendation(s)" to the above list, but at a minimum, it is generally felt that the above elements must be met in order to satisfy the requirement for informed consent [15]. In the typical clinical setting, recommendations are often a part of the information presented to the patient. It should also be appreciated that the above elements imply more than the idea of "shared decision-making" between the physician and the patient. While shared decision-making is an important component of the physician–patient relationship the final step in the process (i.e., consent) requires that the decision and authorization for treatment and intervention be made by the patient, and that it be made in an environment of voluntariness. Just as a patient may decide for the recommended treatment plan (informed consent), the patient may also decide against what is being presented (informed refusal) [15, 16].

The concept of "voluntariness"—while an ethical ideal—has the potential to be one of the weakest links in the consent process. How information and data are presented to the patient, research subject, or blood donor can influence the person's ability to make an informed, voluntary decision [15, 16]. Persuasive use of language, manipulation of data and information, and other types of coercion (knowingly or unknowingly) can undermine the informed consent process. Although not always possible or feasible, an advocate for the patient, research subject, or blood donor can be helpful in situations where there may be conflict of interest concerns with the individual(s) seeking the subjects' informed consent [17, 18]. An advocate is focused on the welfare of the person who is being asked for consent and can be a family member or other surrogate decision-maker or, in cases involving blood donation or transfusion, it might be the transfusion medicine physician or professional who, theoretically, has no direct involvement with the patient or donor [17, 18]. Transfusion medicine professionals are able to put transfusion- and donor-related technology, concepts, and therapeutic interventions into proper perspective; as long as they are not placed in situations where there may be potential conflict of interest concerns.

Informed consent in transfusion medicine

Informed consent thus has both legal and ethical justification and in recent decades, it has achieved a firm foundation in the practice of clinical medicine and in medical research. In this section, I will focus my discussion on the place of informed consent in blood banking and transfusion medicine [19].

The AABB (American Association of Blood Banks) first published a Code of Ethics for its membership in 1957 and it was last revised in 1997 [18, 19]. While the AABB's Code does not specifically address the issue of informed consent, there are references to behavior that could imply upholding it in the context of blood donors and transfusion recipients. The AABB Code states that individual and institutional members pledge to "provide and promote the highest quality of service and care to patients in accordance with current scientific knowledge and established standards for practice. . .Develop and/or support policies that prevent or eliminate the exploitation of donors and patients and oppose those measures that may adversely affect their health. . .[and] to abide by the principles of fair, just, equitable and legal standards of behavior in all relations with the patients and donors they serve..." Providing high quality care, under established legal and medical practice standards, and abiding in fair and just principles of behavior can be interpreted as including and promoting the tenets of informed consent. In 1986, the AABB issued a memorandum that recommended obtaining informed consent from patients prior to blood transfusion [18, 19]. This recommendation became codified in its *Standards for Blood Banks and Transfusion Services* [20]. The AABB *Standards* defines the minimum elements of consent for transfusion recipients, including the "right to accept or refuse transfusion [20]." For the blood donor, the AABB Standards also stipulates that "The consent of all donors shall be obtained before the donation" and delineates elements that should be included in the consent process [20].

The International Society of Blood Transfusion (ISBT) first addressed the issue of informed consent in their Code of Ethics for Blood Donation and Transfusion in 1980, and again in 2000 when the Code was revised [21]. The ISBT Code specifically states that "The donor should provide informed consent to the donation of blood or blood components and ...be advised of the risks connected with the procedure..." and that "Patients should be informed of the known risks and benefits of blood transfusion and/or alternative therapies and have the right to accept or refuse the procedure [21]." Today, many jurisdictions in the United States, as well as other regulatory and policy setting agencies (e.g., Joint Commission on Accreditation of Health Care Organizations, and the World Health Organization), require or recommend that patients undergo informed consent prior to blood transfusion.

Donor informed consent

At the time the American Red Cross Blood Donor Service was inaugurated in 1941 every blood donor was required to sign a "release" before donating blood [22]. This blood donor release was not in place to signify that the donor was making an informed decision and had decided to proceed with donation, but the release was more of a record that the donor was embarking upon blood donation "at his or her own risk," and basically provided absolution for everyone associated with the donation process in the event that harm was suffered by the donor [22].

The informed consent process for blood donation has undergone some changes since the early 1940s but there are virtually no data examining whether or not donors today comprehend the risks of donation any better than they did 60 years ago [18, 19, 23]. The usual donation process in current use involves giving the donor several information sheets to read that may or may not contain comprehensible information on the potential or real risks associated with donation. It is not uncommon that donors may be given only a few minutes to read the information presented to them. In addition, the collection facility staff does not generally sit down with the donor and go over the written information to ensure comprehension. In the author's experience, even "seasoned" donors who have donated many times without any adverse incidents may be surprised to learn that they are still at risk for fainting, or that they could develop a false-positive infectious disease test, or that they are personally responsible for any follow-up medical examinations or testing (including associated costs) that might be incurred or recommended. As compared to the whole blood donor, however, it is more likely that the apheresis or hematopoietic stem cell (HSC) donor will undergo a truly informed consent process because of the level of complexity involved in the collection process and/or because medications may be administered to the donor as part of the donation process [23].

While there have been a number of studies examining the adequacy of informed consent in various areas of medicine, there are virtually no studies of the informed consent process as it applies to blood donation. A recent study on informed consent for umbilical cord blood donation found a concerning lack of comprehension by the women consenting to the donation [24]. One other study on donor comprehension suggested that a donor's level of understanding may be related to how information is presented to him/her [25]. Additional studies on the informed consent process in blood and blood component donation are needed, particularly as blood component collection procedures become more complicated and may involve the administration of drugs to donors, and as new infectious disease screening tests are added (often under research protocols).

The donation of blood and blood components has a long history of being viewed as a safe procedure and this perception may have contributed to a certain "sense of security" for transfusion medicine personnel. In fact, whole blood donation has often been promoted as a possible health benefit for the donor. However, it is only in recent years that scientifically based studies have been performed to examine the risks associated with donating blood. Several studies in recent years have demonstrated that between 7 and 21% of blood donors suffer some sort of reaction or injury [26]. Common reactions include vasovagal symptoms, bruising, fatigue, and arm soreness [26, 27]. Less common reactions are nausea and vomiting, hematoma, or sensory changes [26, 27]. Rarely, arterial puncture, nerve damage, thrombophlebitis, and infection may occur [28, 29]. However, these are real and significant risks that are often not disclosed or explained to the donor prior to donation. Donors undergoing apheresis or HSC procedures have another set of risks, in addition to those common to whole blood donation, which may include exposure to certain medications or "donor enhancement drugs" (e.g., corticosteroids, granulocyte colony-stimulating factor [G-CSF], and/or hydroxyethyl starch) [17, 18, 23].

Transfusion medicine professionals have an obligation to protect donors from harm. This is a moral duty that is central to our profession and that is upheld by The Codes of Ethics of the AABB and the ISBT. A donor "bill of rights" has been advocated by some transfusion medicine professionals to ensure that the protection of donors is kept in the forefront [18, 23].

Informed consent for transfusion

Blood transfusion is a medical intervention that is potentially associated with adverse outcomes. As such, obtaining and documenting the patient's informed consent prior to transfusion therapy is legally and ethically upheld [16, 19]. Transfusion therapy has become embedded as a component of many medical and surgical interventions—sometimes as a life-saving intervention—and it has the potential to be taken for granted by the treating physician, or viewed as just another part of a normal, routine therapeutic plan. But, what might be considered "routine" or intuitive therapy by the physician may not be viewed as such by the patient. The competent, adult Jehovah's Witness patient immediately comes to mind where the principle of individual autonomy is a critical consideration in assessing the alternatives to transfusion before almost any medical or surgical intervention [30]. However, any competent adult has the right to refuse therapy—including potentially life-saving blood transfusion—and physicians have a moral duty to respect the patient's right to self-determination. A significant body of case law and other legal decisions in the United States, Canada, Europe, and other countries uphold the right of competent adults to refuse medical therapy and other life-saving measures including blood transfusion [30–32]. Physicians who do not obtain proper informed consent and adhere to the patient's wishes regarding blood transfusion or other medical interventions can potentially be found liable in civil suits for battery or negligence [33]. In the case of a minor or incompetent Jehovah's Witness patient the courts have generally allowed blood transfusions at the discretion of the treating physician. The pregnant Jehovah's Witness patient and the Jehovah's Witness patient that presents in an emergent situation have their unique aspects [34, 35]. Such ethical and legal dilemmas can be very difficult and disconcerting for the physician whose goal is to preserve their patient's life and, thus, some physicians will refuse to enter into a physician–patient relationship where refusal of care (e.g., a blood transfusion) could potentially result in an adverse outcome. A patient's right to refuse even life-saving therapy—such as a blood transfusion—underscores the fact that informed consent, when properly performed, is a shared decision-making process that involves meaningful discussion between the patient and the physician so that both are in agreement as to the treatment plan and any associated risks [30, 33, 36].

Documentation of informed consent for transfusion in the patient's medical record can take different formats [16]. A written progress note in the medical record by the physician that includes the elements of the informed consent process as it relates to transfusion is sufficient documentation. A separate form for documenting the informed consent process for transfusion is also acceptable, as is incorporating the consent for transfusion into a preoperative informed consent document. It should be understood, however, that simply having a signed note or form in the medical record does not document that the consent was "informed." Simply handing the patient a consent form and asking him to read and sign it is not informed consent. Informed consent is a process—and a process of education—that occurs over time between the physician and the patient or the patient's surrogate decision-maker. Thus, as it relates to transfusion, it is crucial that the person obtaining the patient's informed consent have sufficient knowledge in transfusion medicine in order to provide accurate and timely information as well as the ability to answer potential questions. An important role for the transfusion medicine professional is to provide transfusion medicine education for those health care professionals who participate in the informed consent process [19].

There have been few studies examining the informed consent process for transfusion. A 1993 study performed by Eisenstaedt et al. found that although 62% of the U.S. hospitals surveyed required written informed consent for transfusion there was little indication that true informed choice had been achieved [37]. A 2007 study from Canada showed that in 75% of the cases there was no documentation in the patient's medical record that any discussion about the risks, benefits, and alternatives to blood transfusion had occurred [38]. Although written informed consent for transfusion is not required in Canada this study points to a significant breakdown in the physician–patient relationship. Unpublished data from the author's institution shows that documentation in the patient's medical record of informed consent for transfusion occurs approximately 67–71% of the time; but as noted in other studies, the quality of the informed consent process is unknown. The minimal data available to date is concerning for the lack of documentation for informed consent before transfusion. Just as concerning is the lack of studies examining the adequacy of the informed consent process when it has been documented to have occurred. The difficulties associated with obtaining true informed consent are not limited to transfusion medicine but are evident in all of medicine. This is an important area for further study and research.

Conclusion

The ethical principles underlying autonomy, the individual as having decision-making capacity in health care, and the right for informed consent are relatively recent concepts in medicine and research. This is also true as it relates to informed consent in transfusion medicine. Central to the ethics of informed consent is that it be viewed as a process of education over time and in the context of respect, participation, collaboration, and negotiation.

The transfusion medicine professional is not uncommonly placed in the difficult position of trying to balance the needs of patients, donors, hospital administrators, and physicians. However, the transfusion medicine professional must continue to work and advocate for the ethical treatment of both donors and recipients. This is even more critical as "donor enhancing drugs" are developed to promote cellular collections from otherwise healthy donors, new technologies are developed to harvest blood cells and components, as donors increasingly serve as research subjects for infectious disease testing undergoing development, and adverse risks to transfusion continue to be associated with significant morbidity and mortality. Central to future debates on informed consent in transfusion medicine will be objective studies of its adequacy and efficacy, and how best to realize the ethical principles it reflects. This is an important and desirable ideal for our profession to strive for and to achieve.

References

1. Carrick P. *Medical Ethics in Antiquity*. D. Reidel, Dorbrecht, Holland, 1985, pp. 59–96.
2. Faden RR, Beauchamp TL. *A History and Theory of Informed Consent*. Oxford University Press, New York, NY, 1986, pp. 53–113.
3. Mazur DJ. Influence of the law on risk and informed consent. Brit Med J 2003;731–4.
4. *Schloendorff v. Society of New York Hospital*, 211 NY 125, 105 NE 92 (1914).
5. *Salgo v. Leland Stanford Junior University Board of Trustees*, 154 Cal App 2d 560 (1957).
6. *Canterberry v. Spence*, 150 US App 263, 464 F2d 772 (1972).
7. Cobbs v. Grant, 8 Cal 3d 229, 502 P2d 1, 104 Cal Rptr 505 (1972).
8. *Wilkinson v. Vesey*, 295 A2d 676 (Rhode Island), 1972.
9. Nuremberg Code. http://ohsr.od.nih.gov/guidelines/nuremberg.html (accessed May 19, 2009).
10. Belmont Report. http://ohsr.od.nih.gov/guidelines/belmont.html (accessed May 19, 2009).
11. Declaration of Helsinki. http://www.wma.net/e/policy/b3.htm (accessed May 19, 2009).
12. Mishkin B. Law and public policy in human studies research. Perspect Biol Med 2000; 43:362–72.
13. White BC, Zimbelman J. Abandoning informed consent: an idea whose time has not yet come. J Med Philos 1998;23:477–99.
14. Beauchamp TL, Childress JF. *Principles of Biomedical Ethics*, 5th edn. Oxford University Press, New York, NY, 2001, pp. 57–112.
15. Pellegrino ED, Thomasma DC. *The Virtues in Medical Practice*. Oxford University Press, New York, NY, 1993, pp. 127–43.
16. Domen RE, Smith JL. Confidentiality and informed consent issues in transfusion medicine. In: Macpherson CR, Domen RE, Perlin TM (eds) *Ethical Issues in Transfusion Medicine*. AABB Press, Bethesda, MD, 2000, pp. 39–54.
17. Volk EE, Domen RE, Smith ML. An examination of ethical issues raised in the pretreatment of normal volunteer granulocyte donors with granulocyte colony-stimulating factor. Arch Pathol Lab Med 1999; 123:508–13.
18. Domen RE. Ethical issues in transfusion medicine: the safety of blood and hematopoietic stem cell donation. Curr Hematol Rep 2005;4:465–9.
19. Domen RE. Medical ethics in transfusion medicine: a focus on the issue of informed consent. Blood Ther Med 2000;1:11–16.
20. AABB. *Standards for Blood Banks and Transfusion Services*, 24th edn. AABB Press, Bethesda, MD, 2006, pp. 16–17, 46–7.
21. International Society of Blood Transfusion. A code of ethics for blood donation and transfusion. Vox Sang 2002;82:166.
22. Coates JB Jr, McFetridge EM (eds). *Blood Program in World War II*. Department of the Army, Washington, DC, 1964, pp. 139–41.
23. Domen RE, Sazama K. Informed consent: the donor perspective. In: Stowell CP, Sazama K (eds) *Informed Consent in Blood Transfusion and Cellular Therapies: Patients, Donors, and Research Subjects*. AABB Press, Bethesda, MD, 2007, pp. 113–37.
24. Sugarman J, Kurzberg J, Box TL, Horner RD. Optimization of the informed consent for umbilical cord blood banking. Am J Obstet Gynecol 2002;187: 1642–6.
25. Lindstrøm TC, Røsvik A. Ambiguity leads to uncertainty: ambiguous demands to blood donors. Scand J Caring Sci 2003;17:74–7.
26. Newman BH, Pichette S, Pichette D, Dzaka E. Adverse effects in blood donors after whole-blood donation: a study of 1000 blood donors interviewed 3 weeks after whole-blood donation. Transfusion 2003; 43:598–603.
27. Zervou EK, Ziciadis K, Karabini F, Xanthi E, Chrisostomou E, Tzolou A. Vasovagal reactions in blood donors during or immediately after blood donation. Transfus Med 2005;15:389–94.
28. Newman BH, Waxman DA. Blood donation-related neurologic needle injury: evaluation of 2 years' worth of data from a large blood center. Transfusion 2001; 41:571–2.
29. Newman BH. Arterial puncture phlebotomy in whole-blood donors. Transfusion 2001;41:1390–92.
30. Stowell CP. Informed consent for patients: blood transfusion and cellular therapies. In: Stowell CP, Sazama K (eds) *Informed Consent in Blood Transfusion and Cellular Therapies: Patients, Donors, and Research Subjects*. AABB Press, Bethesda, MD, 2007, pp. 59–112.
31. Ariga T. Refusal of blood by Jehovah's witnesses and the patient's right to self-determination. Leg Med, in press.
32. Sarteschi LM. Jehovah's witnesses, blood transfusions and transplantation. Transplant Proc 2004;499–501.
33. Lo B. *Resolving Ethical Dilemma: A Guide for Clinicians*, 2nd edn. Lippincott Williams & Wilkins, Philadelphia, PA, 2000, pp. 19–29.

34. Schonholz DH. Blood transfusion and the pregnant Jehovah's Witness patient: avoiding a dilemma. Mt Sinai J Med 1999;66:277–9.
35. Woolley S. Jehovah's Witnesses in the emergency department: what are their rights? Emerg Med J 2005; 22:869–71.
36. Rogers DM, Crookston KP. The approach to the patient who refuses blood transfusion. Transfusion 2006;46:1471–7.
37. Eisenstaedt RS, Glanz K, Smith DG, Derstine T. Informed consent for blood transfusion: a regional hospital survey. Transfusion 1993;33:558–61.
38. Rock G, Berger R, Filion D, et al. Documenting a transfusion: how well is it done? Transfusion 2007;47: 568–72.

CHAPTER 44

Blood Transfusions, Jehovah's Witnesses, and the American Patients' Rights Movement[1]

Charles H. Baron
Boston College Law School, Newton Centre, MA, USA

As de Tocqueville observed in the mid-nineteenth century, the United States has been a fertile ground for the growth of an "innumerable multitude" of religious sects.[2] America was founded and settled in great part by persons who were seeking religious freedom in the new world, which had been denied to them in the old world. The constitutions of the 50 states generally protect such religious freedom. And the first article of the Bill of Rights of the Constitution of the United States provides that "Congress shall make no law respecting an establishment of religion, or prohibiting the free exercise thereof...." This language has been interpreted, among other things, to protect all religious beliefs from discriminatory governmental interference.[3] Thus, in theory at least, American law—as well as American history and tradition—encourages individuals and groups to seek after their spiritual well-being in accordance with the creed of their choice.

One of America's most flourishing religious groups is the Watchtower Bible and Tract Society—commonly known as "Jehovah's Witnesses." Born in the early 1870s as a Christian Bible study group in western Pennsylvania, it has grown into a worldwide organization comprising over four million adherents in over 200 countries. A central tenet of the group is a commitment to the Bible as the word of God (Jehovah) representing literal truth. Members of the group devote a great deal of effort to bringing the word of the Bible to nonmembers. In the United States, they distribute literature from house to house and in public places. Because of these proselytizing activities and because their beliefs and practices they are sometimes perceived as disturbingly different from those of the majority (if not harmful); governmental agencies have often tried to regulate them in ways that were contrary to their beliefs. As a result, Witnesses have been involved in a great deal of constitutional litigation in the United States—much of it before the Supreme

---

[1] This paper is an updated English version of two articles that have previously been published in French: Baron, C., Sang Pechè et Mort: les Tèmoins de Jèhovah et le mouvement des droits des malades, in Revue Trimestrielle du ressort de la Cour d'Appel de Versailles, Octobre-Dècembre 1993, p. 93, and Baron, C., Aspects relatifs au mouvement des droits des malades aux Ètats-Unis in S. Gromb & A. Garay (eds.), CONSENTEMENT ÈCLAIRÈ ET TRANSFUSION SANGUINE (1996), p. 30.

[2] De Tocqueville, A., "*Democracy in America* 290" (Mayer, ed., Perennial Library, 1988).

[3] See, for example, *Church of the Lukumi Babalu Aye v. City of Hialeah*, 508 U.S. 520 (1997) (holding unconstitutional a city's ban on "ritual slaughter" of animals that was intended to discriminate against the Santeria religion which engaged in such practices).

Alternatives to Blood Transfusion in Transfusion Medicine, 2nd edition. Edited by A. Maniatis, P. Van der Linden, J.-F. Hardy.

Court of the United States. Indeed, more American constitutional law may have been made by Jehovah's Witnesses than by any other group.[4]

Among the beliefs that set Witnesses apart from most other Americans is their conviction that the Bible forbids them to accept blood transfusions—even to save their lives—because it would constitute the sin of "eating blood." The line of thought that results in this conviction comprises two steps. First, Witnesses read the Bible as prohibiting Christians, as well as Jews, from eating blood. Second, they believe "eating blood" includes not only ingestion by mouth but also ingestion by other means—including blood transfusions.

There are, of course, scriptural provisions regarding the eating of blood that apply only to Jews. At Leviticus 17:10–12, for example, God says to Moses:

> As for any man of the house of Israel or some alien resident who is residing as an alien in their midst who eats any sort of blood, I shall certainly set my face against the soul that is eating the blood, and I shall indeed cut him off from among his people. For the soul of the flesh is in its blood, and I myself have put upon the altar for you to make atonement for your souls, because it is the blood that makes atonement by the soul in it. That is why I have said to the sons of Israel: "No soul of you must eat blood and no alien resident who is residing as an alien in your midst should eat blood."

This provision is part of God's special covenant with Israel, and therefore, applies only to Jews. But the ban on eating blood, the Witnesses point out, antedates Mosaic Law. At Genesis 9:1–4, God says to Noah after the flood:

> Be fruitful and become many and fill the earth. And a fear of you and a terror of you will continue upon every living creature of the earth and upon every flying creature of the heavens, upon everything that goes moving on the ground, and upon all the fishes of the sea. Into your hand they are now given. Every moving animal that is alive may serve as food for you. As in the case of green vegetation, I do give it all to you. Only the flesh with its soul—its blood—you must not eat.

This ban predates the covenant with Israel and is universal. God's ban on eating blood is thus binding on everyone who worships him. It is not contingent upon acceptance of the covenant with Israel, and it applies to Christians as well as Jews.

Further scriptural authority for this is provided by Acts 15:28–29. There the first council of the new Christian church, in response to a question as to whether converts to Christianity were to be circumcised according to Mosaic Law, replies:

> [T]he Holy Spirit and we ourselves have favored adding no further burden to you, except these necessary things, to keep abstaining from things sacrificed to idols and from blood and from things strangled and from fornication. If you carefully keep yourselves from these things, you will prosper.[5]

For the Witnesses, it is clear that God has commanded all his people to abstain from eating blood. And if eating blood is wrong because it is wrong to nourish one's self with the soul of another living being, they contend, how can it matter if the nourishment comes by way of one's mouth or by way of a transfusion directly into one's veins? Of course the Bible does not speak of blood transfusions because there was no thought of them at the time. But the principle is the same. "[T]he decree that Christians must 'abstain from blood' . . . covers the taking of blood into the body, whether through the mouth or directly into the bloodstream."[6]

After World War II, this part of the belief structure of Jehovah's Witnesses began increasingly to come into direct conflict with the belief structure of modern medicine. Until then, doctors and surgeons had not regularly availed themselves of blood transfusions. A Frenchman—Jean Baptiste Denis—is credited with having performed the first

---

[4] Between 1919 and 1988, the Supreme Court of the United States heard 71 cases in which the sect's practices raised important questions of federal substantive or constitutional law. In 47 of them, the Court ruled in favor of the Jehovah's Witnesses.

[5] For other authority to the same effect, see Watchtower Bible and Tract Society, *Jehovah's Witnesses and the Question of Blood*. 1977, pp. 10–17.

[6] Watchtower Bible and Tract Society. *Jehovah's Witnesses and the Question of Blood*. 1977, p.18.

successful blood transfusion in 1667.[7] (It was "successful" in that the 15-year-old boy whom he transfused with a half pint of lamb's blood did not die.) But the foundations of modern transfusion science were not laid until the early 1900s when the four basic blood type groupings were identified.[8] And it was not until several decades later, after other scientific advances had been made and "the concept of blood banks was introduced and the exigencies of World War II stimulated the investigation of methods for blood preservation, that blood became readily available and blood transfusion became popular."[9] Not until that point did modern medicine begin to believe that blood transfusions were essentially benign and that refusal of blood, when "medically necessary," was an irrational act.

The best-known early American court case acting out the conflict between the beliefs of modern medicine and those of Jehovah's Witnesses is *Application of the President and Directors of Georgetown College, Inc.*[10] Mrs. Jesse Jones, a 25-year-old mother of a 7-year-old child, had been brought by her husband to the emergency room of the Georgetown Hospital in the District of Columbia. She had lost two-thirds of her body's blood supply from a ruptured ulcer. The doctors who took charge of her case believed that she had a very good chance of survival with a blood transfusion but that she would die without one. Mr. and Mrs. Jones were Jehovah's Witnesses. They were eager to have the doctors treat Mrs. Jones, but they would not consent to a blood transfusion. The doctors considered this behavior to be medically irrational and wanted to override the Jones' refusal in order to save Mrs. Jones' life. They sought a court order allowing them to do so.

Judge J. Skelly Wright, a highly respected federal appeals court judge, gave them the order they wanted. A lower court judge had refused their request, and counsel for the hospital, a very famous and able attorney by the name of Edward Bennett Williams, had immediately appealed to Judge Wright, asking him for an emergency order to keep the patient alive—at least until the case could be fully heard on its merits. Several months after granting this order, Judge Wright filed an opinion in which he attempted to justify the emergency action he had taken. In it he cites two nineteenth century US Supreme Court decisions which state, in dictum, that First Amendment "free exercise" of religion guarantees do not prevent the government from making religiously-inspired suicide attempts illegal.[11] However, as Judge Wright himself notes, District of Columbia law did not make attempted suicide illegal and Mrs. Jones did not want to kill herself. He also argues that, because she had a 7-year-old child, Mrs. Jones could be forced to stay alive since "[t]he state as *parens patriae* will not allow a parent to abandon a child."[12] However, no statutes or legal precedents could be pointed to suggesting that a parent's medical treatment decisions could be overruled on the ground that they placed a child at risk of abandonment. As a "third set of considerations," Judge Wright pointed to "the position of the doctors and the hospital. Mrs. Jones was their responsibility to treat. The hospital doctors had the choice of administering the proper treatment or letting Mrs. Jones die in the hospital bed, thus exposing themselves, and the hospital, to the risk of civil and criminal liability in either case."[13] However, as is pointed out in a later opinion by one of Judge Wright's fellow judges, Mr. and Mrs. Jones had both "volunteered to sign a waiver to relieve the hospital of any liability for the consequences of failure to effect the transfusion."[14]

---

[7] Hagen P. *Blood: Gift or Merchandise?* 1982, p.12.

[8] Solomon, A history of transfusion medicine, In: Ross A (ed.) *III American Association of Blood Banks, Administrative Manual 2.* 1990.

[9] Wintrobe M. *Clinical Hematology*, 8th edn., 1981.

[10] 331 F. 2d 1000 (D.C. Cir. 1964) (hereinafter "Georgetown I.").

[11] *Late Corporation of the Church of Later Day Saints v. United States* (*Romney v. United States*), 136 U.S. 1, 49–50 (1890); *Reynolds v. United States*, 98 U.S. (8 Otto) 145, 166 (1878). The facts of the cases did not involve suicide. They involved state laws prohibiting the practice of religiously inspired polygamy.

[12] Georgetown I, p.1008.

[13] Georgetown I, p. 1009.

[14] Application of the President and Directors of Georgetown College, Inc., 331 F. 2d 1010, 1015–16 (D.C. Cir. 1964) (hereinafter "Georgetown II.").

The real basis for Justice Wright's opinion seems to be that, like the doctors involved, he found the Jones' position hard to understand and irrational—Mrs. Jones' life was being thrown away for no good reason. At one point, he suggests that "Mrs. Jones was *in extremis* and hardly *compos mentis* at the time in question: she was as little able competently to decide for herself as any child would be."[15] At other points, he raises the possibility that the Jones really wanted someone else to make the decision for them—thus relieving them of their religious obligation.[16] Finally, he describes a confrontation between Mr. Jones and representatives of the hospital in terms that suggest that he felt the latter were being forced to deal with some naive person who simply did not understand the modern world:

> The President of Georgetown University, Father Bunn, appeared and pleaded with Mr. Jones to authorize the hospital to save his wife's life with a blood transfusion. Mr. Jones replied that the Scriptures say that we should not drink blood, and consequently his religion prohibited transfusions. The doctors explained to Mr. Jones that a blood transfusion is totally different from drinking blood in that the blood physically goes into a different part and through a different process in the body. Mr. Jones was unmoved.[17]

Despite all its problems, the *Georgetown* decision came to wield an extraordinary influence in American law. The flaws are evident. No counsel was present to argue the Jones' side of the case. (Although Judge Wright had advised Mr. Jones to seek counsel, he had declined to do so.) Judge Wright himself admitted that the case's emergency circumstances required that he decide it in great haste. And several of Judge Wright's colleagues, when a petition for rehearing was filed a month later, took the opportunity to write opinions critical of what he had done and the reasons he gave for doing it.[18] That the case has been so influential despite all this may have something to do with the eminence of the judge and the lawyer involved in it. But it probably has more to do with the fact that the decision seemed to provide legal endorsement to the growing hegemony of the medical profession in American society. Counsel for the Joneses on their petition for a rehearing had argued: "The precedent created here is a threat to so many other persons that judicial substitution of medical discretion for individual discretion should be examined in principle to see where it is leading."[19] When the court denied the petition for rehearing, its decision could be read as saying for all intents and purposes: "Doctors know best, and doctor's orders (at least when life may be at risk) are to be followed."[20]

In the wake of the decision, other courts made themselves available to order Jehovah's Witnesses to submit to blood transfusions.[21] And even where courts refused to grant requested orders to force transfusions, they tended to accept Judge Wright's analytical framework. Often the decisions turned on whether or not the patient had minor children who would be "abandoned" by the death of a parent.[22] One court, in 1972, refused to order a transfusion for a Witness who was a father of minor children, but it felt compelled to justify its decision on the ground that "a close family relationship existed which went beyond the immediate members, that the children would be well cared for, and that the family business would continue to supply material needs."[23]

---

[15] Georgetown I, p. 1008.

[16] Georgetown I, pp. 1007, 1009.

[17] Georgetown I, p. 1007.

[18] Georgetown II, pp. 1010–1018.

[19] Georgetown II, p. 1013.

[20] In fact, as the court points out, its denial of the petition for rehearing was not meant to suggest any position on the merits of Judge Wright's decision. Georgetown II, p. 1010.

[21] See, for example, *Hamilton v. McAuliffe*, 277 Md. 336, 353 A. 2d 634 (1976); *United States v. George*, 239 F. Supp. 752 (D.C. Conn. 1965); *Raleigh Fitkin-Paul Morgan Memorial Hospital v. Anderson*, 42 N.J. 421, 201 A. 2d 537 (1964).

[22] Compare In Re Brooks' Estate, 32 Ill. 2d 361, 205 N.E. 2d 435 (1965) with *Hamilton v. McAuliffe*, 277 Md. 336, 353 A. 2d 634 (1976) and *Raleigh Fitkin-Paul Morgan Memorial Hospital v. Anderson*, 42 N.J. 421, 201 A. 2d 537 (1964).

[23] In Re Osborne, 294 A. 2d 372, 374 (D.C. Ct. App. 1972).

In 1976, with the celebrated decision of *In Re Quinlan*[24] it might have appeared that the plight of Witness patients who refused blood transfusions had been ameliorated. In that case, the Supreme Court of New Jersey recognized the right of Karen Quinlan, a young woman in a persistent vegetative state, to "die with dignity." The court allowed her family to have her removed from life support despite the unwillingness of her physician to agree to such a measure. The court based its decision upon the unwritten constitutional "right to privacy" which the US Supreme Court had developed in a series of cases—most prominently, the then recent abortion rights case, *Roe v. Wade*.[25] "Presumably," said the court, "this right is broad enough to encompass a patient's decision to decline medical treatment under certain circumstances, in much the same way as it is broad enough to encompass a woman's decision to terminate pregnancy under certain conditions."[26] On the surface, the *Quinlan* decision seemed a great victory for patient's rights. But a close reading of the opinion revealed that the decision was not as great a victory for patients as it had seemed—and that it was not victory at all for Jehovah's Witnesses refusing blood transfusions.

In its opinion, the *Quinlan* court made clear that the right to refuse treatment was not absolute. Two important state interests could outweigh it in appropriate cases. The first was the state's interest in preserving human life. This interest was not strong enough to outweigh the right to choose death in the case before the court because Karen Quinlan's life prospects were so poor and because the medical treatment being forced upon her was so invasive. But where such prospects were better or the treatment being recommended was less intrusive, treatment might still be forced on a patient. The second important interest of the state was that of protecting the professional ethics and discretion of the medical profession. That interest was not strong enough to outweigh the right to choose death in Karen's case because it was not clear that the medical profession as a whole opposed allowing people in Karen's condition to refuse treatment. Karen's physician had said that he was opposed, but many doctors, if not all, were in favor of having patients in a persistent vegetative state removed from life support. And what made some doctors refuse, as Karen's physician had, was fear of legal liability. By its decision in *Quinlan*, the court was removing that fear as a factor. If a particular patient's doctor still refused, the court would not force him or her to comply with the patient's wishes, but it would allow the patient's family to find another doctor who would comply.

Thus, *Quinlan* was less a recognition of patient's rights than of physicians' rights. Treatment could be refused for Karen Quinlan because such a refusal was not "medically irrational." However, patients refusing treatment which the medical profession believed to be life-saving and noninvasive could have treatment forced upon them. That this meant no change in the law for Jehovah's Witnesses who refused blood transfusions was made explicit. A scant 5 years before *Quinlan*, the Supreme Court of New Jersey had decided in *John F. Kennedy Memorial Hospital v. Heston*[27] that blood transfusions could be forced upon a Jehovah's Witness patient even in a case where the patient had no minor children who might be abandoned by her death. The *Quinlan* court took pains to make clear that *Heston* was still good law. The Witness cases in general were approved because the medical procedure involved in them (a blood transfusion) "constituted a minimal bodily invasion and the chances of recovery and return to functioning life were very good."[28] And *Heston* in particular was reaffirmed because it involved "most importantly a patient apparently salvable to long life and vibrant health—a situation not at all like the present case."[29]

But if *Quinlan* did not wreak a revolution for patient's rights—including those of Jehovah's Witnesses—it did provide a foundation upon which

---

[24] 70 N.J. 10, 355 A. 2d 647 (1976).
[25] 410 U.S. 113 (1973).
[26] In Re Quinlan, 70 N.J. 10, 40, 355 A. 2d 647, 663 (1976).
[27] 58 N.J. 576, 279 A. 2d 670 (1971).
[28] 70 N.J. at 41, 279 A. 2d at 664.
[29] 70 N.J. at 39, 279 A. 2d at 663.

such a revolution could be wrought. *Quinlan* had at least recognized patient autonomy as an important right. And its reasoning offered a guide as to how the scope of that right might be expanded. The medical profession and the courts needed to be shown that patient refusal of treatment was not as irrational as it seemed. Even if refusal seemed irrational from the point of view of the medical profession, it was very often, if not always, perfectly rational in terms of the values of the patients involved. And more often than the medical profession and the courts suspected, refusal of treatment was rational from a medical point of view as well.

Since *Quinlan*, the Witnesses have earnestly and persistently worked at establishing their right to refuse blood transfusions by educating the medical profession, the courts, and the public as to the rationality of their views. Education regarding the scriptural basis for their position has, of course, been fundamental—as has education regarding the perceived "invasiveness" of blood transfusions from the point of view of their religious beliefs and the poor spiritual "prognosis" they suffer from having their earthly lives prolonged at the cost of their salvation. (In the words of the family of the patient in one case: "He wants to live in the Bible's promised new world where life will never end. A few hours here would never compare to everlasting life."[30]) However, they have also done a brilliant job of making the case for the medical rationality of their position.

First, they have worked at demonstrating that blood transfusions, from a purely scientific point of view, are not the completely benign treatment modalities they have been thought to be. In this effort, they have been helped, of course, by the advent of the blood-borne scourges of AIDS and Hepatitis B. But as the Witnesses have shown, blood transfusions have always been much riskier than the run-of-the-mill medical practitioner was aware of or was willing to admit. The evidence for this comes entirely from scientific literature—literature which had been largely ignored by the medical profession as a whole. In 1960, an article in one medical journal had warned: "Blood is a dynamite! It can do a great deal of good or a great deal of harm. The mortality from blood transfusion equals that from ether anesthesia or appendectomy. In the London area, there has been reported one death for every 13,000 bottles of blood transfused."[31] In addition to the risk of death from hemolytic reactions (due to improper matching of blood types), there are the risks that result from the suppression of the body's natural immune system caused by a transfusion. And there are the risks of a long list of diseases, in addition to AIDS and hepatitis B that can be carried by transfused blood.

Second, Jehovah's Witnesses have worked with surgeons and physicians to develop and popularize methods of operating upon and treating patients without using blood transfusions. Not only had the run-of-the-mill physician downplayed the risks of blood transfusions, he had also exaggerated their necessity. For decades, anesthesiologists had, for example, routinely transfused patients preoperatively on the grounds of "medical necessity" whenever the patient's hemoglobin had gone below 10 g/dL. They believed this practice had a basis in scientific fact. In reality, it had been based upon myth. "The etiology of the requirement that a patient have 10 grams of hemoglobin (Hgb) prior to receiving an anesthetic," one scientist reported in 1988, "is cloaked in tradition, shrouded in obscurity, and unsubstantiated by clinical or experimental evidence."[32] Members of Jehovah's Witness hospital Liaison Committees, which have been established across the United States (as well as in many other countries, including France), have met with physicians and surgeons, providing them with information that disabuses them of mistaken notions regarding the necessity of transfusions and makes them aware of neglected techniques for treating patients without blood.

[30] In Re Osborne, 294 A. 2d 372, 373 (D.C. Ct. App. 1972).

[31] Unger. Medical-legal aspects of blood transfusion. NY State J Med 1960;60(2):237.

[32] Zauder, "How did we get a "magic number" for preoperative hematocrit, hemoglobin level?" In: *Perioperative Red Cell Transfusion: Program and Abstracts* (June 27–29, 1988).

Through the work of their Hospital Liaison Committees, the Witnesses claim to have secured the cooperation of over 13,000 American doctors in treating Witness patients without blood transfusions. Cooperating surgeons have discovered that even heart surgery can be performed without imposing blood transfusions on the grounds of "medical necessity." The distinguished cardiac surgeon, Michael DeBakey, for example, has reported his experience that "in the great majority of situations [involving Witnesses] the risk of operation without the use of blood transfusions is no greater than in those patients on whom we use blood transfusions."[33] And the techniques learned with Witness patients are often, then, employed with patients generally. One orthopedic surgeon reports: "What we have learned from those (Witness) patients, we now apply to all our patients that we do total hips on."[34]

These gains for the Witnesses within the medical community have helped to produce gains for them within the legal system as well. After *Quinlan*, the development of "right to die" doctrine by American courts began to accelerate. In 1977, the Supreme Judicial Court of Massachusetts, in *Superintendent of Belchertown Hospital v. Salkewicz*,[35] held that a patient had a constitutional right to refuse chemotherapy for cancer—even if the patient was likely to die significantly sooner without treatment than with it. Like *Quinlan*, the case involved a situation where the medical community might not have thought that refusal of treatment was "medically irrational." And like *Quinlan*, the opinion talked of state interests that could outweigh the patient's right to refuse treatment, adding to the interests in preserving human life and in protecting the medical profession the additional interests mentioned in *Georgetown*—preventing suicide and protecting third parties such as minor children. But the tone of the opinion was much more aggressive in asserting the right of patients to exercise their autonomy in medical decision-making. "The constitutional right to privacy, as we conceive it," said the court at one point, "is an expression of the sanctity of individual free choice and self-determination as fundamental constituents of life. The value of life as so perceived is lessened not by a decision to refuse treatment, but by the failure to allow a competent human being the right of choice."[36]

Cases after *Salkewicz* increasingly emphasized the autonomy of patients and allowed them to refuse a wider range of treatments. Courts gradually moved from allowing refusal only of "extraordinary" or "unnatural" or objectively "intrusive" treatment modalities, to allowing refusal of any sort of treatment the patients felt to be intrusive in their particular case.[37] Courts enforced the rights of patients, not only when they wanted mechanical respiration stopped, but also when they wanted hydration and nutrition stopped.[38] But in one respect, nonetheless, the fact patterns of these cases threw into question the extent to which they were truly endorsing patient autonomy. The cases typically involved patients with a grim prognosis. Most of the patients were terminally ill, living with irreversible and degenerative physical conditions, or in a persistent vegetative state. In contrast to most of the Jehovah's Witness patients who refuse blood, they were not likely to be, in the words of *Quinlan*, "a patient apparently salvable to long life and vibrant health."

It is only recently that courts have begun clearly to demonstrate their commitment to patient autonomy by gradually giving full protection to the right of Witness patients to refuse blood transfusions. Although the courts of most jurisdictions have continued to recognize the possibility that state interests—particularly the state's interest in protecting minors from abandonment by parents—can outweigh the right of Witnesses to refuse blood

[33] Dixon, Smalley. Jehovah's Witnesses: the surgical/ethical challenge. JAMA;246:2471.

[34] Watchtower Bible and Tract Society. *How Can Blood Save Your Life?* 1990, p. 16.

[35] 373 Mass. 728, 370 N.E. 2d 417 (1977).

[36] 373 Mass. 728, 370 N.E. 2d 417 (1977) at 742, 370 N.E. 2d at 426.

[37] See *Brophy v. New England Sinai Hospital*, 398 Mass. 417, 497 N.E. 2d 626 (1986).

[38] *Brophy v. New England Sinai Hospital*, 398 Mass. 417, 497 N.E. 2d 626 (1986) and see *Bouvia v. Superior Ct.* 179 Cal. App. 3d 1127 (1986).

transfusions, it is becoming very rare for courts to find the right actually outweighed in any given case. The highest courts of both Massachusetts[39] and Florida[40] have made clear that they will force the state to carry a very heavy burden when it attempts to show that a Witness' right to refuse a blood transfusion should be outweighed by his or her duty to parent minor children. And in 1990, the highest court of one state—New York—rejected wholesale the *Georgetown* device of employing an obligation to support one's children to restrict patient autonomy. "[W]e know of no law in this state prohibiting individuals from participating in inherently dangerous activities or requiring them to take special safety precautions simply because they have minor children," said the court. "There is no indication that the State would take a more intrusive role when the risk the parent has assumed involves a very personal choice regarding medical care. On the contrary, the policy of New York, as reflected in the existing law, is to permit all competent adults to make their own personal health care decisions without interference from the State."[41]

Even in New Jersey, the Witnesses' efforts at educating the courts and medical profession seem to have turned the law around. In 1992, the Appellate Division of the Superior Court of New Jersey handed down *In Re Hughes*,[42] a case involving a Witness patient whose surgeon, despite the patient's earlier instructions to the contrary, had transfused her when complications arose in surgery. When the patient recovered competency, she sought reversal of a judge's order authorizing the transfusions during the time when she had been incompetent. The Appellate Division affirmed the order, but only on the narrow ground that the record before the judge had left doubt as to what the patient would have wanted under the circumstances. And, in very strong language, the court evidenced an attitude toward the rights of Jehovah's Witnesses very different from that of *Heston* and *Quinlan*. "[A] competent Jehovah's Witness or person holding like views," said the court, "has every right to refuse some or all medical treatment, even to the point of sacrificing life... Should a patient decide, with full knowledge of the potential situation, to refuse life-sustaining medical treatment and the patient communicates this decision via clear and convincing oral directives, actions or writings, the patient's desires should be carried out."[43] Unlike the opinions in *Heston* and *Quinlan*, the opinion in *Hughes* is full of language sympathetic to the "rationality" of the Witnesses' position. This is likely to have been because of the excellent *amicus* brief filed in the case by the Watchtower Bible and Tract Society. Much of the court's language was drawn from material contained in that brief.

Since 1993, further progress has been made by the Watchtower Bible and Tract Society in its struggle with American medicine over the issue of whether blood transfusions will be forced upon Jehovah's Witnesses.

In the *Hughes* case, the New Jersey court had ultimately decided in favor of the physician-defendant on the ground that, despite Mrs. Hughes' signing of the hospital's standard written form for refusal of blood and her oral instructions, the physician had had a reasonable basis for doubting that Mrs. Hughes would have continued to refuse blood if she could have been made aware of the life-threatening emergency that followed her surgery. In an earlier case, *Werth v. Taylor*,[44] the Court of Appeals of Michigan had also found in favor of a physician who had been sued under the *Hughes* circumstances. In that case, the Michigan court had set up what seemed an insurmountable legal hurdle for unconscious Witness patients. "[I]n a situation like the present," the court said, "where there is an emergency calling for an immediate decision, nothing less than a fully conscious contemporaneous decision by the patient will be sufficient to override

[39] *Norwood Hospital v. Munoz*, 409 Mass. 116, 4564 N.E. 2d 1017 (1991).

[40] *Public Health Trust v. Wons*, 541 So. 2d 96 (Fla. 1989).

[41] *Fosmire v. Nicoleau*, 74 N.Y. 2d 607, 551 N.E. 2d 77, 84 (1990).

[42] 259 N.J. Super. 193, 611 A. 2d 1148 (1992).

[43] 259 N.J. Super. 193, 611 A. 2d 1148 (1992) at 202–203, 611 A. 2d at 1153.

[44] 190 Mich. App. 141, 475 N.W.2d 426 (1991).

evidence of medical necessity."[45] But in *Hughes*, the New Jersey court had said "Should a patient decide, with full knowledge of the potential situation, to refuse life-sustaining medical treatment and the patient communicates this decision via clear and convincing oral directives, actions, or writings, the patient's desires should be carried out."[46]

Counsel for the Watchtower Society responded to the challenge of *Hughes* by drafting and disseminating advance-directive "writings" which attempt to communicate in "clear and convincing" fashion a refusal of blood transfusions "with full knowledge" of the types of medical emergencies that might arise in the future. Written forms, tailored to conform to the laws of the each of the 51 American jurisdictions, have been made available through the Society's Hospital Liaison Committees in every state and in the District of Columbia. By means of explicit language in such advance directives, the person executing the document informs all health care personnel

> I am one of Jehovah's Witnesses. On the basis of my firmly held religious convictions, see *Acts* 15:28, 29, and on the basis of my desire to avoid the numerous hazards and complications of blood, **I absolutely, unequivocally and resolutely refuse homologous blood** (another person's blood) **and *stored* autologous blood** (my own stored blood) under any and all circumstances, no matter what my medical condition. This means no whole blood, no red cells, no white cells, no platelets, and no blood plasma no matter what the consequences. Even if health-care providers (doctors, nurses, etc.) believe that only blood transfusion therapy will preserve my life or health, I do not want it. Family, relatives or friends may disagree with my religious beliefs and with my wishes as expressed herein. However, their disagreement is legally and ethically irrelevant because it is my subjective choice that controls. Any such disagreement should in no way be construed as creating ambiguity or doubt about the strength or substance of my wishes.[47]

The person executing this directive also informs all health care personnel that "**I accept and request alternative nonblood management** to build up or conserve my own blood, to avoid or minimize blood loss, to replace lost circulatory volume, or to stop bleeding. For example, volume expanders such as dextran, saline or Ringer's solution, or hetastarch would be acceptable to me."[48] The person executing the form may also, (by choosing among options offered on the form), make clear to health care personnel whether or not he consents to the use of products containing minor blood fractions or non-stored autologous blood—blood therapies upon which the Society has taken no position and which it has designated "conscience matters."

A four-page document explaining the use of the advance directive has also been prepared for distribution in each jurisdiction. The informative leaflet which accompanies the combined advance directive/health care proxy designed for use in Massachusetts (whose law authorizes the appointment of a health-care agent or "proxy" to make health-care decisions for an incompetent patient) urges prospective patients to discuss the details of their desires and their advance directives with the person they appoint as their health care agent. It also urges the prospective patient to "discuss with your doctor the same information you discuss with your agent. . . . Be sure to discuss in depth the many medical alternatives for bloodless surgery that are available and acceptable to you .... Let your doctor know that you have thoroughly discussed these matters with your agent. (You may even want to introduce your agent to your doctor.) The better your doctor understands you, the less likely it is that problems

---

[45] 190 Mich. App. 141, 475 N.W.2d 426 (1991) at 147, 475 N.W.2d at 429 [emphasis in the original].

[46] 259 N.J. Super. 193, 202–203, 611 A.2d 1148, 1153 (1992).

[47] "Health Care Proxy" prepared by the Watchtower Bible and Tract Society for use in the Commonwealth of Massachusetts (October, 1994) at p. l. The full four-page form is attached hereto as Appendix A.

[48] "Health Care Proxy" prepared by the Watchtower Bible and Tract Society for use in the Commonwealth of Massachusetts (October, 1994) at p. l. The full four-page form is attached hereto as Appendix A.

will arise."[49] To further avoid problems stemming from misunderstanding, prospective patients are urged to carry on their person at all times an "Advance Medical Directive/Release" card. "Thus, in the event of an emergency in which you are unconscious, the Advance Medical Directive/Release will identify you as one of Jehovah's Witnesses, will make known your refusal of blood, and will identify your emergency contacts."[50] It is also suggested that the emergency contacts be the same people who have been granted health-care agency by means of the health-care proxy.

To the extent that such documents are employed by Jehovah's Witness patients, one would expect to see continuation of the existing trend toward increasing physician compliance with refusals of blood transfusions. Those physicians who do not comply certainly risk running afoul of another developing trend—the increasing tendency of courts to entertain suits for damages against physicians who force transfusions upon unwilling patients. For example, in the 1994 Ohio case of *Perkins v. Lavin*,[51] a Witness patient brought an action for damages against her physician for having administered a blood transfusion while she was unconscious. At the time that she had entered the hospital for treatment of postpartum hemorrhaging, she had given the physician oral notice that she was not to be provided any blood or blood derivatives and had signed a form stating: "I REQUEST THAT NO BLOOD OR BLOOD DERIVATIVES BE ADMINISTERED TO [ME] DURING THIS HOSPITALIZATION, NOTWITHSTANDING THAT SUCH TREATMENT MAY BE DEEMED NECESSARY IN THE OPINION OF THE ATTENDING PHYSICIAN OR HIS ASSISTANTS TO PRESERVE LIFE OR PROMOTE RECOVERY. I RELEASE THE ATTENDING PHYSICIAN, HIS ASSISTANTS, THE HOSPITAL AND ITS PERSONNEL FROM ANY RESPONSIBILITY WHATEVER FOR ANY UNTOWARD RESULTS DUE TO MY REFUSAL TO PERMIT THE USE OF BLOOD OR ITS DERIVATIVES." Nonetheless, the doctor had transfused her to save her life when her blood count dropped dramatically as a result of surgical complications. When the patient brought suit for money damages based upon theories of assault and battery and intentional infliction of emotional distress, the physician defended himself on the ground that he had not intended to inflict personal injury on the plaintiff. Rather, he claimed, he had intended merely to preserve plaintiff's health and life and had, in fact, done so. The court held for the defendant as to the claim for intentional infliction of emotional distress on the ground that defendant's behavior did not rise to the level of "outrageousness" required to make out a claim under that theory. However, as to the assault and battery claim, the court reversed a lower court finding for defendant, stating:

> In arguing that it cannot be held liable for assault and battery if it did not intend to "inflict personal injury," defendant has misapprehended the gist of the tort of battery. Battery not only protects individuals from harmful contact, but protects them from any offensive contact.
>
> "a harmful or offensive contact with a person resulting from an act intended to cause the plaintiff or a third person to suffer such a contact, *** is a battery."
>
> "Battery" includes innocent intentional contact and even intentional contact meant to assist the complainant, if that contact is unauthorized ***.[52]

And, in the 1994 case of *Clark v. Perry*,[53] the North Carolina Court of Appeals entertained a suit for damages against a physician on grounds of malpractice and failure to obtain informed consent where the allegations of plaintiff were not that he had deliberately transfused a Witness patient against the latter's will, but that he had negligently failed to discover that the patient was a Witness

[49] "Questions & Answers about the Health Care Proxy ('Combined Form')," prepared by the Watchtower Bible and Tract Society to accompany the health care proxy form for Massachusetts at p. 2. The full four-page document is attached hereto as Appendix B.

[50] "Questions & Answers about the Health Care Proxy ('Combined Form')," at l.

[51] 648 N.E.2d 839 (Ohio App. 9 Dist. 1994).

[52] 648 N.E.2d 839 (Ohio App. 9 Dist. 1994) at 841 [citations to authority omitted].

[53] 114 N.C. App. 297, 442 S.E.2d 57 (1994).

who had refused all blood and blood products. The patient's principal physician had been made well aware of the patient's religious beliefs, and the patient had taken steps to make sure that his views regarding blood transfusions were made manifest to hospital staff and had been entered in his hospital record. Nonetheless, a staff specialist who claimed to have been unaware of the patient's religious objections ordered a blood transfusion administered at a point when the patient was unconscious or asleep. Ultimately, the court affirmed a dismissal of plaintiff's claim. But it was solely on the ground that insufficient evidence had been introduced to prove that the defendant had been negligent in not knowing of the patient's objection to blood transfusions.

Perkins v. Lavin also highlights another aspect of progress in this field since 1993. The Witness patient in that case refused a life-saving blood transfusion just after having given birth to a child. The child was clearly dependent upon the patient for her care. Nonetheless, the court made no mention of the state's interest in preventing "abandonment of minor children" in discussing whether the plaintiff had a cause of action against her physician. Indeed, no such defense was raised by the physician. Likewise, no mention of such a defense was made in *Werth v. Taylor*, where the Witness patient had two young children at home and had just given birth to twins. This trend against giving critical weight to such an interest of the state is perhaps most manifest in some of the recent cases dealing with attempts to force cesarean births upon women who are experiencing troubled pregnancies. In the 1994 Illinois case of *In Re Baby Boy Doe*,[54] doctors urged a c-section or an induced birth upon a patient on the ground that her 35-week, viable fetus would otherwise die or be born mentally retarded. The patient refused because of her personal religious beliefs and chose instead to await natural childbirth. Her physicians then applied to a court for an order compelling the patient to consent to a c-section. The court refused to grant such an order, and the Appellate Court of Illinois affirmed. "[A] woman's right to refuse invasive medical treatment," said the court, "is not diminished during pregnancy. The woman retains the same right to refuse invasive treatment, even of lifesaving or other beneficial nature, that she can exercise when she is not pregnant. The potential impact upon the fetus is not legally relevant. . . ."[55] However, whether this degree of rejection of the state interest in protecting innocent third parties would extend to cases of refusal of blood was left open. In distinguishing a 1964 New Jersey case[56] which had held that a transfusion could be forced upon a Witness patient so as to protect the fetus she was carrying, the court said: "This and other similar blood transfusion cases are inapposite, because they involve a relatively non-invasive and risk-free procedure, as opposed to the massively invasive, risky, and painful cesarean section. Whether such non-invasive procedures are permissible in Illinois, we leave for another case."[57]

In the past 5 years, the right of adult, competent Jehovah's Witnesses to refuse blood transfusions has become even more clearly established in American law. Case law issuing from state courts has continued the trend toward supporting patient interests in personal autonomy and religious freedom over state interests advanced in favor of forced transfusions. Thus, in 1997, in its opinion in *In re Fetus Brown*,[58] the Appellate Court of Illinois moved beyond its 1994 decision in *In re Baby Boy Doe*[59] to hold that a blood transfusion could not be forced upon a pregnant Witness patient in order to save the life of her fetus. In doing so, the court explicitly rejected the language in the *Baby Boy Doe* opinion that had suggested that a blood transfusion, unlike the caesarean section proposed

---

[54] 198 Ill. Dec. 267, 260 Ill. App.3d 392, 632 N.E.2d 326 (Ill. app., 1st Dist. 1994).

[55] 198 Ill. Dec. 267, 260 Ill. App.3d 392, 632 N.E.2d 326 (Ill. app., 1st Dist. 1994) at 273, 260 Ill. App.3d at 401, 632 N.E.2d at 332.

[56] *Raleigh Fitkin-Paul Memorial Hospital v. Anderson*, 42 N.J. 421, 201 A.2d 537 (1964).

[57] 198 Ill. Dec. at 273, 260 Ill. App.3d at 402, 632 N.E.2d at 333.

[58] 294 Ill. App.3d 159, 689 N.E.2d 397 (1997).

[59] 260 Ill. App.3d 392, 632 N.E.2d 326 (1994).

in *Baby Boy Doe*, was a "relatively noninvasive and risk free procedure."[60] The court held in *Brown* that "a blood transfusion is an invasive medical procedure that interrupts a competent adult's bodily integrity" and concluded that "[u]nder the law of this State... we cannot impose a legal obligation upon a pregnant woman to consent to an invasive medical procedure for the benefit of her viable fetus."[61]

The right of competent Jehovah's Witness to refuse transfusions has become so well established in the law that courts show increasing willingness to entertain actions for money damages against physicians who force transfusions upon unconsenting patients. Despite the difficulties such cases present for convincing juries that substantial damages have been suffered (the physician claims that he is being punished for having saved the life of a patient), large money damage awards are being recovered in a significant number of cases. In the 1994 case of *Sargeant v. New York Infirmary-Beekman Downtown Hospital*,[62] a New York State jury awarded $500,000 to a Witness adult who was transfused against his will.[63] In the 1997 case of *Jones v Wrona*,[64] an Illinois jury awarded the plaintiff $150,000. Between 1991 and 1998, at least 11 similar cases were settled out-of-court for amounts totaling in excess of $480,000.[65] This trend is likely to be helped along by the 1999 decision of the highest court of Massachusetts in *Shine v. Vega*.[66] In that case, the family of a young woman with asthma brought an action for money damages against a physician who claimed to have saved her life by forcibly intubating her when she presented herself at an emergency room suffering from an acute asthma episode. Two years after the forced intubation incident, the patient died as a result of another acute episode because her intense fear of hospitals caused by the earlier experience kept her from again seeking emergency room assistance. The trial court dismissed the family's wrongful death action on the ground that the doctor had acted properly in light of the emergency situation. However, on appeal, the Supreme Judicial Court of Massachusetts reversed the lower court and reinstated the damage suit on the ground that the patient had made very clear to the physician that she would not consent to the intubation, even if, in the physician's opinion, refusal might lead to her death. "In the often chaotic setting of an emergency room," the court observed, "physicians and medical staff frequently must make split-second life-saving decisions. Emergency medical personnel may not have the time necessary to obtain the consent of a family member when a patient is incapable of consenting without jeopardizing the well-being of the patient. *But a competent patient's refusal to consent to medical treatment cannot be overridden whenever the patient faces a life-threatening situation.*"[67]

Even in cases involving minor patients, American courts are demonstrating increased respect for Witnesses' religious objections. In the United States, the statutory age of majority at which children are generally judged to be competent to make decisions for themselves is 18. However, by statute and by case law, children below the age of majority are under certain circumstances considered to be "mature minors" and empowered to make some medical decisions for themselves. The "mature minor" doctrine has begun to be extended by court decision to situations where minor Witness patients refuse blood transfusions for themselves. Thus, in the 1999 case of *In re Rena*,[68] the Appeals Court of Massachusetts reversed a lower court decision ordering the administration of a blood transfusion upon a 17-year-old Witness patient because the lower court had failed to consider the level of

[60] 260 Ill. App.3d 392, 632 N.E.2d 326 (1994) at 402, 632 N.E.2d at 333.

[61] In re Fetus Brown at 171, 689 N.E.2d at 405.

[62] No. 16068/91 (Sup. Ct. N.Y. County, July 25, 1994).

[63] A new trial was ordered in this case on the ground that the judge believed the verdict to be excessive, and it was later settled out-of-court for $75,000.

[64] No. 94 L 2935 (Cir. Ct. Will County [Ill.], November 12, 1997).

[65] Letter dated August 12, 1999, from Donald T. Ridley, Esq., Associate General, Watchtower Bible and Tract Society of Pennsylvania.

[66] 709 N.E.2d 58 (Ma. 1999).

[67] 709 N.E.2d 58 (Ma. 1999) at 65 [emphasis supplied].

[68] 46 Mass. App. Ct. 335, 705 N.E.2d 1155 (1999).

maturity of the patient in issuing its order. The patient's level of maturity was relevant for determining whether or not she was competent to make the decision for herself. It was also relevant for deciding what was truly in her "best interest" even if she was not yet fully competent to make the decision for herself. "Although the judge did consider Rena's wishes and her religious convictions in this matter, he made no determination as to her maturity to make an informed choice," the court said. Pointing to earlier decisions of the Illinois Supreme Court[69] and the Maine Supreme Judicial Court[70] in which the rights of mature minors had been protected under similar circumstances, the court concluded "we think [the trial judge's action] was error particularly in the circumstances of this case where Rena will soon attain the age of 18. In addition, in assessing Rena's preferences and religious convictions, he should not have relied solely on the representations made by her attorney and her parents but should have heard Rena's own testimony on these issues where she apparently had the testimonial capacity to answer questions. Only after evaluating this evidence in light of her maturity could the judge properly determine her best interests."[71]

Where Witness parents wish to refuse blood transfusions for their minor children, American law generally does not permit them to do so if there is no alternative course of acceptable medical treatment. As the US Supreme Court observed in the 1944 case of *Prince v. Massachusetts*,[72] "Parents may be free to become martyrs themselves. But it does not follow that they are free, in identical circumstances, to make martyrs of their children before they have reached the age of full and legal discretion when they can make that choice for themselves." In 1968, the US Supreme Court affirmed, on the authority of *Prince*, a lower court decision that a minor could be transfused over the protest of his Witness parents.[73] However, where alternative acceptable courses of medical treatment are available, cases have recognized the right of parents to make reasonable medical choices for their children different from those which attending physicians believe to be best.[74] In a recent South Carolina decision, *Banks v. Medical University of South Carolina*,[75] that right was explicitly held to apply to situations where Witness parents refuse blood transfusions for their children. In that case, the child died while being provided emergency treatment that included an unconsented-to blood transfusion. The parents sued the hospital and physicians involved for wrongful death and battery and introduced expert evidence that there had been no emergency requiring transfusion of blood plasma. The lower court found for the hospital, but the Supreme Court of South Carolina reversed on appeal. "Banks concedes that she had no authority to withhold necessary medical treatment from her child even if such treatment was contrary to her religious views," the court said. "However, she contends that the transfusions were not necessary and, therefore, her consent was required. She presented testimony of an expert witness... to establish that there was no emergency justifying the transfusion of blood to Phaedra.... We find that Banks has presented an issue of material fact as to whether Phaedra was in a life threatening situation which would have justified the administration of the transfusions without parental consent. Therefore, summary judgment was improperly granted."[76]

The willingness of the *Banks* court to consider the question of the reasonableness of a physician's decision to transfuse in an emergency situation evidences another aspect of the progress being made in the United States by The Watchtower Society. As a result of the extraordinary

---

[69] In re E.G., 133 Ill.2d 98, 549 N.E.2d 322 (1989).

[70] In re Swan, 569 A.2d 1202 (Me. 1990).

[71] In re Rena, 46 Mass. App. Ct. at 337–38, 705 N.E.2d at 1157. For a similar holding, see also, In re W.M., 823 S.W.2d 128 (Mo. Ct. App. 1992).

[72] 321 U.S. 158, 170 (1944).

[73] *Jehovah's Witnesses v. King County Hospital*, 278 F. Supp. 488 (W.D. Wash. 1967), aff'd. per curiam, 390 U.S. 598 (1968).

[74] See, for example, In re Hofbauer, 47 N.Y.2d 648, 393 N.E.2d 1009 (1979).

[75] 444 S.E.2d 519 (S.C. 1994).

[76] 444 S.E.2d 519 (S.C. 1994) at 521–22.

work of the Society's Hospital Liaison Committees, bloodless medical treatment (including bloodless surgery) is gradually becoming the "gold standard" of practice among top physicians and surgeons in the United States. Whereas, 5 years ago, bloodless medicine and surgery programs were established at only about 14 centers in the United States, there are about 100 such centers in the United States today.[77] These centers are liberally distributed across the country. Sites include some of the most prestigious medical institutions in America, such as Ohio's Cleveland Clinic, which has been rated as the top center in the United States for heart surgery. With help from the Hospital Liaison Committees, the American medical community is learning that bloodless medicine and surgery tend to produce better results for patients and significantly reduce medical costs as well. Patients who are treated without transfusions not only avoid the risk of contracting blood-borne diseases such as AIDS and hepatitis, they also recover more quickly from surgical procedures (transfusions tend to depress the body's natural immune system) and spend fewer days in the hospital.[78] A study recently conducted by members of the Cleveland Clinic's anesthesiology department concluded that using a bloodless surgery protocol 50% of the time "could save the healthcare industry up to $3.7 billion dollars a year. That includes savings of about $400 to $1400 for every unit of transfused blood from outside donors, factoring in the extra costs of treating postoperative fevers and infections."[79]

Clearly, it is not only Witness patients who benefit from the work of the Hospital Liaison Committees. "No one wants to get blood," one heart surgeon was recently quoted as saying. "As patients become more informed, they're going to specify they don't want blood products. Maybe not to the extent of dying for it (as do Witnesses), but to reduce risks."[80] One California bloodless surgery center reported this year that "one fifth of the patients requesting bloodless surgery are non-Witnesses."[81] Another California center, Alvarado Hospital, reported that only 35% of its patients in 1998 (compared to 97% in 1997) received blood or other blood products such as plasma. "[T]he heart-lung surgery department at [Alvarado] has cut expenses by 40 percent by reducing transfusions, which cost up to $300 per unit for the blood and its storage and shortening hospital stays for patients," a nurse-specialist stated.[82] Widespread use of bloodless medicine and surgery has been helped along by the development of new procedures for recycling the patient's own blood, for increasing the oxygen-carrying capacity of red blood cells, and for stimulating the body to produce additional red blood cells. "But the most important technique," say practitioners, "is simply good housekeeping—cutting cleanly and stopping the bleeding as it occurs."[83] For this purpose, surgeons will frequently use electro cautery to stop bleeding as they cut or employ new harmonic scalpels, which use ultrasonic vibrations to cut and seal the wound at the same time.

Ironically, through their success in improving surgical and medical techniques for all patients, Witness patients seem to have caused a slight medical backlash against themselves. Now that the medical reasons for refusing blood transfusions have become so well known, attention has been distracted somewhat from the Witnesses' religious objections. Even the Witnesses' "blood refusal card" (carried by members to prevent blood from being administered

---

[77] Mary McGrath. Bloodless surgery answer to some patients' prayers, Omaha World-Herald, August 10, 1999, at pp.. 1, 8.

[78] Article in February 1998 issue of Archives of Pathological Laboratory Medicine and article in February 11, 1999 issue of the New England Journal of Medicine.

[79] Ron Shinkman. More going bloodless, Modern Healthcare, November 9, 1998, at p. 57.

[80] Eric Niiler, Bloodless surgery, San Diego Union-Tribune, February 18, 1999, at pp. E-1 and E-7.

[81] Eric Niiler, Bloodless surgery, San Diego Union-Tribune, February 18, 1999, at p. E-7.

[82] Eric Niiler, Bloodless surgery, San Diego Union-Tribune, February 18, 1999.

[83] Andrew Pollack, "Bloodless" surgery gains new acceptance, The New York Times, April 21, 1998, at p. F8-F9.

to them while unconscious during an emergency) gives among the reasons for refusal "the numerous risks and complications resulting from the use of blood." For this reason, some doctors have suggested that they will not honor the blood refusal card in cases where they believe that the medical benefits of a blood transfusion outweigh its medical "risks and complications." In an article published in 1998,[84] two American physicians alleged that Witness patients who execute the cards do so after having heard only The Watchtower Society's one-sided views of the medical risks of blood transfusions. They urge emergency physicians, as a result, not to comply with wishes expressed in a blood refusal card unless a Witness patient reaffirms them after having had medical choices fully explained to him or her at the time of the emergency. As Donald Ridley, Associate General Counsel for The Watchtower Society points out in an answering article,[85] this line of reasoning, were it to be taken seriously, would put in jeopardy all of the progress in patients' rights made in the United States in the last 25 years. Doctors in the United States do not have legal power to require patients to prove that a decision to refuse treatment is "medically rational" in order to have the refusal respected. And, ultimately, the Witness blood refusal card does not justify refusal on grounds of medical rationality. It relies upon the Witnesses' reading of the Bible's proscription against eating blood and states that the patient is willing to accept death over violation of that proscription.

In the end, assiduous protection of the rights of Witness patients depends at least as much upon the work of lawyers as it does upon the work of doctors. In this respect, The Watchtower Society has come a long way since 1964 when, in the *Georgetown Hospital Case*, Mr. Jones, who had been advised by Judge Wright that he should obtain a lawyer, "went to the telephone and returned in 10 or 15 minutes to advise that he had taken the matter up with his church and that he had decided that he did not want counsel."[86] A growing number of attorneys in the United States now represent Witness patients in blood refusal cases with assistance from the Society. Associate General Counsel Ridley has recently published a very helpful handbook for "Legally Defending Jehovah's Witnesses' Choice of Alternative Nonblood Management" that is made available to such attorneys. Ridley also has appeared as counsel for either Witness patients or The Watchtower Society as *amicus curiae* in the most significant refusal cases heard in the American courts in the last 10 years. And he contributes to journals of law,[87] medicine,[88] and hospital administration[89] scholarly articles that effectively make the case for respecting refusal of blood transfusions on grounds of religious freedom and patient autonomy.

For the moment at least, the efforts of supportive medical and legal personnel have combined to produce a situation in the United States where nonconsensual transfusion of adult Witness patients has become extremely rare. "This is a dramatic change from just five or ten years ago," Ridley reports, "when there was still a great deal of

---

[84] Migden DR, Braen GR, The Jehovah's Witness blood refusal card: ethical and medicolegal considerations for emergency physicians. Acad Emerg Med 1998;5:815.

[85] Donald Ridley. Honoring Jehovah's Witnesses' advance directives in emergencies: a response to Drs. Migden and Braen. Acad Emerg Med 1998;5:824.

[86] Application of the President and Directors of Georgetown College, Inc., 331 F.2d 1000, 1007 (D.C. Cir. 1964).

[87] See, for example, Donald Ridley. In practice: health care law: whose life is it anyway? NJ Law J 1999;156:121, and Donald Ridley. Health care decision making in the family. Family Law Update1997, 237.

[88] See, for example, Donald Ridley. Guest Editorial: Respecting pregnant women's treatment choices, Obstet Gynecol Surv 1999;54:215 and Donald Ridley. Judicial diagnosis: treating children of Jehovah's Witnessses. Med Health RI 1998;81:418.

[89] See, for example, Donald Ridley. Treatment refusals by pregnant women, 15 Hosp. Law Newsletter # 9 (July 1998); Donald Ridley. Accepting patients' refusals of treatment, 13 Hosp. Law Newsletter # 12 (October 1996); Donald Ridley. Working with Jehovah's Witnesses on treatment issues, 12 Hosp. Law Newsletter # 4 (February 1995); and Donald Ridley. Accommodating Jehovah's Witnesses' choice of nonblood management. J Healthc Risk Manag 1990;Winter:17.

uncertainty about the law. Since then, as a result of the law's repeated defense and protection of patient choice, I can only conclude that providers either are rarely going to court to obtain such orders or that courts, when so importuned, are not granting such orders."[90] However, it would be mistaken to conclude that the need for vigilance has ended. Among other things, recent court decisions seem to open the door to greater participation by legislatures and executive agencies in defining rights in this area. Judges have lately shown a preference for avoiding constitutional questions, if possible, by protecting the right to refuse treatment under the common law of informed consent rather than by means of constitutional law.[91] And they have shown as well a propensity to avoid weighing state interests favoring treatment against a patient's right to refuse treatment where the state itself has not entered the case to press such interests.[92] Thus these recent cases leave open the possibility that courts could rule differently if legislation were passed removing some of the protection provided by the common law or if the executive branch were to intervene in a case to press the importance of countervailing state interests. Were legislatures or executive agencies to consider taking such steps, efforts would have to be mounted to oppose them politically and legally. Happily, executive agencies have thus far shown no interest in intervening in such cases. And, to the extent that state legislatures have shown interest in passing legislation in this field, it has been more to add protections to the right to refuse blood transfusions than to take them away.[93]

The Witnesses seem to be successfully recovering from the blow dealt them in *Georgetown*. The days when blood transfusions could be forced upon Witness patients on the ground that refusal was "medically irrational" are, hopefully, over. By dint of cases like *Georgetown*, the American medical profession had achieved something of the status of an established state church. Its dogma regarding the low risk and high benefits of blood transfusions had been forced upon unbelievers by the state. Through education and advocacy, the Witnesses have convinced the state to reconsider its position and to take a more neutral stance between the beliefs of their religion and those of American medicine. They have even managed to get American medicine to reconsider some of its beliefs in the light of further evidence. In the process, all of American society has benefited. Not only Jehovah's Witnesses, but patients in general, are today less likely to be given unnecessary blood transfusions because of the work of the Witnesses' Hospital Liaison Committees. Patients in general enjoy greater autonomy over a whole range of health care decisions because of the work done by the Witnesses as part of an overall patients' rights movement. And the causes of freedom in general and religious freedom in particular have been advanced by the Witnesses' dedicated resistance to efforts to force them to take action inconsistent with their religious beliefs.

---

[90] Letter dated August 12, 1999, from Donald T. Ridley, Esq., Associate General, Watchtower Bible and Tract Society of Pennsylvania.

[91] See, for example, *Stamford Hospital v. Vega*, 236 Conn. 646, 674 A.2d 821 (1996) and see generally James Hankins, The Common Law Right of bodily self-determination in Connecticut: life and death after *Stamford Hospital v. Vega*. Conn L Rev 1997;29:945.

[92] *Stamford Hospital v. Vega*, 236 Conn. 646, 674 A.2d 821 (1996) and *Harrell v. St. Mary's Hospital*, 678 So.2d 455 (D. Ct. App. FL 1996).

[93] See, for example, New York Public Health Law, sec. 2803-c (a): "Every patient's civil and religious liberties, including the right to independent personal decisions and knowledge of available choices, shall not be infringed and the facility shall encourage and assist in the fullest possible exercise of these rights." and (c) "Every patient shall have the right to receive adequate and appropriate medical care, to be fully informed of his or her medical condition and proposed treatment unless medically contraindicated, and to refuse medication and treatment after being fully informed of and understanding the consequences."

Appendix A

Durable Power of Attorney for Health Care
(Pennsylvania Statutes Annotated title 20, §§5601 to 5607)

(1) I, ____,
Print your full name
am of sound mind and I voluntarily make this Durable Power of Attorney for Health Care. There are two parts to this document: Part 1 sets forth my health-care instructions; Part 2 appoints a person to make health-care decisions for me on matters not covered in my instructions. This document shall take effect upon my incapacity.

PART 1–Health-Care Instructions

(2) I am one of Jehovah's Witnesses. On the basis of my firmly held religious convictions, see *Acts* 15:28, 29, and on the basis of my desire to avoid the numerous hazards and complications of blood, **I absolutely, unequivocally and resolutely refuse homologous blood** (another person's blood) **and *stored* autologous blood** (my own stored blood) under any and all circumstances, no matter what my medical condition. This means no whole blood, no red cells, no white cells, no platelets, and no blood plasma no matter what the consequences. Even if health-care providers (doctors, nurses etc.) believe that only blood transfusion therapy will preserve my life or health, I do not want it. Family, relatives or friends may disagree with my religious beliefs and with my wishes expressed herein. However, their disagreement is legally and ethically irrelevant because it is my subjective choice that controls. Any such disagreement should in no way be construed as creating ambiguity or doubt about the strength or substance of my wishes.

Also, because many health-care providers view Jehovah's Witnesses refusal of blood with disapproval and even hostility, I am concerned that someone may claim that I *orally* consented to a blood transfusion. Thus, I hereby state that it is my conscious decision that my absolute refusal of blood transfusion **shall not be revocable by me orally.** If anyone claims that I have orally consented to a blood transfusion, I demand that such claim be ignored unless confirmed in writing signed by me and subscribed by at least two disinterested witnesses.

(3) With respect to **minor blood fractions*** or products containing minor blood fractions, according to my conscience I ACCEPT: [initial <u>one</u> of the three choices below]

_____ (a) <u>NONE.</u>
_____ (b) <u>ALL.</u>
_____ (c) <u>SOME.</u> That is, I ACCEPT: [initial choice(s) below]
_____ Products that may have been processed with or contain small amounts of albumin (e.g., streptokinase, and some recombinant products [such as erythropoietin (EPO) and synthesised clotting factors], and some radionuclide scan preparations may contain albumin).
_____ Immunoglobulins (e.g., Rh immune globulin, gammaglobulin, horse serum, snake bite antivenins).
_____ Clotting factors (e.g., fibrinogen, Factors VII, VIII, IX, XII).
_____ Other: ____

(4) I accept and request alternative nonblood medical management to build up or conserve my own blood, to avoid or minimize blood loss, to replace lost circulatory volume, or to stop bleeding. For example, volume expanders such as dextran, saline or Ringer's solution, or hetastarch would be acceptable to me.

(5) With respect to **non-stored autologous blood*** (my own non-stored blood), according to my conscience I ACCEPT: [initial choice(s) below]

___ (a) DIALYSIS OR HEART-LUNG EQUIPMENT (diversion of my blood within an extracorporeal circuit that *does not involve storage* or more than brief interruption of blood flow and that is constantly linked to my circulatory system, provided any equipment used is not primed with stored blood).
___ (b) HEMODILUTION (dilution of my blood within an extracorporeal circuit *that does not involve storage* or more than brief interruption of blood flow and that is constantly linked to my circulatory system, provided any equipment used is not primed with stored blood).
___ (c) INTRAOPERATIVE OR POSTOPERATIVE BLOOD SALVAGE (contemporaneous recovery and reinfusion of blood lost during or after surgery that *does not involve storage* or more than brief interruption of blood flow, provided any equipment used is not primed with stored blood).
___ (d) NONE.

---

* **Warning:** Consult your doctor regarding potential health risks.

(6) With respect to providing, withholding, or withdrawing life-sustaining treatment at the end of life, and consistent with Pennsylvania Statutes Annotated title 20, § 5404, my declaration, which in no way alters my absolute refusal of blood as directed above, is: [initial one of three choices below]
______ (a) NOT TO PROLONG LIFE*. That is, if to a *reasonable degree of medical certainty my condition is hopeless* (for example, if to a reasonable degree of medical certainty I have an incurable and irreversible condition that will result in my death within a relatively short time, or if am unconscious and to a reasonable degree of medical certainty will not regain consciousness, or if I have brain damage or a brain disease that makes me unable to recognize people or communicate and to a reasonable degree of medical certainty my condition will not improve), I do not want my life to be prolonged. Thus in such situations, I do not want mechanical respiration (ventilation), cardiopulmonary resuscitation (CPR), tube feeding (artificial nutrition or hydration), etc. However, I do want palliative care – treatment for comfort.
______ (b) TO PROLONG LIFE. That is, I want my life to be prolonged as long as possible within the limits of generally accepted health-care standards, although I realize this means that I might be kept alive on machines for years in a hopeless condition.
______ (c) OTHER. [If you do not completely agree with either (a) or (b) above, you can initial here and write your own end-of-life instructions in the space provided. **NOTE:** Unless your agent knows your wishes about artificial nutrition and hydration, your agent may not be able to make decisions about these matters.]

____

____

____

(7) Other health-care instructions (e.g., your wishes regarding organ donation, current medication, allergies, other medical problems, etc.): ______________________________________

____

____

____

(8) I am primarily concerned that my refusal of blood and choice of alternative nonblood management be respected regardless of my medical condition. My rights under the federal and state constitutions and state common law require health-care providers to respect and comply with my treatment decisions. My rights are not dependant on, and do not vary with, my medical condition. Thus my decision to refuse blood and choose nonblood management must be respected even if my life or health is deemed to be threatened by my refusal. *Stamford Hosp. v. Vega*, 674 A.2d 821 (Conn. 1996) (Witness patient's refusal of blood protected by state common law right of bodily self-determination); *In re Dubreuil*, 629 So. 2d 819 (Fla. (1993) (Witness patient's refusal of blood protected by state constitutional rights of personal privacy and religious freedom); *Norwood Hosp. v. Munoz*, 564 N.E.2d 1017 (Mass. 1991) (Witness patient's refusal of blood protected by state common law right of bodily self-determination and federal constitutional right of personal privacy); *Fosmire v. Nicoleau*, 551 N.E.2d 77 (N.Y. 1990) (Witness patient's refusal of blood protected by state common law right of bodily self-determination); *In re E.G.*, 549 N.E.2d 322 (Ill. 1989) (Witness patient's refusal of blood protected by state common law right of bodily self-determination); *Public Health Trust v. Wons*, 541 So. 2d 96 (Fla. 1989) (Witness patient's refusal of blood protected by state constitutional rights of personal privacy and religious freedom); *In re Milton*, 505 N.E.2d 255 (Ohio 1987) (non-Witness patient's religion-based refusal of treatment protected by 1st Amendment guarantee of free exercise of religion; *In re Brown*, 478 So. 2d 1033 (Miss. 1985) (Witness patient's refusal of blood protected by state constitutional rights of personal privacy and religious freedom; *In re Osborne*, 294 A.2d 372 (D.C. 1972) (Witness patient's refusal of blood protected by 1st Amendment guarantee of free exercise of religion); *In re Estate of Brooks*, 205 N.E.2d 435 (Ill. 1965) (Witness patient's refusal of blood protected by 1st Amendment guarantee of free exercise of religion).

---

* [This footnote applies only to pregnant women.] If I am pregnant and there is a reasonable chance my fetus could survice, I want my life to be prolonged for the sake of my fetus, notwithstanding my instructions in Paragraph (6)(a). However, in no way does this change my wishes about nonblood treatment for both myself and my fetus. After any efforts to save my fetus, my instructions in Paragraph (6)(a) shall again control.

The United States Supreme Court has said that "[i]t is settled now . . . that the Constitution places limits on a State's right to interfere with a person's most basic decisions about . . . bodily integrity." *Planned Parenthood v. Casey*, 505 U.S. 833, 849 (1992). In *Cruzan v. Missouri Department of Health*, 497 U.S. 261 (1990), the Supreme Court stated: "It cannot be disputed that the Due Process Clause [of the Fourteenth Amendment to the United States Constitution] protects an interest in life as well as an interest in refusing life-sustaining medical treatment." *Id.* at 281. The Court also said: "The principle that a competent person has a constitutionally protected liberty interest in refusing unwanted medical treatment may be inferred from our prior decisions." *Id.* at 278. In addition, in *Washington v. Harper*, 494 U.S. 210 (1990), the Supreme Court said that prison inmates suffering from mental disorders possess "a significant liberty interest in avoiding the unwanted administration of antipsychotic drugs under the Due Process Clause of the Fourteenth Amendment." *Id.* at 221-22. The Court also observed that "[t]he forcible injection of medical into a nonconsenting person's body represents a substantial interference with that person's liberty." *Id.* at 229.

There is no indication in these Supreme Court cases that a person must be in a terminal, irreversible, incurable or untreatable condition, or in a permanently unconscious or vegetative state in order to exercise his fundamental Fourth Amendment right to refuse treatment or otherwise control what is done to his body. Indeed, Nancy Cruzan herself was not terminally ill. *See* 497 U.S. at 266, n.1. Moreover, implicit throughout the majority opinion in *Cruzan* and expressly stated in Justice O'Connor's concurrence and all the dissents (except Justice Scalia's) is the acceptance of advance written directives as clear and convincing evidence of a formerly competent person's wishes. Therefore, because I have prepared this advance directive while competent, if I become incompetent, my wishes as expressed herein must be respected as if I were competent.

(9) [This paragraph applies only to pregnant women.] In *Planned Parenthood v. Casey*, 505 U.S. 833, 860 (1992), the Supreme Court confirmed that "viability marks the earliest point at which the State's interest in fetal life is constitutionally adequate to justify a legislative ban on therapeutic abortions." Thus, since I have the right to abort my pregnancy before viability I necessarily have the lesser right to refuse blood transfusions before viability. In addition, even if my fetus is viable, the Supreme Court has said that mothers cannot be exposed to increased medical risks for the sake of their fetuses and that the state's interest in the potential life of the fetus is insufficient to override the mother's interest in preserving her own health.

Thornburgh v. American College of Obstetricians & Gynecologists, 476 U.S. 747, 768 –71 (1986); see *Planned Parenthood v. Casey*, 505 U.S. 833, 846 (1992). Also, in the cases of *In re A.C.*, 573 A.2d 1235 (D.C. 1990), and *In re Doe*, 632 N.E.2d 326 (Ill. App. Ct.), *cert. denied*, 114 S. Ct. 1198 (1994), refusals of treatment by women with viable fetuses were upheld. Although both of these cases involved Caesarean sections, as a matter of principle and logic they show that it is the pregnant woman who should decide what is to be done to herself and her fetus. Therefore, I demand that my refusal of blood and choice of alternative nonblood management be followed and that my doctors manage my care and the care of my fetus without transfused blood.

(10) In sum, based on federal and state constitutional law and state common law, I demand that the instructions set forth in this document be followed regardless of my medical condition. Any attempt to administer blood to me contrary to my instructions will be a violation of my Fourteenth Amendment liberty interest in bodily self-determination, my First Amendment right of religious free exercise, my state constitutional rights of personal liberty or privacy and religious freedom, and my state common law rights of bodily self-determination and personal autonomy.

PART 2–Appointment of Health-Care Agent

(11) I hereby appoint the following person as my health-care agent: [**Notice**: You may choose any adult to be your agent, but it is recommended that you not choose your doctor, any of your doctor's employees, or any employee of a hospital or nursing home where you might be a patient, unless the individual is related to you by blood, marriage, or adoption.]

Agent's full name: ______________________________

Agent's address: ______________________________

Work Telephone: (__) ________ Home Telephone: (__) ________ Other: (__) ________

(12) If the agent appointed above is unavailable, unable, or unwilling to serve or continue to serve, then I appoint the following alternative agent to serve with the same powers: [See "Notice" in Paragraph 11 above.]

Alternate agent's full name: ______________________________

Alternate agent's address: ______________________________

Work Telephone: (__) ________ Home Telephone: (__) ________ Other: (__) ________

(13) To the extent this document sets forth my health-care instructions, there is no need or reason to look to my agent for a decision. However, I grant my agent full power and authority to ensure that the wishes expressed in this document are followed by health-care providers. Further, I grant my agent full power and authority to make health-care decisions for me on matters not covered by this document. My agent's authority is effective as long as I am incapable of make my own health-care decisions.

(14) In harmony with the limitations in the preceding paragraph, my agent's authority shall include but not be limited to the following:

(a) To consent to, refuse, or withdraw consent to any or all types of medical care treatment, surgical procedures, diagnostic procedures, medication, and the use of other mechanical or other procedures related to health care. This authorization includes the power to consent to pain-relieving medication for relief of severe and intractable pain.

(b) To request, review, and received any information, oral or written, regarding my physical or mental health, including, but not limited to, medical and hospital records, and to consent to the disclosure of this information.

(c) To employ or discharge my health-care providers; to authorize my admission or discharge from any hospital, nursing home, mental health or other medical care facility; and the take any lawful actions that may be necessary to carry out my wishes, including the granting of releases from liability to health-care providers.

(15) A copy of this document shall be as valid as the original. I ask that a copy of this document be made part of my permanent medical record. I have provided copies of this document to my health-care agent and alternate agent. It is my intention that this document be honored in any jurisdiction in which it is presented and that it be construed liberally to give my agent the fullest discretion in making health-care decisions in my behalf consistent with my instructions.

(16) If my health-care providers cannot respect my wishes as expressed in this document or as otherwise known to my agent and a transfer of care is necessary to effectuate my wishes, I direct my health-care providers to cooperate with and assist my agent in promptly transferring me to another health-care provider that will respect my wishes. In such circumstances, I direct my health-care providers to transfer promptly all my medical records, including a copy of this document, to the other health-care provider.

(17) This document revokes any prior health-care power of attorney or health-care proxy executed by me.

(18) The provisions of this entire document are separable, so that the invalidity of one or more provisions shall not affect any others.

(19) I understand the full import of this document and I am emotionally and mentally competent to execute it.

(20) SIGNED: ______________________________ ______________________________

Your signature   Date

____

Address

(21) STATEMENT BY WITNESSES

I declare that the person who signed this document (the principal) or the person who signed on behalf and at the direction of the principal knowingly and voluntarily signed this writing by signature or mark in my presence. Also, I am not the person appointed as agent or alternate agent by this document.

______________________________	______________________________
Signature of witness 1	Signature of witness 2
______________________________	______________________________
Print name	Print name
______________________________	______________________________
Address	Address

Questions & Answers

about the Durable Power of Attorney for Health Care (DPA*)

What is a Durable Power of Attorney for Health Care (DPA*)? It is a single document designed to serve two functions: (1) to let you put your specific health-care instructions in writing, and (2) to let you appoint someone to make other health-care decisions for you in the event you are unable to do so. Patients could accomplish the above two functions by filling out two separate documents. However, the accompanying DPA form simplifies this by combining these two functions into one form.

What is "Part 1—Health-Care Instructions"? This part of the form sets forth your written instructions to others (doctors, nurses, etc.) about your specific health-care wishes. Your instructions do not take effect unless you become unable to make or communicate your health-care decisions yourself. No one except you can change your written instructions, not even the person that you appoint to make health-care decisions for you.

What is "Part 2—Appointment of Health-Care Agent"? This part of the form is used to appoint another person to make other health-care decisions for you in the event that you are unable to make or communicate such decisions yourself. The person you appoint thus becomes your "health-care agent." (For more details, see the questions and answers under the "HEALTH-CARE AGENT" heading below.)

Do I need a lawyer or doctor to fill out the DPA? No. This question-and-answer guide is designed to enable you to complete the DPA without the assistance of lawyers or doctors. However, you should feel free to consult with anyone you think might be able to help you fill out the form.

Are there instructions or some sort of checklist to help me fill out the DPA? Yes. There is a checklist. (See Figure 1 on the last page of this question-and-answer guide.) However, you should thoroughly read through these questions and answers before using the checklist. Thereafter you may use the checklist when filling out the DPA. The checklist refers to both theocratic articles and specific questions about this guide. Look up the references if you are unsure about the choice or decision to be made.

* The titles of the forms the Society's Legal Department has prepared vary from state to state depending on state law. For example, California calls its form a "Durable Power of Attorney for Health Care," Michigan calls its form a "Health Care Directive and Designation of Patient Advocate," New York calls its form a "Health Care Proxy," etc. However, since the majority of the titles use the words "power of attorney" or "proxy," the Society's Legal Department generally refers to them as either "DPA" (durable power of attorney) or "Proxy" forms.

What should I do with my completed DPA? Make several good, clear photocopies of the completed form. (You may want to note on the photocopies where the original is kept.) Keep the original in a secure yet accessible place–not a safe-deposit box. Give a copy to your health-care agent, alternate agent, your doctor (ask your doctor to make it part of your permanent medical record), and any other family members or close friends you want. You may also want to carry a copy with you and put a copy in the glove box of your car. Also, if you know you are going to be hospitalized, you should give a copy of your form to hospital administration.

How is the DPA different from regular power of attorney? Powers of attorney generally are used for business and financial matters, not health-care matters. The DPA, however, is for health-care matters, *not* for business or financial matters.

If I already have a living will or other advance directive for health-care, why should I execute the DPA? Living wills and other advance directives for health care established by state laws typically limit a person's right to refuse 'life-sustaining' treatment to terminal illnesses. This means that unless your condition is terminal (i.e., you have no hope for recovery and death is imminent), you would not be allowed to refuse blood. Even in state that have laws that do not limit a person's right to refuse treatment to terminal illnesses, their advance directives forms do not address your refusal of blood and choice of alternative nonblood management as thoroughly as the DPA.

Does the DPA replace the "Advance Medical Directive/Release" card? No. These two documents work with each other. The Advance Medical Directive/Release card is small in size so that it can be carried with you at all times. Thus, in the event of an emergency in which you are unconscious, the Advance Medical Directive/Release will identify you as one of Jehovah's Witnesses, will make known your refusal of blood, and will identify your emergency contacts.

The DPA, on the other hand, contains important information that could not be included on the Advance Medical Directive/Release card. Thus, it would be wise to make the emergency contacts on your Advance Medical Directive/Release

CONTENTS

PENNSYLVANIA

the same persons you appoint as health-care agent and alternate agent on your DPA. In this way your health-care agent will be contacted in an emergency and will be able to provide immediately a copy of your DPA to health-care providers, if a copy is not with you. (See Figure 2 on the last page of this guide.)

10. **Should I discuss my instructions and appointment of health-care agent with my doctors?** Yes. Basically, discuss with your doctor the same information you discuss with your agent. (See Question 23.) Be sure to discuss in depth the many medical alternatives for bloodless surgery that are available and acceptable. (See Question 16.) Let your doctor know that you have thoroughly discussed these matters with your agent. (You may even want to introduce your agent to your doctor.) The better your doctor understands you, the less likely it is that problems will arise.

11. **Are my doctor and other health-care personnel protected from legal liability if they honor the wishes expressed in my DPA?** Yes. A doctor or any other health-care provider is protected from legal liability when acting in accordance with your wishes as expressed in your DPA; indeed, they are legally obligated to respect your wishes. They need be more concerned about liability if they were to act contrary to your DPA.

12. **Could my DPA be overridden by my family members or other relatives?** No. You alone have the right to control what is done to your body. A family member's or relative's disagreement with your health-care decisions is legally irrelevant. If you have appointed a health-care agent, only he has the legal authority to make other health-care decisions for you.

13. **Will my DPA be honored with I travel to another state?** It should be. The U.S. Supreme Court has said that the U.S. Constitution gives competent persons the right to refuse medical treatment. Thus, your DPA should be honored in any state. However, because of the potential for uncertainty on this point in some states, there is a thorough discussion of your constitutional rights in the DPA.

14. **What if I want to change or cancel my DPA?** All you need to do is fill out another DPA. Your new form will contain your changes and will automatically cancel your previous DPA. (To be on the safe side, you may want to ask for your old DPAs back from those to whom you gave one. You should discard your old forms and distribute your new ones.) If for some reason you are unable to fill out a new form, you may simply tell your doctor(s), agent or others about your changes (or that you have decided to cancel your existing form altogether.) It is best, however, to put any changes in writing by filling out a new form.

BLOOD RELATED
(DPA, Paragraphs 3-5)

15. **Where can I get information about minor blood fractions?** Information on minor blood fractions can be found in *The Watchtower* of October 1, 1994, page 31, and *The Watchtower* of June 1, 1990, pages 30-31.

16. **Where can I get information about medical alternatives and bloodless surgery?** Information on medical alternatives to blood transfusion and on bloodless surgery techniques can be found in *Awake!* of November 22, 1991, page 10, *How Can Blood Save Your Life?* pages 14-17, 28, and *Jehovah's Witnesses and the Question of Blood*, pages 49-58.

17. **Where can I get information about autologous blood-procedures such as hemodilution and intraoperative blood salvage?** Information on autologous transfusion therapy can be found in *The Watchtower* of March 1, 1989, pages 30-31.

END-OF-LIFE DECISIONS
(DPA, Paragraph 6)

18. **What are end-of-life decisions?** End-of-life decisions are potential life-or-death decisions patients may face because of deteriorating health (perhaps due to old age) or because of a serious accident. For example, if you are hopelessly ill, would you want to be kept alive on a respirator? If you are terminally ill, would you want to be fed intravenously or by other artificial methods? If your situation is hopeless, would you want all financial means available to you or your family to be expended to pay for treatment, perhaps involving transportation to a distant center to receive the most advanced treatment? These and other questions about end-of-life decisions are addressed in *Awake!* of October 22, 1991, pages 3 to 9.

19. **Why should I think about end-of-life decisions now?** Questions about end-of-life care can arise suddenly and unexpectedly. Thus, it only makes sense to think about these matters while you are capable of doing so. Although discussing end-of-life decisions may not be easy for some, imagine the difficulties your spouse or family would face if your wishes were unknown. You can make your wishes known, of course, by recording your instructions in Paragraph 6 of the DPA. You can also make your wishes known by appointing a health-care agent in Paragraph 11 of the DPA and discussing your wishes about end-of-life care with your agent.

20. **Are there any circumstances where a Christian may choose NOT to prolong life?** Yes. For a Christian, questions about whether life should be prolonged or not arise *only* if his medical condition has been *clearly determined to be hopeless*. See *Awake!* of September 8, 1986, pages 20-21. Examples of hopeless situations might include the following: (1) to a

reasonable degree of medical certainty you have an incurable and irreversible condition that will result in your death within a relatively short time, (2) you are unconscious and to a reasonable degree of medical certainty you will not regain consciousness, or (3) you have brain damage or a brain disease that makes you unable to recognize people or communicate and to a reasonable degree of medical certainty your condition will not improve.

HEALTH-CARE AGENT

(DPA, Paragraphs 11-14)

What will my health-care agent do? Your agent will make health-care decisions for you. However, because your written instructions in Part 1 of the DPA set forth your health-care wishes, your agent will make decisions only on matters *not* covered by your instructions.

To illustrate, if you are unconscious but your doctor, who knows that you are one of Jehovah's Witnesses, wonders if you will refuse blood in a life-threatening situation, your written instructions in Part 1 clearly answer this, so your agent has no authority in the matter. However, your agent can direct the doctor to your instructions and ensure that your wishes are respected. On the other hand, if you are in a coma and the doctor wants to know what kind of treatment to give you, your agent would make decisions for you if your written instructions in Part 1 do not cover this.

For decisions your agent makes that are not covered by your instructions, your agent will be guided by your personal beliefs and values. As you might well imagine, acting as a health-care agent is an extremely serious matter since the agent could be required to make life-or-death decisions for you.

Whom should I appoint as my health-care agent? Your agent should be someone you trust and are close to, someone who understands your personal beliefs and values, such as a close family member or a good friend. Before appointing an agent, ask yourself:

(1) If questions arise about my health care that are not covered by the instructions set forth in my DPA, can I trust that my agent will make decisions consistent with my beliefs and values as a true Christian?

(2) If someone challenges my written instructions, is my agent capable of taking steps to see that my wishes are upheld? How would my agent react to a hospital or courtroom setting in which my instructions are questioned?

Thus, before appointing an agent, it would be good to talk with the person you have in mind to make sure he understands your wishes and is willing to assume the responsibility of acting as your agent.

What should I discuss with my prospective health-care agent? You should discuss your personal beliefs and values, and you should be sure you prospective health-care agent understands you.

Discuss the health-care instructions that appear in Part 1 of the DPA. The discussion should review your specific instructions about homologous blood, minor blood fractions, nonblood alternatives, and autologous blood. Also, discuss your instructions about end-of-life decisions, since doctors will look to your agent if questions arise that are not addressed in your written instructions. In addition to discussing and explaining the instructions in Part 1 of your DPA, express your general feelings about medical treatment and explain WHY you feel the way you do.

Discuss Part 2 on the DPA. That is, the responsibilities (described in the form) and decisions your prospective agent may be faced with in the event your instructions in Part 1 do not cover a situation that arises.

Why is it so important that I talk with my health-care agent in advance? It is important to talk to your agent because the guidelines set forth in your instructions (especially with regard to end-of-life decisions) cannot cover every situation. If you fail to discuss such matters with your agent, serious problems could arise. Obviously, if you avoid thinking about these matters it does not mean different situations will not come up. It only means that someone else will have to decide without the benefit of your general views and feelings on the matter. Therefore, meaningful discussions you have with your agent can guide him in the event a situation comes up that is not covered in your written instructions.

If I became unable to communicate or make decisions myself, would my doctor be obligated to consult with my health-care agent? Yes. Your health-care agent has legal authority to make medical decisions for you in harmony with your wishes as stated in your DPA. Your doctor is therefore legally obligated to consult with your health-care agent and to respect his decisions as if they were your own.

Could my health-care agent be held legally liable for decisions he makes for me? No, your health-care agent will not be liable for treatment decisions made in good faith on your behalf. Also, he cannot be held liable for the costs of your care.

Checklist for Filling out Durable Power of Attorney for Health Care
(check off each box below as section is completed)

☑	What To Do	Reference(s)
☐ Paragraph (1)	•Print your full name..	self-explanatory
	PART 1–Health-Care Instructions	
☐ Paragraph (3)	•Initial one of the three choices regarding *minor blood fractions.**...............	w94 10/1 p.31, w90 6/1 pp. 30-1
☐ Paragraph (5)	•Initial choices(s) regard *autologous blood.**...	w89 3/1 pp. 30-1
☐ Paragraph (6)	•Initial one of the three choices regarding *end-of-life* decisions....................	q&a #18-20, g91 10/22 pp. 3-9, g86 9/8 pp. 20-1
	PART 2–Appointment of Health-Care Agent	
☐ Paragraph (11)	•Name a health-care agent, list address, and telephone numbers..................	q&a #3, 21-26
☐ Paragraph (12)	•Name an alternate health-care agent, etc.	self-explanatory
☐ Paragraph (20)	•Sign your name in the presence of two witnesses, etc.	self-explanatory
☐ Paragraph (21)	•Your two witnesses sign, etc.	self-explanatory

Abbreviations: w = *The Watchtower*; g = *Awake!*; q&a = Refers to this 4-page guide with its questions and answers.
*This is a conscience matter and may not be acceptable to some of Jehovah's Witnesses. PA 1/97

(You may wish to type or write in the language indicated below on your Advance Medical Directive/Release to indicate that you have executed a health-care power of attorney. –See question and answer #9 on first page of this guide.)

Allergies:________________________
Current medication:__________________
Medical problems:___________________
____

MEDICAL DIRECTIVE
(Signed document inside)
➡ `I have also executed a health-care power of attorney (or proxy).`
NO BLOOD

IN CASE OF EMERGENCY,
PLEASE CONTACT:
Name:____________________________
`(health-care agent)` ⬅
Telephone:________________________
Address:__________________________
____

ALTERNATE CONTACT:
Name:____________________________
`(alternate health-care agent)` ⬅
Telephone:________________________
Address:__________________________
____
Open to signed document ⬇

PART 9
Cost Issues

CHAPTER 45

The Cost and Cost-Effectiveness of Allogeneic and Autologous Blood

Brian Custer
Blood Systems Research Institute, San Francisco, USA

Introduction

The previous edition of this chapter in *Alternatives to Blood Transfusion in Transfusion Medicine* raised important issues [1]. Unfortunately, in the intervening years relatively little additional research has been conducted on the economics of allogeneic versus autologous blood. Some of the hypotheses discussed in the previous edition are yet to be verified. The cost and cost-effectiveness of allogeneic and autologous blood remain important questions without overwhelming evidence in support of one option over the other, although a deeper understanding of the contributors to the cost of each type of blood is emerging. The risks and costs of allogeneic transfusion that broadly range over several different types of adverse outcomes from transfusion of the wrong blood type through transfusion-related immunomodulation (TRIM) to transfusion-transmitted infection remain the most important hazards of allogeneic transfusion. For autologous blood, the primary benefits remain the elimination of many, but not all, such adverse events. The cost-effectiveness of each of these approaches to blood transfusion varies on the basis of the transfusion indication and patient population. Also, because autologous blood is not always a viable substitute for allogeneic blood even within the same surgical category, such as orthopedic arthroplasty, studies that compare these transfusion approaches can be severely limited by confounding by indication based on the underlying patient characteristics. Therefore, while this chapter will focus on general economic evidence related to allogeneic and autologous blood, it is important to recognize that available evidence may not always be applicable to specific settings or patients.

Alternatives to Blood Transfusion in Transfusion Medicine, 2nd edition. Edited by A. Maniatis, P. Van der Linden, J.-F. Hardy.

Part I—cost of blood

In developing countries, economic factors seem insurmountable, for example, in countries such as Haiti, Guatemala, and Honduras [and many other developing countries], the cost of processing a unit of donated blood exceeds the annual per capita budget allocation for health care [2]. In most developed countries, the cost of blood and transfusion represents approximately 1% of the entire health care budget. In the United States in 2003, blood and blood components comprised less than 1% of hospital expenses equaling about $3 billion out of $500 billion in total hospital expenses [3] and in a typical hospital laboratory, the largest single budget item is blood products for transfusion [4]. While the percentage of total health care expenditures that blood and transfusion comprises in developed countries is relatively small, blood transfusion costs remain a relevant consideration and target for resource allocation scrutiny due to recent increases in the per-unit cost of blood procurement and testing and because overutilization of blood and the associated costs incurred are preventable. Moreover, there is potential for substantial resource saving of not only

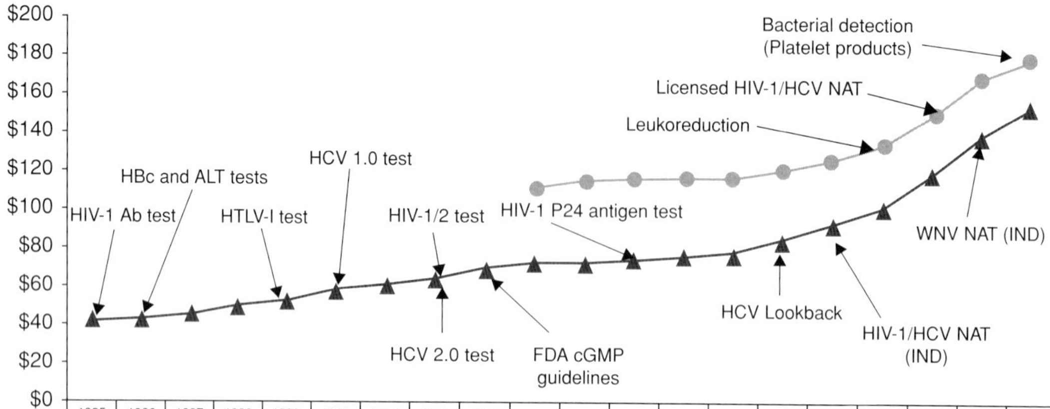

	1985	1986	1987	1988	1989	1990	1991	1992	1993	1994	1995	1996	1997	1998	1999	2000	2001	2002	2003	2004
	543	43	45	49	53	58	61	64	68	73	73	75	76	77	85	92	101	110	140	154
										111	115	116	117	117	121	125	134	151	153	175

Figure 45.1 Average per unit red cell blood charge to hospitals by America's Blood Centers members in the last 20 years with the date of implementation of additional safety measures indicated and adjusted to 2006 USD. The dark line represents nonleukoreduced red blood cells and the gray line represents leukoreduced red blood cells. Reproduced with permission from America's Blood Centers.

money but also blood itself. Each of these potential savings is increasingly relevant because the eligible donor pool may not be as large as previously estimated [5] and as the blood donor population ages without replacement by younger donors, the potential for reduced blood availability places a new emphasis on improved utilization. Potential for further increases in the cost of blood also contributes to the need to reconsider the trade-offs between allogeneic and autologous blood.

For allogeneic blood, the societal perspective attempts to capture all costs that are incurred from the donor to the recipient, including the cost of adverse events. A blood bank's cost of procuring and supplying blood is the first component of the overall cost of blood from the societal perspective. These costs are the easiest to measure because they are reflected in the blood center charges that hospitals pay for obtaining blood. Based on a survey of over 1400 hospitals and blood centers in 2001 in the United States, the mean cost of 1 unit of leukoreduced (nonirradiated, non-CMV-negative) packed RBC was $154 representing a 26% increase over the 1999 cost [6]. Similarly, the mean cost of a unit of aphaeresis platelets was $475 representing a 4.6% decrease from 1999, and for FFP, the mean cost of unit was $52 representing a 4% increase over the same time period [6]. Unfortunately, the lag time for the publication of this type of data is years, and so the reported results may not be reflective of the current procurement cost of blood from a hospital perspective. The costs of additional safety measures for allogeneic blood over the last 20 years are reflected in the steady increase in blood charges at US hospitals (Figure 45.1), as evident by the transition to near-universal leukoreduction and expanding infectious disease testing (NAT for HIV, HCV, and WNV, and now serological screening for Chagas disease in 2007). Each new safety measure can be linked to an increase in the fees charged to hospitals by blood centers. Internationally blood cost publications over the last decade have shown a steady increase in the cost of blood, with substantial increases ranging between 26 and 170% over the period from the middle 1990s to middle 2000s evident in Canada, the United States, and the United Kingdom [7].

Consensus cost elements

Reports on the cost of blood are limited by the cost categories used in each analysis. The seemingly simple question of "What is the cost of blood?"

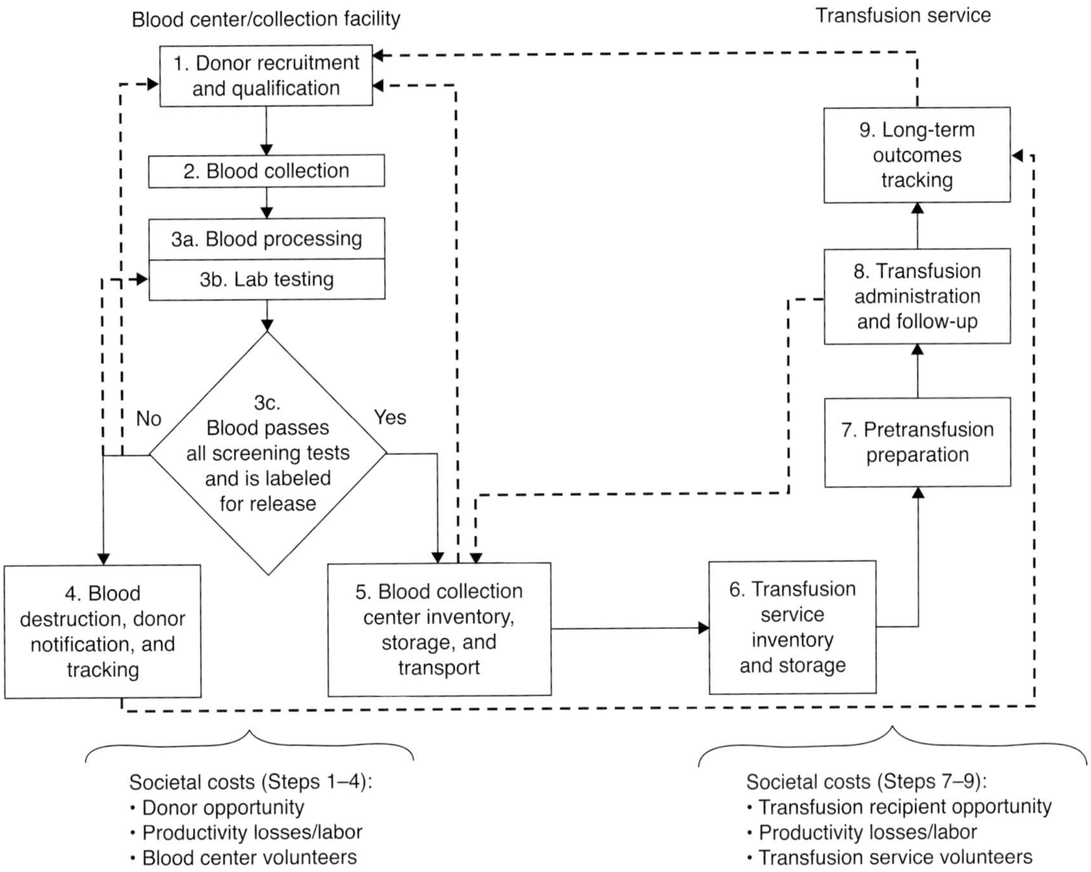

Figure 45.2 Cost elements or cost centers that contribute to the overall societal cost of allogeneic blood, solid arrows show direct cost dependencies and dashed arrows show indirect dependencies and feedback influences. Reprinted from Transfusion Medicine Reviews, 19(1), The Cost of Blood: Multidisciplinary Consensus Conference for a Standard Methodology, 66–78, Copyright 2005, with permission from Elsevier.

turns out to be not so simple. A new approach has begun, which works by defining the cost contributors to be included in an assessment of the overall cost of blood (Figure 45.2). Two research projects have sought to define the cost elements that should be included by convening experts and developing consensus recommendations, followed by work to develop activity based cost accounting methods to capture the costs of transfusion more rigorously [8, 9].

Blood cost literature

Detailing the elements that should be included and actually measuring these elements are separate activities. A small number of studies have assessed the cost of blood from the societal perspective in different developed countries. In a systematic review done in 1999, the cost of blood (adjusted to constant 1990 USD) was $155 for allogeneic transfusion in the United Kingdom, $187 in Canada, and $341 in the United States [7].

At least two studies in the United States have sought to estimate the societal cost of procuring blood in the nation [10, 11]. Each of these studies focused on whole blood and red cell procurement and only the costs of obtaining blood for transfusion, not the cost of transfusion or adverse events. The societal cost of procuring whole blood was between $154 and $218, depending on the region of the country. Blood costs in the United States have been estimated as part of other economic evaluation studies, but infrequently from a societal perspective. The reported cost of a unit of red cells ranges from as low as $67 to as high as $398 [12–16]. Each of these studies assessed cost from the hospital perspective (purchasing and transfusing blood). Some of these cost estimates include the cost of unintended consequences of transfusion-transmitted infections.

A comprehensive societal cost perspective should include the following broad categories: donors' opportunity cost (the value of forgone benefits because a resource is not available for its best alternative use [17] in the case of blood donation, this is the cost of the donor's time spent donating because the donor could have chosen to do something else with his or her time.), cost of collecting blood, blood center processing and testing, distribution, delivery (hospital transfusion service processing and patient administration), transfusion reaction and adverse events management, and blood wastage. Wastage of autologous (and allogeneic) blood should be included because resources are consumed in collecting, processing, and storage of every unit of autologous blood regardless of whether it is transfused and each of these represents an opportunity cost for the healthcare sector in any setting or country. The unit cost estimate from Canada for allogeneic red cell transfusion was $265 in 2002 USD [18]. Increases in costs compared with previous studies were attributed to additional safety measures such as the adoption of nucleic acid testing and leukoreduction, closely paralleling the cost increases seen in the United States. A study from Sweden estimated the cost of transfusion of 2 units of leukoreduced allogeneic red cells, which was €702 (€373 for the first unit and €329 for the second unit); similarly, the societal cost for 2 units of autologous blood was €598 (€304 for the first unit and €294 for the second unit) [19].

Limitations of blood cost studies

In most settings, a unit of donated allogeneic whole blood is processed into red cell, platelet, and plasma components. The issue of component production requires consideration of joint costs, which are costs incurred in a single process that results in 2 or more distinct outputs. The relevance of this issue for allogeneic blood has been noted for years [20, 21]. However, although the need to account for joint costs has been clearly established and discussed in the blood procurement literature [10] and blood cost literature [22], few studies have actually used joint cost methodologies to appropriately estimate the cost of procurement of allogeneic red cells and other components. From a societal perspective, the donors' opportunity cost to donate, the cost of collection, processing, and testing, all should be distributed across all products that are produced from a unit of donated whole blood. Distributing these costs across the relevant component produced in a given setting would lower the procurement cost for a unit of packed allogeneic red cells.

Other elements that contribute to the overall cost of blood have received little consideration. The costs of insurance premiums and litigation resulting from adverse transfusion outcomes, and the cost of organizing and maintaining national or multinational hemovigilance systems have not been included in previous estimates of the societal cost of blood [9]. Incorporating these additional elements will result in increased cost estimates for both allogeneic and autologous blood. Although the relative increase is likely to be larger for allogeneic blood, ethical, legal, and liability issues are present for autologous blood especially because in most settings, autologous blood is not tested for infectious markers before transfusion [23–25].

The most important cost for autologous blood is wastage. The cost of autologous blood increases substantially when wastage is included. In a study that modeled the use of autologous blood in surgical procedures, up to 66% of the preoperative collected autologous blood was wasted resulting in an increased cost of up to $4783 from $68 per unit, at the time when autologous blood was used instead of allogeneic blood depending on the surgery and amount of blood wasted [26]. In the United States, autologous unit wastage continues to be approximately 50% [27].

When costs of allogeneic and autologous blood are compared, an implicit assumption is that they are complete substitutes for one another. Clearly this is not true and clinicians recognize that autologous blood is only appropriate for the subset of patients having elective or planned procedures in which there is appropriate time to store blood and for which the patient is in sufficient health to be able to provide preoperative blood [28].

Part II—cost effectiveness of allogeneic and autologous blood

Although trends indicate a decline in preoperative autologous donation, overall, autologous blood remains the standard of care in the United States for patients undergoing total joint replacement surgery [29] with autologous transfusion accounting for 2.6% of all transfused units in 2001 [6]. However, recent efforts to establish more consistent blood utilization and transfusion practices across hospitals in the United States have focused on many changes including reducing autologous transfusion because of the costs and potential health implications of this procedure. The use of autologous predonation is being discouraged in favor of intraoperative blood donation (acute normovolemic hemodilution) and the use of algorithms that employ selective preoperative epoetin alfa and the use of evidence-based transfusion guidelines [30]. In other countries, autologous blood is not as available as an alternative to allogeneic transfusion. For example, in Sweden, autologous donations accounted for 0.13% of transfused units in 2002 [19] and in the United Kingdom, the standard practice is allogeneic blood [31].

Overview of methods

In health and medicine, cost-effectiveness analysis (CEA) is a methodology that assesses both the costs and medical outcomes of health care interventions. CEA studies provide results as a ratio of costs and effects in terms of natural units such as deaths prevented or infections avoided and are explicitly incremental analyses comparing one intervention with another. In some analyses, the comparator intervention is a "do nothing" or "no intervention" strategy. However, in analyses of preoperative autologous donation, the comparator intervention is most often the allogeneic blood and sometimes intraoperative cell salvage. Cost utility analysis (CUA) is the same methodology as CEA but includes either disability-adjusted life years (DALYs) or quality-adjusted life years (QALYs). In developed countries, QALYs is the preferred measure of outcome because the QALY includes not only mortality but also morbidity and decreased quality of life that occur in the health states before and after the use of each intervention. The major advantage of CUA studies is that cost/QALY results allow for the comparison of interventions within and across different health care disciplines. Because of the variable types and severity of adverse outcomes that are possible from transfusion, it is almost always appropriate to use CUA methods to compare alternatives. Overall economic evidence and the limitations of these analyses in blood safety and transfusion medicine have been discussed in the literature [32, 33]. Discussion of economic evaluation methods for blood transfusion from a hospital perspective focuses on cost-minimization [30, 34] which is not as useful for assessing the overall health achieved by the use of different transfusion alternatives.

CUA of autologous compared with allogeneic blood

Assessments of the cost utility of autologous blood compared with allogeneic blood mainly come from studies conducted and published in the 1990s. The publication dates are important because with the adoption of leukoreduction and screening tests such as nucleic acid testing for HIV and HCV in allogeneic blood, the current viral marker risk profile of allogeneic blood is much lower than what it was at the time of these studies and on the other hand, the current cost of allogeneic blood is significantly higher as a result of such safety measures.

Within the available published studies, there is wide variability in the cost utility profile of autologous blood because of the assumptions made by the researchers, the infectious risks included, the estimated risk of infection acquisition from allogeneic blood, and disease penetrance with consequent

Table 45.1 Cost utility of autologous compared to allogeneic blood. Each results provides the cost utility of autologous blood compared to allogeneic blood in terms of $USD/QALY.

		Surgical procedure				
Analysis year	Perspective	Total joint replacement (hip or knee)	Coronary artery bypass graft	Gynecologic surgery (hysterectomy or tumor removal	Prostatectomy	Author and reference(s)
1992	Hospital	235,000	508,000			Birkmeyer [35, 36]
1992	Societal	235,000	494,000	1,358,000	23,643,000	Etchason [37]
1992	Societal	725 net saving				Healy [38]
1997	Third-party payer	2470				Sonnenerg [14, 39]
(2000)		(2750)	(532)			
1994	Hospital	1043 net saving	1470			Blumberg [40]
1998	Healthcare payer		1,785,000			Marchetti [41]
1998	Not stated			2,208,000		Horowitz [42]
1992	Societal				1,813,000	Goodnough [43]

costs of care and reduced life expectancy. The results of these analyses vary from autologous blood being a dominant strategy (costs less and is more effective) to having very poor cost utility (Table 45.1). The fact that the economic evidence remains conflicted is somewhat surprising. A brief review of these studies will help place the results in context. First studies have not examined the same surgical procedures. Etchason and colleagues evaluated four surgical procedures: hip replacement, coronary artery bypass grafting (CABG), hysterectomy, and prostatectomy [37]. Birkmeyer and colleagues, Etchason and colleagues, Sonnenberg and colleagues, Healy and colleagues, and Blumberg and colleagues included hip or knee replacement surgery as a surgical intervention, thus allowing for the most direct comparison of results between these studies with base case results of $557,000/QALY, $235,000/QALY, $2470/QALY, and cost savings in two studies, respectively. Each of the studies that found autologous blood to be cost savings used a CEA as opposed to CUA methodology. In addition, Sonnenberg, Etchason, and another Birkmeyer study report results for CABG with results of $1470/QALY, $494,000/QALY, and $508,000/QALY, respectively. In a study from Italy, Marchetti reported results for CABG of $1,785,000/QALY.

Limitations of cost-effectiveness and cost utility studies

An effort to examine the reason for the variability in results highlights the importance of the analytical approach [32]. For hip or knee replacement, three studies have similar increased incremental costs [14, 35, 37] and two other studies suggest that autologous blood is cost saving [38, 40]. In comparison, three studies have similar increased incremental effectiveness [35, 37, 38], with the other study having a much larger incremental effectiveness result [14]. The results for the two CABG studies that provide incremental cost and effectiveness results are similar to each other [36, 37].

Several factors contribute to the variability of hip or knee replacement results. First, the analysis perspective is not consistent—two studies were conducted from a hospital perspective [35, 44], two studies conducted from a third party payer perspective [14, 38], and the other from a societal perspective [37]. Each perspective leads to the inclusion of different cost categories. Second, the assumptions in each analysis are different. For hip or knee replacement, the most critical difference between the studies was whether bacterial infection risk resulting from TRIM effects of allogeneic blood is included in the analysis. TRIM encompasses the laboratory immune aberrations that occur after allogeneic transfusion and the established or purported clinical effects that could be beneficial or deleterious [45]. The purported postoperative bacterial infections caused by TRIM are related to immune modulatory or suppressive effects allowing recipient sepsis to develop from endogenous sources. However, evidence of the role and consequences of TRIM resulting from allogeneic transfusion remains controversial. The three economic analyses that included bacterial infection risk suggest that preoperative autologous blood donation is either a dominant strategy [38], cost saving strategy [40], or a highly cost-effective strategy [14] compared with allogeneic blood. Meta-analysis of multiple studies indicates that the risk of postoperative infection is over 2 times greater in persons who receive allogeneic blood compared with autologous blood [46]. Neither of the two studies that reported relatively poor cost utility of autologous blood for CABG included bacterial infection risk. However, the risk of bacterial contamination is most critical for platelets as opposed to red cells, and bacterial contamination is not reserved only for allogeneic blood; autologous blood can also have bacterial contamination [47].

More recently published studies have sought to assess current cost utility profiles of allogeneic and autologous blood in different patient populations and different countries, including countries with different developmental status. One of the previous cost-effectiveness studies of autologous blood was updated with new risk estimates [39]. In the updated analysis, the cost utility of autologous blood for hip replacement was $2750/QALY in year 2000 USD, a result only slightly less cost-effective than from the original study conducted 3 years earlier. On the other hand, a study of the use of autologous blood in gynecologic patients undergoing hysterectomy or related surgical procedures found the cost-effectiveness of autologous blood exceeded $1,000,000/QALY for the procedures considered [42]. In developing countries where the risk of transfusion-transmitted infection remains high, autologous blood, although logistically complex, may be a highly cost-effective intervention [48]. However while conceptually attractive from the standpoint of reducing the risk of viral infection acquisition, the operational feasibility of preoperative autologous collection and storage until needed in developing countries has not been carefully evaluated.

The most extensive systematic reviews and meta-analyses of preoperative autologous blood have been conducted under the sponsorship of the Cochrane Collaboration for the National Health Service by the Health Technology Assessment program in the United Kingdom [31, 49]. The evidence from randomized trials comparing autologous blood with allogeneic blood consistently show that autologous blood significantly reduces the risk of exposure to allogeneic, with meta-analysis of studies with sufficient quality further demonstrating this relationship [31, 49]. However, while autologous blood reduces the likelihood of exposure to allogeneic blood, preoperative autologous blood donation increases the risk of exposure to any type of blood (autologous or allogeneic) [31, 49]. Evidence from some randomized clinical trials suggests that autologous blood is better than allogeneic blood [50], whereas other studies have not found a benefit. Nonetheless, these are effectiveness questions and are addressed elsewhere in *Alternatives to Blood Transfusion in Transfusion Medicine* (see Chapter 7 The Benefits of Allogeneic Erythrocyte Transfusion: What Evidence Do We Have?). Very few randomized trials have measured costs as part of the trial. The lack of cost estimates makes it difficult to determine whether autologous blood provides a measurable economic benefit. Long-term studies of accumulated health care costs between allogeneic and autologous blood are not available. In at least one randomized study with a short-term time horizon where costs were collected at the time of the trial, costs were higher by $758 per patient in the autologous blood arm because of the wastage of autologous units [51].

Summary

Closely related to preoperative autologous donation is the use of intraoperative cell savage. The use of this procedure is increasingly common and may have more favorable cost-effectiveness than preoperative autologous donation [34]. Unfortunately, there are too few published studies of the health economics of this topic from which to draw conclusions. The next chapters of *Alternatives to Blood Transfusion in Transfusion Medicine* address. The economic data on preoperative autologous blood compared with allogeneic blood remain limited and conflicting. The cost of collecting and processing allogeneic blood exceeds the cost of collecting autologous blood, and the cost of adverse events are higher for allogeneic blood. However, autologous blood donation results in significant blood wastage and increases the chances of receiving any type of blood. Each of these factors increases the cost of each unit of autologous blood. The relative cost-effectiveness of autologous blood compared with allogeneic blood continues to hinge on the existence and sequelae of TRIM. If TRIM is a true phenomena associated with allogeneic blood that leads to increased risk of clinical complications such as bacterial sepsis and cancer recurrence and other perturbations of a blood recipient's immune system, beyond those associated with the effects of blood storage alone which occur for both allogeneic and autologous blood, the cost utility of autologous blood is likely favorable. As stated in 1999 and reiterated in 2006, until more definitive data are available on the magnitude and costs of the risk of TRIM-induced bacterial infection, the cost-effectiveness of preoperative autologous blood donation remains debatable [14, 31].

References

1. Blumberg N, Heal JM. Cost issues: cost effectiveness of allogeneic versus autologous blood. In: *NATA: Transfusion Medicine and Alternatives to Blood Transfusion*. 2000.
2. Vinelli E. Taking a closer look at blood donation in Latin America. Dev Biol 2005;120:139–44.
3. Centers AB. Blood services: cost, reimbursement and billing. Blood Counts 2005;4(1):1–4.
4. Sumwalt D. Don't let blood products attract budget vampires. Hosp Mater Manage 1997;22(11):9, 12–13.
5. Riley W, Schwei M, McCullough J. The United States' potential blood donor pool: estimating the prevalence of donor-exclusion factors on the pool of potential donors. Transfusion 2007;47(7):1180–88.
6. Sullivan MT, Cotten R, Read EJ, Wallace EL. Blood collection and transfusion in the United States in 2001. Transfusion 2007;47(3):385–94.
7. Amin M, Fergusson D, Aziz A, Wilson K, Coyle D, Hebert P. The cost of allogeneic red blood cells–a systematic review. Transfus Med 2003;13(5):275–85.
8. The cost of blood: multidisciplinary consensus conference for a standard methodology. Transfus Med Rev 2005;19(1):66–78.
9. Shander A, Hofmann A, Gombotz H, Theusinger OM, Spahn DR. Estimating the cost of blood: past, present, and future directions. Best Pract Res 2007;21(2): 271–89.
10. Custer B, Johnson ES, Sullivan SD, et al. Community blood supply model: development of a new model to assess the safety, sufficiency, and cost of the blood supply. Med Decis Making 2005;25(5):571–82.
11. Madden E, Murphy EL, Custer B. Modeling red cell procurement with both double-red-cell and whole-blood collection and the impact of European travel deferral on units available for transfusion. Transfusion 2007;47(11):2025–37.
12. Roberts WA, Kirkley SA, Newby M. A cost comparison of allogeneic and preoperatively or intraoperatively donated autologous blood. Anesth Analg 1996; 83(1):129–33.
13. Cantor SB, Hudson DV, Jr, Lichtiger B, Rubenstein EB. Costs of blood transfusion: a process-flow analysis. J Clin Oncol 1998;16(7):2364–70.
14. Sonnenberg FA, Gregory P, Yomtovian R, et al. The cost-effectiveness of autologous transfusion revisited: implications of an increased risk of bacterial infection with allogeneic transfusion. Transfusion 1999; 39(8):808–17.
15. Goh M, Kleer CG, Kielczewski P, Wojno KJ, Kim K, Oesterling JE. Autologous blood donation prior to anatomical radical retropubic prostatectomy: is it necessary? Urology 1997;49(4):569–73.
16. Cremieux PY, Barrett B, Anderson K, Slavin MB. Cost of outpatient blood transfusion in cancer patients. J Clin Oncol 2000;18(14):2755–61.
17. Gafni A, Birch S. NICE methodological guidelines and decision making in the National Health Service in England and Wales. PharmacoEconomics 2003;21(3): 149–57.
18. Amin M, Fergusson D, Wilson K, et al. The societal unit cost of allogenic red blood cells and red blood cell transfusion in Canada. Transfusion 2004;44(10): 1479–86.

19. Glenngard AH, Persson U, Soderman C. Costs associated with blood transfusions in Sweden–the societal cost of autologous, allogeneic and perioperative RBC transfusion. Transfus Med 2005;15(4):295–306.
20. Jacobs P, Turner AR, Kopetsky D. Joint costs in health care: application to blood component production. J Ambulatory Care Manage 1992;15(1):48–55.
21. Trenchard PM, Dixon R. Blood product costing: relationship to price and clinical efficacy. Transfus Med 1995;5(3):231–40.
22. Jidell E, Norda R, Berseus O, Sward-Nilsson AM. Regarding the article "costs associated with blood transfusion in Sweden—the societal cost of autologous, allogeneic and perioperative RBC transfusion". Transfus Med 2006;16(2):151–2; author reply 3.
23. Brooks JP, Ferrell JE. Legal and ethical considerations in the transfusion of infected or untested autologous blood. Am J Clin Pathol 2007;128(1):135–42.
24. Shulman IA, Osby M. Storage and transfusion of infected autologous blood or components: a survey of North American laboratories. Arch Pathol Lab Med 2005;129(8):981–3.
25. Domen RE. Preoperative autologous blood donation: clinical, economic, and ethical issues. Cleve Clin J Med 1996;63(5):295–300.
26. Keating EM, Meding JB, Faris PM, Ritter MA. Predictors of transfusion risk in elective knee surgery. Clin Orthop 1998; 357: 50–59.
27. Brecher ME, Goodnough LT. The rise and fall of preoperative autologous blood donation (editorial). Transfusion 2001;41:1459–62. Transfusion 2002; 42(12):1618–22.
28. Laupacis A, O'Connor AM, Drake ER, et al. A decision aid for autologous pre-donation in cardiac surgery–a randomized trial. Patient Educ Couns 2006;61(3): 458–66.
29. Goodnough LT. Autologous blood donation. Crit Care 2004;8(Suppl. 2): S49–52.
30. Boucher BA, Hannon TJ. Blood management: a primer for clinicians. Pharmacotherapy 2007;27(10): 1394–411.
31. Davies L, Brown TJ, Haynes S, Payne K, Elliott RA, McCollum C. Cost-effectiveness of cell salvage and alternative methods of minimising perioperative allogeneic blood transfusion: a systematic review and economic model. Health Technol Assess 2006;10(44): iii–iv, ix–x, 1–210.
32. Custer B. Economic analyses of blood safety and transfusion medicine interventions: a systematic review. Transfus Med Rev 2004;18(2):127–43.
33. van Hulst M, de Wolf JT, Staginnus U, Ruitenberg EJ, Postma MJ. Pharmaco-economics of blood transfusion safety: review of the available evidence. Vox Sang 2002;83(2):146–55.
34. Pape A, Habler O. Alternatives to allogeneic blood transfusions. Best Pract Res 2007;21(2):221–39.
35. Birkmeyer JD, Goodnough LT, AuBuchon JP, Noordsij PG, Littenberg B. The cost-effectiveness of preoperative autologous blood donation for total hip and knee replacement. Transfusion 1993;33(7):544–51.
36. Birkmeyer JD, AuBuchon JP, Littenberg B, et al. Cost-effectiveness of preoperative autologous donation in coronary artery bypass grafting. Ann Thorac Surg 1994;57(1):161–8.
37. Etchason J, Petz L, Keeler E, et al. The cost effectiveness of preoperative autologous blood donations. N Engl J Med 1995;332(11):719–24.
38. Healy JC, Frankforter SA, Graves BK, Reddy RL, Beck JR. Preoperative autologous blood donation in total-hip arthroplasty. A cost-effectiveness analysis. Arch Pathol Lab Med 1994;118(4):465–70.
39. Sonnenberg FA. Autologous transfusion—a reasonable measure under the principles of health economics? Anasthesiol Intensivmed Notfallmed Schmerzther 2003;38(1):54–8.
40. Blumberg N, Kirkley SA, Heal JM. A cost analysis of autologous and allogeneic transfusions in hip-replacement surgery. Am J Surg 1996;171(3):324–30.
41. Marchetti M, Barosi G. Cost-effectiveness of epoetin and autologous blood donationin reducing allogeneic blood transfusions incoronary artery bypass graft surgery. Transfusion 2000;40(6):673–81.
42. Horowitz NS, Gibb RK, Menegakis NE, Mutch DG, Rader JS, Herzog TJ. Utility and cost-effectiveness of preoperative autologous blood donation in gynecologic and gynecologic oncology patients. Obstet Gynecol 2002;99(5 Pt 1):771–6.
43. Goodnough LM, Grishaber JE, Birkmeyer JD, Monk TG, Catalona WJ. Efficacy and cost-effectiveness of autologous blood predeposit in patients undergoing radical prostatectomy procedures. Urology 1994; 44(2):226–31.
44. Blumberg N. Allogeneic transfusion and infection: economic and clinical implications. Semin Hematol 1997;34(3 Suppl. 2):34–40.
45. Vamvakas EC, Blajchman MA. Transfusion-related immunomodulation (TRIM): an update. Blood Rev 2007;21(6):327–48.

46. Duffy G, Neal KR. Differences in post-operative infection rates between patients receiving autologous and allogeneic blood transfusion: a meta-analysis of published randomized and nonrandomized studies. Transfus Med 1996;6(4):325–8.
47. Carson JL, Altman DG, Duff A, et al. Risk of bacterial infection associated with allogeneic blood transfusion among patients undergoing hip fracture repair. Transfusion 1999;39(7):694–700.
48. Nnodu OE, Odunukwe N, Odunubi O, Ekanem E, Njoku OS. Cost effectiveness of autologous blood transfusion–a developing country hospital's perspective. West Afr J Med 2003;22(1):10–12.
49. Henry DA, Carless PA, Moxey AJ, et al. Pre-operative autologous donation for minimising perioperative allogeneic blood transfusion. Cochrane Database Syst Rev 2002 (2):CD003602.
50. Heiss MM, Mempel W, Jauch KW, et al. Beneficial effect of autologous blood transfusion on infectious complications after colorectal cancer surgery. Lancet 1993;342(8883):1328–33.
51. Billote DB, Glisson SN, Green D, Wixson RL. A prospective, randomized study of preoperative autologous donation for hip replacement surgery. J Bone Joint Surg 2002;84-A(8):1299–304.

CHAPTER 46

Autologous Blood Predonation in Cardiac Surgery

Wulf Dietrich

Institute for Research in Cardiac Anesthesia and Working Group of Perioperative Hemostasis, Departments of Anesthesiology and Transfusion Medicine, University of Munich, Munich, Germany

Autologous blood donation is one of the oldest methods of avoiding allogeneic blood transfusion. It gained high popularity during the AIDS crisis in the 1980s. A contemporary editorial in *New England Journal of Medicine* was entitled "The patient's blood is the safest blood" [1]. It is commonly practiced in a variety of noncardiac procedures; but it was demonstrated repeatedly also prior to elective cardiac surgery to be an effective practice to reduce the exposure of patients to allogeneic blood [2–4]. Other studies did not completely confirm these results [5].

Perioperative bleeding presents still a problem in cardiac surgery [6]. Transfusion medicine has changed considerably over the past years. However, transfusion of allogeneic blood still is associated with inherent risks. Recently, the risk of transfusion of allogeneic blood products on short- [7, 8] and long-term [9] outcome was emphasized [10, 11].

An extended guideline evaluated the effectiveness of autologous predonation [6] and concluded that predonation of as much as two units autologous blood is reasonable for blood conservation in carefully selected patients before routine cardiac operation. This was a class I recommendation with a level A evidence.

A systematic review from the Cochrane Library published in the year 2001 found an overall reduction of the risk receiving allogeneic blood transfusion by a relative 63%. The absolute reduction was 44%. But the risk of receiving any transfusion (autologous and/or allogeneic) was even increased in patients who predonated. The authors concluded that, since allogeneic blood is safe nowadays, the true benefit of predonation is questionable [12]. The overall quality of the investigated studies in this review was poor. This review was not updated until now.

In the early days there were concerns about the safety of this method, especially about an increase in the risk of myocardial infarction due to the loss of hemoglobin. But today there is an increasing body of publications documenting the safety of this technique. However, the cost-effectiveness has been questioned. Recent investigations examined the cost-effectiveness of autologous blood donation and presumed a low cost-effectiveness of this practice [13, 14]. In these studies effectiveness was defined as quality-adjusted years of life saved (QALY) by the avoidance of transfusion-transmitted viral infections like HIV, hepatitis or HTLV. The extremely low per-unit probability of these infections [15] resulted in cost-effectiveness values ranging from 235,000 USD up to 1,190,000 USD per QALY for autologous blood donation in elective cardiac surgery [14]. From these results it has been concluded that autologous blood donation is not cost-effective [16].

The high costs of autologous predonation are mainly the result of high personnel costs and unnecessary predonation resulting in discarding

Alternatives to Blood Transfusion in Transfusion Medicine, 2nd edition. Edited by A. Maniatis, P. Van der Linden, J.-F. Hardy.

predonated blood units. The personnel costs can be reduced by optimal organization of the predonation unit, while tailoring the predonation program to the specific needs of a specific hospital and/or a defined patient population, can lower the discarding rate. A prerequisite for this is the thorough information about the transfusion practice within the hospital.

The cost-effectiveness model of autologous blood donation based solely on the avoidance of viral infections excludes several aspects from consideration: potential risks associated with allogeneic transfusion like posttransfusion infections [17–21] or long-term mortality [22] could change the estimates of cost-effectiveness substantially. Other studies also reported an unfavorable effect of allogeneic blood-product transfusion [7, 23, 24]. Further, the emergence of new diseases is likely to place considerable additional cost to allogeneic transfusion by the implementation of new testing or inactivation strategies [25, 26]. Neither patient's preferences nor quality of life related to transfusion practices are weighted against the cost of autologous blood donation. Finally, there are repeated serious shortages of blood supply, placing increasing attention to the development of blood conservation strategies.

Experiences and results of a center with organized autologous predonation program

We analyzed the practice and results of the autologous predonation program at our hospital [27]. The aim of that study was to assess transfusion practice and costs in cardiac surgery with and without autologous blood donation and to develop a diagnosis- and gender-based decision model for the optimization of autologous blood donation. The costs of autologous predonation and transfusion were calculated. We studied 4878 patients undergoing elective open-heart surgery with and without autologous blood donation. Out of these, 868 patients (18%) underwent autologous blood donation while 4010 (82%) did not. Allogeneic blood transfusion was recorded as primary end point.

Autologous blood donation was carried out on an outpatient basis in the German Heart Center Munich by an anesthesiologist experienced in blood donation and the respective surgical intervention. There was at least one session and a maximum of three sessions depending on diagnosis, gender, and available time before the operation. To utilize the capacity of the staff effectively, as far as possible, at least four patients donated blood in parallel. Within each session 6 to 8 mL/kg of whole blood were taken and processed to one unit of packed red cells (PRC) and one unit of fresh frozen plasma (FFP). Since 2003 the majority of donated units was stored as whole blood. The removed blood volume was simultaneously substituted by crystalloids. The last session of autologous blood donation was carried out no later than 5 days before admission to the hospital for surgery. All patients were routinely substituted with oral iron. This technique of autotransfusion and the incidence was not changed after the withdrawal of aprotinin, which was routinely used in almost all patients, in 2006.

Demographic and clinical data of patients were documented prospectively according to a standardized database. The preoperative cardiovascular state of patients was assessed according to the NYHA classification and the Cleveland Clinic risk stratification [28]. Perioperative transfusion was indicated if the hematocrit was less than 21% in female and less than 24% in male patients or less than 18% during ECC or if clinical signs of insufficient oxygen supply were apparent. Intravenous anesthesia with sufentanil, midazolam, and pancuronium was used in all patients. A high dose aprotinin regime (approximately 6 million KIU per patient) was part of the routine protocol.

To estimate the number of autologous blood donations necessary to avoid the transfusion of one unit of allogeneic blood a decision-model was developed. Calculation basis was a decision tree. Decision tree analysis was conducted for the whole population and for coronary artery bypass grafting (CABG) and aortic valve replacement (AVR) patients, separately for male and female patients. Patients who were classified NYHA IV were excluded, since most of them were not eligible for autologous blood donation (Figure 46.1).

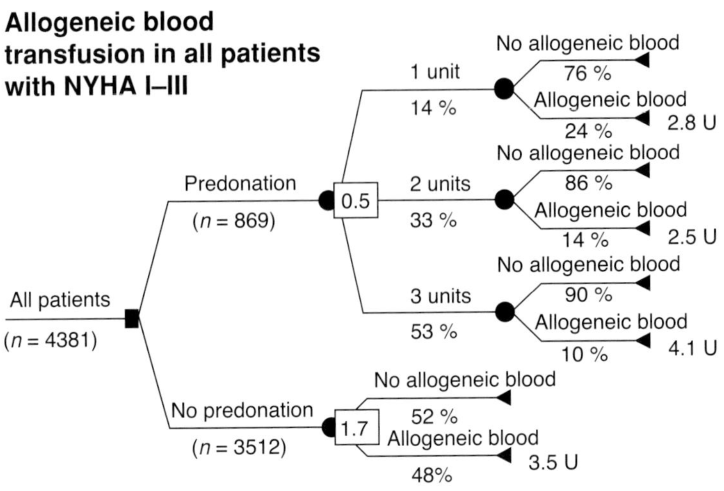

Figure 46.1 Decision tree analysis of all patients. While 48% of patients without predonation received allogeneic blood transfusion, only 24, 14, or 10%, respectively, of patients with predonation received allogeneic blood. This figure shows that the predonation of two units autologous blood caused the best blood saving effect (U = units of allogeneic blood). In total, the donation of three units was no more effective. However, in the subgroup of female patients the predonation of three units was more effective compared to two units. The autologous program must be tailored to the specific needs of patients and operation.

Costs were calculated from the hospital perspective, which differs from the patients or the national economic perspective. Only expenses arising for the hospital were calculated and included. Acquisition costs for allogeneic blood units and laboratory material were obtained from the hospitals price lists, staff costs, and the controlling department provided costs for investments and maintenance. Since the discarding of autologous units donated, but not transfused, has been suggested to be a main cost driver in autologous blood donation in recent studies, the costs of predonated autologous units were taken into consideration regardless of whether transfused or not. Further, the costs for the predonation of one autologous unit include one autologous FFP. Since for every patient, not undergoing autologous blood donation, two units of allogeneic blood were procured before surgery, the resulting costs of procurement were taken into consideration, even if the units were not transfused, because the costs of allocation incurred regardless whether the unit was used in another patient.

Results

In the whole study population, 20% (849 of 4325), in the CABG group 16% (437 of 2742) and in the AVR group 26% (184 of 717) underwent autologous blood donation. No adverse events due to donation were observed. Of all patients undergoing autologous blood donation 13% received allogeneic blood during their hospital stay, while 48% of the patients without predonation received transfusion (CABG: 15% vs 46%; AVR: 12% vs 50%, $p < 0.05$ each). Patients without predonation received 1.68 ± 3.35 (mean ± SD) allogeneic units, patients in the autologous group 0.42 ± 1.76 units ($p < 0.05$) (CABG patients 1.53 ± 2.88 vs 0.50 ± 1.88 and AVR patients 1.45 ± 2.32 vs 0.25 ± 0.80 units, respectively; all $p < 0.05$). Patients with predonation received a higher total number of any transfusion (autologous and allogeneic) compared to patients without predonation (2.38 vs 1.68 units, $p < 0.05$). The discarding rate of unused autologous blood units was 32% in male and 19% in female patients. This appears fairly high at first sight. However, the respective control group without predonation had a transfusion rate of roughly 50%, i.e., 50% of the procured allogeneic units were not utilized.

In the group with atrial septum defect (ASD) closure 57% of patients underwent autologous blood donation, none of them receiving allogeneic blood. Female patients, regardless of whether undergoing autologous blood donation or not, were more frequently and to a higher extent transfused than male patients. Accordingly, the residual probability to receive allogeneic blood could not be reduced to the same degree as in male patients. Due to the lower discarding rate, costs for female patients predonating two units were equal or even lower than for female patients without predonation.

Is autologous predonation efficacious and cost-effective?

This study demonstrates that the predonation of autologous blood is an effective practice to reduce allogeneic blood transfusion with an acceptable cost load. The decision model shows that the predonation of two autologous units keeps the best balance between the reduction of the risk probability to receive allogeneic transfusion and associated costs, whereas the predonation of three units increases costs substantially. The reduction of transfusion risk to 11% in the whole study population was similar or even superior compared to other blood conservation strategies. This technique was neither effective nor cost-effective in operations with a relatively low transfusion rate like closure of an ASD.

The costs for one autologous unit (80 USD) in this study amounted to 77% of those for one allogeneic unit (103 USD). These costs were calculated on the basis of the costs in year 2000. The lower costs for one autologous unit are the result of low collection costs resulting from predonation at the same institution, where surgery takes place. In a department specialized on autologous predonation personnel costs can be cut dramatically by simultaneous donation of several patients.

In accordance with previous studies, autologous predonation patients received a higher number of any transfusion (autologous and allogeneic) than patients without predonation, supporting previous findings that autologous blood donors are more likely than nondonors to receive any transfusion [2, 29]. Despite a lower preoperative hematocrit a higher hematocrit at discharge was found in patients with predonation. This fact must be interpreted as "over-transfusion" or a more liberal transfusion indication for autologous compared to allogeneic units. However, a more restrictive transfusion regimen alone would not alter cost estimates in this model, since costs of predonated autologous units were taken into consideration regardless of whether transfused or not.

The numbers of predonated autologous units necessary to avoid one allogeneic unit were chosen as end point to express the potential of autologous predonation to save allogeneic blood. Overall, the donation of 1.5 autologous units saved one allogeneic unit for additional cost of 19 USD. At the same time the residual risk to receive allogeneic blood is reduced from almost 50–11%. This suggests a good relationship between costs and clinical benefit.

Conclusion

The higher the probability of transfusion the better is efficacy and cost-effectiveness of autologous predonation. In view of latest results about the detrimental effects of allogeneic blood transfusion [10, 11], efforts to reduce transfusion incidence must be undertaken. Autologous predonation is one tool to reduce allogeneic transfusion. Admittedly, in times of short or even no waiting lists this technique is only applicable in a limited number of patients. But since cardiac surgery still remains a high-transfusion area [30, 31], it offers ideal conditions for autologous blood donation. The fact that, compared to other blood conservation strategies, lower costs are generated to save one allogeneic unit demonstrates, that autologous blood donation today still remains a promising and cost-effective alternative in the attempt to reduce allogeneic blood transfusion in elective cardiac surgery, even in times with no or only short waiting lists [32].

References

1. Surgenor DM: The patient's blood is the safest blood. N Engl J Med 1987;316:542–4.
2. Dupuis JY, Bart B, Bryson G, Robblee J. Transfusion practices among patients who did and did not predonate autologous blood before elective cardiac surgery. Can Med Assoc J 1999;160:997–1002.

3. Dzik WH, Fleisher AG, Ciavarella D, et al. Safety and efficacy of autologous blood donation before elective aortic valve operation. Ann Thorac Surg 1992;54:1177–81.
4. Gandini G, Franchini M, Bertuzzo D, et al. Preoperative autologous blood donation by 1073 elderly patients undergoing elective surgery: a safe and effective practice. Transfusion 1999;39:174–8.
5. Waters JH, Lee JS, Klein E, O'Hara J, Zippe C, Potter PS. Preoperative autologous donation versus cell salvage in the avoidance of allogeneic transfusion in patients undergoing radical retropubic prostatectomy. Anesth Analg 2004;98:537–42.
6. Ferraris VA, Ferraris SP, Saha SP, et al. Perioperative blood transfusion and blood conservation in cardiac surgery: the society of thoracic surgeons and the society of cardiovascular anesthesiologists clinical practice guideline. Ann Thorac Surg 2007;83:S27–86.
7. Spiess BD, Royston D, Levy JH, et al. Platelet transfusions during coronary artery bypass graft surgery are associated with serious adverse outcomes. Transfusion 2004;44:1143–8.
8. Koch CG, Li L, Duncan AI, et al. Morbidity and mortality risk associated with red blood cell and blood-component transfusion in isolated coronary artery bypass grafting. Crit Care Med 2006;34:1608–16.
9. Koch CG, Li L, Duncan AI, et al. Transfusion in coronary artery bypass grafting is associated with reduced long-term survival. Ann Thorac Surg 2006;81:1650–57.
10. Rawn JD: Blood transfusion in cardiac surgery: a silent epidemic revisited. Circulation 2007;116:2523–4.
11. Murphy GJ, Reeves BC, Rogers CA, et al. Increased mortality, postoperative morbidity, and cost after red blood cell transfusion in patients having cardiac surgery. Circulation 2007;116:2544–52.
12. Henry DA, Carless PA, Moxey AJ, et al. Pre-operative autologous donation for minimising perioperative allogeneic blood transfusion. Cochrane Database Syst Rev 2001;CD003602.
13. Birkmeyer JD, Aubuchon JP, Littenberg B, et al. Cost-Effectiveness of preoperative autologous donation in coronary artery bypass grafting. Ann Thorac Surg 1994;57:161–9.
14. Etchason J, Petz L, Keeler E, et al. The cost effectiveness of preoperative autologous blood donations. N Engl J Med 1995;332:719–24.
15. Dodd RY. The risk of transfusion-transmitted infection. N Engl J Med 1992;327:419–21.
16. Brecher ME, Goodnough LT. The rise and fall of preoperative autologous blood donation. Transfusion 2001;41:1459–62.
17. Chelemer SB, Prato BS, Cox PM, Jr, O'Connor GT, Morton JR. Association of bacterial infection and red blood cell transfusion after coronary artery bypass surgery. Ann Thorac Surg 2002;73:138–42.
18. Kuehnert MJ, Roth VR, Haley NR, et al. Transfusion-transmitted bacterial infection in the United States, 1998 through 2000. Transfusion 2001;41:1493–9.
19. Leal-Noval SR, Rincon-Ferrari MD, Garcia-Curiel A, et al. Transfusion of blood components and postoperative infection in patients undergoing cardiac surgery. Chest 2001;119:1461–8.
20. Murphy PJ, Connery C, Hicks GL, Blumberg N. Homologous blood transfusion as a risk factor for postoperative infection after coronary artery bypass graft operations. J Thorac Cardiovasc Surg 1992;104:1092–9.
21. Sonnenberg FA, Gregory P, Yomtovian R, et al. The cost-effectiveness of autologous transfusion revisited: implications of an increased risk of bacterial infection with allogeneic transfusion. Transfusion 1999;39:808–17.
22. Engoren MC, Habib RH, Zacharias A, et al. Effect of blood transfusion on long-term survival after cardiac operation. Ann Thorac Surg 2002;74:1180–86.
23. Hebert PC, Wells G, Blajchman MA, et al. A multicenter, randomized, controlled clinical trial of transfusion requirements in critical care. N Engl J Med 1999;340:409–17.
24. Rao SV, Jollis JG, Harrington RA, et al. Relationship of blood transfusion and clinical outcomes in patients with acute coronary syndromes. JAMA 2004;292:1555–62.
25. Pealer LN, Marfin AA, Petersen LR, et al. Transmission of West Nile virus through blood transfusion in the United States in 2002. N Engl J Med 2003;349:1236–45.
26. Goodnough LT, Shander A, Brecher ME. Transfusion medicine: looking to the future. Lancet 2003;361:161–9.
27. Dietrich W, Thuermel K, Heyde S, Busley R, Berger K. Autologous blood donation in cardiac surgery: reduction of allogeneic blood transfusion and cost-effectiveness. J Cardiothorac Vasc Anesth 2005;19:589–96.
28. Higgins TL, Estafanous FG, Loop FD, et al. Stratification of morbidity and mortality outcome by preoperative risk factors in coronary artery bypass patients. A clinical severity score. JAMA 1992;267:2344–8.

29. Forgie MA, Wells PS, Laupacis A, Fergusson D. Preoperative autologous donation decreases allogeneic transfusion but increases exposure to all red blood cell transfusion: results of a meta-analysis. Arch Intern Med 1998;158:610–16.
30. Nuttall GA, Stehling LC, Beighley CM, Faust RJ. Current transfusion practices of members of the American society of anesthesiologists: a survey. Anesthesiology 2003;99:1433–43.
31. Stover EP, Siegel LC, Parks R, Levin J, et al. Variability in transfusion practice for coronary artery bypass surgery persists despite national consensus guidelines: a 24-institution study. Anesthesiology 1998;88:327–33.
32. Dietrich W, Busley R, Kriner M. Preoperative autologous blood donation in cardiac surgery. Reduction of allogeneic blood requirements. Anaesthesist 2006;55:753–9.

CHAPTER 47

Cost-Effectiveness of Pharmacological Alternatives

Dean Fergusson & Brian Hutton
Ottawa Health Research Institute, University of Ottawa Faculty of Medicine, Ottawa, Ontario, Canada

Introduction to economic evaluation in healthcare

Economic evaluations in healthcare are an important element of decision making and patient management, particularly as new technologies emerge. The purpose of an economic evaluation is to ensure that the benefits from a given treatment are greater than their opportunity costs, which aids decision makers in determining the optimal way to allocate funds to different healthcare programs. Economic evaluations in healthcare can take on varying forms; comprehensive economic analyses can be categorized as (1) cost-effectiveness analyses,) cost-utility analyses, (3) cost-benefit analyses, or (4) cost-minimization analyses, while partial economic analyses may consist of (1) cost descriptions, (2) cost of illness studies, or (3) cost comparison studies. Cost-effectiveness studies evaluate the ratio of the cost of the intervention to a relevant measure of its effect. Conversely, cost-utility analyses combine the consideration of quantity and quality of life, using quality adjusted life years (QALYs) as the outcome measure of interest in the analysis. Cost-benefit analyses measure both the costs and consequences of treatment alternatives in terms of dollars, while cost-minimization analyses seek to determine the least expensive treatment alternative.

Alternatives to Blood Transfusion in Transfusion Medicine, 2nd edition. Edited by A. Maniatis, P. Van der Linden, J.-F. Hardy.

Given that there are demonstrated effective pharmacological alternatives each with their own risk profile, we require full economic evaluations in the form of cost-effectiveness studies to best guide clinical use. Cost-effectiveness analyses are a particular type of epidemiologic study that compare two or more interventions (be it drugs, care programs, or other such therapies) by comparing the ratio of costs (measured in monetary value) to benefits (measured by outcomes such as number of patients not transfused, years of life saved, transfusion-related infections avoided, or reoperations avoided) achieved with each of the treatments under consideration. The commonly employed measure used for comparing two treatments, denoted here as A and B, is referred to as the *incremental cost-effectiveness ratio* (ICER), which is of the form:

$$\text{ICER} = \frac{(\text{Cost of A} - \text{Cost of B})}{(\text{Effectiveness summary A} - \text{Effectiveness summary B})}$$

Costs of the interventions are often and preferably gathered in the context of a randomized trial or a large, representative cohort study. Estimates of effectiveness used in economic evaluations are typically gathered from published meta-analyses of previously performed groups of appropriately chosen randomized controlled trials (RCTs). While there is no consensus, if a technology costs (or saves) less than $20,000 per QALY, it is considered to be cost-effective whereas if it costs more than $100,000 per QALY it is considered cost-prohibitive [1]. Technologies with costs per QALY between $20,000 and $100,000 fall within a gray zone and require consideration on a case-by-case basis. As an example, the costs per QALY of dalteparin versus warfarin prophylaxis for venous thrombolic events in major orthopedic surgery is less than CDN 10,000 for hip and knee replacement surgeries as well as hip fractures [2].

Pharmacologic treatment alternatives in cardiac and orthopedic surgery

A number of pharmacologic alternatives are available to minimize blood loss and transfusion requirements during cardiac surgery. Antifibrinolytic agents (aprotinin, tranexamic acid, epsilon-aminocaproic acid) have all been proven effective in reducing allogeneic exposure in cardiac surgery when compared to placebo or no active control. Meta-analyses of RCTs concluded that antifibrinolytic drugs decrease allogeneic red blood cell (RBC) exposure, with aprotinin also decreasing the rates of reoperation for major bleeding [3–5]. Desmopressin has also been used in cardiac surgery yet its effectiveness has not been demonstrated and its use is not common [3]. Erythropoietin has also been evaluated in clinical trials in cardiac surgery. While demonstrating a reduction in blood loss and transfusion requirements, concerns regarding serious adverse events have not led to its use [6, 7].

In orthopedic surgery, erythropoietin has been shown to be effective at reducing blood loss and transfusion requirements when used alone or in combination with preoperative autologous donation (PAD) [7]. The antifibrinolytics, aprotinin, and tranexamic acid, have also proven effective in reducing blood loss and transfusion requirements in orthopedic surgery [4].

The majority of clinical trials assessing the pharmacological alternatives in orthopedic and cardiac surgery have focused on allogeneic red blood cell transfusion avoidance and blood loss as the primary measures of effectiveness. While these measures are important, more clinically meaningful outcomes include prevention of massive bleeding or transfusion, the need for rethoracotomy, and death due to hemorrhage. Given the safety of the blood supply in developed countries, it is important that we demonstrate that the effectiveness of pharmacological alternatives extends beyond a reduction of one unit of red blood cells or a blood loss of 100 mL. To date, only one trial in cardiac surgery has evaluated such measures [8]. Because cost-effectiveness analyses incorporate risks as well as benefits of treatments, we also need to consider possible serious adverse events such as thromboses, renal dysfunction, stroke, myocardial infarction, and mortality.

Systematic review of published economic evaluations

To identify economic evaluations, we performed a systematic review of all published economic evaluations that compared the costs of two or more perioperative strategies published between 1966 and 2006 and indexed in Medline, EMBASE, or identified in a personal electronic library of >8500 transfusion medicine articles. Specific eligibility criteria for inclusion in the review required the use of allogeneic blood alone in one of the study arms, and that the performance of an economic evaluation was a primary aim of the study. Results of this literature search revealed that until 1998, no comprehensive economic evaluation and only one partial economic evaluation [7] had been published, even though the clinical effectiveness of a number of treatments (e.g., aprotinin, tranexamic acid, erythropoietin) had been well established for several years. Since 1998, an additional 11 evaluations have been published [8–18]. Thus a total of 12 economic evaluations including 10 in cardiac surgery (6 aprotinin versus usual care, 2 erythropoietin plus PAD, 1 aprotinin versus tranexamic acid versus epsilon-aminocaproic acid, 1 aprotinin vs epsilon-aminocaproic acid), and two in orthopedic surgery (1 erythropoietin plus PAD, 1 erythropoietin plus PAD versus erythropoietin alone) (Table 47.1). Among the set of 12 economic evaluations, only 4 were considered full evaluations (all of which involved assessment of erythropoietin), and all were set in developed countries (Table 47.1).

Table 47.1 Characteristics of economic evaluations.

Primary author and year of publication	Surgery population	Interventions compared	Country	Journal	Type of economic analysis
Coyle (1999) [10]	Orthopedic	EPO + PAD and EPO	Canada	*Transfusion Medicine*	Full
Woronoff-Lemsi (1999) [11]	Orthopedic	EPO + PAD	France	*Transfusion*	Full
Lazzara (1997) [9]	Cardiac	Aprotinin vs no treatment	United States	*Archives of Surgery*	Partial
Able (1998) [12]	Cardiac	Aprotinin vs no treatment	United States	*Clinical Therapeutics*	Partial
Ray (1999) [13]	Cardiac	Aprotinin vs no treatment	Australia	*Annals of Thoracic Surgery*	Partial
Dignan (2001) [14]	Cardiac	Aprotinin vs no treatment	Australia	*Annals of Thoracic Surgery*	Partial
Robinson (2002) [15]	Cardiac	Aprotinin vs no treatment	United Kingdom	*Clinical Therapeutics*	Partial
Smith (2004) [16]	Cardiac	Aprotinin vs no treatment	United States	*Annals of Thoracic Surgery*	Partial
Marchetti (2000) [17]	Cardiac	EPO + PAD	Italy	*Transfusion*	Full
Coyle (2000) [18]	Cardiac	EPO + PAD	Canada	*Pharmacoeconomics*	Full
Casati (1999) [19]	Cardiac	Aprotinin vs TXA vs EACA	Italy	*Annals of Thoracic Surgery*	Partial
Bennett-Guerrero (1997) [20]	Cardiac	Aprotinin vs EACA	United States/Argentina	*Anesthesiology*	Partial

Abbreviations: EPO, erythropoietin; PAD, preoperative autologous donation; TXA, tranexamic acid; EACA, epsilon-aminocaproic acid.

Economic evaluations in orthopedic surgery

Only two studies in the field of orthopedic surgery met eligibility criteria [10, 11]. In a 1999 economic evaluation performed by Coyle et al., combination of erythropoietin with PAD of red blood cells was compared to no intervention. Investigators identified a cost of CDN $329 million per life year gained with the use of erythropoietin and PAD, and the intervention was found to add only 0.000006 of years of life compared to no treatment; costs of the interventions were estimated as $2904 for erythropoietin versus $968 for no intervention, respectively [10]. Findings from the study led the investigators to conclude that use of erythropoietin was not cost-effective for minimization of blood loss and transfusions in orthopedic surgery. In a 1999 study of erythropoietin with PAD, Woronoff-Lemsi et al. estimated that the incremental cost of one prevented hepatitis C infection was $US 888 million, with 0.31 cases per 100,000 being prevented [11]. With regard to use of erythropoietin alone in comparison to no intervention, Coyle et al. estimated an incremental cost per life year gained of $CDN 66 million, found that only 0.000024 life years were gained with the intervention, and estimated costs of $1857 versus $269 for the two modalities. Again erythropoietin alone was not considered to be cost-effective.

While erythropoietin was found to be clinically effective in randomized trials in terms of reducing the need for transfusion, it was cost-ineffective in rigorously conducted economic evaluations. This was a result of multiple issues, namely (1) the significantly increased safety of the blood supply; (2) the significant cost of erythropoietin; (3) the adverse event profile of erythropoietin compared to blood transfusion; and (4) while the number of patients transfused is decreased, the savings in terms of mean number of units transfused is marginal (approximately ¾ of a unit).

Economic evaluations in cardiac surgery

Ten studies in the field of cardiac surgery met eligibility criteria for inclusion in this systematic review of cost-effectiveness studies. A total of six studies comparing aprotinin with no intervention were identified (Table 47.1). All were cost comparison studies that made use of institutional (hospital) charges and considered only perioperative costs. Most studies were single center evaluations, with four employing data from clinical trials and two incorporating data from institutional cohorts.

Smith et al. carried out a lifetime cost comparison of aprotinin versus no intervention that accounted for costs of stroke, myocardial infarction, reoperation and in-hospital death [16]. Findings in patients undergoing primary CABG and receiving a typical full dose of aprotinin reduced total lifetime costs by $US186 per patient as compared to only $US51 for those receiving half-dose; in patients undergoing repeat CABG, full dosing reduced total lifetime costs by $US6044 as compared to $US4483 with a half dose.

In 1999, Casati et al. randomized a total of 210 patients undergoing elective cardiac surgery to receive aprotinin, tranexamic acid, or epsilon-aminocaproic acid (EACA). Investigators examined the costing of both drugs and blood used in the trial, and noted the lower costs with tranexamic acid ($58 ± $105) and EACA ($101 ± 159) compared to aprotinin ($433 ± 119) [19]. The costs of adverse events were not incorporated into the cost comparison.

In 1997, Bennett-Guerrero et al. performed a multicenter, randomized trial enrolling 204 patients to either aprotinin or EACA, and considered elements of both effectiveness and costs related to bleeding (including RBCs, platelets, frozen plasma, and cryoprecipitate) in a repeat surgery population [20]. Aprotinin was shown to be associated with lesser postoperative thoracic drainage and fewer platelet transfusions, while no differences between groups were observed for red blood cell transfusions or closure time. In regard to aspects of cost, EACA was associated with median hospital costs of $1088 (range $511–2057), while aprotinin was associated with median costs of $1813 (range $1476–2605).

Two studies evaluating the use of erythropoietin in cardiac surgery were identified, both in combination with PAD of red cells. In 2000, Coyle et al. reported a cost-effectiveness analysis of the use of erythropoietin with PAD of blood before elective cardiac surgery [18]. While its use led to a 60% decline in the requirement of allogeneic transfusions (31.6% down to 12.7%), this change was associated with a gain of only 0.000035 life years, as well as an incremental cost per life year gained of $CDN 44.6 million. This result was largely a consequence of the high costs of erythropoietin ($CDN2579) compared with PAD ($CDN1019). In 2000, a US-based cost-effectiveness study reported by Marchetti et al. indicated an incremental cost per QALY gained of $US 5 million [17]. The use of erythropoietin to augment PAD was found to save only an additional 0.000146 years of life compared to PAD alone. The authors claimed that neither strategy was cost-effective for reducing the health effects associated with RBC transfusions, but concluded that incorporation of bacterial complications associated with transfusion into the model would make both modalities cost-effective. In an assessment of erythropoietin alone, Marchetti et al. identified a cost per QALY of $US 7 million, again an excessively large cost, but further indicated that this amount was reduced to $6288 per QALY if bacterial complications were considered [17]. As was the case for its use in orthopedic surgery, erythropoietin is not a cost-effective treatment alternative either alone or to augment PAD. This is a consequence of the high cost of the drug, its minimal reduction of the mean number of units given to those still requiring transfusion (1.35 vs 0.61 units), and the safety of the blood supply.

Summary of findings

For the antifibrinolytic therapies, no economic evaluations have been published in orthopedic surgery despite evidence from clinical trials demonstrating effectiveness at reducing blood loss and transfusion requirements. As for antifibrinolytic therapies in cardiac surgery, the increase in mortality associated with aprotinin compared to the lysine analogs would suggest that the use of the lysine analogs over aprotinin is warranted [8]. However, rigorous economic evaluations of lysine analogs are warranted given the cost discrepancy between these two agents. The use of erythropoietin with or without PAD has not been shown to be cost-effective in both cardiac and orthopedic surgery [10, 18].

The majority of economic evaluations reported in our review suffer from serious limitations. Of the 12 economic evaluations we identified, only 4 (33%) were full economic evaluations where both costs and benefits of treatment and alternatives were assessed [10, 11, 17, 18]. While the clinical effectiveness of each of the pharmacological therapies has been well documented in the context of randomized trials and systematic reviews, the acquisition of true costs (not charges) of both transfusion and adverse events associated with both transfusion and therapies have rarely been performed. Furthermore, economic evaluations require a variety of clinical and geographic settings to ensure their robustness and generalizability. Future economic evaluations in this area must move beyond considering transfusion avoidance as the single clinical outcome of interest, as this outcome is may be no longer considered as clinically important to patients, caregivers, institutions, or payers alike; this is a consequence of the greatly improved safety of blood systems since the 1980s, as well as improved approaches to surgery and anesthesia that serve to minimize blood loss such as the adoption of restrictive transfusion triggers. For example, the latter decrease the use of RBC more effectively than PAD, erythropoietin, or antifibrinolytics at no cost, assuming that morbidity and mortality remain the same [21]. Thus, given the safety of the blood supply in developed countries and the costs associated with blood sparing pharmaceutical agents, moving beyond blood loss and transfusion requirements as outcomes to include serious morbidity and mortality must be considered. To be clear, demonstrating differences in the need for massive transfusion and massive bleeding are clinically and economically important whereas minimal blood loss and the saving of $^1/_2$ a unit to 1 unit of RBCs are not. Efforts to incorporate additional relevant risks, including those associated with anesthesia, the surgical procedure itself, post-surgical care and the combination of multiple interventions during care (and potentially harmful effects resulting from their interaction) is a clinically important next step that must be pursued. Many pharmacologic technologies of past years have been adopted into clinical practice based largely on beliefs and often minimal and weak published evidence that they reduce major adverse events beyond blood loss. However, in many cases, such drugs have not been definitively demonstrated to reduce clinically important outcomes such as need for reoperation, length of hospital stay, quality of life or even death. The BART trial demonstrates the importance of measuring clinically important benefits and potential harms instead, rather than blood loss and the proportion of patients transfused. Moreover, in the presence of established efficacy among several agents, we need large head-to-head RCTs to evaluate the most beneficial, less harmful, and cost-effective blood-sparing agents [8].

Finally, all potential serious adverse events associated with blood sparing interventions (including hypersensitivity, renal dysfunction, myocardial infarction, and thromboses) as well as those associated with blood products used (including febrile reactions, hemolytic reactions, bacterial contaminations, transfusion related acute lung injury, viral contamination, and the impact of blood shortages) merit consideration. Inclusion of these additional factors in economic models will provide more accurate and informative evidence on the cost-effectiveness of pharmacologic alternatives in cardiac and orthopedic surgery.

References

1. Laupacis A, Feeny D, Detsky AS, Tugwell PX. How attractive does a new technology have to be to warrant adoption and utilization? Tentative guidelines for using clinical and economic evaluations. CMAJ 1992;146(4):473–81.
2. Dranitsaris G, Stumpo C, Smith R, Bartle W. Extended dalteparin prophylaxis for venous thromboembolic events: cost-utility analysis in patients undergoing major orthopedic surgery. Am J Cardiovasc Drugs 2009;9(1):45–58.
3. Laupacis A, Fergusson D. Drugs to minimize perioperative blood loss in cardiac surgery: meta-analyses using perioperative blood transfusion as the outcome. Anesth Analg 1997;85:1258–67.
4. Henry DA, Carless PA, Moxey AJ, et al. Antifibrinolytic use for minimising perioperative allogeneic blood transfusion. Cochrane Database Syst Rev 2007;(4):CD001886.
5. Levi M, Cromheecke ME, de Jonge E, et al. Pharmacological strategies to decrease excessive blood loss in cardiac surgery: a meta-analysis of clinically relevant endpoints. Lancet 1999;354:1940–47.
6. Alghamdi AA, Albanna MJ, Guru V, Brister SJ. Does the use of erythropoietin reduce the risk of exposure to allogeneic blood transfusion in cardiac surgery? A systematic review and meta-analysis. J Card Surg 2006;21(3):320–26.
7. Laupacis A, Fergusson D. Erythropoietin to minimize perioperative blood transfusion: a systematic review of randomized trials. The international study of perioperative transfusion (ISPOT) investigators. Transfus Med 1998;8(4):309–17.
8. Fergusson DA, Hébert PC, Mazer CD, et al. BART investigators. A comparison of aprotinin and lysine analogues in high-risk cardiac surgery. N Engl J Med 2008;358(22):2319–31.
9. Lazzara RR, Kidwell FE, Kraemer MF, Wood JA, Starr A. Reduction in costs, blood products, and operating time in patients undergoing open heart surgery. Arch Surg 1997;132(8):858–60.
10. Coyle D, Lee KM, Fergusson DA, Laupacis A. Economic analysis of erythropoietin use in orthopaedic surgery. Transfus Med 1999;9(1):21–30.
11. Woronoff-Lemsi MC, Arveux P, Limat S, et al. Erythropoietin and preoperative autologous blood donation in the prevention of hepatitis C infection: necessity or luxury? Transfusion 1999;39(9):933–7.
12. Able ME, Tilly DA. The effect on costs of the use of half-dose aprotinin for first-time reoperative coronary artery bypass patients. Clin Ther 1998;20(3):581–91.
13. Ray MJ, Brown KF, Burrows CA, O'Brien MF. Economic evaluation of high-dose and low-dose aprotinin therapy during cardiopulmonary bypass. Ann Thorac Surg 1999;68(3):940–45.
14. Dignan RJ, Law DW, Seah PW, et al. Ultra-low dose aprotinin decreases transfusion requirements and is cost effective in coronary operations. Ann Thorac Surg 2001;71(1):158–63.
15. Robinson D, Bliss E. A model of the direct and indirect effects of aprotinin administration on the overall costs of coronary revascularization surgery in a university teaching hospital cardiothoracic unit. Clin Ther 2002;24(10):1677–89.
16. Smith PK, Datta SK, Muhlbaier LH, et al. Cost analysis of aprotinin for coronary artery bypass patients: analysis of the randomized trials. Ann Thorac Surg 2004;77(2):635–42.
17. Marchetti M, Barosi G. Cost-effectiveness of epoetin and autologous blood donation reducing allogeneic blood transfusions incoronary artery bypass graft surgery. Transfusion 2000;40(6):673–81.
18. Coyle D, Lee KM, Fergusson DA, Laupacis A. Cost effectiveness of epoetin-alpha to augment preoperative autologous blood donation in elective cardiac surgery. Pharmacoeconomics 2000;18(2):161–71.
19. Casati V, Guzzon D, Oppizzi M, et al. Hemostatic effects of aprotinin, tranexamic acid and epsilon-aminocaproic acid in primary cardiac surgery. Ann Thorac Surg 1999;68(6):2252–6.
20. Bennett-Guerrero E, Sorohan JG, Gurevich ML, et al. Cost-benefit and efficacy of aprotinin compared with epsilon-aminocaproic acid in patients having repeated cardiac operations: a randomized, blinded clinical trial. Anesthesiology 1997;87(6):1373–80.
21. Hébert PC, Wells G, Blajchman MA, et al. A multicenter, randomized, controlled clinical trial of transfusion requirements in critical care. Transfusion requirements in critical care investigators, Canadian critical care trials group. N Engl J Med 1999;340(6):409–17. Erratum in: N Engl J Med 1999; 340(13):1056.

Index

Note: Page numbers with f and t refer to figures and tables respectively.